PRIMER ON MULTIPLE SCLEROSIS

EDITED BY

BARBARA S. GIESSER, MD, FAAN
Department of Neurology
David Geffen School of Medicine at UCLA
Los Angeles, CA

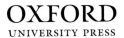

OXFORD
UNIVERSITY PRESS

2011

Oxford University Press, Inc., publishes works that further
Oxford University's objective of excellence
in research, scholarship, and education.

Oxford New York
Auckland   Cape Town   Dar es Salaam   Hong Kong   Karachi
Kuala Lumpur   Madrid   Melbourne   Mexico City   Nairobi
New Delhi   Shanghai   Taipei   Toronto

With offices in
Argentina   Austria   Brazil   Chile   Czech Republic   France   Greece
Guatemala   Hungary   Italy   Japan Poland   Portugal   Singapore
South Korea   Switzerland   Thailand   Turkey   Ukraine   Vietnam

Published by Oxford University Press, Inc.
198 Madison Avenue, New York, New York 10016
www.oup.com

Library of Congress Cataloging-in-Publication Data
Primer on multiple sclerosis / edited by Barbara S. Giesser.
    p. ; cm.
  Includes bibliographical references and index.
  ISBN 978-0-19-536928-1 (alk. paper)
  1. Multiple sclerosis.   I. Giesser, Barbara S.
  [DNLM: 1. Multiple Sclerosis. WL 360 P953 2011]
  RC377.P747 2011
  616.8'34—dc22
                                                2010000644
_____ISBN-13 9780195369281_____

The science of medicine is a rapidly changing field. As new research and clinical
experience broaden our knowledge, changes in treatment and drug therapy occur.
The author and publisher of this work have checked with sources believed to be
reliable in their efforts to provide information that is accurate and complete, and in
accordance with the standards accepted at the time of publication. However, in
light of the possibility of human error or changes in the practice of medicine, neither the author, nor the publisher, nor any other party who has been involved in the
preparation or publication of this work warrants that the information contained
herein is in every respect accurate or complete. Readers are encouraged to confirm
the information contained herein with other reliable sources, and are strongly
advised to check the product information sheet provided by the pharmaceutical
company for each drug they plan to administer.

9 8 7 6 5 4 3 2 1
Printed in China
on acid-free paper

This is dedicated to our patients and their families, and to the end of multiple sclerosis, when such books will no longer be necessary.

Foreword

Finally, an excellent and comprehensive text on multiple sclerosis (MS) developed by a clinical neurologist who has specialized in the care of patients with MS for almost 30 years! So much has changed in MS care during that time and this primer attempts to reflect the advances in basic research, clinical understanding, diagnosis, therapeutics, and psychosocial issues that have occurred.

The editor of this book, Barbara Giesser, began her training at the MS Care Center at the Albert Einstein College of Medicine in 1982 and has had an unparalleled career in MS care, education, and research. The chapter authors are some of the very best in their fields and provide comprehensive yet practical information in a clear and well-focused manner.

There is detailed information on the genetics, epidemiology, immunology, and neuropathology of MS. An excellent chapter on neuroimaging demonstrates how magnetic resonance imaging (MRI) plays a pivotal role in diagnosis and management.

The book comprises a number of chapters on MS-related symptoms, including some that have traditionally been largely overlooked, such as pain, cognitive and mood disorders, and sexual dysfunction. MS is becoming increasingly recognized in pediatric clinics, and this too is well covered. There are excellent discussions of disease-modifying therapies, other immunomodulatory and immunosuppressive strategies, novel compounds in development, and complementary and alternative treatments. Perhaps the two chapters that really illustrate the uniqueness and comprehensiveness of this book, however, are those dealing with employment considerations and legal planning issues. This text is a masterful production—one that will undoubtedly benefit a wide range of MS practitioners and quickly become indispensable to their bedside and office decision-making.

Jody Corey-Bloom, MD, PhD
University of California, San Diego

Preface

Persons with multiple sclerosis (MS) turn to their neurologist for help in managing a chronic, incurable, unpredictable, and often frightening illness. However, management of persons with MS has increasingly become more complex and sophisticated. Whereas a generation ago they might only be offered ACTH and an assistive device, persons with MS can now discuss multiple treatment options with their health-care professionals. These treatment strategies, including pharmacologic and rehabilitative modalities, can impact disease natural history, ameliorate or prevent many symptoms, and significantly improve function and quality of life. Ideally, the neurologist and other health-care professionals from many disciplines can collaborate to provide optimal patient care.

Similarly, research in MS is proceeding at a rapid pace. Thanks to technological improvements, and significant gains in knowledge in immunology, genetics, and pathology, to name just a few key disciplines, scientists are getting closer to elucidating the molecular underpinnings of MS, and thus closer to developing even more definitive therapies.

Therefore, in order to effectively manage persons with MS, the practicing neurologist has to have an understanding of the basic science behind the disease, as well as the most current "best practice" treatment guidelines. In this book, we have attempted to provide the theory and the practice of providing comprehensive care to persons with MS.

The book begins with a fascinating review of the history of MS, beginning in the fourteenth century, and then moves into the twenty-first century with the latest information concerning genetics, immunology, pathology, and epidemiology. The chapters on diagnosis include both the clinical and paraclinical parameters for diagnosing what may initially be an elusive disease, for which there is currently no pathognomonic sign, symptom, or lab assay. The clinical chapters cover the range of common signs and symptoms of MS and their treatment, as well as offer comprehensive discussions of areas that may be less familiar, including disorders of sleep, cognitive disorders, and pain. Additionally, we have provided information to help neurologists assist their patients in dealing with some of the often devastating psychosocial and vocational consequences of MS. There is a chapter on employment, as well as a chapter that discusses issues such as legal planning, insurance coverage, and discrimination in the workplace. Because of the widespread interest in nonallopathic therapies, there is a chapter on complementary and alternative medicine in MS. Finally, there are chapters devoted to an overview of the current state of clinical and basic science research directions, and a chapter on commonly used outcome measures in such trials.

Our goal is to have compiled a broad and practical guide to the basic information that a clinical neurologist may need to access in delivering care to persons with MS. We hope that this book may also be useful to other health-care professionals, as well as trainees.

I would like to acknowledge the very gracious and expert assistance and guidance of our editors at Oxford University Press: Craig Panner, who developed the concept of a primer on MS, and David D'Addona. This book would never have happened without the incomparable mentorship of the late Dr. Labe Scheinberg. I am indebted to Lynn, for her advice and encouragement, and to Phil, David, Marisa, Mark, Jody and Harold, for their unconditional love and support.

Barbara S. Giesser
Los Angeles, CA

Contents

Contributors

Alon Y. Avidan, MD, MPH
UCLA Sleep Disorders Center
Department of Neurology
David Geffen School of Medicine at UCLA
Los Angeles, CA

Allen C. Bowling, MD, PhD
Multiple Sclerosis Service and
Complementary and Alternative
Medicine Service
Colorado Neurological Institute (CNI)
Englewood, CO

Tiffany Braley, MD
Multiple Sclerosis Center
Department of Neurology
University of Michigan Health System
Ann Arbor, MI

Erik V. Burton, MD
Department of Neurology
University of Texas Southwestern Medical Center
Dallas, TX

Dorothee E. Chabas, MD, PhD
UCSF Regional Pediatric MS Center
University of California-San Francisco
San Francisco, CA

Tanuja Chitnis, MD
Partners Pediatric MS Center
Partners Pediatric Multiple Sclerosis Center
Massachusetts General Hospital for Children
Harvard Medical School
Boston, MA

Christopher Christodoulou, PhD
Department of Neurology
State University of New York at Stony Brook
Stony Brook, New York

Laura D. Cooper, Esq.
Attorney at Law
Eugene, OR

Anne H. Cross, MD
Department of Neurology
Washington University School of Medicine
St. Louis, MO

Frederick W. Foley, PhD
Department of Neuropsychology &
Psychosocial Research
Holy Name Hospital Multiple Sclerosis Center
Teaneck, NJ

Elliot M. Frohman, MD, PhD, FAAN
Departments of Neurology and Ophthalmology
University of Texas
Southwestern Medical Center
Dallas, TX

Barbara S. Giesser, MD, FAAN
Department of Neurology
David Geffen School of Medicine at UCLA
Los Angeles, CA

Wendy Gilmore, PhD
Department of Neurology
Keck School of Medicine of the University of
Southern California
Los Angeles, CA

Erica Grazioli, DO
Northshore Neurosciences
Erie, PA

Jodie K. Haselkorn, MD, MPH
MS Center of Excellence West
Department of Veteran Affairs
Department of Rehabilitation Medicine
Department of Epidemiology
University of Washington School of Medicine
Seattle, WA

Robert M. Herndon, MD, FAAN
Department of Neurology
University of Mississippi Medical Center
Jackson, MS

Rosalind C. Kalb, PhD
Vice President, Professional Resource Center
National Multiple Sclerosis Society
New York, NY

Ja-Hong Kim, MD
Clark Urology Clinic
Ronald Reagan UCLA Medical Center
Los Angeles, CA

George H. Kraft, MD, MS
Department of Rehabilitation Medicine and
Neurology
Western Multiple Sclerosis Clinical Center
University of Washington Medical Center
Seattle, WA

Stephen Krieger, MD
Corinne Goldsmith Dickinson Center for
Multiple Sclerosis
Mount Sinai Medical Center
New York, NY

Lauren Krupp, MD
National Pediatric MS Center
Department of Neurology
Stony Brook University Medical Center
Stony Brook, NY

Nancy Kuntz, MD
Division of Child Neurology
Children's Memorial Hospital
Northwestern Feinberg School of Medicine
Chicago, IL

Nicholas G. LaRocca, PhD
Vice President, Health Care Delivery and
Policy Research
National Multiple Sclerosis Society
New York, NY

Claudia F. Lucchinetti, MD, FAAN
Department of Neurology
Mayo Clinic
Rochester, MN

Angeli S. Mayadev, MD
MS Center at Swedish Neuroscience Institute
Swedish Medical Center
Seattle, WA

Thomas E. McNalley, MD
Department of Rehabilitation Medicine
University of Washington School of Medicine
Seattle, WA

Cornelia Mihai, MD
Department of Neurology
Syracuse VA Medical Center
Syracuse, NY

Aaron Miller, MD, FAAN
Corinne Goldsmith Dickinson Center for
Multiple Sclerosis
Mount Sinai Medical Center
New York, NY

T. Jock Murray, MD, FAAN
Dalhousie MS Research Unit
Halifax, Canada

Norman S. Namerow, MD, MS, FAAN
Department of Neurology
David Geffen School of Medicine at UCLA
Los Angeles, CA

Jayne M. Ness, MD, PhD
Center for Pediatric Onset Demyelinating Disease
Children's Hospital of Alabama
University of Alabama at Birmingham
Birmingham, AL

Steven W. Nissen, MS, CRC
Senior Director, Employment and Community
Programs
National Capital Chapter
National Multiple Sclerosis Society
Washington, DC

Marc R. Nuwer, MD, PhD, FAAN
Department of Neurology
David Geffen School of Medicine at UCLA
Department of Clinical Neurophysiology
UCLA Medical Center
Los Angeles, CA

Svenja Oynhausen, MD
Corinne Goldsmith Dickinson Center for
Multiple Sclerosis
Mount Sinai Medical Center
New York, NY

Yashma Patel, MD
Department of Neurology
Stony Brook University Medical Center
Stony Brook, NY

Laura Piccio, MD, PhD
Department of Neurology
Washington University School of Medicine
St. Louis, MO

Sreeram V. Ramagopalan, DPhil
Wellcome Trust Centre for Human Genetics
Department of Clinical Neurology
University of Oxford
Oxford, UK

Loren A. Rolak, MD, FAAN
The Marshfield Multiple Sclerosis Center
Marshfield, WI

Phillip D. Rumrill, Jr., PhD, CRC
Director of the Center for Disability Studies
School of Lifespan Development and
Educational Sciences
Kent State University
Kent, OH

A. Dessa Sadovnick, PhD
Department of Medical Genetics
Faculty of Medicine, Division of Neurology
University of British Columbia
Vancouver, Canada

Lawrence M. Samkoff, MD, FAAN
Department of Neurology
University of Rochester
School of Medicine and Dentistry
Rochester, NY

Nancy L. Sicotte, MD, FAAN
Department of Neurology
Division of Brain Mapping
David Geffen School of Medicine at UCLA
Los Angeles, CA

Jefferson C. Slimp, PhD
Department of Rehabilitation Medicine
University of Washington School of Medicine
Seattle, WA

Wallace W. Tourtellotte, MD, PhD
Neurology Service
VA West Los Angeles Healthcare Center
Distinguished Professor of Neurology
David Geffen School of Medicine at UCLA
Los Angeles, CA

Rhonda Voskuhl, MD
Director of UCLA Multiple Sclerosis
Program
Department of Neurology
David Geffen School of Medicine at UCLA
Los Angeles, CA

Emmanuelle L. Waubant, MD, PhD
UCSF Regional Pediatric MS Center
University of California-San Francisco
San Francisco, CA

Leslie P. Weiner, MD
Department of Neurology
Keck School of Medicine of the University of
Southern California
Los Angeles, CA

Bianca Weinstock-Guttman, MD
Department of Neurology
Jacobs Neurological Institute
Baird Multiple Sclerosis Center
SUNY University at Buffalo
Buffalo, NY

E. Ann Yeh, MD
Women and Children's Hospital of Buffalo
Pediatric MS Center of the JNI
SUNY University at Buffalo
Buffalo, NY

PRIMER ON MULTIPLE SCLEROSIS

Part I **Historical Background**

1

The History of Multiple Sclerosis: From the Age of Description to the Age of Therapy

T. Jock Murray

The story of knowledge of multiple sclerosis is like a history of medicine in miniature.
—*Tracy J. Putnam, Centenary of Multiple sclerosis. Arch Neurol Psych 1938;40(4):806–813*

There are many stages in the story of multiple sclerosis (MS). In the centuries before the disorder had a name and was clearly characterized, individuals were noted to develop a form of nervous disease that was particularly resistant to any known therapies. After it was characterized and named in the mid-nineteenth century, clinicians attempted to understand why the disorder happened to young adults, and many cases were reported in the medical literature showing the diversity of clinical pattern and course. In the twentieth century, research focused on the pathophysiology of the disease, exploring the underlying biochemical, immunological, genetic, geographical, and environmental aspects of the disease. This was supported by remarkable advances in laboratory sciences, imaging, genetics, immunology, and pathology. These periods were a prelude to the most recent and most dramatic stage, the therapeutic era, which began with arrival of the first agents that significantly affected the outcome of the disease in the 1990s (Murray, 2005). This chapter will describe the path through these periods that reflect primarily on the struggle to find therapies.

We may be tempted to think the therapeutic era began in recent decades when the disease-modifying therapies (DMTs) arrived, but therapies were always offered to people with MS, and in some periods even in more profusion than today. The therapeutic imperative of physicians, a pressure and need to always try to do something for their patient, has always been there and was just as strong for the eighteenth-century physician as it is now for the twentieth-century neurologist. We always want to do something for the distressed patient in front of us.

In the last two decades we have entered a new era of hope and promise, with insights from basic science, clinical trials, and personal experience that tell us we can effectively alter the prognosis and outcome in most cases, confident we will see dramatic advances and improvements in the next few years.

In the following chapters a group of leaders in the field will outline the dramatic advances in knowledge and therapeutics of MS. This initial chapter will provide an overview of how we came to this new therapeutic era, and the slow and steep steps necessary to achieve each milestone.

THE PRE-CLASSIFICATION ERA

In the late eighteenth and early nineteenth centuries, there was an enthusiasm about classifying disease, led by prominent clinician scientists such as William Cullen in Scotland and John Hunter in London. They had seen the marvelous results of the botanists in classifying the plant and animal kingdom and thought this could be achieved in medicine as well. The rise of medical journals assisted and accelerated the spread of knowledge internationally when a new disease was separated, described, and named. There was a triple reward for recognizing a new disease—making a contribution, receiving the attention of the profession, and having your name linked to the disorder into posterity (for example, Parkinson, Addison, Hodgkin, Bright, and Tourette).

Rosenberg indicated that the frame of a disease was more than its biology. It includes the beliefs about cause, social and personal reactions to the disorder, response of the health-care system, and a range of other concepts that not only determine how we treat the patients but how we direct research and ultimately how the patients will experience the disease (Rosenberg and Golden, 1992). If the disease is framed differently, the experience of the patient will differ as well.

There are cases of a progressive neurological disease in the past which we now suspect may have been multiple sclerosis before the disease had a name. These unfortunate people were thought to have a nervous disorder, often diagnosed as "paraplegia," creeping palsy, or some other general category. St. Ludwina of Scheiden (1380–1433) was well described in the Church records of her canonization (Murray, 2005). The progressive neurological disease causing loss of balance, lancinating facial pain, blindness in one eye, facial weakness, and progressive weakness was recognized as untreatable by the prominent court physician Godfried de la Haye in 1396. He said attempts to treat her would just impoverish her father. He added, "Believe me, there is no cure for this illness; it comes directly from God." (Thurston HJ and Attwater D, 1990:95).

Other early cases suspicious of MS before it was clearly named and framed were described in my book on the history of MS; they include Halla, the drummer Bock, Will Coffin, Margaret of Myddle, William Brown of the Hudson's Bay Company, Alan "Lighthouse" Stevenson, Heinrich Heine, and the Victorian novelist and botanist Margaret Gatty (Murray, 2005).

Perhaps the best documented case, because of his detailed journals, is Augustus d'Este, the grandson of King George III. There is no doubt of the diagnosis in his case. His physicians, the most prominent in the land, such as Sir Ashley Cooper, Sir Benjamin Brodie, and Sir Richard Bright, all recognized he had a progressive "paraplegia." Such a paraplegia was of the passive phase, which could remain for a long time in the "functional" form, which meant it could recover but would be expected to later transition to an "organic" and progressive form. If a paraplegia were thought to be complete, it was classified as a paraplexia. The various treatments offered him were herbal remedies, steel

waters, beef steaks twice a day, London porter beer, Sherry, and Madiera wines. He was given massages with liniments of camphorated alcohol, opium, and Florence oil. He felt these were making him stronger. He was later given blistering plasters over his back, baths and washes with sulphate of zinc and aqua plantaginis, doses of flowers and herbs, and valerian twice a day mixed in the herbs. He noted that his "connections" with a young woman he met at the seaside lacked a "wholesome vigor" and sought help for his impotence. He later lost faith in all these treatments and looked to the founder of hydrotherapy, Vincent Priessnitz, in Gräfenberg. He was a very regular exerciser and kept a separate journal of his measured exercise and timing. He tried horseback riding, a course of mercury, and the new electricity therapy, which he thought made him worse. As his disease slowly progressed, he accessed fewer consultants and fewer therapies, but he kept up his regular exercises, limited as they were, and died unhappy, not so much about his disease but because of his inability to link his name with the Royal family, as he was made illegitimate by the annulment of his parents marriage after he had been born. His record is a remarkable account of MS management and the courageous struggle of a person with the disease before it was named and fully framed.

In the early nineteenth century it was thought that the disorders of the nervous system might be due to accumulation of toxins as the humeral theory was only slowly leaving the medical belief system. Nervous diseases might also be due to over- or under-stimulation of the nerves. There were complex remedies concocted according to diagnostic features of the diseases, and whether the condition was characterized as hot or cold, moist or dry, and by complex astrological measurements. Medicines administered contained such substances as musk, castor, asafetida, valerian, garlic, oil of amber, skunk cabbage, coffee, and a long list of other "cerebral stimulants" such as henbane, deadly nightshade, and extract of hemp (Murray, 2005). Approaches thus tended to deplete the system of noxious humors by vomiting, purging, bleeding, scarification, cupping, or other procedures. Also stimulation of the nerves could be done with chemical, herbals, electricity, and various physical methods such as rough massage, horseback riding, cold water therapy, or irritating plasters. The Brounian system defined conditions as hyperexcitable (sthenic) or lowered excitability (asthenic), and treatments would attempt to address this imbalance. Paralysis required excitation and stimulation, so a person diagnosed with "paraplegia" would be subjected to stimulation by Galvanic or Faradic charges, moxibuxtion, counter-irritation, wrapping in cold sheets, or hosed by torrents of icy water. Even when more and more neurological diseases were separated and named during the nineteenth century, treatment remained much the same. Even though physicians would have their favored approaches and remedies, their general approach to a neurological patient did not vary much.

THE DESCRIPTION OF CHARCOT

In the early nineteenth century, a number of clinicians who were examining the pathology of their cases of neurological disease were becoming aware that there was a progressive disorder of young adults characterized by scattered gray patches of softening and scarring in the nervous system. The French were particularly active in assessing the clinical and pathological features of neurological disease; among the most active were Edme Vulpian and Jean-Martin Charcot at the Salpêtrière, the huge Paris hospital housing over 5000 sick and poverty-stricken persons, mostly women. Vulpian and Charcot presented some early cases of a condition they called *la sclérose en plaque disseminée* to a local medical society and published, with Vulpian as first author, in a hospital gazette, but it was a series of lectures, subsequently published that clarified the disease for the medical world and forever associated Charcot with the disorder we now call multiple sclerosis. When Charcot stepped on his lecture stage in 1868 and delivered three lectures on the disease he was aware of the work on the condition by Charles Prosper Ollivier d'Angers, Robert Carswell, Jean Cruveilhier, Friedrich Theodor von Frerich, Ludwig Türck, Eduard Rindfleisch, E. Leyden, Carl Frommann, and his friend and colleague Edme Vulpian. Charcot mentioned these contributions and never claimed to be first (Charcot, 1868). Charcot's contribution was to so clearly define the features of the disease and give it a

name, so that others around the world could now recognize and diagnose cases. As he concluded his description of the clinical features, the pathology, the course, and prognosis, he came to the discussion of treatment and sadly concluded, "After what has preceded, need I detain you long over the question of treatment? The time has not yet come when such a subject can be seriously considered" (Charcot, 1881, p. 221).

THE TWENTIETH CENTURY: MORE THEORIES AND POLYPHARMACY

Despite Charcot's nihilistic conclusion, over the next 60 years many remedies and techniques would be tried, and even those who were as skeptical as Charcot would still have their various procedures and list of medicines for their MS patients. William Gowers said that "even less can be done than for other degenerative diseases of the nervous system," but he still used nerve tonics such as arsenic, nitrate of silver, and quinine, as well as hydrotherapy and electricity, coupled with advice about healthy living and avoidance of stress and pregnancy (Gowers, 1893). Others administered many medications to their patients, including strychnine, ergot, barium chloride, and phosphorus. Tremor was treated with toxic doses of solanine, veratrum, and intramuscular hyocyamine and arsenic. Ataxia was treated with a suspension apparatus that hung the patient aloft by straps under the chin and axillae, a Russian invention, but one that was losing favor by the end of the nineteenth century, although Charcot and his students employed it at the Salpêtrière.

By 1900 little was added to Charcot's outline of the clinical and pathological picture of MS. Some observations of familial cases and of a geographic pattern of incidence were made but were not generally accepted. The same therapies were still being used, and that became even harsher when all the antisyphilitic remedies were applied to MS. Clinicians knew MS was not syphilis but both had widespread brain and spinal cord changes so it seemed logical to apply therapies from one disease to another, and we still see this jump in logic applied to MS today. (What major therapy of cancer, rheumatoid arthritis, and other immunological disease has not been applied to MS?) Perhaps the most disturbing antisyphilitic treatment applied to MS patients was the attempt to create fever by various means, whether in a Turkish bath-like fever box, injection of various vaccines or even milk, and most surprising, purposely giving the MS patient malaria to induce recurrent fevers. All these must have made MS patients worse, at least in the short term, as most are temperature sensitive and develop generalized weakness and increased symptoms when subjected to heat or fever. It does remind us that physicians may sometimes overlook the objective signs of distress, side effects, or worsening because of an overriding belief that the patient will somehow be better. As Sir William Gowers put it in 1893, "When more is known of the causes and essential pathology of the disease in different cases, more rational methods may brighten the therapeutic prospect" (Gowers, 1893, p. 544).

When the magical X-ray made its appearance at the end of the nineteenth century, it was soon being directed to the spinal cords of MS patients as a form of radiation therapy. Those who believed MS was due to a toxin used many methods of "detoxification," an approach that still has some current adherents. Most accepted Pierre Marie's strong opinion that MS was due to infection and hoped there would soon be a vaccine for MS, and in the meantime gave any new anti-infection medicine to MS patients, and this still occurs. McAlpine in 1925 recommended removal of any source of infection, and MS patients often were subjected to removal of their teeth, tonsillectomy, and sinus drainage, as well as anti-infection remedies in this preantibiotic era (McAlpine, 1925).

The list of remedies and procedures was growing in the early decades of the twentieth century, but a young perceptive neurologist at the London Hospital, Russell Brain (later Lord Brain), reviewed the vast array of therapies administered to hopeful MS patients in 1930 and concluded:

> No mode of therapy is successful enough to achieve, at the most, a greater improvement than might have occurred spontaneously …. The multiplication of remedies is eloquent of their inefficacy. (Brain, 1930, p. 381)

That did not diminish the therapeutic attempts of neurologists and in 1936 Brickner published a 29-page list evaluating 158 different therapies applied to MS patients (Brickner, 1935–36). Perhaps it is not surprising that he concluded that the best approach was his own treatment, known as "Brickner's quinine treatment for MS." Tracy Putnam, a prominent New York neurologist, did a primitive statistical analysis of the Brickner list against the results of the treatments on 1407 of his own patients and concluded that half of the patients had profited from the various therapies (Tally, 1998).

Another approach in the 1940 was the treatment of MS with anticoagulants. It had been noted since the observations of Eduard Rindfleisch in 1863 that there are blood vessels in the center of a plaque (Rindfleisch, 1863). It was then logical to hypothesize that the scattered lesions in MS were due to local ischemia, emboli, or vascular disease, so when warfarin became available it was widely used in MS, fostered by the enthusiasm of Tracey Putnam for this approach.(Putnam et al., 1947; Tally, 1998).

In 1950 George Schumacher was asked by the newly formed Advisory Board of the National MS Society to prepare a report on the state of MS therapy (Schumacher, 1950). He indicated that the prognosis in MS was not as gloomy as most believed, but the disease had significant medical and social impact. He suggested a means of codifying the diagnostic criteria, which became known as the Schumacher Criteria, later superceded by the Poser and McDonald Criteria.

Turning to therapy, Schumacher dispensed with approaches he thought useless, such as arsenic, fever therapy, vaccines and sera, autohemotherapy, lecithin, X-ray therapy, sympathectomy, belladonna, endocrine therapies, and penicillin. He thought general measures could be helpful to the patient, such as good nutrition, avoidance of stress and pregnancy, and moderate physical therapy. He reviewed the list of therapies that appeared on the scene since Brickner's 1936 review, but he concluded that no patient had been cured by anticoagulants, circulatory stimulants, vitamins, drugs to affect the immune state, and enzymes like Cytochrome C. He also dismissed the transfusion therapies of Lehoczky, Tschabitscher, and Leo Alexander, and the various hemolytic and vaccine therapies. In his final remarks he was as somber and negative as Russell Brain 20 years earlier:

> In summary of the drug treatment of multiple sclerosis it may be said that the outlook for cure of the disease by use of drugs is unpromising and that the outlook for symptomatic relief by drugs is less optimistic than would appear from the large number of reports which make claims of favorable effects. (Schumacher, 1950, p. 1249)

Again the wet blanket thrown over the therapeutic field by a prominent neurologist did not dampen the therapeutic enthusiasm of neurologists. Many new therapies were suggested in the 1950s. Most popular was the histamine desensitization approach fostered by Bayard Horton at the Mayo Clinic (Horton et al., 1944) and adapted by a general practitioner, Hinton Jonas of Tacoma, Washington, who said he had personally administered 150,000 large doses of histamine "without a single bad result" (Jonas, 1952).

There was some excitement over the news that the Russians had a vaccine for MS in the 1950s. All was under suspicion during the Cold War and the late Richard Masland was approached by two physicians associated with the CIA who wanted him to test serum from a Russian patient who had been treated with the vaccine. Later it would be revealed that the Russian vaccine for MS was rabies vaccine, and not surprisingly, made MS patients worse (personal communication, 1990).

THE MODERN ERA: 1950 AND BEYOND

After the 1950s the field began to brighten. More scientists were exploring aspects of the disease and the immunological relationships. Epidemiological observations confirmed the odd geographical distribution of the disease. Efforts were being made to better classify the disease. Steroids appeared on the scene as the first convincing therapy for attacks of MS. Early MS clinics were appearing in Montreal, Newcastle, and Atlanta. Perhaps most promising, Sylvia Lawry was using her considerable personal energy and chutzpah to construct a National MS Society, which would catalyze an international movement in support of patients and of research.

Therapies at this time looked very much like those used a century before, with many remedies recommended by neurologists who had little confidence that these would have much effect. The favored remedy and approach would change every few years as the initial enthusiasm over the latest medication faded. Perhaps we should remember the comment of Sir William Osler, who described the first three MS cases in Canada a century earlier and was skeptical and sanguine about unbridled enthusiasm for the latest drug, stating, "One should treat as many patients as possible with a new drug while it still has the power to heal."

Although all neurologists gave some medications to their MS patients, virtually all who published on the disease in the 1950s and 1960s stated that therapy had little effect on the disease. Sadly, many neurologists regarded MS as a hopeless situation and often delivered the bad news about the diagnosis along with the message that there was little reason to return as there was nothing that could be done. Prominent neurologists such as Houston Merritt and Foster Kennedy stated that they avoided giving the patient the diagnosis because it was such a "death sentence," although the family might be told (Murray, 2005).

Although some therapies came and went during these decades, George Schumacher concluded that no patient had been cured by any therapy and symptomatic therapy was also ineffective (Schumacher, 1950). Thygesen felt those who were encouraged by a therapeutic response had forgotten that the disease was characterized by spontaneous remissions, and that most people with MS "are amiable people who hate to disappoint their doctor" and gave responses their doctor wished to hear (Thygeson, 1953).

THE ERA OF STEROIDS AND CLINICAL TRIALS

Cortisone and ACTH were initially thought to be a cure for rheumatoid disease, and in the 1950s they were being used in MS patients. Although some reports suggested improvement, the first double-blind clinical trial in MS was carried out by Henry Miller in Newcastle in his Demyelinating Disease Unit, suggesting improvement in MS, especially in optic neuritis (Miller et al., 1961). Although subsequent trials, including the 1970 ACTH trial headed by Augustus Rose, showed marginal effect (Rose et al., 1970) and negative trials with oral steroids, these became the mainstay of MS therapy during these years. The approach of Leo Alexander with long-term ACTH (the Alexander regimen) was widely used in MS therapy (Alexander and Cass, 1963). Subsequently recommendations would confine steroid therapy to high doses of intravenous steroid for acute attacks or optic neuritis, although comparable high doses of oral steroid are currently under study.

Miller's incorporation of the recently developed concepts of randomized clinical trials was an important step in the subsequent evaluation of therapies for MS (Miller et al., 1961). Design concepts for trials in other areas of medicine were incorporated in subsequent MS trials. In 1974 a National Advisory Commission on Multiple Sclerosis put forward the idea of trials that were preliminary, pilot, and full studies, and this later was changed to Phase I–IV studies by the Department of Health Education and Welfare (HEW) in 1977. In 1979 a committee under Joe Brown outlined suggestions for the design of a clinical trial in MS (Brown et al., 1979). Clinicians were now aware that the natural history of MS required that trials have large numbers of patients and be longer in duration than they were previously.

OTHER THERAPEUTIC ATTEMPTS

Some alteration of diet was a part of the therapeutic regime for most illnesses in the past, but specific dietary recommendations for MS began with Roy Swank in Montreal in the 1940s when he was working in the MS clinic there with Bert Cosgrove. Swank's diet primarily reduces animal fat and increases vegetable oils and was fostered by him for over half a century (Swank, 1950). The diets developed by others usually incorporated the lowering of animal fats as well but added other elements that they often said were more important such as the elimination diets, low-gluten diet, MacDougall diet, Shatin diet, Evers diet, and so many others, all with little scientific basis, much enthusiasm and publicity, and usually a short

time before obscurity. Swank's diet is an exception because it continues to circulate, and the basic concept of lowered animal fat/increased vegetable oils has some theoretical logic and clinical evidence.

Since the late nineteenth century when Pierre Marie's made his enthusiastic prediction that MS was an infection that would soon be eliminated by a vaccine, every attempt has been made to treat MS as an infection (Marie, 1895). When antisyphilitic treatments failed, the new antibiotics were tried, and since the 1960s almost every new antibiotic and antiviral medication has been tried in MS. William Mervyn Crofton, a Dublin pathologist, claimed he had a vaccine. Dr. P. LeGac in France developed an antirickettsia treatment that was popular in the 1960s. Blood transfusions, serotherapy, and plasma transfusions had proponents and then faded from view as did anticoagulant therapy, antihistamines, snake venom, colonic irrigation, hyperbaric oxygen, magnetism, and removal of dental amalgam.

THE ERA OF IMMUNOSUPPRESSANTS

Since 1935 there was evidence that MS was characterized by an immune reaction, and when immunology advanced rapidly as a field in the 1960s, each new immunologically active agent was tried in MS patients with mostly disappointing results. Although these were commonly used up until the 1990s, most therapies faded due to disappointing or uncertain results in the face of serious side effects and long-term concerns. There have been trials of azathioprine, cyclophosphamide, cyclosporine, sulphinpyrazone, total lymphoid irradiation, methotrexate, cladribine, levamisole, linomide, transfer factor, myelin basic protein, T-cell vaccination, azathioprine, cyclophosphamide, and techniques such as plasmapheresis. Some are used in specific clinical situations, and a few are still under study. Greater interest recently has been in stem cell transplantation, monoclonal antibodies, and a list of other agents that affect the immune system.

THE MODERN THERAPEUTIC ERA

In 1980 a number of meetings centered on the need for new approaches to MS therapy, better designs for trials, and collaborations that would foster clinical trials. Interferons were discovered by two independent groups in the 1950s, and in 1964 Wheelock and Sibley noted interferon in the serum after infection (Wheelock and Sibley, 1964). During the 1970s Merrigan and Oldstone were studying the effects of interferons in mice and were interested in the idea of a trial of interferon in MS. By an odd trick of fate, some interferon returned by a purchaser was offered to Larry Jacobs of Buffalo, who considered using it to treat amyotrophic lateral sclerosis (ALS) but chose MS because there were more patients available (Jacobs and Johnson, 1994). At the same time Byron Waksman stimulated interest in interferon studies in MS, and Kenneth Johnson joined Merrigan and Oldstone in studies of interferons. Through a series of trials and developments of techniques and dosages, three commercially available interferons were available to MS patients: Betaseron, Avonex, and Rebif. After a 27-year saga, copolymer-I was developed in Israel and marketed as glatiramer acetate (Copaxone).

After a decade of clinical studies to demonstrate the place of these four drugs in the treatment of MS, two new agents have been approved for MS: mitoxantrone (Novantrone) and natalizumab (Tysabri). Unfortunately, soon after the release of Tysabri some cases of progressive multifocal leukoencephalopathy (PML) developed in patients on the drug and it was voluntarily withdrawn, then reintroduced with new restrictions and monitoring.

THE FUTURE

More clinical trials for MS occur each year, and many new agents are on the horizon. As the search for therapies that alter the outcome of the disease continues, there is also progress in developing better symptomatic therapies. There are also early steps in the evaluation of the many alternative therapies used by MS patients. The important basis for new therapies, however, will come from increasing basic research that reveals the underlying processes and mechanisms in the disease. Promising results with bone marrow transplantation, fingolomide, cladribine, fampridine, laquinimod, teriflunomide, rituximab, and many other agents under study show the promise for the future.

The therapeutic era of MS is just beginning.

ACKNOWLEDGMENT

This brief article is adapted from T. Jock Murray's *Multiple Sclerosis: The History of a Disease* (New York: Demos, 2005, chapter 15, pp. 391–503). This chapter has 272 references to the history of therapy.

REFERENCES

Alexander L, Cass LJ. The present status of ACTH therapy in multiple sclerosis. *Ann In Med.* 1963;58:454–471.

Brain WR. Critical review. Disseminated sclerosis. *Quart J Med.* 1930;23:343–391.

Brickner RM. A critique of therapy in multiple sclerosis. *Bull Neurol Inst NY.* 1935–36; 4:665–698.

Brown JR, Beebe GW, Kurtzke JF, Loewenso RB, Silberberg DH, Tourtellotte WW. The design of clinical studies to assess therapeutic efficacy in multiple sclerosis. *Neurology.* 1979;29:3–23.

Charcot JM. *Lectures on the Diseases of the Nervous System.* Vol. 2. Sigurdson G, trans-ed. London: New Sydenham Society; 1881.

Gowers WR. *A Manual of Diseases of the Nervous System.* Vol. 2. 2nd ed. London: J&A Churchill; 1893:557.

Horton BT, Waegener HP, Aita JA, Woltman HW. Treatment of multiple sclerosis by intravenous administration of histamine. *JAMA.* 1944;124:800–812.

Jacobs L, Johnson KP. A brief history of the use of interferons as treatment of multiple sclerosis. *Arch Neurol.* 1994;51:1245–1252.

Jonas HD. *My Fight to Conquer Multiple Sclerosis.* New York: Julian Messner; 1952.

Marie P. *Lectures on Diseases of the Spinal Cord.* Lubbock M, trans. London: New Sydenham Society; 1895:134–136.

McAlpine D. The treatment of disseminated sclerosis. *Lancet.* 1925;2:82–83.

Miller HG, Newell DJ, Ridley A. Treatment of multiple sclerosis with corticotrophin (ACTH). *Lancet.* 1961; 2:1361–1362.

Murray TJ. Multiple Sclerosis: The History of a Disease. New York: Demos; 2005.

Putnam TJ. Centenary of Multiple sclerosis. *Arch Neurol Psych.* 1938;40(4):806–813.

Putnam TJ, Chiavacci LV, Hoff H, et al. Results of treatment of multiple sclerosis with dicoumarin. *Arch Neurol.* 1947;57:1–13.

Rindfleisch E. Histologische Detail zu der Grauen Degeneration von Gehirn and Rückenmark. *Virhow Arch Path Anat Physiol.* 1863;26:474–483.

Rose AS, Kuzma JW, Kurtzke JF, Namerow NS, Sibley WA, Tourtellotte WW. Cooperative study in the evaluation of therapy in multiple sclerosis: ACTH vs placebo—final report. *Neurology.* 1970;20:1–59.

Rosenberg CE, Golden J, eds. *Framing Disease Studies in Cultural History.* New Brunswick, NJ: Rutgers University Press; 1992.

Schumacher GA. Multiple sclerosis and its treatment. *JAMA.* 1950;143:1059–1065, 1146–1154, 1241–1250.

Swank RL. Multiple sclerosis: a correlation of its incidence with dietary fat. *Am J M Sc.* 1950;220:421–430.

Tally C. A History of Multiple Sclerosis and Medicine in the United States. 1870–1960 [dissertation]. San Francisco: University of California; 1998.

Thurston HJ, Attwater D, eds. *Butler's Lives of the Saints.* Vol II, Westminister, Christian Classics, 1990:95.

Thygesen P. *The Course of Disseminated Sclerosis: A Close-up of 105 Attacks.* Copenhagen, Denmark: Rosenkilde and Bagger; 1953.

Wheelock EF, Sibley WA. Interferon in human serum during clinical viral infections. *Lancet.* 1964;1: 382–385.

Part 2 **Basic Science**

2 Genetics and Epidemiology of Multiple Sclerosis

Sreeram V. Ramagopalan and A. Dessa Sadovnick

The etiology of multiple sclerosis (MS) remains elusive. Genes, environment, and the interactions thereof all have important roles and there is increasing evidence for epigenetics. While it is clear that risks for relatives to develop MS are directly related to the amount of DNA sharing, environmental factors (other than intrafamilial ones) continue to warrant important consideration.

GLOBAL DISTRIBUTION OF MULTIPLE SCLEROSIS

Multiple sclerosis is a relatively common disease in Europe, the United States, Canada, New Zealand, and parts of Australia. Multiple sclerosis is rare in Asia as well as in the tropics and subtropics (Pugliatti et al., 2002). Some of the highest prevalence rates in the world are reported for Northern Scotland; the Orkney Islands report a prevalence of 270 per 100,000 (Pugliatti et al., 2002).

More complex patterns of disease distribution do however exist within some countries and continents. To illustrate, while continental Italy and Sicily report prevalence estimates of approximately 50 per 100,000, the prevalence in Malta is one-tenth of this. Within regions of temperate climate, MS incidence and prevalence increase with latitude (distance from the equator); see Figure 2-1. The clearest example of this effect is seen in Australia (Hammond et al., 1988). The prevalence of MS in Hobart (South Australia; temperate climate) is 75.6 per 100,000 compared with a prevalence of 11 per 100,000 in Northern Queensland (Northern Australia, tropical climate). A similar latitude effect on MS prevalence has been documented in North America (Kurtzke et al., 1979). Some of the geographical distribution can

be explained on the basis of ethnicity and genetic factors (e.g., African Americans have a lower MS risk) (Sadovnick and Ebers, 1993), but latitude remains the strongest factor for risk after controlling for ethnicity (Wallin et al., 2004). However, of interest, the latitude effect does seem to be decreasing to some extent over the last few decades (Wallin et al., 2004).

Migration Studies

The effects of migration between high- and low-risk geographic regions for MS have been examined in several populations (e.g., UK immigrants to South Africa, or Asian and Caribbean immigrants to the United Kingdom). Although there is potential for migration bias, these studies consistently show that MS risk is influenced at least to some extent by the migrant's country of origin (Dean and Elian, 1997). Despite the limits of small sample sizes, a "critical age" has been hypothesized: immigrants who migrate before adolescence acquire the risk of their new country, while those who migrate after retain the risk of their home country (Dean, 1967). However, an Australian migration study has now suggested that this critical age may extend into the twenties (Hammond et al., 2000).

Temporal Trends

A female-specific increase in the incidence of MS has been documented (Barnett et al., 2003; Wallin et al., 2004; Grytten et al., 2006). A recent Canadian study was able to show that this increase was real and not an artefact related to changes in ascertainment (Orton et al., 2006). Year of birth

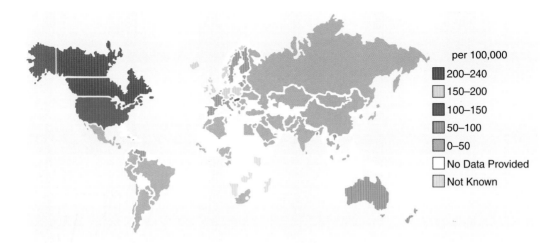

Figure 2-1 Global prevalence of multiple sclerosis. (Maps courtesy of the Atlas of MS database; available at http://www.atlasofms.org/index.aspx)

was shown to be a significant predictor of the female: male (F:M) sex ratio of MS over the period 1931–1980, with the ratio increasing from 1.9 to 3.2 during this time (Orton et al., 2006). There was no evidence to suggest decreasing incidence in males (Orton et al., 2006) and this female-specific increasing incidence of MS has since been confirmed in a number of other populations (Debouverie et al., 2007; Alonso and Hernan, 2008; Hirst et al., 2009).

Month of Birth

A pooled analysis of over 40,000 patients from Canada, Great Britain, Denmark, and Sweden showed that significantly fewer people with MS were born in November and significantly more were born in May (Willer et al., 2005). The finding of a birth pattern suggests that the origins of the disease date to very early in life, but it does not reveal specifically when during pregnancy the seasonal factor occurs. Candidate factors that may be responsible for month of birth effects include maternal/fetal folate and vitamin D levels and infection, all of which vary seasonally (Willer et al., 2005). These factors may interact with disease predisposing genes as the month-of-birth effect was more pronounced in familial cases.

GENETIC EPIDEMIOLOGY

The importance of genetic factors in susceptibility to MS has been demonstrated by genetic epidemiological studies (Dyment et al., 2004a). Family studies assessing risks to relatives of MS probands have revealed a marked familial aggregation of the disease. First-degree relatives are generally at a 15–35 times greater risk of developing MS compared to the rest of the population. This risk correlates with degree of kinship (Sadovnick et al., 1988; Willer et al., 2003) (see Fig. 2-2). However fundamental familial clustering of a trait (or disease) is not sufficient to infer the importance of genetics, since environmental influences also aggregate in families. The importance of the environment in familial risk is highlighted by the observation that twin concordance for MS depends on place of birth (Islam et al., 2006).

A number of strategies have been employed to dissect the environmental from the genetic components underlying MS susceptibility. Studies of MS in conjugal pairs (Robertson et al., 1997; Ebers et al., 2000) have shown that spouses (sexual partners) of index cases develop MS no more often than the background general population. Together with data from half-siblings (Ebers et al., 2004), step siblings (Dyment et al., 2006), and adoptees (Ebers et al., 1995), these studies provide

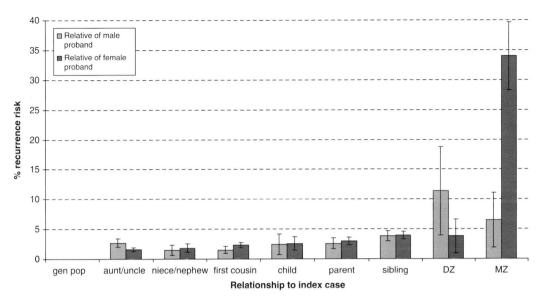

Figure 2-2 Age-adjusted percentage recurrence risks for relatives of Canadian male and female multiple sclerosis probands. DZ, dizygotic; MZ, monozygotic.

no evidence for a transmissible factor or other environmental factors operative within the familial microenvironment, either in childhood or adulthood. Thus, genetics (the sharing of DNA identical by descent [IBD]) is responsible for most, if not all, of the familial aggregation of MS.

The half-sibling studies found that the risk for maternal half-sibs (common mother, different father, 25% genetic sharing) was 2.35% compared to 1.31% for paternal half-sibs (common father, different mother, 25% genetic sharing). These findings are taken to implicate a maternal effect in disease susceptibility, despite the mothers not having MS (Ebers et al., 2004). This has since been confirmed in a Dutch extended pedigree (Hoppenbrouwers et al., 2008), a study of avuncular pairs (Herrera et al., 2008), and an investigation of interracial matings (Ramagopalan et al., 2009c). The maternal effect in MS is substantial. Risk for MS in siblings who share only a mother (25% genetic sharing) compared with risk in full siblings (i.e. those who share a mother and a father, hence 50% genetic sharing) does not differ significantly (2%–35% vs 3%–11%, $p = 0.1$). This finding indicates that maternal effects might even be the major component of familial aggregation.

Epidemiological data suggest that genetic factors may also affect the phenotypic expression of the disease. Studies have found that age of onset has a tendency to cluster in families, with the effect being most pronounced in monozygotic twins (Bulman et al., 1991). In sibling pairs with MS, modest but significant concordance for disease course exists (Runmarker and Andersen, 1993; Hensiek et al., 2007). It has been shown that the rate of acquisition of disability is also similar in sibling pairs (Brassat et al., 1999; Chataway et al., 2001), but the evidence is conflicting (Hensiek et al., 2007). Taken together, these observations highlight the fact that genetic factors are likely to influence clinical outcome.

ENVIRONMENTAL FACTORS IN MULTIPLE SCLEROSIS

Although genetic susceptibility explains the clustering of MS within families (Ebers et al., 1995), it cannot fully explain either the geographic variations in MS prevalence or the changes in risk that occur with migration. The relevant environmental factor(s) in MS susceptibility, which must act at a broad population level, remain unknown but strong candidates include vitamin D and infectious agents.

Infectious Agents

One hypothesis is that MS is caused by a pathogen that is more common in geographic regions of high MS prevalence, but is so ubiquitous that no evidence of transmissibility is seen in disease manifestation, a later consequence of prior infection (Kurtzke, 1993). There is no genetic epidemiological data that can exclude this possibility, which nevertheless maintains focus on host factors. Early investigations attempted to uncover the responsible agent, resulting in many viruses, including measles (Sibley and Foley, 1965), mumps (Millar et al., 1971), rubella (Horikawa et al., 1973), varicella-zoster (Ross et al., 1965), and Epstein-Barr (EBV) (Sumaya et al., 1980) being implicated as causative for MS. However, associations of viral antibodies with MS have not been consistently replicated (Ascherio and Munger, 2007).

Several studies have investigated whether childhood viral illnesses such as measles, rubella, varicella, and mumps increase the risk to subsequently develop MS. There have been many reports suggesting an association between one or more of these infectious diseases and MS (Tarrats et al., 2002; Pekmezovic et al., 2004), but these were not confirmed in a larger registry-based study (Bager et al., 2004). However, evidence is growing that a history of infectious mononucleosis ("EBV") is associated with susceptibility to MS (Lindberg et al., 1991; Marrie et al., 2000; Nielsen et al., 2007; Zaadstra et al., 2008), especially in those developing infectious mononucleosis after the age of 15 years old (Thacker et al., 2006). A systematic review and meta-analysis of 14 case-control and cohort studies reported a combined relative risk for MS after infectious mononucleosis of 2.3 ($p < 10^{-8}$). The epidemiological data associating EBV infection with MS stand on their own for replication. A consistent finding is that almost all patients with MS (>99%) are infected with EBV, compared with only about 90% of control individuals (Ascherio and Munch, 2000).

High population exposure to EBV makes for difficulty in resolving any disease-related effect. The association of clinically apparent EBV infection with MS may be causally related. However, EBV infection could also be a ubiquitous cofactor in disease initiation or represent a co-association between MS and this clinical viral infection determined by a risk factor common to both. The observation that EBV has been linked to other putative autoimmune diseases (James et al., 1997) may suggest a role as an important nonspecific trigger in the autoimmune cascade. The exact role, if any, of EBV in MS remains to be elucidated, although molecular mimicry has been suggested (Lang et al., 2002) and evidence of EBV infection in brain-infiltrating B cells in MS postmortem tissue has been found (Serafini et al., 2007).

Vitamin D

In accordance with the disease geography, vitamin D has been proposed as a key environmental factor for MS (Acheson et al., 1960). At high latitudes, circulating vitamin D fluctuates with seasonal ultraviolet (UV) light exposure. During the winter in Northern Canada, the levels of circulating vitamin D in pregnant women and newborns is low (Newhook et al., 2009). Given this seasonal fluctuation in vitamin D, decreased concentrations in utero could potentially explain the month of birth effect in MS. Vitamin D interacting with MS susceptibility genes may explain the correlation between latitude of birth and twin concordance rates.

Levels of past sun exposure are inversely related to MS susceptibility but only for the period between the ages of 6 and 15 years old (adjusted odds ratios [ORs] for high summer sun exposure 0.31 [0.16–0.59]) (van der Mei et al., 2003). This relationship held true in a subgroup who did not believe that sun exposure was related to risk of MS and was also confirmed by showing correlation with skin damage, a time-insensitive but nevertheless objective measure of sun exposure. Further evidence for the role of childhood sun exposure came from discordant MS monozygotic twin pairs, in which the affected twin was more likely to report decreased sun exposure as a child (Islam et al., 2007). Together, these findings argue persuasively that sun exposure in childhood and adolescence is inversely related to MS susceptibility.

Whether or not sun exposure reflects the effects of vitamin D is not clear. However, high serum levels of 25-hydroxyvitamin D, 25(OH)D$_2$, a precursor to the active form of vitamin D, were shown to be protective against MS (OR 0.38 [0.19-0.75]) (Munger et al., 2006). This relationship was particularly marked when the 25(OH)D$_2$ levels were measured prior to age 20 years. Correlation does not necessarily mean causation, but the growing knowledge of the pleiotropic actions of vitamin D, including immunomodulatory functions (Correale et al., 2009), lends strong support to this vitamin as being important in etiology.

Smoking

Smoking has been implicated in several ways with respect to MS. One issue is whether smoking is a risk factor (Hernan et al., 2001; Mikaeloff et al., 2007; Jafari et al., 2009). Smoking can be a risk factor to the person who is actually smoking and/ or smoking could also be a risk factor through second-hand exposure. However, in both scenarios, age of exposure (including prenatal), dosage, and duration must be considered. The "critical" time of exposure to any risk factor for MS is still unclear, but data have shown that it may be as early as gestation (e.g., Ebers et al., 2004) or well into adulthood (e.g., Hammond et al., 2000). The second issue is whether smoking (or exposure to second-hand smoke) can influence the course of MS (time to progress from CIS to MS, number of relapses, severity, etc.) once a patient has expressed the first clinical sign or symptom (e.g., DiPauli et al., 2008; Sundstrom and Nystrom, 2008; Montgomery et al, 2008; Healy et al., 2009; Pittas et al., 2009) There is also the question of whether an individual who smokes *(1)* increases his/her risk to develop MS and *(2)* influences the clinical course of the disease. Despite several studies, it still remains unclear whether smoking (or exposure to second-hand smoke) is indeed a definitive risk factor or a modifier of disease course.

GENETICS

Until recently, the standard approach for identifying susceptibility alleles for complex traits has been to use linkage studies or association analysis of candidate loci.

Linkage

Genetic linkage assesses the cotransmission of alleles and disease within families. According to Mendel's laws, if two alleles are situated on different chromosomes or are separated by a large distance on a single chromosome (in the presence of recombination), they will segregate and assort independently at meiosis. The nonindependent assortment of alleles may therefore be used to measure the distance between two loci (Dawn Teare and Barrett, 2005).

In the mid-1990s, the first generation of genomic screens for linkage in MS were performed using a variety of methodologies and family types. Microsatellite-based studies from the United Kingdom (Sawcer et al., 1996), the United States (Haines et al., 1996), Canada (Ebers et al., 1996), and Finland (Kuokkanen et al., 1997) employing between 200 and 400 families implicated many distinct regions, although with little consensus. The one exception was the major histocompatibility complex (MHC) on chromosome 6p21, which was identified in each of these genome scans as either a positive linkage (Ebers et al., 1996; Haines et al., 1996; Sawcer et al., 1996) or as a region of interest (Kuokkanen et al., 1997). Despite extensive follow-up of each of these genome scans with additional markers and/or additional families (Chataway et al., 1998; Haines et al., 2002; Saarela et al., 2002; Hensiek et al., 2003; Dyment et al., 2004b; Kenealy et al., 2004), no other consistent linkage was found. Even the most powerful MS linkage study performed to date using single nucleotide polymorphism (SNP) markers in 730 multiplex families (Sawcer et al., 2005) found significant linkage only for the MHC.

While linkage provides adequate power to detect major susceptibility loci, it is less powerful when genetic effects are small (Risch and Merikangas, 1996). In addition, because linkage within families is only interrupted by recombination, linkage is a poor tool for fine-mapping in small genomic regions. The MS linkage screens highlight that the MHC is the locus with the strongest genetic effect in MS and any other genes must make considerably weaker contributions to disease risk. Future linkage studies aimed at identifying susceptibility loci for MS will therefore require larger sample sizes and more powerful methods (Risch and Merikangas, 1996).

Association

In contrast to linkage, genetic association is sensitive to differences in allele frequencies between cases and controls at the population level (Cordell and Clayton, 2005). While association may be useful for identifying loci with weak genetic effects, a large number of polymorphic markers is required and an adequate sample size is needed to thoroughly interrogate a particular genomic region (Hattersley and McCarthy, 2005). In the absence of a solid understanding of the mechanisms that underlie MS, there are no compelling a priori candidate genes for MS; hence, the list of genes that have been investigated for MS susceptibility is long and continually expanding. Nearly all have failed replication attempts. This may be due to population stratification (where population substructure may produce spurious associations), publication bias, and/or inadequate sample sizes (Colhoun et al., 2003).

Genome-Wide Association Studies

Until recently, genome-wide association studies (GWAS) have not been technically feasible due to the large number of polymorphisms that must be typed. With recent advances in high-throughput single nucleotide polymorphism (SNP) genotyping technology, GWAS have become a reality. It is now possible to genotype up to 1 million SNPs per sample. A consortium of more than 50 British groups, known collectively as the Wellcome Trust Case Control Consortium (WTCCC), examined genetic variation at 500,000 SNPs within the genomes of 17,000 individuals to identify genes for rheumatoid arthritis, hypertension, Crohn disease, coronary artery disease, bipolar disorder, and type 1 and type 2 diabetes (The Wellcome Trust Case Control Consortium, 2007). This was a landmark study, and it set the benchmark for GWAS in terms of sample size, genotyping quality control, and statistical analysis.

The International Multiple Sclerosis Genetics Consortium published the first whole-genome association study for MS in 2007 (Hafler et al., 2007). The group screened more than 300,000 SNPs in 931 MS trios (two unaffected parents and one affected offspring). About 100 SNPs were followed up on the basis of statistical significance and biological candidacy in another cohort of more than 3000 patients with MS. No SNP outside the MHC reached genome-wide significance in the screening phase of the study. Significant association overall was found with the interleukin 7 receptor alpha gene or *IL7RA*. This gene was previously associated to MS using a candidate gene approach by groups in Sweden (Zhang et al., 2005) and Australia (Booth et al., 2005), and thus the genome-wide study confirms this as an MS susceptibility gene. *IL7RA* has a disease odds ratio of approximately 1.2; see Figure 2-3 for a comparison of odds ratios to the MHC. *IL7RA* has since been shown to be expressed differentially between patients and controls (Lundmark et al., 2007) and the allele associated with MS results in increased exon skipping, producing more soluble *IL7R* than membrane-bound *IL7R*, potentially important for immune function (Gregory et al., 2007).

GWAS also provided evidence of association for a number of other genes, including the interleukin 2 receptor alpha (*IL2RA*), the C-type lectin domain family 16, member A (*CLEC16A*), and the CD58 genes (Hafler et al., 2007). Because several hundreds of thousands of comparisons are made in GWAS, the potential for false-positive results is high, and the 95% false-positive rate of genetic association studies (Colhoun et al., 2003) is expected to be improved upon by statistical stringency. *IL2RA, CD58, CLEC16A* did not achieve genome-wide significance and hence, further work was needed on these loci. Consistent replication in different populations would provide evidence of causality (Chanock et al., 2007), and this was provided by the International Multiple Sclerosis Genetics Consortium and other independent groups (Ramagopalan et al., 2007a; De Jager et al., 2009), with differences in expression of these genes between patients and controls also being found (see Fig. 2-3).

The Major Histocompatibility Complex

Located on chromosome 6p21, the MHC region spans 3.5 megabases (Mb), including the class I

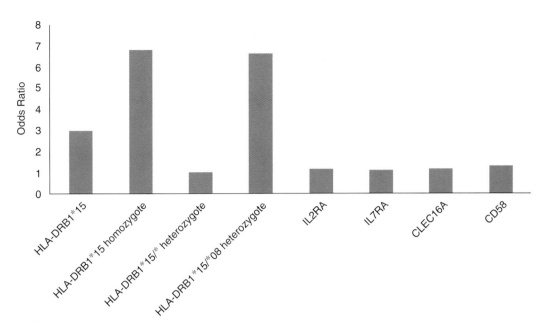

Figure 2-3 Percentage risk increase with genes conclusively associated with multiple sclerosis.

and class II subregions. This has more recently been expanded to a concept of the extended MHC region spanning 7.6 Mb and comprising at least 252 expressed genes, many of which are related to and involved in immune development, maturation, and function (Horton et al., 2004).

Associations of MS with alleles of the MHC were among the earliest reported associations in MS genetics. The first such associations identified were with the HLA class I alleles *HLA-A*03* (Jersild et al., 1972; Naito et al., 1972) and *HLA-B*07* (Compston et al., 1976). Associations with the HLA class II alleles HLA-DR2 were subsequently shown (Jersild et al., 1973; Winchester et al., 1975; Terasaki et al., 1976). This class II association has been fine-mapped to the *HLA-DRB5*0101—HLA-DRB1*1501—HLA-DQA1*0102—HLA-DQB1*0602* extended haplotype (Fogdell et al., 1995). This HLA class II haplotype confers a relative risk of approximately 3 and homozygosity for this haplotype increases risk by over six-fold (Dyment et al., 2004a). Intense linkage disequilibrium in the class II region makes it difficult to identify the specific susceptibility factor(s) involved in the Northern European population, as the *HLA-DRB1*1501, HLA-DQA1*0102,* and *HLA-DQB1*0602*

alleles almost always occur together (Dyment et al., 2004a).

HLA-DR or HLA-DQ?

Intense linkage disequilibrium in the class II region makes it difficult to identify the specific susceptibility factor(s) involved in the Northern European population, as the *HLA-DRB1*1501, HLA-DQA1*0102,* and *HLA-DQB1*0602* alleles are almost always present together on the DR2 haplotype (Dyment et al., 2004a). Evidence for a primary association of *HLA-DRB1* came from a study of African Americans with MS (Oksenberg et al., 2004). African Americans have greater haplotypic diversity and patterns of linkage disequilibrium that are distinct from those in Northern Europeans; in particular, *HLA-DRB1*1501* and *HLA-DQB1*0602* are not always found on the same haplotype. In African American patients, a selective association with *HLA-DRB1*15* was revealed, independent of *HLA-DQB1*0602* (Oksenberg et al., 2004). Conclusions from this study are at odds with data from African Brazilian MS patients, where association was with *HLA-DQB1*0602* rather than *HLA-DRB1*15* (Caballero et al., 1999; Alves-Leon et al., 2007). More recently, it has been shown that *HLA-DRB1* cannot be the sole susceptibility locus for this region, and it is likely that the *haplotype* determines risk or protection (Chao et al., 2008).

HLA-DRB1 Allelic Heterogeneity

While MS is associated with the HLA-DRB1*1501—HLA-DQA1*0102—HLA-DQB1*0602 haplotype in Northern European populations (Fogdell et al., 1995), in other populations, for example Sardinia, MS is associated with the *HLA-DRB1*0301—HLA-DQA1*0501—HLA-DQB1*0201* and *HLA-DRB1*0405—HLA-DQA1*0501—HLA-DQB1*0301* haplotypes (Marrosu et al., 1997). The HLA association was recently revisited in an exceptionally large Canadian MS population (Dyment et al., 2005), and results shifted the paradigm. *HLA-DRB1*15* was shown not to be the sole risk-increasing allele. Similar to previous studies in Sweden (Masterman et al., 2000; Modin et al., 2004), the *HLA-DRB1*17* (03) allele was shown to be associated in the Canadian population, but increased risk to a lesser extent than *HLA-DRB1*15* (1.7-fold risk increase as compared to 3). Furthermore, a hierarchy of disease-associated alleles was uncovered, with indications of alleles that protect against disease, in particular, *HLA-DRB1*14* (Dyment et al., 2005) and *HLA-DRB1*11* (Ramagopalan et al., 2007b). *HLA-DRB1*14* has the most dominant role in MS MHC genetics and completely abrogates any risk associated with *HLA-DRB1*15* when they are inherited together (Ramagopalan et al., 2007b). The effect of this allele may be part of the reason why the prevalence of MS in Asia is low, where the frequency of this allele is high (Ramagopalan et al., 2007b). Interestingly, *HLA-DRB1*14* is also strongly protective against type 1 diabetes (Erlich et al., 2008), perhaps hinting at common mechanisms to disease protection.

HLA-DRB1 Epistasis

A more compelling observation from the Canadian study was the discovery of epistatic interactions between *HLA-DRB1* haplotypes. On its own, *HLA-DRB1*08* modestly increases the risk of MS but when present with *HLA-DRB1*15* on the other parental haplotype, it more than doubles the risk associated with a single copy of *HLA-DRB1*15*

(Dyment et al., 2005). Additionally, *HLA-DRB1*01* and *HLA-DRB1*10* protect against MS but only in the presence of *HLA-DRB1*15* in trans (Dyment et al., 2005; Ramagopalan et al., 2007b; Ramagopalan and Ebers, 2009), although reports from Sweden suggest that *HLA-DRB1*01* may be protective on its own (Brynedal et al., 2007). Nevertheless, it is clear that the net effect of the two parental haplotypes in combination, which can be called the *diplotype*, is what determines an individual's MS risk. Epistasis of haplotypes is the key determinant of MS risk.

MHC Class II: Structure and Function

MHC class II molecules present antigen to CD4$^+$ T helper cells and are integral to successful maintenance of self-tolerance by the immune system and the adaptive immune response to invading pathogens figure 2-4 (Watts, 2004). Each *HLA-DRB1* allele forms, by the presence of defined amino acid anchors, a number of specific pockets comprising a peptide-binding groove (Jones et al., 2006). Different *HLA-DRB1* alleles may thus have different binding affinities for disease-related peptides as determined by their protein sequence, subsequently influencing composition of T cell repertoires, ultimately resulting in *HLA-DRB1* alleles having varying effects on disease risk. Protein sequence analysis has failed to provide unequivocal support for this hypothesis. Class II alleles in MS patients are structurally no different to those in healthy controls (Cowan et al., 1991). While some studies have suggested that variable residues in the DR beta chain may determine MS susceptibility (Ghabanbasani et al., 1995), others could not find any evidence to show that MS pathogenesis is mediated by allele-overlapping antigen binding sites (Zipp et al., 2000). More recently, Barcellos et al. (2006) have suggested that the amino acid at position 60 of the *HLA-DRB1* protein sequence determines the effect of a *HLA-DRB1* allele on MS susceptibility. However, the purported disease risk–increasing codon at this amino acid is also seen in *HLA-DRB1*01*, which is not a susceptibility allele (Dyment et al., 2005; Ramagopalan et al., 2007b). In conclusion, no sequence variant of *HLA-DRB1* can fully explain the risk attributable to all disease associated alleles, suggesting that other risk factors are

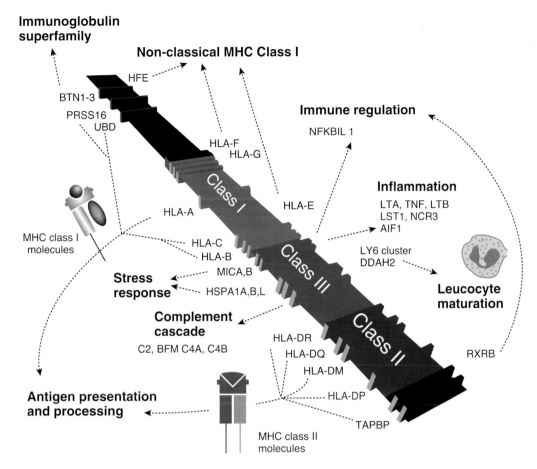

Figure 2-4 The major histocompatibility complex.

present on *HLA-DRB1* haplotypes (Ramagopalan et al., 2009b), and this perhaps detracts away from antigen presentation as the sole mechanism of the MHC association in MS (Hiremath et al., 2008).

Other MHC Loci?

In addition to the established HLA class II association, several groups have suggested that additional MHC loci may influence MS susceptibility, but these reports remain controversial. Originally thought to be secondary to a stronger HLA class II association, it has now been suggested that HLA class I may also play a primary role in MS. A recent report suggests that *HLA-A*02* has a protective

effect independent of *HLA-DRB1*15* (Brynedal et al., 2007), while another has proposed that *HLA-C*05* plays a similar role (Yeo et al., 2007). These investigations were largely based on case-control data raising the possibility that population stratification and linkage disequilibrium produced these results. The recent Wellcome Trust Case Control Consortium study, which analyzed the DNA of 17,000 individuals of similar ancestry in Great Britain showed that allele frequencies in the MHC vary considerably across the country (The Wellcome Trust Case Control Consortium, 2007), highlighting the potential unreliability of using case-control methodology for this region. Additionally, observations of association at the MHC region must be considered in the context of the extensive linkage disequilibrium present in this area; haplotype-based analysis could find no effect of the HLA class I loci independent of *HLA-DRB1* (Chao et al., 2007). Furthermore, a study using over 1100 Canadian and Finnish MS families genotyped for over 650 SNP markers spanning the whole MHC showed no evidence for additional association independent of *HLA-DRB1*, implying that HLA-associated MS susceptibility is determined by HLA class II alleles or closely located variants (Lincoln et al., 2005).

It has recently been shown that *HLA-DRB1*15 haplotypes are heterogeneous and not all *HLA-DRB1*15 haplotypes are associated with MS susceptibility (Chao et al., 2008). Transmission analysis of HLA class I and II haplotypes revealed at least three populations of *HLA-DRB1*15 haplotypes, including those that are overtransmitted (susceptible) and those that are neutral-transmitted/under-transmitted (nonsusceptible). This observation, in conjunction with the finding that linkage is present in *HLA-DRB1*15-negative families, which cannot be explained by other *HLA-DRB1* alleles (Ligers et al., 2001; Dyment et al., 2005), suggests that an additional MHC class II-linked susceptibility element (s) exists. The identity and location of putative variants are unknown but undoubtedly include *HLA-DQ*, and they may extend to epigenetic modifications or regulatory elements in the class II region in tight linkage disequilibrium with MS susceptibility and resistance *HLA-DRB1* haplotypes (Lincoln et al., 2005; Chao et al., 2008).

GENES AND ENVIRONMENT

There may be interactions of EBV and vitamin D with the HLA, which would add further support to a role of these environmental factors in MS.

Although the exact mechanism, if any, of EBV in MS pathogenesis remains to be elucidated, molecular mimicry has been suggested to be involved as a T cell receptor from an MS patient was shown to recognize both a *HLA-DRB1*1501-restricted myelin basic protein (MBP) and *HLA-DRB5*0101-restricted EBV peptide (Lang et al., 2002).

Early studies also provided evidence for an effect of vitamin D on HLA gene expression (Rigby et al., 1990; Skjodt et al., 1990), although no specific mechanism had been characterized. Recently, sequence analysis localized a single

MHC vitamin D response element (VDRE) to the promoter region of *HLA-DRB1*, which was completely conserved in *HLA-DRB1*15 haplotypes but variant to some extent in all others. Functional studies showed that the VDRE present in the *HLA-DRB1* promoter influenced gene expression and imparted 1,25-dihydroxyvitamin D3 sensitivity to *HLA-DRB1*15. The variant VDRE present on other, non-MS-associated *HLA-DRB1* haplotypes was not responsive to 1,25-dihydroxyvitamin D3 (Ramagopalan et al., 2009a). This result perhaps goes some way in explaining why twin concordance is latitude dependent.

Genes and Outcome

As the association between *HLA-DRB1* and MS susceptibility is definite, several studies have focussed on the part *HLA-DRB1* alleles may play on modifying disease expression. Surprisingly, the results trying to relate HLA class II alleles to disease outcome have been inconsistent and contradictory. This is epitomized by studies from the United States. The initial investigation of DR2 by Barcellos and colleagues did not find any effect of the haplotype on disease course (Barcellos et al., 2002), although the group did later discover a dose effect wherein individuals homozygous for DR2 were noted to have more severe disease (Barcellos et al., 2003). Afterward, the same group could not find evidence to support their findings of DR2 homozygosity predisposing to severe disease in a large U.S. and European cohort (Barcellos et al., 2006). Most recently, the group has now suggested that *HLA-DRB1*15 influences disease severity as inferred by magnetic resonance (MR) spectroscopy and magnetic resonance imaging (MRI) measures (Okuda et al., 2008).

It has been suggested that discrepancies between reports have arisen from disease heterogeneity, ethnic variation, and the ascertainment of non-population-based cases that fail to capture extremes of clinical outcome (Kantarci et al., 2002; Ramagopalan et al., 2008). A recent study has attempted to deal with these issues and take advantage of the lessons learned from previous studies. DeLuca and colleagues compared *HLA-DRB1* genotypes in Canadian and Sardinian benign and malignant MS patients lying at opposite extremes of the distribution of *long-term* outcome using stringent clinical criteria (DeLuca et al., 2007). Benign patients were defined as where minimal disability (i.e., EDSS ≤ 3) was attained over a period of greater than 20 years from disease onset. In contrast, malignant cases acquired significant disability (i.e., EDSS > 6) within 5 years of disease onset. The influence on statistical power of this approach is profound (Risch and Zhang, 1995; DeLuca et al., 2007). *HLA-DRB1*01* was significantly underrepresented in malignant compared with benign cases at least in part resulting from an epistatic interaction with *HLA-DRB1*1501*. This allele appears to attenuate the progressive disability that characterizes MS in the long term.

SUMMARY

In summary, the etiology of MS is still unclear but it is now recognized that the degree of complexity is beyond what was believed even up to 10–15 years ago. The complexity comes from the realization that one cannot predict the expression of the phenotype from knowledge of the individual effects of the individual factors considered alone. Genes, environment, postgenomic modifications, and chance all interact.

ACKNOWLEDGMENTS

The Canadian collaborative Project on Genetic Susceptibility to MS (CCPGSMS) is funded mainly by the MS Society of Canada Scientific Research Foundation. Professors A. Dessa Sadovnick and George C. Ebers are the principal investigators.

The Multiple Sclerosis Society of the United Kingdom provided partial support and studentship support.

The authors would like to thank all patients who generously participated in this study and physicians participating in the CCPGSMS. Experiments performed for this investigation comply with current guidelines and ethics.

The authors gratefully acknowledge collaborators of the CCPGSMS: T. Traboulsee, V. Devonshire, S. A. Hashimoto, J. Hooge, J. Oger (Vancouver), L. Metz (Calgary), S. Warren (Edmonton), W. Hader, K. Knox (Saskatoon), R. A. Marrie (Winnipeg), M. Freedman (Ottawa), D. Brunet (Kingston), M. Kremenchutzky (London), P. O'Connor, T. Gray, M. Hohol (Toronto), P. Duquette, Y. Lapierre (Montreal), V. Bhan, C. Maxner (Halifax), and M. Stefanelli (St. Johns).

REFERENCES

Acheson ED, Bachrach CA, Wright FM. Some comments on the relationship of the distribution of multiple sclerosis to latitude, solar radiation, and other variables. *Acta Psychiatr Scand Suppl.* 1960;35:132–147.

Alonso A, Hernan MA. Temporal trends in the incidence of multiple sclerosis: a systematic review. *Neurology.* 2008;71:129–135.

Alves-Leon SV, Papais-Alvarenga R, Magalhaes M, Alvarenga M, Thuler LC, Fernandez y Fernandez O. Ethnicity-dependent association of HLA DRB1-DQA1-DQB1 alleles in Brazilian multiple sclerosis patients. *Acta Neurol Scand.* 2007;115:306–311.

Ascherio A, Munch M. Epstein-Barr virus and multiple sclerosis. *Epidemiology.* 2000;11:220–224.

Ascherio A, Munger KL. Environmental risk factors for multiple sclerosis. Part I: the role of infection. *Ann Neurol.* 2007;61:288–299.

Bager P, Nielsen NM, Bihrmann K, et al. Childhood infections and risk of multiple sclerosis. *Brain.* 2004; 127:2491–2497.

Barcellos LF, Kamdar BB, Ramsay PP, et al. Clustering of autoimmune diseases in families with a high-risk for multiple sclerosis: a descriptive study. *Lancet Neurol.* 2006;5:924–931.

Barcellos LF, Oksenberg JR, Begovich AB, et al. HLA-DR2 dose effect on susceptibility to multiple sclerosis and influence on disease course. *Am J Hum Genet.* 2003;72:710–716.

Barcellos LF, Oksenberg JR, Green AJ, et al. Genetic basis for clinical expression in multiple sclerosis. *Brain.* 2002;125:150–158.

Barnett MH, Williams DB, Day S, Macaskill P, McLeod JG. Progressive increase in incidence and prevalence of multiple sclerosis in Newcastle, Australia: a 35-year study. *J Neurol Sci.* 2003;213:1–6.

Booth DR, Arthur AT, Teutsch SM, et al. Gene expression and genotyping studies implicate the interleukin 7 receptor in the pathogenesis of primary progressive multiple sclerosis. *J Mol Med.* 2005;83:822–830.

Brassat D, Azais-Vuillemin C, Yaouanq J, et al. Familial factors influence disability in MS multiplex families. French Multiple Sclerosis Genetics Group. *Neurology.* 1999;52:1632–1636.

Brynedal B, Duvefelt K, Jonasdottir G, et al. HLA-A confers an HLA-DRB1 independent influence on the risk of multiple sclerosis. *PLoS ONE.* 2007;2:e664.

Bulman DE, Sadovnick AD, Ebers GC. Age of onset in siblings concordant for multiple sclerosis. *Brain.* 1991;114(Pt 2):937–950.

Caballero A, Alves-Leon S, Papais-Alvarenga R, Fernandez O, Navarro G, Alonso A. DQB1*0602 confers genetic susceptibility to multiple sclerosis in Afro-Brazilians. *Tissue Antigens.* 1999;54:524–526.

Chanock SJ, Manolio T, Boehnke M, et al. Replicating genotype-phenotype associations. *Nature.* 2007;447: 655–660.

Chao MJ, Barnardo MC, Bu GZ, et al. Transmission of class I/II multi-locus MHC haplotypes and multiple sclerosis susceptibility: accounting for linkage disequilibrium. *Hum Mol Genet.* 2007;16:1951–1958.

Chao MJ, Barnardo MC, Lincoln MR, et al. HLA Class I Alleles Tag HLA-DRB1*1501 Haplotypes for Differential Risk in Multiple Sclerosis Susceptibility. *Proc Natl Acad Sci USA.* 2008;105(35):13069–13074.

Chataway J, Feakes R, Coraddu F, et al. The genetics of multiple sclerosis: principles, background and updated results of the United Kingdom systematic genome screen. *Brain.* 1998;121(Pt 10):1869–1887.

Chataway J, Mander A, Robertson N, et al. Multiple sclerosis in sibling pairs: an analysis of 250 families. *J Neurol Neurosurg Psychiatry.* 2001;71:757–761.

Colhoun HM, McKeigue PM, Davey Smith G. Problems of reporting genetic associations with complex outcomes. *Lancet.* 2003;361:865–872.

Compston DA, Batchelor JR, McDonald WI. B-lymphocyte alloantigens associated with multiple sclerosis. *Lancet.* 1976;2:1261–1265.

Cordell HJ, Clayton DG. Genetic association studies. *Lancet.* 2005;366:1121–1131.

Correale J, Ysrraelit MC, Gaitan MI. Immunomodulatory effects of Vitamin D in multiple sclerosis. *Brain.* 2009;132:1146–1160.

Cowan EP, Pierce ML, McFarland HF, McFarlin DE. HLA-DR and -DQ allelic sequences in multiple sclerosis patients are identical to those found in the general population. *Hum Immunol.* 1991;32:203–210.

Dawn Teare M, Barrett JH. Genetic linkage studies. *Lancet.* 2005;366:1036–1044.

De Jager PL, Jia X, Wang J, et al. Meta-analysis of genome scans and replication identify CD6, IRF8 and TNFRSF1A as new multiple sclerosis susceptibility loci. *Nat Genet.* 2009;41:776–782.

Dean G. Annual incidence, prevalence, and mortality of multiple sclerosis in white South-African-born and in white immigrants to South Africa. *Br Med J.* 1967; 2:724–730.

Dean G, Elian M. Age at immigration to England of Asian and Caribbean immigrants and the risk of developing multiple sclerosis. *J Neurol Neurosurg Psychiatry.* 1997;63:565–568.

Debouverie M, Pittion-Vouyovitch S, Louis S, Roederer T, Guillemin F. Increasing incidence of multiple sclerosis among women in Lorraine, Eastern France. *Mult Scler.* 2007;13:962–967.

DeLuca GC, Ramagopalan SV, Herrera BM, et al. An extremes of outcome strategy provides evidence that multiple sclerosis severity is determined by alleles at the HLA-DRB1 locus. *Proc Natl Acad Sci USA.* 2007;104:20896–20901.

Di Pauli F, Reindl M, Ehling R, et al. Smoking is a risk factor for early conversion to clinically definite multiple sclerosis. *Mult Scler.* 2008;14:1026.

Dyment DA, Ebers GC, Sadovnick AD. Genetics of multiple sclerosis. *Lancet Neurol.* 2004a;3:104–110.

Dyment DA, Herrera BM, Cader MZ, et al. Complex interactions among MHC haplotypes in multiple sclerosis: susceptibility and resistance. *Hum Mol Genet.* 2005;14:2019–2026.

Dyment DA, Sadovnick AD, Willer CJ, et al. An extended genome scan in 442 Canadian multiple sclerosis-affected sibships: a report from the Canadian Collaborative Study Group. *Hum Mol Genet.* 2004b;13:1005–1015.

Dyment DA, Yee IM, Ebers GC, Sadovnick AD. Multiple sclerosis in stepsiblings: recurrence risk and ascertainment. *J Neurol Neurosurg Psychiatry.* 2006;77:258–259.

Ebers GC, Kukay K, Bulman DE, et al. A full genome search in multiple sclerosis. *Nat Genet.* 1996;13: 472–476.

Ebers GC, Sadovnick AD, Dyment DA, Yee IM, Willer CJ, Risch N. Parent-of-origin effect in multiple sclerosis: observations in half-siblings. *Lancet.* 2004;363: 1773–1774.

Ebers GC, Sadovnick AD, Risch NJ. A genetic basis for familial aggregation in multiple sclerosis. Canadian Collaborative Study Group. *Nature.* 1995;377:150–151.

Ebers GC, Yee IM, Sadovnick AD, Duquette P. Conjugal multiple sclerosis: population-based prevalence and recurrence risks in offspring. Canadian Collaborative Study Group. *Ann Neurol.* 2000;48:927–931.

Erlich H, Valdes AM, Noble J, et al. HLA DR-DQ haplotypes and genotypes and type 1 diabetes risk: analysis of the type 1 diabetes genetics consortium families. *Diabetes.* 2008;57:1084–1092.

Fogdell A, Hillert J, Sachs C, Olerup O. The multiple sclerosis- and narcolepsy-associated HLA class II haplotype includes the DRB5*0101 allele. *Tissue Antigens.* 1995;46:333–336.

Ghabanbasani MZ, Gu XX, Spaepen M, et al. Importance of HLA-DRB1 and DQA1 genes and of the amino acid polymorphisms in the functional domain of DR beta 1 chain in multiple sclerosis. *J Neuroimmunol.* 1995; 59:77–82.

Gregory SG, Schmidt S, Seth P, et al. Interleukin 7 receptor alpha chain (IL7R) shows allelic and functional association with multiple sclerosis. *Nat Genet.* 2007; 39(9):1083–1091.

Grytten N, Glad SB, Aarseth JH, Nyland H, Midgard R, Myhr KM. A 50-year follow-up of the incidence of multiple sclerosis in Hordaland County, Norway. *Neurology.* 2006;66:182–186.

Hafler DA, Compston A, Sawcer S, et al. Risk alleles for multiple sclerosis identified by a genomewide study. *N Engl J Med.* 2007;357:851–862.

Haines JL, Bradford Y, Garcia ME, et al. Multiple susceptibility loci for multiple sclerosis. *Hum Mol Genet.* 2002;11:2251–2256.

Haines JL, Ter-Minassian M, Bazyk A, et al. A complete genomic screen for multiple sclerosis underscores a role for the major histocompatability complex. The Multiple Sclerosis Genetics Group. *Nat Genet.* 1996;13:469–471.

Hammond SR, English DR, McLeod JG. The age-range of risk of developing multiple sclerosis: evidence from a migrant population in Australia. *Brain.* 2000;123 (Pt 5):968–974.

Hammond SR, McLeod JG, Millingen KS, et al. The epidemiology of multiple sclerosis in three Australian cities: Perth, Newcastle and Hobart. *Brain.* 1988;111 (Pt 1):1–25.

Hattersley AT, McCarthy MI. What makes a good genetic association study? *Lancet.* 2005;366:1315–1323.

Healy BC, Ali EN, Guttmann CRG, et al. Smoking and disease progression in multiple sclerosis. *Arch Neurol.* 2009;66:858–864.

Hensiek AE, Roxburgh R, Smilie B, et al. Updated results of the United Kingdom linkage-based genome screen in multiple sclerosis. *J Neuroimmunol.* 2003;143:25–30.

Hensiek AE, Seaman SR, Barcellos LF, et al. Familial effects on the clinical course of multiple sclerosis. *Neurology.* 2007;68:376–383.

Hernan MA, Oleky MJ, Ascherio A. Cigarette smoking and incidence of Multiple Sclerosis. *Am J Epi.* 2001; 154:69–74.

Herrera BM, Ramagopalan SV, Lincoln MR, et al. Parent-of-origin effects in MS. Observations from avuncular pairs. *Neurology.* 2008;71:799–803.

Hiremath MM, Chen VS, Suzuki K, Ting JP, Matsushima GK. MHC class II exacerbates demyelination in vivo independently of T cells. *J Neuroimmunol.* 2008; 203:23–32.

Hirst C, Ingram G, Pickersgill T, Swingler R, Compston DA, Robertson NP. Increasing prevalence and incidence of multiple sclerosis in South East Wales. *J Neurol Neurosurg Psychiatry.* 2009;80:386–391.

Hoppenbrouwers IA, Liu F, Aulchenko YS, et al. Maternal transmission of multiple sclerosis in a dutch population. *Arch Neurol.* 2008;65:345–348.

Horikawa Y, Tsubaki T, Nakajima M. Rubella antibody in multiple sclerosis. *Lancet.* 1973;1:996–997.

Horton R, Wilming L, Rand V, et al. Gene map of the extended human MHC. *Nat Rev Genet.* 2004;5:889–899.

Islam T, Gauderman WJ, Cozen W, Hamilton AS, Burnett ME, Mack TM. Differential twin concordance for multiple sclerosis by latitude of birthplace. *Ann Neurol.* 2006;60:56–64.

Islam T, Gauderman WJ, Cozen W, Mack TM. Childhood sun exposure influences risk of multiple sclerosis in monozygotic twins. *Neurology.* 2007;69:381–388.

Jafari N, Hoppenbrouwers IA, Hop WC, Breteler MB, Hintzen RQ. Cigarette smoking and riks of MS in multiplex families. *Mult Scler.* 2009;15:1363.

James JA, Kaufman KM, Farris AD, Taylor-Albert E, Lehman TJ, Harley JB. An increased prevalence of Epstein-Barr virus infection in young patients suggests a possible etiology for systemic lupus erythematosus. *J Clin Invest.* 1997;100:3019–3026.

Jersild C, Fog T, Hansen GS, Thomsen M, Svejgaard A, Dupont B. Histocompatibility determinants in multiple sclerosis, with special reference to clinical course. *Lancet.* 1973;2:1221–1225.

Jersild C, Svejgaard A, Fog T. HL-A antigens and multiple sclerosis. *Lancet.* 1972;1:1240–1241.

Jones EY, Fugger L, Strominger JL, Siebold C. MHC class II proteins and disease: a structural perspective. *Nat Rev Immunol.* 2006;6:271–282.

Kantarci OH, de Andrade M, Weinshenker BG. Identifying disease modifying genes in multiple sclerosis. *J Neuroimmunol.* 2002;123:144–159.

Kenealy SJ, Babron MC, Bradford Y, et al. A second-generation genomic screen for multiple sclerosis. *Am J Hum Genet.* 2004;75:1070–1078.

Kuokkanen S, Gschwend M, Rioux JD, et al. Genomewide scan of multiple sclerosis in Finnish multiplex families. *Am J Hum Genet.* 1997;61:1379–1387.

Kurtzke JF. Epidemiologic evidence for multiple sclerosis as an infection. *Clin Microbiol Rev.* 1993;6:382–427.

Kurtzke JF, Beebe GW, Norman JE, Jr. Epidemiology of multiple sclerosis in U.S. veterans: 1. Race, sex, and geographic distribution. *Neurology.* 1979;29:1228–1235.

Lang HL, Jacobsen H, Ikemizu S, et al. A functional and structural basis for TCR cross-reactivity in multiple sclerosis. *Nat Immunol.* 2002;3:940–943.

Ligers A, Dyment DA, Willer CJ, et al. Evidence of linkage with HLA-DR in DRB1*15-negative families with multiple sclerosis. *Am J Hum Genet.* 2001;69:900–903.

Lincoln MR, Montpetit A, Cader MZ, et al. A predominant role for the HLA class II region in the association of the MHC region with multiple sclerosis. *Nat Genet.* 2005;37:1108–1112.

Lindberg C, Andersen O, Vahlne A, Dalton M, Runmarker B. Epidemiological investigation of the association between infectious mononucleosis and multiple sclerosis. *Neuroepidemiology.* 1991;10:62–65.

Lundmark F, Duvefelt K, Iacobaeus E, et al. Variation in interleukin 7 receptor alpha chain (IL7R) influences risk of multiple sclerosis. *Nat Genet.* 2007;39: 1108–1113.

Marrie RA, Wolfson C, Sturkenboom MC, et al. Multiple sclerosis and antecedent infections: a case-control study. *Neurology.* 2000;54:2307–2310.

Marrosu MG, Murru MR, Costa G, et al. Multiple sclerosis in Sardinia is associated and in linkage disequilibrium with HLA-DR3 and -DR4 alleles. *Am J Hum Genet.* 1997;61:454–457.

Masterman T, Ligers A, Olsson T, Andersson M, Olerup O, Hillert J. HLA-DR15 is associated with lower age at onset in multiple sclerosis. *Ann Neurol.* 2000; 48:211–219.

Mikaeloff Y, Caridade G, Tardieu M, Suissa S and on behalf of the KIDSEP study group. Parental smoking at home and the risk of childhood-onset multiple sclerosis in children. *Brain.* 2007;130(10):2589–2595.

Millar JH, Fraser KB, Haire M, Connolly JH, Shirodaria PV, Hadden DS. Immunoglobulin M specific for measles and mumps in multiple sclerosis. *Br Med J.* 1971;2:378–380.

Modin H, Olsson W, Hillert J, Masterman T. Modes of action of HLA-DR susceptibility specificities in multiple sclerosis. *Am J Hum Genet.* 2004;74:1321–1322.

Montgomery SM, Bahmanyar S, Hillert J, Ekbom A, Olsson T. Maternal smoking during pregnancy and multiple sclerosis amongst offspring. *European Journal of Neurology.* 2008;15: 1395–1399.

Munger KL, Levin LI, Hollis BW, Howard NS, Ascherio A. Serum 25-hydroxyvitamin D levels and risk of multiple sclerosis. *JAMA.* 2006;296:2832–2838.

Naito S, Namerow N, Mickey MR, Terasaki PI. Multiple sclerosis: association with HL-A3. *Tissue Antigens.* 1972;2:1–4.

Newhook LA, Sloka S, Grant M, Randell E, Kovacs CS, Twells LK. Vitamin D insufficiency common in newborns, children and pregnant women living in Newfoundland and Labrador, Canada. *Matern Child Nutr.* 2009;5:186–191.

Nielsen TR, Rostgaard K, Nielsen NM, Koch-Henriksen N, Haahr S, Sorensen PS, Hjalgrim H. Multiple sclerosis after infectious mononucleosis. *Arch Neurol.* 2007;64:72–75.

Oksenberg JR, Barcellos LF, Cree BA, et al. Mapping multiple sclerosis susceptibility to the HLA-DR locus in African Americans. *Am J Hum Genet.* 2004;74:160–167.

Okuda DT, Srinivasan R, Oksenberg JR, et al. Genotype-phenotype correlations in multiple sclerosis: HLA genes influence disease severity inferred by 1HMR spectroscopy and MRI measures. *Brain.* 2008;132(1):250–259.

Orton SM, Herrera BM, Yee IM, et al. Sex ratio of multiple sclerosis in Canada: a longitudinal study. *Lancet Neurol.* 2006;5:932–936.

Pekmezovic T, Jarebinski M, Drulovic J. Childhood infections as risk factors for multiple sclerosis: Belgrade case-control study. *Neuroepidemiology.* 2004;23:285–288.

Pittas F, Ponsonby AL, van der Mei IA, et al. Smoking is associated with progressive disease course and increased progression in clinical disability in a prospective cohort of people with multiple sclerosis. *J Neurol.* 2009;256: 577–585.

Pugliatti M, Sotgiu S, Rosati G. The worldwide prevalence of multiple sclerosis. *Clin Neurol Neurosurg.* 2002;104:182–191.

Ramagopalan SV, Anderson C, Sadovnick AD, Ebers GC. Genomewide study of multiple sclerosis. *N Engl J Med* 2007a;357:2199–2200; author reply 2200–2191.

Ramagopalan SV, Deluca GC, Degenhardt A, Ebers GC. The genetics of clinical outcome in multiple sclerosis. *J Neuroimmunol.* 2008;(201–202):183–199.

Ramagopalan SV, Ebers GC. Epistasis: multiple sclerosis and the major histocompatibility complex. *Neurology.* 2009;72(6):566–567.

Ramagopalan SV, Maugeri N, Handunnetthi L, et al. Expression of the multiple sclerosis associated MHC class II allele HLA-DRB1*1501 is regulated by vitamin D. *PLoS Genet.* 2009a;5(2)e1000369.

Ramagopalan SV, McMahon R, Dyment DA, Sadovnick AD, Ebers GC, Wittkowski KM. An extension to a statistical approach for family based association studies provides insights into genetic risk factors for multiple sclerosis in the HLA-DRB1 gene. *BMC Med Genet.* 2009b;10:10.

Ramagopalan SV, Morris AP, Dyment DA, et al. The Inheritance of Resistance Alleles in Multiple Sclerosis. *PLoS Genet.* 2007b;3:e150.

Ramagopalan SV, Yee IM, Dyment DA, et al. Parent-of-origin effect in multiple sclerosis. Observations from interracial matings. *Neurology.* 2009c;73:602–606.

Rigby WF, Waugh M, Graziano RF. Regulation of human monocyte HLA-DR and CD4 antigen expression, and antigen presentation by 1,25-dihydroxyvitamin D3. *Blood.* 1990;76:189–197.

Risch N, Merikangas K. The future of genetic studies of complex human diseases. *Science.* 1996;273: 1516–1517.

Risch N, Zhang H. Extreme discordant sib pairs for mapping quantitative trait loci in humans. *Science.* 1995;268:1584–1589.

Robertson NP, O'Riordan JI, Chataway J, et al. Offspring recurrence rates and clinical characteristics of conjugal multiple sclerosis. *Lancet.* 1997;349:1587–1590.

Ross CA, Lenman JA, Rutter C. Infective Agents and Multiple Sclerosis. *Br Med J.* 1965;1:226–229.

Runmarker B, Andersen O. Prognostic factors in a multiple sclerosis incidence cohort with twenty-five years of follow-up. *Brain.* 1993;116(Pt I):117–134.

Saarela J, Schoenberg Fejzo M, Chen D, et al. Fine mapping of a multiple sclerosis locus to 2.5 Mb on chromosome 17q22-q24. *Hum Mol Genet.* 2002;11: 2257–2267.

Sadovnick AD, Baird PA, Ward RH. Multiple sclerosis: updated risks for relatives. *Am J Med Genet.* 1988; 29:533–541.

Sadovnick AD, Ebers GC. Epidemiology of multiple sclerosis: a critical overview. *Can J Neurol Sci.* 1993;20: 17–29.

Sawcer S, Ban M, Maranian M, et al. A high-density screen for linkage in multiple sclerosis. *Am J Hum Genet.* 2005;77:454–467.

Sawcer S, Jones HB, Feakes R, et al. A genome screen in multiple sclerosis reveals susceptibility loci on chromosome 6p21 and 17q22. *Nat Genet.* 1996;13: 464–468.

Serafini B, Rosicarelli B, Franciotta D, et al. Dysregulated Epstein-Barr virus infection in the multiple sclerosis brain. *J Exp Med.* 2007;204:2899–2912.

Sibley WA, Foley JM. Infection and immunization in multiple sclerosis. *Ann N Y Acad Sci.* 1965;122: 457–466.

Skjodt H, Hughes DE, Dobson PR, Russell RG. Constitutive and inducible expression of HLA class II determinants by human osteoblast-like cells in vitro. *J Clin Invest.* 1990;85:1421–1426.

Sumaya CV, Myers LW, Ellison GW. Epstein-Barr virus antibodies in multiple sclerosis. *Arch Neurol.* 1980;37:94–96.

Sundstrom P, Nystrom L. Smoking worsens the prognosis of multiple sclerosis. *Mult Scler.* 2008;14:1031.

Tarrats R, Ordonez G, Rios C, Sotelo J. Varicella, ephemeral breastfeeding and eczema as risk factors for multiple sclerosis in Mexicans. *Acta Neurol Scand.* 2002;105:88–94.

Terasaki PI, Park MS, Opelz G, Ting A. Multiple sclerosis and high incidence of a B lymphocyte antigen. *Science.* 1976;193:1245–1247.

Thacker EL, Mirzaei F, Ascherio A. Infectious mononucleosis and risk for multiple sclerosis: a meta-analysis. *Ann Neurol.* 2006;59:499–503.

The Wellcome Trust Case Control Consortium. Genome-wide association study of 14,000 cases of seven common diseases and 3,000 shared controls. Nature. 2007;447:661–678.

van der Mei IA, Ponsonby AL, Dwyer T, et al. Past exposure to sun, skin phenotype, and risk of multiple sclerosis: case-control study. *BMJ.* 2003;327:316.

Wallin MT, Page WF, Kurtzke JF. Multiple sclerosis in US veterans of the Vietnam era and later military service: race, sex, and geography. *Ann Neurol.* 2004;55:65–71.

Watts C. The exogenous pathway for antigen presentation on major histocompatibility complex class II and CD1 molecules. *Nat Immunol.* 2004;5:685–692.

Willer CJ, Dyment DA, Risch NJ, Sadovnick AD, Ebers GC. Twin concordance and sibling recurrence rates in multiple sclerosis. *Proc Natl Acad Sci USA.* 2003; 100:12877–12882.

Willer CJ, Dyment DA, Sadovnick AD, Rothwell PM, Murray TJ, Ebers GC. Timing of birth and risk of multiple sclerosis: population based study. *BMJ.* 2005;330:120.

Winchester R, Ebers G, Fu SM, Espinosa L, Zabriskie J, Kunkel HG. B-cell alloantigen Ag 7a in multiple sclerosis. *Lancet.* 1975;2:814.

Yeo TW, De Jager PL, Gregory SG, et al. A second major histocompatibility complex susceptibility locus for multiple sclerosis. *Ann Neurol.* 2007;61: 228–236.

Zaadstra B, Chorus A, van Buuren S, Kalsbeek H, van Noort J. Selective association of multiple sclerosis with infectious mononucleosis. *Mult Scler.* 2008; 14:307–313.

Zhang Z, Duvefelt K, Svensson F, et al. Two genes encoding immune-regulatory molecules (LAG3 and IL7R) confer susceptibility to multiple sclerosis. *Genes Immun.* 2005;6:145–152.

Zipp F, Windemuth C, Pankow H, et al. Multiple sclerosis associated amino acids of polymorphic regions relevant for the HLA antigen binding are confined to HLA-DR2. *Hum Immunol.* 2000;61:1021–1030.

3   Neurophysiology of Multiple Sclerosis

Jefferson C. Slimp

The fundamental injury in multiple sclerosis has long been considered to be inflammatory mediated demyelination of the central nervous system, caused by altered immune system function. The loss of myelin leads to a disruption of communication among the neurons of the brain and spinal cord. Specifically, conduction of action potentials along axons may be slowed or completely blocked, consequently disrupting information processing and information transfer. While destruction of myelin may be disrupting in and of itself, MS patients now are also known to have significant degeneration of axons and loss of cell bodies (Lumsden, 1970; Bo et al., 2003; Geurts and Barkhof, 2008). Recent work has even raised the question of whether the fundamental problem in MS may be initially one of neurodegeneration with a secondary inflammatory demyelination (Trapp and Nave, 2008).

To understand the symptomatology as well as gain insights into the underlying pathology requires a basic understanding of neurophysiology. This chapter will present the basic principles of neurophysiology with respect to those relevant to multiple sclerosis.

CELLS OF THE BRAIN

Neurons and glia compose the two cell types of the brain. Both of these types of cells are involved in the pathological process of MS. Glia are 10 times more numerous than neurons, but neurons are considered more functional because of their signaling and information-processing capabilities. Neurons are involved in conveying sensory messages from the environment to the brain, linking information from different areas of the brain, and

delivering signals to create responses to this information. Glial cells are classified as astrocytes, oligodendrocytes, or microglia. Glia have a supportive role, providing insulation and influencing signal propagation, maintaining ionic balance, modulating synaptic action, and guiding neural development.

A typical neuron consists of a soma (cell body) with a number of processes (neurites) emanating from the soma that make the neuron a unique cell in the body (Fig. 3-1). During development, a neuron will begin with multiple neurites, one of which will elongate rapidly and become an axon and the others forming shorter branches called dendrites. Dendrites and the soma are covered with synapses, which receive information from other neurons. Most neurons have an axon, which originates from an area on the soma called the axon hillock. The first part of the axon is called the initial segment and is the site of generation of the action potential. The length of the axon varies depending on the type of neuron and on the distance the destination is away from the soma. Axons often branch forming collaterals. There also exist neurons that lack axons such as may be found in the retina, olfactory bulb, and certain areas of cerebral cortex (Meyer, 1983; Meyer et al., 1984; Peichl and Gonzalez-Soriano, 1994; Egger et al., 2003).

As one of the types of glial cells, astrocytes are numerous and are found throughout the brain. Astrocytes may communicate with neurons as well as other glial cells. Their processes extend to neuronal synapses, to nodes of Ranvier, and to the blood–brain barrier. They appear to have an essential role in regulating the chemical environment of neurons, such as potassium from the extracellular space and glutamate from around synapses.

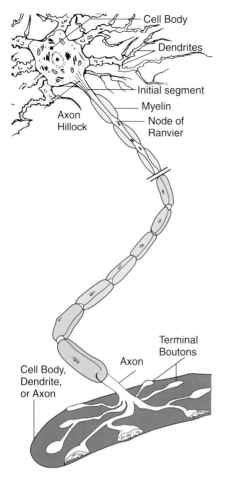
Cell Body
Dendrites
Initial segment
Myelin
Node of
Ranvier
Axon
Hillock
Terminal
Boutons
Axon
Cell Body,
Dendrite,
or Axon

Figure 3-1 Typical neuron with cell body and neurites (dendrites and axon). Myelin sheaths are shown as a series of wraps around the axon separated by nodes of Ranvier. At its termination an axon may branch before making contact with another cell's dendrites, axons, or cell body.

With respect to MS, astrocytes have been ignored for the most part over the years, but recently interest in the role of astrocytes in demyelination and remyelination has revived (Williams et al., 2007). Astrocytes seemingly have a role in both demyelination through regulation of the passage of T cells through the blood brain–barrier, the migration of immune cells through brain tissue, and the activation of inflammatory cells and remyelination through the migration and proliferation of oligodendrocytes precursor cells (see Williams et al., 2007).

Microglia are considered to be the sole representative cell of the immune system residing in the brain (Smith, 2001). Normally, microglia are quiescent, but when activated by substances or signals associated with disease or injury, they can serve as phagocytes removing cellular debris from dead or degenerating neurons or glia. Microglia are part of the pathological process of inflammation and demyelination in MS, working in concert with T lymphocytes, macrophages, and peripheral dendritic cells.

Oligodendrocytes have a crucial role in the propagation of electrical signals along the axons of projection neurons. These cells provide the lipid dense myelin sheaths that encompass the axon and that are the focus of the pathology of MS (Fig. 3-1). Myelin sheaths are insulating layers formed by extensions of an oligodendrocyte that are wrapped around the axon like paper around a tube. Oligodendrocyte precursor cells differentiate into mature oligodendrocytes with astrocytes involved in the signaling process for differentiation and proliferation (Williams et al., 2007). Additionally, oligodendrocytes myelinate not one but several axons, all of which means that there is a plethora of molecular factors involved in these multiple cell interactions.

To assist in understanding this physiological disorder, it will be helpful to explore the concept of an electrically excitable membrane and conduction of impulses along such a membrane. The discussion will pertain to excitable membranes, in general, such as both nerve and muscle membranes, but the focus will be on neuronal activity. The key to understanding excitable membranes and nerve conduction lies in the membrane structure of lipids and proteins and the fluids bathing the membrane. This unique relationship allows the formation of electrical potentials that are the basis for conduction of action potentials along nerve fibers, which is the basic mechanism for transfer of information among nerve cells. When an electrically excitable membrane is at rest it demonstrates an electrical charge across its membrane that is electrically negative on the inside compared to the outside. When an action potential occurs, the transmembrane potential becomes temporarily reversed so that the inside becomes positive with respect to the outside. This process is regenerative and propagates an impulse along the membrane outward from the site of activation. These events find their basis in the composition of the fluids that are present on each side of the membrane, the characteristics of the membrane, and the proteins that form channels or pores through the membrane.

FLUIDS AROUND THE NERVE MEMBRANE

Water is the main constituent of the fluids surrounding the nerve membrane. The salient property of water is its uneven distribution of charge. The oxygen atom has a greater affinity for electrons than hydrogen, and thus by capturing the shared electrons becomes negatively charged, whereas the hydrogen atoms become positively charged. Water is considered to be a polar molecule and, as such, an effective solvent. The important ions for electrical excitability that are dissolved in water are sodium, potassium, calcium, and chloride. Sodium (Na^+) and potassium (K^+) are called monovalent cations, because they are positively charged and

have one less electron than protons. Calcium (Ca^+) is a divalent cation because it is positively charged and has two less electrons than protons. Chloride (Cl^-) is a monovalent anion because it is negatively charged and has one more electron than protons.

THE NERVE MEMBRANE

The nerve (and muscle) membrane is a phospholipid bilayer (see Fig. 3-2, quaternary). Phospholipids, like other lipids, are long nonpolar chains of carbon atoms bonded to hydrogen atoms with the distinction of a polar phosphate group attached to one end. The nonpolar chains of carbon and hydrogen are hydrophobic and point toward the middle of the membrane. The polar phosphate end is hydrophilic and points outward from the membrane. As a result, the lipid bilayer of the nerve membrane is impenetrable to water and separates the water of the outside from that of the

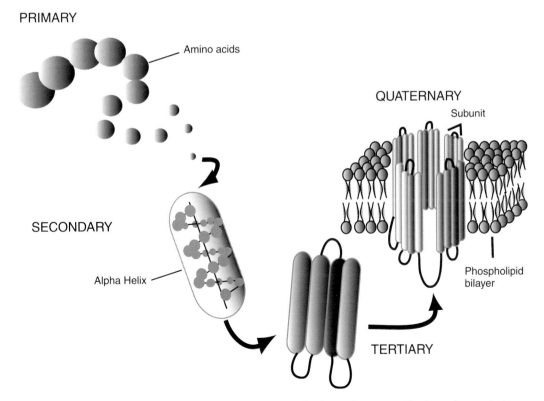

Figure 3-2 Levels of protein structure. Primary, a polypeptide chain of amino acids. Secondary, spiral organization of polypeptide. Tertiary, folded configuration of a polypeptide. Quaternary, multiple polypeptide chains bonded together and shown here embedded in a phospholipid bilayer membrane.

inside of the cell. Only lipid-soluble entities, such as carbon dioxide and oxygen, may pass through such a membrane. Water-soluble entities, such as the ions associated with nerve cells, must pass through specialized pores or channels. Different channels are selective for different ions. The difference in channels is a function of the protein configurations specific to each channel.

TRANSMEMBRANE PROTEINS

As with other cells, nerve cells are unique with respect to the types and distribution of proteins they make. Depending on how the protein is synthesized it may form a single polypeptide chain (primary structure), a spiral configuration of the polypeptide chain (secondary structure), a folded configuration of the proteins (tertiary structure), or multiple polypeptide chains bonded together (quaternary structure) (Fig. 3-2). Each separate polypeptide chain in a quaternary structure is called a subunit. Some examples of proteins in a neuron are the enzymes for chemical reactions, receptors that combine with various entities such as neurotransmitters, and proteins that span the nerve membrane.

CHANNELS

One such quaternary structure that spans the nerve membrane is an ion channel. Channels may contain a number of subunits. One such transmembrane subunit is called the alpha subunit in which most of the functional properties reside. There are other subunits that may extend outside of the membrane or exist across or within the membrane; these are called beta, gamma, and delta subunits.

The transmembrane alpha subunit is a collection of proteins, sometimes depicted like staves of a barrel, which form a pore-like configuration that spans the membrane (Fig. 3-3 and also Fig. 3-2, quaternary structure). Each protein in a transmembrane subunit may contain a nonpolar portion within the membrane that favors the lipid membrane and a polar portion on each end that favors water. The diameter of the pore and the configuration of the amino acids lining the pore confer ion selectivity to the channel.

There may also be a portion of the alpha subunit structure (Fig. 3-3) that is voltage sensitive and will demonstrate different conformational configurations depending on the transmembrane voltage. Changing the voltage can result in a rearrangement of the proteins that will alter the permeability of a channel and, thus, the flow of ions through the pore. These channels are referred to as voltage-dependent channels.

Moreover, within an ion selective channel type or family, such as potassium or sodium channels, there can be variations in gene expression controlling the formation of channel proteins, rendering a number of subfamilies and isoforms. For example, there is considerable diversity in potassium channels with over 30 different isoforms identified (Judge et al., 2007). For sodium channels, nine different isoforms have been characterized. Not all of these subunits have implications for neural functioning as some are associated with skeletal and cardiac muscle function. Interestingly, recent evidence has shown that two potassium channel isoforms called $K_v1.3$ and $K_v1.5$, upregulate when T lymphocytes, macrophages, microglia, and dendritic cells are activated during the inflammatory disease process, although the exact role of this upregulation is yet to be determined (Judge et al., 2006). Blocking these potassium channels may have potential therapeutic effects through an immunosuppressive action (Judge et al., 2006).

Similarly, sodium channel isoforms, $Na_v1.4$ and $Na_v1.5$, are found in skeletal and cardiac muscle, respectively. For those isoforms associated with neural function, different isoforms both within the potassium and sodium families are found differentially distributed on the neuron and within the nervous system. So, for example, sodium channel isoforms, $Na_v1.1$, $Na_v1.2$, $Na_v1.3$, and $Na_v1.6$, are found in the brain, whereas $Na_v1.7$, $Na_v1.8$, and $Na_v1.9$ are found outside of the brain primarily in dorsal root ganglion neurons (Catterall et al., 2005). Within these sets, some are found on axons, whereas others are found on dendrites or interneurons. Subunit variation also determines the particular properties or type of ion flow through the channel.

As with potassium channels, sodium channels are not confined to neurons. Sodium channels, particularly the $Na_v1.6$ isoform, may be found in and

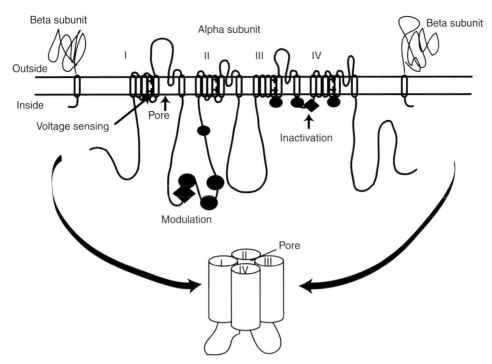

Figure 3-3 Schematic representation of sodium channel subunits showing the alpha unit as four repetitions or domains (I–IV) of six transmembrane folded subunits. The pore of sodium channel is formed by the arrangement of the domains and the configuration of the loop between the fifth and sixth portion of each domain. The voltage-sensitive portion is indicated as the fourth folded member in each domain. The inactivation gate is shown as an intracellular loop between domains III and IV. The extracellular beta subunits and intracellular loops are also indicated.

apparently regulate microglia and macrophages. Both of these inflammatory cells are closely associated with the disease process in MS. Moreover, it appears that $Na_v1.6$ expression is upregulated in acute lesions in MS (Craner et al., 2005).

In addition to transmembrane alpha subunits, which form the core portion of the channel, the protein complexes of channels also have beta subunits and loops either on the outside or inside of the membrane (Fig. 3-3). A major function of beta subunits and loops is gating or controlling the flow of the ions specific for the channel. The channel may be deactivated (closed to ion passage), activated (open to ion passage), or inactivated (block ion passage). Inactivation is thought to be due to a tethered plug on the inside of the membrane that blocks the channel after it has been activated.

ION PUMPS

Another transmembrane macromolecular protein complex, separate from the channel complex, is the ion pump. These pumps use ATP, formed in the cell's mitochondria, as the energy to transport ions across the membrane. They serve to maintain the concentration differences of ions across the nerve membrane, namely a high concentration of K^+ inside and a high concentration of Na^+ and Ca^{2+} outside the cell. One pump transports Na^+ and K^+. It is an enzyme that breaks down ATP in the presence of internal Na^+ and exchanges an internal Na^+ for an external K^+. A second pump is a calcium pump that transports Ca^{2+} out of the cell. Both of these pumps perform work to move the ions against their concentration gradient, consuming ATP in the process. Their function of maintaining the concentration differences of Na^+, K^+, and Ca^{2+} is essential to neural activity. Without the action of these pumps, neural activity can carry on for a period of time but eventually an imbalance of ions will occur and neuronal function will fail.

THE MEMBRANE AND ION MOVEMENT

As mentioned previously, nerve and muscle cell membrane have an electrical potential across the membrane. Typically, when a nerve cell is not activated, it shows a 65 mV difference across its membrane with the inside negative with respect to the outside (usually denoted –65 mV). This transmembrane potential is called the resting membrane potential and must exist in order for a nerve to function normally. The explanation for basis of the resting membrane potential relies on understanding the ions involved and their distribution across the membrane.

Imagine a neuronal cell filled with water in which K^+ and an anion (A^-) are placed. After a period of time, the ions will become equally distributed throughout the cell by the process of diffusion. If measured, no electrical potential difference will exist across the solution in the cell because the positive and negative charges are equal in number.

Assume that the cell has an impermeable membrane, such as phospholipid bilayer that separates the fluid of the cell from the fluid surrounding it. Furthermore, assume the K^+ and an anion (A^-) concentration on the inside is much higher than the concentration of the K^+ and an anion (A^-) on the outside. No electrical potential difference can be measured across the membrane because the number of cations and anions on each side will be equal and no electrical difference will be present.

Now assume that the phospholipid bilayer contains channels that are selectively permeable to K^+. Potassium ions will be free to move through the channels, but the anions will not move through due to the selectivity of the channel. The movement of the K^+ will be governed by two forces: concentration gradient and electrical potential. On the one hand, K^+ will move down its concentration gradient from the high concentration inside of the cell to the low concentration outside

of the cell, resulting in fewer cations within the cell. Since A^- will not be able to cross the membrane, an electrical difference will develop across the membrane with the inside negative because of the decreasing number of cations. The movement of K^+ will continue to move down its concentration gradient from inside to outside, but this movement will be counterbalanced by the increasing negative electrical force inside the cell, which will draw the K^+ back to the inside. Eventually, an equilibrium potential will be reached in which movement of K^+ out will be balanced by movement of K^+ in.

Knowing the electrical charge of an ion and its concentration difference across a membrane, the equilibrium potential can be calculated exactly using the Nernst equation:

$$E = 2.303 \frac{RT}{zF} \log \frac{[ion]_o}{[ion]_i}$$

where E is the equilibrium potential, R is the gas constant, T is absolute temperature, z is the charge of the ion, F is the Faraday constant, and log is base 10 logarithm for the concentration of the ion outside the cell $[ion]_o$, and inside the cell $[ion]_i$. From this equation, it should be apparent that if the ion concentration is higher inside the cell, such as is the case for K^+, then the potential difference will be negative, and if the concentration is higher outside the cell the potential difference will be positive. Thus, for K^+ in neurons, E is –80mV. Sodium and calcium are found in highest concentration outside the cell and, therefore, their equilibrium potentials will be positive. For Na^+, it is +62 mV, and for Ca^+ it is +123 mV. This, of course, means that for K^+ the concentration gradient will move K^+ from inside to outside and the electrical force will serve to move K^+ from outside to inside in a counteractive manner. For Na^+ and Ca^+, the concentration gradient will move the ions from outside to inside.

The actual measurement of –65 mV is less than the –80 mV equilibrium potential for K^+ and suggests that the resting membrane potential is not due solely to K^+ but to a combination of ion flows. The relatively high permeability of K^+ accounts for most of the resting membrane potential, but there exists a steady leakage of Na^+ into the cell as well.

THE NEURAL IMPULSE

The action potential, sometimes referred to as a neural impulse or a spike, transmits information over distances in the nervous system. During an action potential, the neural membrane briefly reverses polarity and becomes positive inside before returning to the resting condition (Fig. 3-4). This polarity reversal spreads outward from its point of origin and propagates along the axon. In many neurons, but not all, the action potential begins at the axon hillock, near the cell body and conducts the length of the axon. In sensory neurons, the action potential begins at the end of the neurite that terminates in the sensory structure and propagates along the axon toward the brain. An important characteristic is that the action potential maintains its size as it propagates along the axon, indicating a regenerative quality.

The shape of an action potential as displayed in a voltage-time dimension consists of a rapid rise in potential or depolarization from the resting level of –65 mV to +40 mV followed by a fall in voltage or repolarization that overshoots the original resting membrane potential for a short time, a hyperpolarization.

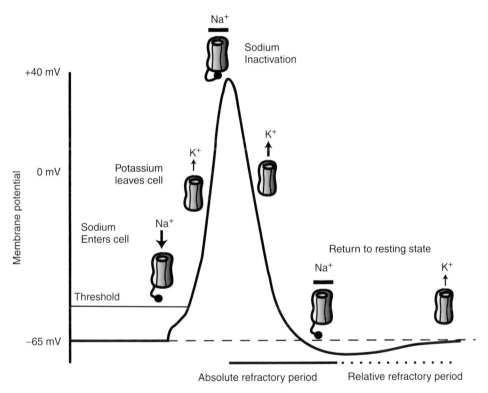

Figure 3-4 Schematic diagram of a recording of an action potential, showing the sequence of changes in membrane potential and the corresponding sodium and potassium channel changes. When the membrane potential reaches threshold, the sodium channel opens and sodium rapidly enters the cell driving the membrane potential in a positive direction. Potassium channels simultaneously open but more slowly, allowing efflux of potassium. The inactivation gate of the sodium channel slowly closes stopping the influx of sodium. With sodium conduction stopped and potassium exiting the cell, the membrane potential returns to baseline overshooting for a brief period. While the inactivation gate is closed the membrane is absolutely refractory to further activation. During the overshoot it is relatively refractory meaning a larger stimulus would be needed to reach the threshold for activation. The time course of an action potential is about 3 milliseconds.

The initiation of an action potential is a depolarization of the resting membrane potential from −65mV to the threshold for an action potential (approximately −40 to −50 mV), a value that depends on the particular neuron in question. The events that can depolarize a membrane to threshold are several and include the action of a neurotransmitter when it combines with its specific receptor, mechanical events that stretch a nerve ending and open gated sodium channels, chemical events that either directly or indirectly affect sodium channels through second messengers.

When threshold is reached, the voltage-sensitive segments of both sodium and potassium channels are activated. The voltage-sensitive segment of the sodium channel alters the configuration of the pore region and the configuration of the gating subunit. As a result of the rapid change in pore configuration, sodium rushes into the cell, driven by the concentration and electrical gradients for sodium. The membrane potential proceeds toward the equilibrium potential for sodium. At this time, the membrane potential is showing its rapid rise due to the influx of sodium. The configuration change in the gating subunit takes slightly longer to complete and, when it does, it blocks or inactivates the sodium channel. The rise in membrane potential is terminated by the closure of the gating subunit, preventing further sodium movement through the channel, which leads to a fall of the action potential back toward resting levels. Simultaneously, the potassium channel is also undergoing a configuration change, which opens the potassium channels, increasing the permeability of the membrane to potassium. This action takes place more slowly than the rapidly acting sodium channel, occurring about 1 msec later. The effect of potassium ions leaving the cell is to drive the membrane potential more negative, that is, toward potassium's equilibrium potential. The potassium channels remain open to the point that the membrane potential falls beyond the resting level, forming a hyperpolarization that lasts 1–2 milliseconds.

As the voltage declines below activation threshold, the voltage-sensitive regions of the sodium and potassium channels are no longer activated and the pore and gating subunits return to the resting condition; that is, the sodium pore configuration is no longer permeable to sodium, the inactivating gating subunit opens again, and the potassium channel's pore configuration becomes less permeable to potassium.

While the inactivation gating subunit is engaged, the sodium channel is incapable of passing sodium, even in the presence of an activating threshold or greater voltage level. This time is referred to as the absolute refractory period. Once the inactivation gating subunit opens in response to membrane potentials more negative than threshold, the sodium channel is capable of being activated again. However, during the hyperpolarization phase of the action potential, which is due to the open potassium channels, a stronger depolarizing current is needed to open sodium channels. This time is referred to as the relative refractory period.

ACTION POTENTIAL CONDUCTION

Propagation of the action potential along an axon is a function of the influx of positive charge, carried by the sodium ions. This internal positive charge spreads along the inside of the axon, in the form of a local current. This local current depolarizes the adjacent membrane and activates the adjacent voltage-sensitive sodium and potassium channels, thus spreading the action potential along the axon membrane. The spread of positive charge along the axon is a passive spread of ionic current, meaning that the current falls in value exponentially with distance from its origin. The action potential, on the other hand, does not diminish amplitude over distance because it is an active process, whose energy is derived from the stored energy of the concentration gradients for sodium and potassium provided by the ion pumps and the selective permeable membrane.

The speed of conduction of an action potential along an axon depends on the anatomy of the axon. The passive spread of the local current, like the spread of any current, depends on the resistance. The current will flow down the axon through the cytosol and through the membrane. The resistance of the cytosol is proportional to the diameter of the axon, and the resistance of the membrane is proportional to the thickness and structure of the membrane. Thus, the lower the resistance of the cytosol the greater the current flow down the axon and, consequently, the faster the conduction along the axon.

As a rule, the larger the diameter of an axon, the more rapid is the conduction. A classic example is the giant axon of the squid, which is used by the squid to perform escape maneuvers. The axon is about 1 mm in diameter, huge by vertebrate standards, and has been much used for research on membrane biophysics. Many of the principles of resting membrane function and action potentials were based on squid axon research. The squid giant axon also serves as a model for unmyelinated axons in vertebrates. The spread of the action potential is supported by a nearly uniform distribution of sodium channels across the membrane (isoform $Na_v1.2$).

Conduction in unmyelinated axons in vertebrates is not particularly fast not only because unmyelinated axons are small in diameter but also because the action potentials spread from one sodium channel to the next. The solution to increase conduction velocity solely by increasing axon diameter, as it is done in squid, is not an option in vertebrates because their many neurons would mean an inordinately huge and impractical amount of territory devoted to large axons. Instead, vertebrates developed the system of myelin to increase conduction speed.

The myelin sheaths, formed by either oligodendrocytes in the central nervous system (CNS) or by Schwann cells in the periphery, serve to insulate the axons, thereby increasing the overall resistance across the membrane. The myelin does not coat the axon entirely along its length but is broken periodically at regions called the nodes of Ranvier. The length of myelin or the intermodal distance varies from 0.2 to 2 mm, with larger diameter axons having longer internodal distances.

The function of the myelin sheaths is to insulate the axon, which allows the passive spread of the internal positive charge to extend farther down the axon. This happens in part because of the increased resistance across the membrane, forcing the charge down the less resistant axon but mainly because of the lower capacitance of a thicker membrane and the lower amount of charge used to develop the capacitance, leaving more charge to spread further down the axon.

Another significant structural characteristic of the myelinated nerve membrane is distribution of sodium and potassium channels. Sodium channels are densely expressed at the nodes of Ranvier with much fewer sodium channels found in the internodal regions (Ritchie and Rogart, 1977). Specifically, the sodium channel subfamily, $Na_v1.6$, is densely expressed at the nodes of Ranvier in mature individuals. Interestingly, during maturation $Na_v1.2$ channels are found at nodes of Ranvier but are eclipsed by $Na_v1.6$. $Na_v1.6$ is also present at the initial segment of the axon in conjunction with $Na_v1.1$ (Vacher et al., 2008). Potassium channels similarly concentrate in the nodal and paranodal regions (Judge et al., 2006).

The effect of myelin on passive spread of the local current and the focal density of sodium channels at the nodes of Ranvier means the action potential develops at the node of Ranvier and not in the internodal space, lending a saltatory quality to conduction in myelinated axons. The depolarization does not need to be continuous as in unmyelinated fibers but can skip from one node of Ranvier to the next. The overall effect is one of greater speed of conduction but with less ionic conductance, and hence with greater efficiency and less energy consumption.

NEUROPHYSIOLOGICAL CHANGES WITH MULTIPLE SCLEROSIS

The generally accepted notion of MS as an inflammatory mediated demyelinating disease implies alteration in axonal conduction. Conduction may be completely blocked, it may be delayed, or it may conduct intermittently. The early course of MS of a relapsing-remitting pattern suggests a process leading to conduction impairment followed by a mechanism(s) for recovery of function. For patients that later develop the secondary progressive or those who have a primary progressive pattern, this suggests a second process of conduction impairment.

RELAPSE: LOSS OF FUNCTION, DEMYELINATION, AND CONDUCTION BLOCK

As was demonstrated experimentally several years ago, conduction block in axons is a consequence of demyelination (McDonald and Sears, 1969; McDonald and Sears, 1970). Using a model of diphtheria toxin–induced demyelination in cat spinal cord, these studies showed three principal abnormalities. First, conduction block occurred in severe demyelination. Second, conduction slowing was characteristic of smaller lesions. Third, there was an inability of demyelinated fibers to faithfully conduct trains of impulses. Moreover, these effects occurred specifically in the demyelinated region and not in the unaffected portions of the axon.

The loss of a single internode is sufficient to cause conduction block. One explanation is the changes in the passive electrical properties of the internodal myelin (Rasminsky and Sears, 1972). Internodal capacitance is increased and internodal transverse resistance is decreased with demyelination, both of which would absorb more of the longitudinal local current, preventing sufficient current from reaching the next node. A second, and not mutually exclusive, explanation is the observation that Na^+ channels are found in high density at the nodes of Ranvier and in low density in the internodal membrane (Ritchie and Rogart, 1977; Waxman, 1977). As explained earlier, this scenario is ideal for efficient and rapid salutatory conduction in normal axons, but with demyelination it leaves the exposed internodal membrane incapable of conduction due to the lack of sufficient Na^+ channels.

If demyelination is less extensive and confined only to the paranodal region causing nodal widening, a condition that may occur in MS (Wolswijk and Balesar, 2003), conduction may still fail. The failure occurs first, because the increased membrane capacitance consumes more of the local current to fulfill the capacitance, and second because the widened node disperses the local current. Thus, the local current cannot depolarize the membrane sufficiently to open Na^+ channels at the next node of Ranvier.

If the lesion is smaller and has not completely demyelinated the axon, conduction may continue, but conduction velocity is slowed through the demyelinated region but not through normal part of the axon (McDonald and Sears, 1970). Much variability occurs in the conduction velocity of various neurons.

Temporary neurological deficits may occur in MS that are not easily explained by demyelination. While there may be other factors associated with inflammation, the most promising and intriguing is nitric oxide. Nitric oxide has been shown to block conduction in axons (Redford et al., 1997; Shrager et al., 1998) and is known to be prevalent in MS plaques (Smith and Lassmann, 2002). While the mechanism is not known, it may interfere with sodium channels or the sodium pump or inhibit mitochondrial metabolism causing membrane depolarization (see Smith, 2007).

REMISSION AND RESTORATION OF AXONAL CONDUCTION IN DEMYELINATED AXONS

The presence of silent demyelinating lesions found at autopsy in patients with no clinical correlates suggests that conduction may be restored or present in demyelinated segments (O'Riordan et al., 1998; Lebrun et al., 2008). Based on brain imaging studies, it has been estimated that inflammatory lesions occur nearly 10 times as often as clinical relapses occur (Miller et al., 1993; Filippi et al., 1998). Recovery of function in MS may occur for several reasons, such as the cessation of inflammation or plasticity within remaining functioning parts of the nervous system, but at the axon level there is clear evidence that restoration of conduction occurs in persistently demyelinated axons as well as remyelinated axons (Felts et al., 1997).

As mentioned earlier, demyelinated axons fail to conduct because of the paucity of sodium channels in the internodal nerve membrane that render the membrane inexcitable. Restoration of conduction relies on the insertion of new sodium channels distributed along the demyelinated membrane. Studies in rodent experimental allergic encephalomyelitis (EAE) models of MS showed upregulation of $Na_v1.2$ and $Na_v1.6$ isoforms of sodium channels in demyelinated regions (Craner et al., 2003; Craner et al., 2004a). Acute lesions in MS show a similar pattern of expression of $Na_v1.2$ and $Na_v1.6$ isoforms along demyelinated segments (Craner et al., 2004b). The presence of $Na_v1.6$ has been associated with axonal loss (see later discussion), but the expression of $Na_v1.2$ isoforms along extended segments of demyelinated axon is comparable to the diffuse pattern of $Na_v1.2$ in developing premyelinated axons and unmyelinated axons (see Waxman, 2006).

Conduction in these recovered axons is not on par with normal axons. Conduction velocity may be substantially reduced on the order of

0.5–2.5 m/sec (Smith and McDonald, 1999), compared to a normal velocity of 40–50 m/sec. The reduction in conduction velocity, even though restricted to the demyelinated area, is sufficient to reduce conduction velocity over the length of the axon. The latency increase, particularly if accrued over multiple demyelinated segments, is most likely the basis for increased latencies seen in clinical somatosensory, visual, and auditory evoked potentials.

What may be more important functionally than changes in conduction velocity is the inability of demyelinated fibers to conduct a second impulse in the normal time frame or to conduct trains of impulses faithfully. Normal axons may conduct a second impulse within 0.5–1.4 msec following the first, whereas demyelinated axons take 1.0 to 6.0 msec before being able to conduct a second impulse. The failure to conduct a second impulse is related to prolongation of the refractory period (Felts et al., 1997). Instead of conducting trains of impulse steadily up to 1000/sec as is normal, demyelinated axons show intermittent periods of failure to conduct action potentials with the overall rate reduced by severalfold. The periods of conduction block are associated with membrane hyperpolarization caused by activation of the Na^+/K^+ ATPase, or sodium pump induced by the increased intracellular sodium from the preceding neural activity (Bostock and Grafe, 1985).

Under normal conditions, the amount of local current at a node of Ranvier is more than sufficient to depolarize the membrane, on the order of three to five times that which is necessary to cause action potentials (Tasaki, 1953). In demyelinated axons, the safely factor is reduced to near unity, which means depolarization of the membrane may fail (Smith, 1994). Two factors cause the amount of current at the node of Ranvier to be reduced. First, the lack of myelin increases the capacitance of the membrane, which absorbs more charge as it charges the membrane capacitor, and second, the lack of myelin disperses current along the internode, reducing the effective amount at the node.

Even subtle changes in the environment may have major effects on conduction. One such factor is temperature. Many MS patients report disturbing loss of function with seemingly small increases in temperature. Symptoms may worsen while taking a hot shower (Waxman and Geschwind, 1983), sitting in the sun (Berger and Sheremata, 1985), exercising (Smith and McDonald, 1999), and, in one case, using a hair dryer (Brickner, 1950). While heating may worsen or lead to symptoms, cooling may have the opposite effect and may encourage nonfunctional axons to activation. The duration of the action potential is a function of temperature. The chemical processes at work in the sodium channel, namely the opening of the sodium channel pore and the closing of the inactivation gate, proceed faster with increased temperature, rendering a short duration. Because the temperature coefficient for sodium inactivation is larger than that for sodium activation (Schauf and Davis, 1974; Davis and Schauf, 1981), cooling has the distinct effect of increasing the action potential duration, thereby providing more local current for depolarization at the next node.

Prolongation of an action potential may also be achieved with potassium channel blockers, such as scorpion venom, 4-aminopyridine (4-AP), and 3-4 diaminopyridine (3,4-DAP). Recall that potassium channels are opened in a delayed fashion during an action potential, which contributes to the cessation of the action potential and restoration of the membrane current to resting levels. Blocking potassium channels would prolong the action potential by decreasing the effect of potassium current to restore the membrane potential to its resting level. Experimentally, restoration of conduction in animal peripheral nerve models of demyelinated axons was demonstrated originally using scorpion venom (ref), and then later using 4-AP (Bostock et al., 1978; Sherratt et al., 1980; Bostock et al., 1981). Clinical trials of 4-AP in MS patients showed clear neurological benefits (Jones et al., 1983; Stefoski et al., 1987; Davis et al., 1990; Stefoski et al., 1991; Van Diemen et al., 1993; Bever et al., 1994; Schwid et al., 1997). Widespread use, however, was limited because 4-AP and 3,4-DAP are potent convulsants with a narrow toxic to therapeutic ratio and, therefore, induced seizures in some patients. Because these adverse events correlated with peak serum concentrations, whereas efficacy of treatment correlated with total dose (Bever et al., 1994), sustained-release forms of 4-AP have been tested and found beneficial and has received FDA approval (Schwid et al., 1997; Goodman et al., 2007; Goodman et al., 2009).

Interestingly, the mechanism of action of potassium channel blockers in MS may have as much to do with improvement in synaptic transmitter release (Felts and Smith, 1994; Fujihara and Miyoshi, 1998) as it does prolongation of the action potential in demyelinated axons (Shi and Blight, 1997).

Some MS patients experience tingling sensation or neuropathic pain, sometimes called positive symptoms in contrast to loss of function, referred to as negative symptoms. These positive symptoms may be related to hyperexcitability of the demyelinated nerve membrane leading to spontaneous activity that conducts bidirectionally. The impulses reaching the brain are interpreted as tingling sensations or flashes of light (see Smith and McDonald, 1999; Smith, 2007). The impulses may be continuous or bursting in character. Regular discharges may be related to slow, inward sodium current (Rizzo et al., 1996; Kapoor et al., 1997), while bursting discharges may be due to prolonged, inward potassium current (Kapoor et al., 1993; Felts et al., 1995). The role of potassium currents is less certain, but circumstantially potassium concentrations may be relevant since astrocytes, which are reduced in numbers in MS lesions, regulate extracellular potassium levels.

In some MS patients, body movements elicit sensations such as the radiating shock-like sensations that occur with flexing the neck (Lhermitte sign) or flashes of light that occur with eye movements. In these cases, hyperexcitable, demyelinated axons have likely become mechanosensitive, such that slight deformation or stretching of the axon produces action potentials. Microneurographic recording in patients with Lhermitte sign show bursts of action potentials with neck flexion (Nordin et al., 1984) and experimentally demyelinated central axons demonstrate mechanosensitivity (Smith and McDonald, 1982).

REMISSION AND REMYELINATION

In addition to restoration of conduction in demyelinated axons, remission is likely advanced by remyelination. In order for remyelination to occur, the denuded axons must acquire new myelin sheaths. While much is understood about the origin, the activity, and the fate of oligodendrocytes, the reason for loss of these cells in the MS lesion is still uncertain, with arguments for both apoptosis and a cytolytic process having merit (Raine, 1997; Cudrici et al., 2006). Multiple sclerosis lesions are notably devoid of oligodendrocytes. If present, as they can be in acute inflammatory lesions, they are without their processes and myelin sheathings of axons and, seemingly, do not participate in remyelination (Raine, 1997). Current evidence suggests that remyelination begins with oligodendrocyte precursor cells. Normally quiescent, oligodendrocyte precursor cells may become activated, migrate into lesioned areas, differentiate, and eventually mature to form myelin sheaths (Smith et al., 1979; Smith et al., 1981; Keirstead and Blakemore, 1999; Franklin and ffrench-Constant, 2008). A plethora of molecular factors influence this process, including growth factors, adhesion molecules, cytokines, and transcription factors. Possibly because these many and varied factors are not precisely the same in remyelination as in development may explain the observation that the newly regenerated myelin is thinner than original layering and has a shorter internode length (Blakemore, 1974; Franklin and ffrench-Constant, 2008).

One important reason for remyelination is restoration of efficient conduction. Conduction in demyelinated axons, which is slower and nonsaltatory, requires the action of many sodium channels, consuming more energy. Remyelination presumable returns the axon to a more efficient mode. Support for efficient conduction comes from the observation that sodium and potassium channels undergo reorganization so that higher concentrations of these channels are again found at the new nodes of Ranvier (Black et al., 2006). Also, from experimental studies, it is known that remyelinated axons will conduct axon potentials, but this remains to be demonstrated in MS at the axonal level, although evoked potential data are suggestive that electrophysiological measures may improve with remyelination (Matthews and Small, 1979; Frederiksen and Petrera, 1999; Jones and Brusa, 2003; Klistorner et al., 2007). Experimentally formed lesions left to spontaneously remyelinate clearly conduct action potentials over the remyelinated segments (Smith et al., 1979; Smith et al., 1981). Moreover, remyelination has been associated with restoration of behavior (Jeffery and Blakemore, 1997). While remyelination may be expected to improve conduction, it must be remembered that remyelination is not necessary for restoration of function as that may be attained by conduction in demyelinated axons.

A second important reason for remyelination is that neurons may be protected from degeneration through trophic support from the oligodendrocyte. Support for this concept is from experiments with a knockout mouse model for the gene encoding a nucleotide phosphodiesterase enzyme specific to oligodendrocytes. These mice show a late developing axon degeneration even in the presence of normal appearing myelin (Griffiths et al., 1998; Lappe-Siefke et al., 2003).

AXONAL DEGENERATION AND PROGRESSION OF MULTIPLE SCLEROSIS

Axonal degeneration has been a descriptor of MS even since the early studies by Charcot in the 1800s. Ample histological and postmortem studies have demonstrated axonal loss in MS, and axonal degeneration is likely at the heart of secondary progressive and primary progressive forms of MS (Kuhlmann et al., 2002; Trapp and Nave, 2008). Several mechanisms may account for axon loss but recent thought has been directed to the imbalance of energy supply and demand and the roles of sodium channels, calcium, and nitric oxide (for reviews, see Stys, 2005; Smith, 2007; Franklin and ffrench-Constant, 2008; Gonsette, 2008).

During inflammation several substances are produced that may lead to neurodegeneration, one of which is iNOS, an enzyme involved in the production of nitric oxide (NO). iNOS is upregulated in MS producing large amounts of nitric oxide (Smith and Lassmann, 2002). Nitric oxide has both beneficial and destructive roles in the nervous system. On the deleterious side, nitric oxide and its derivative peroxynitrite inhibit mitochondrial function, reducing the production of ATP (Gonsette, 2008). A consequence of reduced ATP production is impairment of the sodium pump.

Failure of the sodium pump means that normal neural activity, or certainly if there is increased neural activity, will raise the internal sodium concentration. Moreover, the accumulation may be greater than normal because NO may alter the

sodium channel and cause it to pass a persistent current, leading to a continual influx of sodium (Ahern et al., 2000). It should also be remembered that demyelinated but functional axons rely on the continuous distribution of $Na_v1.2$ and $Na_v1.6$ isoforms along demyelinated segments and that $Na_v1.6$ supports high, persistent sodium flow, thus further exacerbating the high internal sodium concentrations (Craner et al., 2004a).

Failure to return sodium to the extracellular space by the sodium pump results in high internal sodium concentrations that can lead to a detrimental influx of calcium. The high intracellular sodium concentration reverses the Na^+–Ca^{2+} exchanger, allowing influx of Ca^{2+} (Stys, 1998). Furthermore, intracellular calcium may be released from intracellular stores such as mitochondria and endoplasmic reticulum under certain conditions like ischemia (Nikolaeva et al., 2005). High internal calcium initiates a variety of enzyme systems (calpain, phospholipase, protein kinase) that lead to axonal injury (Stys, 2005).

Another consequence of high intracellular sodium concentration is the release of glutamate into the extracellular space through alteration of the sodium/glutamate transporter. This transporter normally brings glutamate and sodium into the cell in exchange for potassium, but in high sodium loads the transporter may release glutamate. Indeed, glutamate and aspartate levels are increased MS patients (Stover et al., 1997; Srinivasan et al., 2005). Glutamate excitotoxicity may be widespread in white matter as glutamate receptors may be found on oligodendrocytes, myelin, axons, and astrocytes, all of which have shown damage experimentally by glutamate (for review, see Trapp and Nave, 2008).

CONCLUSION

Understanding the normal physiology of neurons as well as the specifics of the pathomechanisms affecting nerve cells leads to clearer and more effective methods of therapy. To be sure, therapies targeting inflammation are foremost not only in resolving the inflammation but also in stemming the subsequent demyelination and neurodegeneration. Neuroprotection with sodium channel blockers has been shown recently to be therapeutically effective (see Waxman, 2008). Also of interest are therapies directed at blocking potassium channels (see Judge and Bever, 2006), reducing the effect of glutamate (see Sheldon and Robinson, 2007), and reversing mitochondrial defects (see Mahad et al., 2008).

REFERENCES

Ahern GP, Hsu SF, Klyachko VA, Jackson MB. Induction of persistent sodium current by exogenous and endogenous nitric oxide. *J Biol Chem.* 2000;275 (37):28810–28815.

Berger JR, Sheremata WA. Reply to letter by F.A. Davis. *J Am Med Assoc.* 1985;253:203.

Bever CT, Jr., Young D, Anderson PA, et al. The effects of 4–aminopyridine in multiple sclerosis patients: results of a randomized, placebo-controlled, double-blind, concentration-controlled, crossover trial. *Neurology.* 1994;44(6):1054–1059.

Black JA, Waxman SG, Smith KJ. Remyelination of dorsal column axons by endogenous Schwann cells restores the normal pattern of Nav1.6 and Kv1.2 at nodes of Ranvier. *Brain.* 2006;129(pt 5):1319–1329.

Blakemore WF. Pattern of remyelination in the CNS. *Nature.* 1974;249(457):577–578.

Bo L, Vedeler CA, Nyland HI, Trapp BD, Mork SJ. Subpial demyelination in the cerebral cortex of multiple sclerosis patients. *J Neuropathol Exp Neurol.* 2003;62 (7):723–732.

Bostock H, Grafe P. Activity-dependent excitability changes in normal and demyelinated rat spinal root axons. *J Physiol.* 1985;365:239–257.

Bostock H, Sears TA, Sherratt RM. The effects of 4-aminopyridine and tetraethylammonium ions on normal and demyelinated mammalian nerve fibres. *J Physiol.* 1981;313:301–315.

Bostock H, Sherratt RM, Sears TA. Overcoming conduction failure in demyelinated nerve fibres by prolonging action potentials. *Nature.* 1978;274(5669):385–387.

Brickner RM. The significance of localised vasoconstriction in multiple sclerosis. *Res Publ Assoc Res Nerv Ment Dis.* 1950;28:236–244.

Catterall WA, Goldin AL, Waxman SG. International Union of Pharmacology. XLVII. Nomenclature and structure-function relationships of voltage-gated sodium channels. *Pharmacol Rev.* 2005;57(4):397–409.

Craner MJ, Damarjian TG, Shujun L, et al. Sodium channels contribute to microglia/macrophage activation and function in EAE and MS. *Glia.* 2005;49(2):220–229.

Craner MJ, Hains BC, Lo AC, Black JA, Waxman SG. Co-localization of sodium channel Nav1.6 and the sodium-calcium exchanger at sites of axonal injury in the spinal cord in EAE. *Brain.* 2004a;127(pt 2): 294–303.

Craner MJ, Lo AC, Black JA, Waxman SG. Abnormal sodium channel distribution in optic nerve axons in a model of inflammatory demyelination. *Brain.* 2003; 126(pt 7):1552–1561.

Craner MJ, Newcombe J, Black JA, Hartle C, Cuzner ML, Waxman SG. Molecular changes in neurons in multiple sclerosis:altered axonal expression of Nav1.2 and Nav1.6 sodium channels and Na$^+$/Ca2$^+$ exchanger. *Proc Natl Acad Sci USA.* 2004b;101(21):8168–8173.

Cudrici C, Niculescu T, Niculescu F, Shin ML, Rus H. Oligodendrocyte cell death in pathogenesis of multiple sclerosis: protection of oligodendrocytes from apoptosis by complement. *J Rehabil Res Dev.* 2006; 43(1):123–132.

Davis FA, Schauf CL. Approaches to the development of pharmacological interventions in multiple sclerosis. *Adv Neurol.* 1981;31:505–510.

Davis FA, Stefoski D, Rush J. Orally administered 4-aminopyridine improves clinical signs in multiple sclerosis. *Ann Neurol.* 1990;27(2):186–192.

Egger V, Svoboda K, Mainen ZF. Mechanisms of lateral inhibition in the olfactory bulb: efficiency and modulation of spike-evoked calcium influx into granule cells. *J Neurosci.* 2003;23(20):7551–7558.

Felts PA, Baker TA, Smith KJ. Conduction in segmentally demyelinated mammalian central axons. *J Neurosci.* 1997;17(19):7267–7277.

Felts PA, Kapoor R, Smith KJ. A mechanism for ectopic firing in central demyelinated axons. *Brain.* 1995;118 (pt 5):1225–1231.

Felts PA, Smith KJ. The use of potassium channel blocking agents in the therapy of demyelinating diseases. *Ann Neurol.* 1994;36(3):454.

Filippi M, Rocca MA, Martino G, Horsfield MA, Comi G. Magnetization transfer changes in the normal appearing white matter precede the appearance of enhancing lesions in patients with multiple sclerosis. *Ann Neurol.* 1998;43(6):809–814.

Franklin RJ, ffrench-Constant C. Remyelination in the CNS: from biology to therapy. *Nat Rev Neurosci.* 2008;9(11):839–855.

Frederiksen JL, Petrera J. Serial visual evoked potentials in 90 untreated patients with acute optic neuritis. *Surv Ophthalmol.* 1999;44(suppl 1):S54–S62.

Fujihara K, Miyoshi T. The effects of 4-aminopyridine on motor evoked potentials in multiple sclerosis. *J Neurol Sci.* 1998;159(1):102–106.

Geurts JJ, Barkhof F. Grey matter pathology in multiple sclerosis. *Lancet Neurol.* 2008;7(9):841–851.

Gonsette RE. Oxidative stress and excitotoxity: a therapeutic issue in multiple sclerosis? *Mult Scler.* 2008; 14(1):22–34.

Goodman AD, Brown TR, Krupp LB, et al. Sustained-release oral fampridine in multiple sclerosis: a randomised, double-blind, controlled trial. *Lancet.* 2009;373(9665):732–738.

Goodman AD, Cohen JA, Cross A, et al. Fampridine-SR in multiple sclerosis: a randomized, double-blind, placebo-controlled, dose-ranging study. *Mult Scler.* 2007;13(3):357–368.

Griffiths I, Klugmann M, Anderson T, et al. Axonal swellings and degeneration in mice lacking the major proteolipid of myelin. *Science.* 1998;280(5369):1610–1613.

Jeffery ND, Blakemore WF. Locomotor deficits induced by experimental spinal cord demyelination are abolished by spontaneous remyelination. *Brain*. 1997;120(pt 1): 27–37.

Jones RE, Heron JR, Foster DH, Snelgar RS, Mason RJ. Effects of 4-aminopyridine in patients with multiple sclerosis. *J Neurol Sci*. 1983;60(3):353–362.

Jones SJ, Brusa A. Neurophysiological evidence for long-term repair of MS lesions: implications for axon protection. *J Neurol Sci*. 2003;206(2):193–198.

Judge SI, Bever CT, Jr. Potassium channel blockers in multiple sclerosis: neuronal Kv channels and effects of symptomatic treatment. *Pharmacol Ther*. 2006; 111(1):224–259.

Judge SI, Lee JM, Bever CT, Jr., Hoffman PM. Voltage-gated potassium channels in multiple sclerosis: overview and new implications for treatment of central nervous system inflammation and degeneration. *J Rehabil Res Dev*. 2006;43(1):111–122.

Judge SI, Smith PJ, Stewart PE, Bever CT, Jr. Potassium channel blockers and openers as CNS neurologic therapeutic agents. *Recent Pat CNS Drug Discov*. 2007;2(3):200–228.

Kapoor R, Li YG, Smith KJ. Slow sodium-dependent potential oscillations contribute to ectopic firing in mammalian demyelinated axons. *Brain*. 1997;120 (pt 4):647–652.

Kapoor R, Smith KJ, Felts PA, Davies M. Internodal potassium currents can generate ectopic impulses in mammalian myelinated axons. *Brain Res*. 1993;611(1): 165–169.

Keirstead HS, Blakemore WF. The role of oligodendrocytes and oligodendrocyte progenitors in CNS remyelination. *Adv Exp Med Biol*. 1999;468:183–197.

Klistorner A, Graham S, Fraser C, et al. Electrophysiological evidence for heterogeneity of lesions in optic neuritis. *Invest Ophthalmol Vis Sci*. 2007;48(10):4549–4556.

Kuhlmann T, Lingfeld G, Bitsch A, Schuchardt J, Brück W. Acute axonal damage in multiple sclerosis is most extensive in early disease stages and decreases over time. *Brain*. 2002;125(pt 10):2202–2212.

Lappe-Siefke C, Goebbels S, Gravel M, et al. Disruption of Cnp1 uncouples oligodendroglial functions in axonal support and myelination. *Nat Genet*. 2003;33(3):366–374.

Lebrun C, Bensa C, Debouverie M, et al. Unexpected multiple sclerosis: follow-up of 30 patients with magnetic resonance imaging and clinical conversion profile. *J Neurol Neurosurg Psychiatry*. 2008;79(2):195–198.

Lumsden CE. The Neuropathology of Multiple Sclerosis. New York, Elsevier; 1970.

Mahad D, Lassmann H, Turnbull D. Review: mitochondria and disease progression in multiple sclerosis. *Neuropathol Appl Neurobiol*. 2008;34(6):577–589.

Matthews WB, Small DG. Serial recording of visual and somatosensory evoked potentials in multiple sclerosis. *J Neurol Sci*. 1979;40(1):11–21.

McDonald WI, Sears TA. Effect of demyelination on conduction in the central nervous system. *Nature*. 1969;221(5176):182–183.

McDonald WI, Sears TA. The effects of experimental demyelination on conduction in the central nervous system. *Brain*. 1970;93(3):583–598.

Meyer G. Axonal patterns and topography of short-axon neurons in visual areas 17, 18, and 19 of the cat. *J Comp Neurol*. 1983;220(4):405–438.

Meyer G, Castaneyra-Perdomo A, Ferres-Torres R. A type of apparently axonless granule cell in the cat auditory cortex. *Anat Embryol (Berl)*. 1984;170(3):319–320.

Miller DH, Barkhof F, Nauta JJ. Gadolinium enhancement increases the sensitivity of MRI in detecting disease activity in multiple sclerosis. *Brain*. 1993;116 (pt 5):1077–1094.

Nikolaeva MA, Mukherjee B, Stys PK. Na$^+$-dependent sources of intra-axonal Ca2$^+$ release in rat optic nerve during in vitro chemical ischemia. *J Neurosci*. 2005;25(43):9960–9967.

Nordin M, Nyström B, Wallin U, Hagbarth KE. Ectopic sensory discharges and paresthesiae in patients with disorders of peripheral nerves, dorsal roots and dorsal columns. *Pain*. 1984;20(3):231–245.

O'Riordan JI, Losseff NA, Phatouros C, et al. Asymptomatic spinal cord lesions in clinically isolated optic nerve, brain stem, and spinal cord syndromes suggestive of demyelination. *J Neurol Neurosurg Psychiatry*. 1998; 64(3):353–357.

Peichl L, Gonzalez-Soriano J. Morphological types of horizontal cell in rodent retinae: a comparison of rat, mouse, gerbil, and guinea pig. *Vis Neurosci*. 1994;11(3): 501–517.

Raine CS. The Norton Lecture: a review of the oligodendrocyte in the multiple sclerosis lesion. *J Neuroimmunol*. 1997;77(2):135–152.

Rasminsky M, Sears TA. Internodal conduction in undissected demyelinated nerve fibres. *J Physiol*. 1972; 227(2):323–350.

Redford EJ, Kapoor R, Smith KJ. Nitric oxide donors reversibly block axonal conduction: demyelinated axons are especially susceptible. *Brain*. 1997;120(pt 12): 2149–2157.

Ritchie JM, Rogart RB. Density of sodium channels in mammalian myelinated nerve fibers and nature of the axonal membrane under the myelin sheath. *Proc Natl Acad Sci USA*. 1977;74(1):211–215.

Rizzo MA, Kocsis JD, Waxman SG. Mechanisms of paresthesiae, dysesthesiae, and hyperesthesiae: role of Na$^+$ channel heterogeneity. *Eur Neurol*. 1996;36(1): 3–12.

Schauf CL, Davis FA. Impulse conduction in multiple sclerosis: a theoretical basis for modification by temperature and pharmacological agents. *J Neurol Neurosurg Psychiatry*. 1974;37(2):152–161.

Schwid SR, Petrie MD, McDermott MP, Tierney DS, Mason DH, Goodman AD. Quantitative assessment of sustained-release 4-aminopyridine for symptomatic treatment of multiple sclerosis. *Neurology*. 1997; 48(4):817–821.

Sheldon AL, Robinson MB. The role of glutamate transporters in neurodegenerative diseases and potential opportunities for intervention. *Neurochem Int.* 2007;51(6–7):333–355.

Sherratt RM, Bostock H, Sears TA. Effects of 4-aminopyridine on normal and demyelinated mammalian nerve fibres. *Nature.* 1980;283(5747):570–572.

Shi R, Blight AR. Differential effects of low and high concentrations of 4-aminopyridine on axonal conduction in normal and injured spinal cord. *Neuroscience.* 1997;77(2):553–562.

Shrager P, Custer AW, Kazarinova K, Rasband MN, Mattson D. Nerve conduction block by nitric oxide that is mediated by the axonal environment. *J Neurophysiol.* 1998;79(2):529–536.

Smith KJ. Conduction properties of central demyelinated and remyelinated axons, and their relation to symptom production in demyelinating disorders. *Eye.* 1994; 8(pt 2):224–237.

Smith KJ. Sodium channels and multiple sclerosis: roles in symptom production, damage and therapy. *Brain Pathol.* 2007;17(2):230–242.

Smith KJ, Blakemore WF, McDonald WI. Central remyelination restores secure conduction. *Nature.* 1979; 280(5721):395–396.

Smith KJ, Blakemore WF, McDonald WI. The restoration of conduction by central remyelination. *Brain.* 1981; 104(2):383–404.

Smith KJ, Lassmann H. The role of nitric oxide in multiple sclerosis. *Lancet Neurol.* 2002;1(4):232–241.

Smith KJ, McDonald WI. Spontaneous and evoked electrical discharges from a central demyelinating lesion. *J Neurol Sci.* 1982;55(1):39–47.

Smith KJ, McDonald WI. The pathophysiology of multiple sclerosis: the mechanisms underlying the production of symptoms and the natural history of the disease. *Philos Trans R Soc Lond B Biol Sci.* 1999;354(1390): 1649–1673.

Smith ME. Phagocytic properties of microglia in vitro: implications for a role in multiple sclerosis and EAE. *Microsc Res Tech.* 2001;54(2):81–94.

Srinivasan R, Sailasuta N, Hurd R, Nelson S, Pelletier D. Evidence of elevated glutamate in multiple sclerosis using magnetic resonance spectroscopy at 3 T. *Brain.* 2005;128(pt 5):1016–1025.

Stefoski D, Davis FA, Faut M, Schauf CL. 4-Aminopyridine improves clinical signs in multiple sclerosis. *Ann Neurol.* 1987;21(1):71–77.

Stefoski D, Davis FA, Fitzsimmons WE, Luskin SS, Rush J, Parkhurst GW. 4-Aminopyridine in multiple sclerosis: prolonged administration. *Neurology.* 1991; 41(9):1344–1348.

Stover JF, Pleines UE, Morganti-Kossmann MC, Kossmann T, Lowitzsch K, Kempski OS. Neurotransmitters in cerebrospinal fluid reflect pathological activity. *Eur J Clin Invest.* 1997;27(12):1038–1043.

Stys PK. Anoxic and ischemic injury of myelinated axons in CNS white matter: from mechanistic concepts to therapeutics. *J Cereb Blood Flow Metab.* 1998;18(1):2–25.

Stys PK. General mechanisms of axonal damage and its prevention. *J Neurol Sci.* 2005;233(1–2):3–13.

Tasaki I. *Nervous Transmission.* Springfield, IL: Charles C. Thomas; 1953.

Trapp BD, Nave KA. Multiple sclerosis: an immune or neurodegenerative disorder? *Annu Rev Neurosci.* 2008; 31:247–269.

Vacher H, Mohapatra DP, Trimmer JS. Localization and targeting of voltage-dependent ion channels in mammalian central neurons. *Physiol Rev.* 2008;88(4): 1407–1447.

Van Diemen HA, Polman CH, Koetsier JC, Van Loenen AC, Nauta JJ, Bertelsmann FW. 4-Aminopyridine in patients with multiple sclerosis: dosage and serum level related to efficacy and safety. *Clin Neuropharmacol.* 1993;16(3):195–204.

Waxman SG. Conduction in myelinated, unmyelinated, and demyelinated fibers. *Arch Neurol.* 1977;34(10): 585–589.

Waxman SG. Axonal conduction and injury in multiple sclerosis: the role of sodium channels. *Nat Rev Neurosci.* 2006;7(12):932–941.

Waxman SG. Mechanisms of disease: sodium channels and neuroprotection in multiple sclerosis-current status. *Nat Clin Pract Neurol.* 2008;4(3):159–169.

Waxman SG, Geschwind N. Major morbidity related to hyperthermia in multiple sclerosis. *Ann Neurol.* 1983; 13(3):348.

Williams A, Piaton G, Lubetzki C. Astrocytes—friends or foes in multiple sclerosis? *Glia.* 2007;55(13):1300–1312.

Wolswijk G, Balesar R. Changes in the expression and localization of the paranodal protein Caspr on axons in chronic multiple sclerosis. *Brain.* 2003;126(pt 7): 1638–1649.

4 Immunology of Multiple Sclerosis

Laura Piccio and Anne H. Cross

Multiple sclerosis (MS) is characterized by inflammation, demyelination, and axonal loss within the central nervous system (CNS), and it is thought to be mediated by autoimmune processes. The first clinical-pathologic description of MS was in 1868 by Charcot, who reported the presence of perivascular inflammatory infiltrates in the CNS of patients with intermittent episodes of neurologic dysfunction (Charcot, 1868). The finding in 1933 by Thomas Rivers that a CNS inflammatory demyelinating disease similar to MS could be induced in animals after immunization with CNS myelin supported the hypothesis that MS is secondary to an autoimmune response to self-antigens (Rivers, 1933). This has become the most commonly used animal model of MS, and it is called experimental autoimmune encephalomyelitis (EAE). However, while EAE can be induced in animals, MS is a spontaneous disease in humans. Current thought is that MS develops in genetically susceptible subjects with a critical environmental contribution. Microbial infections (virus or bacteria) are the main candidates as environmental triggers, but noninfectious environmental factors such as vitamin D levels may also be important (Ascherio and Munger, 2007a, 2007b). Although attempts to isolate a microbial agent from MS patients have not been consistently positive, the role of infections could be transient, allowing breakdown of immune self-tolerance against CNS self-antigen. The main aspects of MS autoimmunity and disease mechanisms will be discussed in this chapter.

THE NORMAL IMMUNE SYSTEM

Adaptive and Innate Immunity

The immune system protects the individual from foreign organisms, such as viruses, bacteria, and fungi. The two main branches of the immune system are the innate and the adaptive. The innate immune system is nonspecific. This branch is the frontline of defense against foreign invaders such as viruses and bacteria. The innate immune system is comprised of macrophages, neutrophils and other polymorphonulear cells, natural killer cells, mast cells, and dendritic cells.

Adaptive immunity is the specific branch of the immune system whereby B and T lymphocytes are educated to specifically recognize foreign antigens. Adaptive immunity was discovered by Edward Jenner about 200 years ago, when he recognized in the late 1790s that exposure to cowpox protected people from the often-fatal smallpox. When the adaptive immune system targets "self-antigens," autoimmune disease can be the result (Janeway et al., 2005).

Both the adaptive and the innate immune systems are implicated in MS, as well as in EAE pathogenesis. The adaptive immune system is believed to initiate pathological myelin-reactive autoimmune responses leading to CNS damage in MS and EAE. The innate immune system is implicated in triggering and modulating those adaptive immune responses. This is demonstrated by the usual requirement for adjuvants (commonly Freunds's adjuvant containing *M. tuberculosis*) that activate cells of the innate immune system when inducing EAE by immunization (Staykova et al., 2008).

T lymphocytes, which express the CD3 surface molecule, are believed to be critical to the development of MS and EAE. T cell lineages and their development are extremely complex and are still being investigated. CD4$^+$ and CD8$^+$ T cells are two main types of T cells bearing the $\alpha\beta$ T cell receptor (TCR). CD4$^+$ and CD8$^+$ T cells recognize their antigenic targets only as processed peptide antigens that are presented in context of major histocompatibility complex (MHC) class II or MHC class I molecules on antigen presenting cells (APCs), respectively. T cells of CD4 and CD8 subtypes can be further classified by function as effector, memory, and regulatory subtypes. CD4$^+$ T cells can also be subdivided into subtypes defined by the cytokines they secrete and their functions. T-helper (Th) 1, Th2, Th17, and T-regulatory (T$_{reg}$) are the main CD4$^+$ T cell subtypes. Th1 cells, which secrete IL-2, IFN-γ and TNFα, and Th17 cells, which secrete IL-17 and IL-22, can each induce EAE. Th2 cells secrete IL-4 and do not induce EAE except under atypical circumstances. T-regulatory cells are protective against autoimmune processes such as EAE. T-regulatory cells express the transcription factor Foxp3, and some of them secrete IL-10. Generally, T-regulatory cells inhibit autoimmunity (Janeway et al., 2005).

Important cells in shaping T cell responses are dendritic cells (DCs). Although not antigen specific themselves, DCs form a bridge between the adaptive and the innate immune systems by presenting processed antigens to T cells, leading to T cell activation and proliferation. Immature DCs are located throughout the body, poised to take up foreign antigens. Once this happens, DCs travel to the lymphoid tissues, where they express high levels of MHC class II and costimulatory molecules (B7-1, B7-2), as well as the processed antigen. In lymphoid tissue, DCs encounter naïve T lymphocytes, and if any of these bears the corresponding TCR that recognizes the antigen-MHC complex expressed by the DC, that T cell will be activated and proliferate.

Mechanisms of Self-Tolerance

A remarkable property of the immune system is its ability to recognize, respond to, and eliminate many foreign (non "self") antigen while not reacting harmfully to self-antigens. This nonresponsiveness to self is called tolerance. Immunologic tolerance to an antigen can be induced by exposure to that antigen during T cell development or under certain conditions after T cell development. Abnormalities in the induction or maintenance of self-tolerance lead to immune responses against self-antigens, often resulting in autoimmune diseases. Tolerance to self-antigens is maintained by several mechanisms, including clonal deletion of self-reactive T cells in the thymus (central tolerance) and induction of T-cell anergy, the latter leading to T cell functional inactivation in periphery after encountering the antigen (peripheral tolerance) (Abbas et al., 2003). These processes alone do not explain the maintenance of immunologic self-tolerance in some cases, as potentially pathogenic autoreactive T cells are present in the periphery of healthy individuals (Ota et al., 1990). Thus, other regulatory mechanisms exist such as active suppression of T cells reactive with self-antigens by regulatory T cells, which play a key role in the control and in the induction of peripheral tolerance in vivo (Hafler et al., 2005).

MULTIPLE SCLEROSIS AS AN AUTOIMMUNE DISEASE

The etiology of MS, particularly the initial inciting event, remains unknown. Multiple sclerosis is considered a CD4$^+$ T cell–mediated autoimmune disease in which the immune response targets CNS antigens. This view is based on the association of the disease with HLA class II molecules (presumably via their role as APC to pathogenic T cells), the cellular composition of CNS infiltrates, and similarities with EAE (McFarland and Martin, 2007). Although strong evidence implicates an abnormal immune response in the pathogenesis of MS, formal proof that MS is an autoimmune disease is lacking.

Pathology Suggests an Autoimmune Etiology

The CNS pathology of MS suggests an immune-driven reaction to a CNS antigen (see Chapter 5). In addition to mononuclear inflammatory cell infiltration, most active MS lesions contain antibodies, complement, and soluble immune mediators such as cytokines and chemokines (Hofman et al., 1989; Selmaj et al., 1991; Cannella and Raine, 1995). Central nervous system pathology reveals injury to myelin, but injury to axons and oligodendrocytes is often seen as well. That several different CNS components are the focus of injury in MS makes the primary "self" target of the presumed autoimmune process unclear. Likewise, whether the autoantigenic target is the same for different patients with MS is not known. Moreover, the pathology in active MS lesions is heterogeneous

(Lucchinetti et al., 1996), suggesting either variation in the immune response(s) and/or the inciting event(s) among individual patients.

Candidates for the Multiple Sclerosis Antigen

For decades, investigators have searched to identify the MS autoantigen. Because of the similarities with EAE and because MS pathology mainly affects CNS white matter, the greatest focus has been on myelin proteins. T cells reactive to myelin proteins, including myelin basic protein (MBP), myelin associated glycoprotein (MAG), myelin oligodendrocyte glycoprotein (MOG), and proteolipid protein (PLP), have been found in MS patients. However, healthy controls harbor myelin-reactive T cells in their peripheral blood in frequencies similar to MS patients (Sun et al., 1991a, 1991b; Markovic-Plese et al., 1995). Thus, differences between MS patients and controls in the activation status or other properties of these myelin-reactive T cells have been sought. Supported by several lines of investigation, it has indeed been shown that myelin-reactive T cells have been activated in many MS patients. For example, Zhang et al. (1994) reported an increased frequency of activated T cells that expressed the IL-2 receptor and recognized MBP and PLP in peripheral blood of MS patients compared with controls. Genetic mutations are a marker of previous activation and proliferation in T cells, because with each cell division, the chance of a genetic mutation increases. One such mutation, in the hypoxanthine-guanine phosphoribosyl transferase gene, allows T cells to live in the presence of normally-toxic 6-thioguanine (Allegretta et al., 1990). T cells recognizing both MBP (Lodge et al., 1994; Lodge et al., 1996) and PLP (Trotter et al., 1997) and that do not die when exposed to toxic levels of 6-thioguanine are found at significantly higher frequency in MS patients than controls. Another group found that T cells reactive with MOG, MBP, or PLP from MS patients expressed far more Kv1.3 channels per cell, a marker of effector memory T cells, than did T cells from control subjects (Wulff et al., 2003). Taken together, data from these studies strongly indicate that MS patients harbor more previously activated memory T cells directed against myelin antigens than do controls. That these activated T cells are reactive with at least three different myelin self-antigens suggests that their presence may be a secondary phenomenon due to the liberation of myelin antigens upon myelin damage. Autoimmunity directed against many other potential CNS antigens could contribute to MS pathogenesis. Non-myelin antigens, such as the small heat-shock protein α-B-crystallin, have been implicated as well (Ousman et al., 2007).

Perhaps the strongest evidence that MS is an autoimmune disease and that myelin proteins are relevant antigens in MS derived from a clinical trial attempting to induce anergy in myelin-reactive T cells (Bielekova et al., 2000). Instead, the trial directly linked disease activity with an enhanced T cell response to MBP. This trial tested an altered peptide ligand (APL) of the major immunogenic epitope of human MBP. Treatment with a high dose of APL led to expansion of myelin-directed T cells in three of eight subjects. Moreover, these three patients all had dramatic increases in magnetic resonance imaging (MRI) contrast-enhancing lesions and all had clinical relapses (Bielekova et al., 2000). The trial was halted.

Humoral Immunity as Indirect Evidence for Autoimmunity in Multiple Sclerosis

The humoral arm of the adaptive immune system has been implicated in MS pathogenesis for decades, due to the findings of oligoclonal bands (OCBs) and increased levels of cerebrospinal fluid (CSF) immunoglobulins (Igs) in more than 90% of MS patients (Paty and Ebers, 1998). B cells, plasma cells, and Igs are typically present in MS lesions and have at times been identified in normal-appearing white matter of MS patients (Esiri, 1977; Prineas and Wright, 1978). Immunoglobulin and immune complexes have been consistently observed in early stages of disease, suggesting a role for the humoral immune system from MS onset (Gay et al., 1997). The neuropathology of active MS lesions most commonly involves Igs and complement deposition in addition to mononuclear cells (Lucchinetti et al., 1996).

Moreover, studies have linked antibody levels to prognosis. Increased concentrations of antibodies in CSF of MS patients correlate with episodes of MS worsening (Olsson and Link, 1973). Excessive CSF free kappa light chains, a byproduct of Ig production, is also correlated with poor prognosis (Rudick et al., 1995; Rinker et al., 2006). IgM and IgG in the CSF typically demonstrate a pattern of limited clonality, referred to as OCBs because of the banding pattern observed when concentrated CSF is electrophoresed (Trotter, 1989). Patients with MS lacking CSF OCBs typically have a more benign course (Zeman et al., 1996). Similarly, higher numbers of CSF OCBs at MS onset are associated with poorer clinical outcome (Avasarala et al., 2001).

Molecular studies indicate that production of antibodies in the CNS of MS patients is antigen driven, making an indirect case for autoimmunity. The complementarity-determining regions (CDR) of antibodies are the antigen-binding sites, and include the Ig heavy-chain variable (VH) region. Somatic hypermutations occur in the CDR when B cells are exposed to their antigen; these mutations often lead to amino acid substitutions that enhance Ig affinity for target antigen. In antigen-driven responses, mutations accumulate in Ig gene regions that contact antigen at a higher rate than in regions that have no antigen contact, and greater numbers of mutations resulting in amino acid substitutions accumulate in comparison to "silent" mutations. Several different laboratories have independently reported Ig mutations characteristic of antigen-driven responses in MS CSF and in MS lesions, bolstering the autoimmune hypothesis of MS pathogenesis (Smith-Jensen et al., 2000).

MOG is a minor protein component of CNS myelin, comprising less than 0.05% of myelin protein. However, this glycoprotein elicits a strong B cell response (Kerlero de Rosbo et al., 1993), perhaps because MOG localizes to the outer surface of myelin and oligodendroglia. Humans can develop both a cellular and a humoral immune response to MOG (Sun et al., 1991b). B cell and antibody responses to MOG (Xiao et al., 1991) are more prevalent in MS patients than in controls. Nonetheless, these antibodies may be the result rather than the cause of CNS pathology.

If anti-myelin antibodies are critical to MS pathogenesis, they should be present at onset. Investigators have reported that in patients with a single isolated clinical demyelinating syndrome suggestive of MS, the presence of myelin-reactive IgM antibodies in serum may predict the development of clinically definite MS. Serum samples from 103 patients who initially presented with neurologic symptoms suggesting demyelination, and who had lesions typical of demyelination on brain MRI, and OCBs in the CSF, were tested for antibodies to MOG and MBP. Not all patients displayed anti-myelin antibodies, but those that did were more likely than the seronegative patients to have a second attack within 2 years. Those initially exhibiting both anti-MOG and anti-MBP antibodies were most likely to have an early relapse (Berger et al., 2003). However, another study failed to demonstrate an association between ant-myelin antibodies and progression to MS in patients who had a first attack (Kuhle et al., 2007).

Axonal damage is a common component of MS plaques. Neurofilaments are cytoskeletal proteins of axons. CSF antibodies against the light neurofilament subunit have been reported in the progressive forms of MS (Silber et al., 2002). Their presence in the CSF of MS patients has also been correlated with cerebral atrophy, as detected by MRI (Eikelenboom et al., 2003). Cerebral atrophy in MS patients is thought to reflect diffuse axonal loss.

These data constitute circumstantial evidence for the humoral immune response being important in MS pathogenesis. However, humoral immunity may not be completely detrimental in MS. Antibodies might also mediate CNS repair, as suggested by one group of investigators who have identified antibodies directed against oligodendrocytes that appear to promote remyelination (Warrington et al., 2001).

Infections as Triggers of Multiple Sclerosis

Epidemiologic studies support an environmental component in triggering MS. The well-known latitudinal gradient whereby those raised further from the equator are at higher risk for developing MS, and the occasional observations of pockets of high MS prevalence have supported the involvement of environmental risk factors. That identical twins are usually discordant for MS (~30% concordance rate) also supports factors other than genetics as triggers for MS. These factors are typically interpreted as environmental. However, recent evidence indicates the latitudinal gradient may be decreasing (Ascherio and Munger, 2007a, 2007b; Alonso and Hernan, 2008).

Through the decades, evidence in favor of various infectious agents as triggers for MS has been reported, only to be later discounted. Distemper, measles, herpes simplex, hepatitis B and Epstein-Barr viruses, and Chlamydia pneumoniae are among several of the infectious organisms that have been suggested to be causative in MS (Giovannoni et al., 2006).

Several current lines of research link infection with Epstein-Barr virus to increased risk of MS. Risk of developing MS is statistically greater in persons with evidence of prior infection with EBV, especially those with clinical history of mononucleosis (Thacker et al., 2006). In pediatric MS, the rate of prior infection with EBV was reported to be double that of age-matched controls. In the same study, no differences in antibody positivity to another infectious agent (CMV) were observed (Alotaibi et al., 2004). It should be noted that these studies report statistical associations and stronger evidence is required before considering EBV as a *causative* factor.

Two main mechanisms have been proposed to explain how infectious agents could induce MS despite lack of evidence for a continuing infection: *(1)* molecular mimicry, involving the activation of autoreactive T and B cells by cross-reactivity between self-antigen and foreign agents (Fig. 4-1 and Table 4-1); and *(2)* bystander activation, meaning that autoreactive cells are activated because of nonspecific inflammatory events that occur during infection. Another possibility is that a combination of these two mechanisms could induce MS after an infection (Sospedra and Martin, 2005).

MECHANISMS OF MS PATHOGENESIS

Overview

In MS, similar to what has been described in EAE, it is believed that autoreactive CD4+ T cells are generated in periphery and subsequently gain access into the CNS by trafficking through the blood brain barrier (BBB). Additionally, focal changes in BBB permeability or focal increase in expression in cell adhesion molecules are believed to be necessary for disease activity (Fig. 4-1 and Table 4-1). Supporting this hypothesis is the profound effect in decreasing MRI lesion activity and

clinical relapses of natalizumab, a monoclonal antibody directed against $\alpha 4$ integrin, a critical adhesion molecule mediating lymphocyte migration through the BBB (Sospedra and Martin, 2005).

Evidence indicates that effector mechanisms causing CNS damage in MS include antibody- and complement-mediated damage, the formation of free radicals, glutamate-mediate excitotoxicity, inflammatory cytokine secretion, and cell-mediated damage either through CD8+ T cells or through Fc receptors and monocytes, macrophages and microglia (McFarland and Martin, 2007). The main cell types implicated in MS immunopathology and the roles of other important immune mediators, including cytokines, adhesion molecules, and chemokines, will be reviewed in this section. An overview of the hypothetical mechanisms underlying MS development are given in Figure 4-1 and Table 4-1.

T Cell Subsets and Their Roles in Multiple Sclerosis Pathogenesis

As previously discussed, current evidence favors CD4+ autoreactive T cells as a central factor in MS pathogenesis. Like many other autoimmune diseases, MS was traditionally thought to be mediated by CD4+ T cells with a Th1 phenotype, characterized by the production of IFN-γ and thus proinflammatory. However, recent evidence indicates that the critical T cells for inducing inflammation and disease, at least in the EAE model, are characterized by the production of IL-17, named Th17, which represent a lineage distinct from the Th1 and Th2 phenotypes (Langrish et al., 2005; Bettelli et al., 2006). Interleukin IL-6, TGF-β, IL-21, and IL-23 are important for the differentiation and/or activation and expansion of Th17 cells (Tesmer et al., 2008). Th1 or Th17 cells are independently capable of inducing EAE (Kroenke et al., 2008). Recently it has been proposed that a first wave of Th17 cells enter the CNS in EAE through the choroid plexus and trigger the entry of a second wave of T cells that migrate in large numbers into CNS by crossing activated parenchymal vessels (Reboldi et al., 2009). This would suggest that Th17 and Th1 cells could both play critical, but different roles in EAE pathogenesis.

The role of IL-17 in the neuropathology of MS is beginning to be elucidated. Recent work

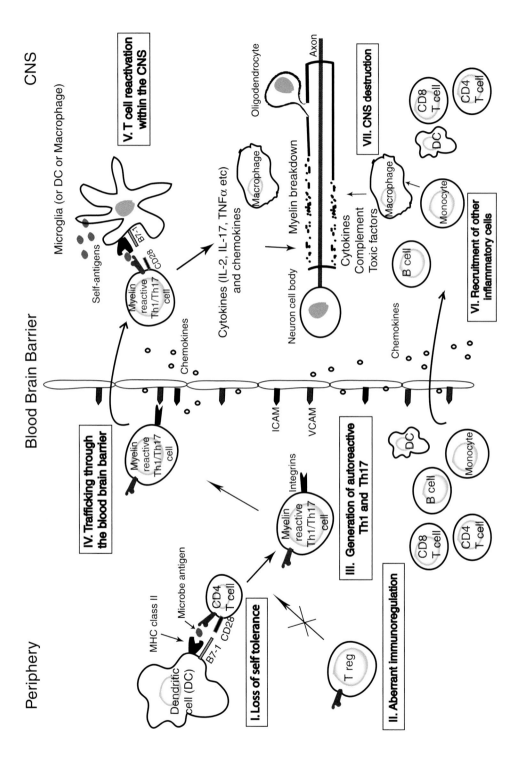

Figure 4-1 Hypothetical mechanisms leading to multiple sclerosis onset and development. These processes are exemplified from I to VII here and in Table 4-1. They include generation of myelin reactive T cells in periphery, trafficking through the blood brain barrier, reactivation of auto-reactive T cell in the central nervous system (CNS) and tissue damage.

Table 4-1 Immunological Processes Thought to Be Implicated in the Development of Multiple Sclerosis Lesions

Immune Processes	Site	Cells or Molecules Implicated	Mechanisms
I. Loss of self-tolerance	Periphery	APCs (dendritic cells) and T cells	Common microbes containing protein sequences cross-reactive with myelin self-antigens lead to the generation of autoreactive T cells
II. Aberrant immune regulation	Periphery	Regulatory T cells	Immunoregulatory defects (e.g., decreased T regulatory cells in the circulation) could favor activation of myelin reactive T cells
III. Generation of myelin-reactive T cells	Periphery	T h1 and Th17 cells	Activated self-reactive T cells differentiate into the pro- inflammatory subsets Th1 and Th17
IV. Trafficking through the blood brain barrier	BBB	Adhesion molecules and chemokines	Activated myelin-reactive T cells migrate into the CNS by interacting with adhesion molecules and chemokines at the BBB
V. T cell reactivation	CNS	Myelin-reactive T cells and APCs in the CNS	Reactivation of myelin-specific T cells, which recognize the self-antigen presented by local APCs (microglia)
VI. Recruitment of other inflammatory cells	BBB/CNS	T cells, B cells, monocytes, dendritic cells; adhesion molecules and chemokines	Immune and inflammatory cells are recruited into the CNS through the BBB. Recruited APCs (macrophages, DC, B cells) perpetuate T cell re-activation in the CNS and may also directly mediate damage.
VII. CNS destruction	CNS	T cells, B cells, macrophages, antibodies, cytokines/ chemokines, free radicals, other toxic factors	Myelin breakdown and axon damage is sustained by cell-mediated cytotoxic mechanisms and soluble factors including inflammatory cytokines (e.g., TNFα), antibodies, complement, nitric oxide, peroxynitrite, etc.

APCs, antigen presenting cells; BBB, blood brain barrier; CNS, central nervous system.

demonstrated the presence of IL-17 in MS lesions (Tzartos et al., 2008). Another study showed that human Th17 cells migrate across the BBB, releasing granzyme B, which can lead to neuronal death (Kebir et al., 2007). Additionally, it has been suggested that high serum IL-17 concentrations identify a subset of relapsing-remitting MS patients with a primarily Th17-mediated disease that is not responsive to therapy with IFN-β (Axtell et al., 2010). Overall, the significance of Th17 pathways in MS pathogenesis needs further characterization.

Despite the focus on and evidence of the importance of CD4$^+$ T cells in MS, the potential involvement of CD8$^+$ T cells cannot be dismissed. CD8$^+$ T cells are present in inflammatory MS lesions (Traugott et al., 1983). Also, examination of MS lesions had shown clonal expansion of CD8$^+$ T cells based on T cell receptor analysis (Babbe et al., 2000). One hypothesis would be that MS lesion formation is initiated by Th1 and Th17 cells, while amplification and damage are mediated by CD8$^+$ T cells (McFarland and Martin, 2007).

Regulatory T cells (T$_{reg}$) are another important subset of T cells implicated in the regulation of autoimmune and inflammatory responses in MS. Several populations of T$_{reg}$ have been described and the most extensively studied is characterized as CD4$^+$CD25^{high} and express the transcription factor Foxp3 (Walker et al., 2003; von Boehmer, 2005). Their mechanisms of suppression are poorly understood and may involve processes of cell–cell interaction and suppression mediated by the production of IL-10 and TGF-β. In MS it is not known if T$_{reg}$ cells exert their effect in periphery or within the CNS (Viglietta et al., 2004).

Role of Microglia and Macrophages

Microglia are considered the resident macrophages of the CNS and are quickly activated by injury or pathogens (Nimmerjahn et al., 2005). Microglia provide functions similar to other tissue macrophages, including phagocytosis, antigen presentation and production of cytokines, eicosanoids, complement components, excitatory amino acids (glutamate), proteinases, oxidative radicals, and nitric oxide (Benveniste, 1997). Currently, there are no unique histochemical markers that distinguish intrinsic microglia from macrophages which have invaded the brain during inflammation (Guillemin and Brew, 2004). Based on the pathology of active lesions, macrophages/microglia actively participate in myelin breakdown during MS; phagocytosis of myelin proteins in the lesions by these cells is a reliable indicator of ongoing demyelinating activity.

In addition, activated microglia and macrophages express molecules critical for antigen presentation to T cells, including MHC class II and B7-1 and B7-2 molecules. Activated microglia produce a wide range of factors, such as chemokines, prostaglandins, nitric oxide, and the cytokines IL-1β and TNFα. Many of these microglial products are pro-inflammatory, but some may also have neuroprotective roles (Benveniste, 1997).

Role of Dendritic Cells

Dendritic cells (DCs) are absent from the normal brain parenchyma, but they are present in normal meninges, choroid plexus, and CSF, where they likely play a key role in immune surveillance in the CNS (Matyszak and Perry, 1996). Inflammation

is accompanied by recruitment and/or development of DCs in the affected brain tissue. Important concepts have emerged lately regarding DCs in MS. Dendritic cells accumulate in the CSF and CNS during MS and EAE, and in this context they are thought to be involved in the regulation of autoimmune responses directed against myelin antigens (Serafini et al., 2000; Pashenkov et al., 2003). The presence of DCs has been demonstrated in parenchymal lesions and meninges of MS patients with evidence of engulfment of myelin components and interaction with T cells. These findings suggest that CNS-infiltrating DCs may be important for sustaining local T cell activation and expansion (Serafini et al., 2006). Besides their role in adaptive immunity, DCs have several innate functions, such as the production of large amounts of cytokines and the response to a spectrum of environmental cues by extensive differentiation and maturation (Mellman and Steinman, 2001).

Role of Cytokines

Cytokines are soluble proteins that play important roles in all phases of immune responses and inflammatory reactions by acting in complex networks. Secreted by a variety of cell types, cytokines act on cells expressing the appropriate receptor. Typically, cytokines have the capacity to elicit different biological activities depending upon their target cells. Pro-inflammatory cytokines are believed to play roles in MS pathogenesis in several ways, including (1) peripheral immune activation; (2) enhancement of trafficking of activated immune cells into the CNS; and (3) direct damage to oligodendrocytes, myelin, and/or axons. Anti-inflammatory cytokines are considered beneficial in MS (Navikas and Link, 1996; Ozenci et al., 2002; Sospedra and Martin, 2005). Altered cytokine profiles have been found in the CNS (Brosnan et al., 1995) and peripheral mononuclear cells of MS patients compared to healthy individuals (Comabella et al., 1998; Balashov et al., 2000; Karni et al., 2002). Here we summarize the main findings related to MS on pro-inflammatory cytokines (IFN-γ, IL-17, TNF-α), anti-inflammatory cytokines (IL-10, TGF-β), and one with mixed activities (IL-6).

IFN-γ is both produced by Th1 cells and critical in the differentiation of Th1 cells. Thus, IFN-γ is the principal marker of a Th1 response. Its functions include activation of mononuclear cells as well as differentiation of cells of Th1 phenotype (Imitola et al., 2005). A small clinical trial in the late 1980s showed that administration of recombinant IFN-γ to MS patients resulted in disease exacerbation (Panitch et al., 1987). IFN-γ has been shown to have regulatory functions (described mainly in animal systems), including anti-T cell proliferative activity (Badovinac et al., 2000; Konieczny et al., 1998) and induction of T cell apoptosis (Liu and Janeway, 1990; Willenborg et al., 1999).

IL-17 is the signature cytokine of Th17 cells. Accumulating evidence indicates Th17 cells are the initiating T cell subset in autoimmune diseases, including potentially in MS. In EAE studies, Th17 cells were sufficient to induce disease in adoptive transfer experiments (Langrish et al., 2005), suggesting that IL-17 may also be a critical pathogenic factor in MS. Elevated levels of IL-17 were detected in the blood and cerebrospinal fluid of MS patients compared to healthy controls (Matusevicius et al., 1999). An in vitro study indicated that human Th17 cells traverse endothelial cells of a BBB model more efficiently than Th1 cells (Kebir et al 2007). The latter result suggested that one role of Th17 cells in MS may be to breach the BBB, allowing the influx of other immune and inflammatory cells (Kebir et al., 2007).

TNF-α is another pro-inflammatory cytokine that plays a role in MS pathogenesis. TNF-α effects include induction of B7-1 (CD80) and MHC class II expression, and stimulation of IL-12 production, which in turn induces IFN-γ production (Ozenci et al., 2002). Numerous studies have reported elevation of TNF-α in CSF of MS patients compared to controls, especially in patients with active disease (Sharief and Hentges, 1991). Also, the numbers of blood cells expressing TNF-α mRNA (Navikas et al., 1996), serum TNF-α levels (Hohnoki et al., 1998), and levels of TNF-α-secreting blood mononuclear cells (Ozenci et al., 2000) are reported to be higher in MS patients than controls. Because of its potent pro-inflammatory proprieties, it was hypothesized that TNF-α would be detrimental to patients with MS, but strikingly, drugs that block TNF-α actually lead to worsening of MS (The Lenercept Multiple Sclerosis Study Group and the University of British Columbia MS/MRI

Analysis Group, 1999). The reason for this is unclear, but perhaps within the context of the CNS, TNF-α has neuroprotective or anti-inflammatory properties (Turrin and Rivest, 2006).

Elevated levels of pro-inflammatory cytokines must be regulated by the human body. IL-10 is the most important anti-inflammatory cytokine described to date and its main effect is to inhibit pro-inflammatory cytokine production. IL-10 does this by suppressing expression of MHC class II, adhesion molecules, and costimulatory molecules on monocytes/macrophages and dendritic cells (Ozenci et al., 2002). A number of studies have evaluated IL-10 in MS, with partly contradictory results. Decreased numbers of PBMC secreting IL-10 and lower serum levels of IL-10 have been reported in MS (Huang et al., 1999). However, investigators have also described elevated numbers of IL-10 mRNA-expressing blood mononuclear cells (Navikas et al., 1995). Therefore the role of IL-10 in MS is currently not known. Of note, IL-10 levels were increased after initiation of the immunomodulatory drug, interferon-beta (Rudick et al., 1996).

TGF-β is a cytokine that may be involved in suppression of inflammation late in the chronic stages of disease. However, in the relapsing-remitting early phase of MS, TGF-β may heighten inflammation, as it does in EAE models of MS (Luo et al., 2007). TGF-β expression together with IL-6 may drive a Th17 response, perpetuating chronic tissue damage (Bettelli et al., 2007).

Increased levels of IL-6, a cytokine which exhibits both pro- and anti-inflammatory effects, have been shown in MS patient serum (Ozenci et al., 2000). IL-6 induces B cell differentiation and it is important for antibody production. It is also involved in T cell activation, growth, and differentiation (Hirano, 1998). On the other hand, IL-6 has potent anti-inflammatory effects, including inhibition of the pro-inflammatory cytokines IL-1β and TNF-α and inhibition of metalloproteinases (Tilg et al., 1997).

Role of Adhesion Molecules and Chemokines in Lymphocyte Trafficking into the Central Nervous System

In MS, circulating cells of the immune system gain access to the CNS and cause inflammation, demyelination, axonal injury, and gliosis, all leading to the clinical manifestations of the disease (Fig. 4-1 and Table 4-1). Therefore leukocyte migration through the BBB represents an important step in MS pathogenesis. This multistep process occurs in an ordered fashion and is governed by sequential interactions of different adhesion molecules and chemokines at postcapillary venules. The multistep interaction starts with an initial transient contact of a circulating leukocyte with the endothelium (step 1), mediated by adhesion molecules of the selectin family (E and P selectin) and their respective carbohydrate ligands, or by integrins. After the initial tether, the cell rolls along the endothelium and this slows its velocity. If the cell expresses the correct chemokine receptor, this slowing allows it to bind its chemokine ligand, presented on the endothelial surface. This receptor–ligand interaction at the leukocyte surface results in G protein–mediated integrin activation (step 2). Once activated, integrins mediate firm adhesion (step 3) to the vascular endothelium by binding to ligands of the immunoglobulin superfamily on endothelium. This ultimately leads to leukocyte diapedesis (step 4) into the CNS (Engelhardt, 2008). The dramatic effectiveness of the anti-$\alpha4$ monoclonal antibody in MS (Polman et al., 2006), natalizumab, demonstrated that $\alpha4$ integrins are especially critical to this process in MS.

Chemokines play a crucial role in regulating leukocyte migration into the brain. When presented on the surface of the brain endothelium, they mediate leukocyte firm arrest through integrin activation. Additionally, through chemoattractant gradients they drive leukocyte transendothelial migration and locomotion within the tissue (Man et al., 2007).

SUMMARY

Multiple sclerosis is considered an autoimmune disease of the CNS targeting myelin, and it is mediated by cells of the adaptive and innate immune systems. T cells of the Th1 and Th17 subtypes are believed critical to its initiation, based primarily on studies involving the animal model for MS, EAE. Whether MS is truly autoimmune—and, if so, the target(s) of the autoimmunity—is yet unproven.

REFERENCES

Abbas A, Lichtman A, Prober JS. *Cellular and Molecular Immunology.* 5th ed. Philadelphia: W.B. Saunders Company; 2003.

Allegretta M, Nicklas JA, Sriram S, Albertini RJ. T cells responsive to myelin basic protein in patients with multiple sclerosis. *Science.* 1990;247(4943):718–721.

Alonso A, Hernan MA. Temporal trends in the incidence of multiple sclerosis: a systematic review. *Neurology.* 2008;71(2):129–135.

Alotaibi S, Kennedy J, Tellier R, Stephens D, Banwell B. Epstein-Barr virus in pediatric multiple sclerosis. *JAMA.* 2004;291(15):1875–1879.

Ascherio A, Munger KL. Environmental risk factors for multiple sclerosis. Part I: the role of infection. *Ann Neurol.* 2007a;61(4):288–299.

Ascherio A, Munger KL. Environmental risk factors for multiple sclerosis. Part II: noninfectious factors. *Ann Neurol.* 2007b;61(6):504–513.

Avasarala JR, Cross AH, Trotter JL. Oligoclonal band number as a marker for prognosis in multiple sclerosis. *Arch Neurol.* 2001;58(12):2044–2045.

Axtell RC, de Jong BA, Boniface K., et al. T helper type 1 and 17 cells determine efficacy of interferon-β in multiple sclerosis and experimental encephalomyelitis. *Nat Med.* 2010;16(4):406–412.

Babbe H, Roers A, Waisman A, et al. Clonal expansions of CD8(+) T cells dominate the T cell infiltrate in active multiple sclerosis lesions as shown by micromanipulation and single cell polymerase chain reaction. *J Exp Med.* 2000;192(3):393–404.

Badovinac VP, Tvinnereim AR, Harty JT. Regulation of antigen-specific CD8+ T cell homeostasis by perforin and interferon-gamma. *Science.* 2000;290(5495):1354–1358.

Balashov KE, Comabella M, Ohashi T, Khoury SJ, Weiner HL. Defective regulation of IFNgamma and IL-12 by endogenous IL-10 in progressive MS. *Neurology.* 2000;55(2):192–198.

Benveniste EN. Role of macrophages/microglia in multiple sclerosis and experimental allergic encephalomyelitis. *J Mol Med.* 1997;75(3):165–173.

Berger T, Rubner P, Schautzer F, et al. Antimyelin antibodies as a predictor of clinically definite multiple sclerosis after a first demyelinating event. *N Engl J Med.* 2003;349(2):139–145.

Bettelli E, Carrier Y, Gao W, et al. Reciprocal developmental pathways for the generation of pathogenic effector TH17 and regulatory T cells. *Nature.* 2006;441(7090):235–238.

Bettelli E, Oukka M, Kuchroo VK. T(H)-17 cells in the circle of immunity and autoimmunity. *Nat Immunol.* 2007;8(4):345–350.

Bielekova B, Goodwin B, Richert N, et al. Encephalitogenic potential of the myelin basic protein peptide (amino acids 83–99) in multiple sclerosis: results of a phase II clinical trial with an altered peptide ligand. *Nat Med.* 2000;6(10):1167–1175.

Brosnan CF, Cannella B, Battistini L, Raine CS. Cytokine localization in multiple sclerosis lesions: correlation with adhesion molecule expression and reactive nitrogen species. *Neurology.* 1995;45(suppl 6):S16–S21.

Cannella B, Raine CS. The adhesion molecule and cytokine profile of multiple sclerosis lesions. *Ann Neurol.* 1995;37(4):424–435.

Charcot J. Histologic de la sclerose en plaque. *Gazette des Hopitaux.* 1868;41:554–566.

Comabella M, Balashov K, Issazadeh S, Smith D, Weiner HL, Khoury SJ. Elevated interleukin-12 in progressive multiple sclerosis correlates with disease activity and is normalized by pulse cyclophosphamide therapy. *J Clin Invest.* 1998;102(4):671–678.

Eikelenboom MJ, Petzold A, Lazeron, RH, et al. Multiple sclerosis: neurofilament light chain antibodies are correlated to cerebral atrophy. *Neurology.* 2003;60(2):219–223.

Engelhardt B. Immune cell entry into the central nervous system: involvement of adhesion molecules and chemokines. *J Neurol Sci.* 2008;274(1–2):23–26.

Esiri MM. (Immunoglobulin-containing cells in multiple-sclerosis plaques. *Lancet.* 1977;2(8036):478.

Gay FW, Drye TJ, Dick GW, Esiri MM. The application of multifactorial cluster analysis in the staging of plaques in early multiple sclerosis. Identification and characterization of the primary demyelinating lesion. *Brain.* 1997;120(pt 8):1461–1483.

Giovannoni G, Cutter GR, Lunemann J, et al. Infectious causes of multiple sclerosis. *Lancet Neurol.* 2006;5(10):887–894.

Guillemin GJ, Brew BJ. Microglia, macrophages, perivascular macrophages, and pericytes: a review of function and identification. *J Leukoc Biol.* 2004;75(3):388–397.

Hafler DA, Slavik JM, Anderson DE, O'Connor KC, De Jager P, Baecher-Allan C. Multiple sclerosis. *Immunol Rev.* 2005;204:208–231.

Hirano T. Interleukin 6 and its receptor: ten years later. *Int Rev Immunol.* 1998;16(3–4):249–284.

Hofman FM, Hinton DR, Johnson K, Merrill JE. Tumor necrosis factor identified in multiple sclerosis brain. *J Exp Med.* 1989;170(2):607–612.

Hohnoki K, Inoue A, Koh CS. Elevated serum levels of IFN-gamma, IL-4 and TNF-alpha/unelevated serum levels of IL-10 in patients with demyelinating diseases during the acute stage. *J Neuroimmunol.* 1998;87(1–2):27–32.

Huang WX, Huang P, Link H, Hillert J. Cytokine analysis in multiple sclerosis by competitive RT - PCR: a decreased expression of IL-10 and an increased expression of TNF-alpha in chronic progression. *Mult Scler.* 1999;5(5):342–348.

Imitola J, Chitnis T, Khoury SJ. Cytokines in multiple sclerosis: from bench to bedside. *Pharmacol Ther.* 2005;106(2):163–177.

Janeway CA, Walport M, Shlomchik MJ. *Immunobiology. The Immune System in Health and Disease.* 6th ed. New York: Garland Science; 2005.

Karni A, Koldzic DN, Bharanidharan P, Khoury SJ, Weiner HL. IL-18 is linked to raised IFN-gamma in multiple sclerosis and is induced by activated CD4(+) T cells via CD40-CD40 ligand interactions. *J Neuroimmunol.* 2002;125(1–2):134–140.

Kebir H, Kreymborg K, Ifergan I, et al. Human TH17 lymphocytes promote blood-brain barrier disruption and central nervous system inflammation. *Nat Med.* 2007;13(10):1173–1175.

Kerlero de Rosbo N, Milo R, Lees MB, Burger D, Bernard CC, Ben-Nun A. Reactivity to myelin antigens in multiple sclerosis. Peripheral blood lymphocytes respond predominantly to myelin oligodendrocyte glycoprotein. *J Clin Invest.* 1993;92(6):2602–2608.

Konieczny BT, Dai Z, Elwood ET, et al. IFN-gamma is critical for long-term allograft survival induced by blocking the CD28 and CD40 ligand T cell costimulation pathways. *J Immunol.* 1998;160(5):2059–2064.

Kroenke MA, Carlson TJ, Andjelkovic AV, Segal BM. IL-12- and IL-23-modulated T cells induce distinct types of EAE based on histology, CNS chemokine profile, and response to cytokine inhibition. *J Exp Med.* 2008;205(7):1535–1541.

Kuhle J, Pohl C, Mehling M, et al. Lack of association between antimyelin antibodies and progression to multiple sclerosis. *N Engl J Med.* 2007;356(4):371–378.

Langrish CL, Chen Y, Blumenschein WM, et al. IL-23 drives a pathogenic T cell population that induces autoimmune inflammation. *J Exp Med.* 2005;201(2):233–240.

The Lenercept Multiple Sclerosis Study Group and The University of British Columbia MS/MRI Analysis Group. TNF neutralization in MS: results of a randomized, placebo-controlled multicenter study. *Neurology.* 1999;53(3):457–465.

Liu Y, Janeway CA, Jr. Interferon gamma plays a critical role in induced cell death of effector T cell: a possible third mechanism of self-tolerance. *J Exp Med.* 1990;172(6):1735–1739.

Lodge PA, Allegretta M, Steinman L, Sriram S. Myelin basic protein peptide specificity and T-cell receptor gene usage of HPRT mutant T-cell clones in patients with multiple sclerosis. *Ann Neurol.* 1994;36(5):734–740.

Lodge PA, Johnson C, Sriram S. Frequency of MBP and MBP peptide-reactive T cells in the HPRT mutant T-cell population of MS patients. *Neurology.* 1996;46(5):1410–1415.

Lucchinetti CF, Bruck W, Rodriguez M, Lassmann H. Distinct patterns of multiple sclerosis pathology indicates heterogeneity on pathogenesis. *Brain Pathol.* 1996;6(3):259–274.

Luo J, Ho PP, Buckwalter MS, et al. Glia-dependent TGF-beta signaling, acting independently of the TH17 pathway, is critical for initiation of murine autoimmune encephalomyelitis. *J Clin Invest.* 2007;117(11):3306–3315.

Man S, Ubogu EE, Ransohoff RM. Inflammatory cell migration into the central nervous system: a few new twists on an old tale. *Brain Pathol.* 2007;17(2):243–250.

Markovic-Plese S, Fukaura H, Zhang J, et al. T cell recognition of immunodominant and cryptic proteolipid protein epitopes in humans. *J Immunol.* 1995;155(2): 982–992.

Matusevicius D, Kivisakk P, He B, et al. Interleukin-17 mRNA expression in blood and CSF mononuclear cells is augmented in multiple sclerosis. *Mult Scler.* 1999;5(2):101–104.

Matyszak MK, Perry VH. The potential role of dendritic cells in immune-mediated inflammatory diseases in the central nervous system. *Neuroscience.* 1996;74(2): 599–608.

McFarland HF, Martin R. Multiple sclerosis: a complicated picture of autoimmunity. *Nat Immunol.* 2007;8(9):913–919.

Mellman I, Steinman RM. Dendritic cells: specialized and regulated antigen processing machines. *Cell.* 2001; 106(3):255–258.

Navikas V, He B, Link J, et al. Augmented expression of tumour necrosis factor-alpha and lymphotoxin in mononuclear cells in multiple sclerosis and optic neuritis. *Brain.* 1996;119(pt 1):213–223.

Navikas V, Link H. Review: cytokines and the pathogenesis of multiple sclerosis. *J Neurosci Res.* 1996; 45(4):322–333.

Navikas V, Link J, Palasik W, et al. Increased mRNA expression of IL-10 in mononuclear cells in multiple sclerosis and optic neuritis. *Scand J Immunol.* 1995; 41(2):171–178.

Nimmerjahn A, Kirchhoff F, Helmchen F. Resting microglial cells are highly dynamic surveillants of brain parenchyma in vivo. *Science.* 2005;308(5726):1314–1318.

Olsson JE, Link H. Immunoglobulin abnormalities in multiple sclerosis. Relation to clinical parameters: exacerbations and remissions. *Arch Neurol.* 1973; 28(6):392–399.

Ota K, Matsui M, Milford EL, Mackin GA, Weiner HL, Hafler DA. T-cell recognition of an immunodominant myelin basic protein epitope in multiple sclerosis. *Nature.* 1990;346(6280):183–187.

Ousman SS, Tomooka BH, van Noort JM, et al. Protective and therapeutic role for alphaB-crystallin in autoimmune demyelination. *Nature.* 2007;448(7152):474–479.

Ozenci V, Kouwenhoven M, Huang YM, Kivisakk P, Link H. Multiple sclerosis is associated with an imbalance between tumour necrosis factor-alpha (TNF-alpha)- and IL-10-secreting blood cells that is corrected by interferon-beta (IFN-beta) treatment. *Clin Exp Immunol.* 2000;120(1):147–153.

Ozenci V, Kouwenhoven M, Link H. Cytokines in multiple sclerosis: methodological aspects and pathogenic implications. *Mult Scler.* 2002;8(5):396–404.

Panitch HS, Hirsch RL, Schindler J, Johnson KP. Treatment of multiple sclerosis with gamma interferon: exacerbations associated with activation of the immune system. *Neurology.* 1987;37(7):1097–1102.

Pashenkov M, Teleshova N, Link H. Inflammation in the central nervous system: the role for dendritic cells. *Brain Pathol.* 2003;13(1):23–33.

Paty DW Ebers G. (1998). *Multiple Sclerosis.* Philadelphia: F. A. Davis; 1998.

Polman CH, O'Connor PW, Havrdova E, et al. A randomized, placebo-controlled trial of natalizumab for relapsing multiple sclerosis. *N Engl J Med.* 2006;354(9):899–910.

Prineas JW, Wright RG. Macrophages, lymphocytes, and plasma cells in the perivascular compartment in chronic multiple sclerosis. *Lab Invest.* 1978;38(4): 409–421.

Reboldi A, Coisne C, Baumjohann D, et al. C-C chemokine receptor 6-regulated entry of T(H)-17 cells into the CNS through the choroid plexus is required for the initiation of EAE. *Nat Immunol.* 2009;10(5):514–523.

Rinker JR, II, Trinkaus K, Cross AH. Elevated CSF free kappa light chains correlate with disability prognosis in multiple sclerosis. *Neurology.* 2006;67(7):1288–1290.

Rivers T. Observation on attempts to produce acute disseminated encephalomyelitis in monkeys. *J Exp Med.* 1933;58:39–53.

Rudick RA, Medendorp SV, Namey M, Boyle S, Fischer J. Multiple sclerosis progression in a natural history study: predictive value of cerebrospinal fluid free kappa light chains. *Mult Scler.* 1995;1(3):150–155.

Rudick RA, Ransohoff RM, Peppler R, VanderBrug Medendorp S, Lehmann P, Alam J. Interferon beta induces interleukin-10 expression: relevance to multiple sclerosis. *Ann Neurol.* 1996;40(4):618–627.

Selmaj K, Raine CS, Cannella B, Brosnan CF. Identification of lymphotoxin and tumor necrosis factor in multiple sclerosis lesions. *J Clin Invest.* 1991;87(3):949–954.

Serafini B, Columba-Cabezas S, Di Rosa F, Aloisi F. Intracerebral recruitment and maturation of dendritic cells in the onset and progression of experimental autoimmune encephalomyelitis. *Am J Pathol.* 2000; 157(6):1991–2002.

Serafini B, Rosicarelli B, Magliozzi R, et al. Dendritic cells in multiple sclerosis lesions: maturation stage, myelin uptake, and interaction with proliferating T cells. *J Neuropathol Exp Neurol.* 2006;65(2):124–141.

Sharief MK, Hentges R. Association between tumor necrosis factor-alpha and disease progression in patients with multiple sclerosis. *N Engl J Med.* 1991; 325(7):467–472.

Silber E, Semra YK, Gregson NA, Sharief MK. Patients with progressive multiple sclerosis have elevated antibodies to neurofilament subunit. *Neurology.* 2002;58(9): 1372–1381.

Smith-Jensen T, Burgoon MP, Anthony J, Kraus H, Gilden DH, Owens GP. Comparison of immunoglobulin G heavy-chain sequences in MS and SSPE brains reveals an antigen-driven response. *Neurology.* 2000; 54(6):1227–1232.

Sospedra M, Martin R. Immunology of multiple sclerosis. *Annu Rev Immunol.* 2005;23:683–747.

Staykova MA, Linares D, Fordham SA, Paridaen JT, Willenborg DO. The innate immune response to adjuvants dictates the adaptive immune response to autoantigens. *J Neuropathol Exp Neurol.* 2008;67(6): 543–554.

Sun JB, Olsson T, Wang WZ, et al. Autoreactive T and B cells responding to myelin proteolipid protein in multiple sclerosis and controls. *Eur J Immunol.* 1991a; 21(6):1461–1468.

Sun J, Link H, Olsson T, et al. T and B cell responses to myelin-oligodendrocyte glycoprotein in multiple sclerosis. *J Immunol.* 1991b;146(5):1490–1495.

Tesmer LA, Lundy SK, Sarkar S, Fox DA. Th17 cells in human disease. *Immunol Rev.* 2008;223:87–113.

Thacker EL, Mirzaei F, Ascherio A. Infectious mononucleosis and risk for multiple sclerosis: a meta-analysis. *Ann Neurol.* 2006;59(3):499–503.

Tilg H, Dinarello CA, Mier JW. IL-6 and APPs: anti-inflammatory and immunosuppressive mediators. *Immunol Today.* 1997;18(9):428–432.

Traugott U, Reinherz EL, Raine CS. Multiple sclerosis: distribution of T cell subsets within active chronic lesions. *Science.* 1983;219(4582):308–310.

Trotter JL, Damico CA, Cross AH, et al. HPRT mutant T-cell lines from multiple sclerosis patients recognize myelin proteolipid protein peptides. *J Neuroimmunol.* 1997;75(1–2):95–103.

Trotter JL, Rust RS. Human cerebrospinal fluid immunology. In: Brumbach R. Herndon R, eds. *Cerebrospinal Fluid.* Amsterdam, Netherlands: Martinus Nijhoff; 1989:179–226.

Turrin NP, Rivest S. Tumor necrosis factor alpha but not interleukin 1 beta mediates neuroprotection in response to acute nitric oxide excitotoxicity. *J Neurosci.* 2006; 26(1):143–151.

Tzartos JS, Friese MA, Craner MJ, et al. Interleukin-17 production in central nervous system-infiltrating T cells and glial cells is associated with active disease in multiple sclerosis. *Am J Pathol.* 2008;172(1):146–155.

Viglietta V, Baecher-Allan C, Weiner HL, Hafler DA. Loss of functional suppression by CD4+CD25+ regulatory T cells in patients with multiple sclerosis. *J Exp Med.* 2004;199(7):971–979.

von Boehmer H. Mechanisms of suppression by suppressor T cells. *Nat Immunol.* 2004;6(4):338–344.

Walker MR, Kasprowicz DJ, Gersuk VH, et al. Induction of FoxP3 and acquisition of T regulatory activity by stimulated human CD4+CD25- T cells. *J Clin Invest.* 2003;112(9):1437–1443.

Warrington AE, Bieber AJ, Ciric B, et al. Immunoglobulin-mediated CNS repair. *J Allergy Clin Immunol.* 2001; 108(suppl 4):S121–125.

Willenborg DO, Fordham SA, Staykova MA, Ramshaw IA, Cowden WB. IFN-gamma is critical to the control of murine autoimmune encephalomyelitis and regulates both in the periphery and in the target tissue: a possible role for nitric oxide. *J Immunol.* 1999; 163(10):5278–5286.

Wulff H, Calabresi PA, Allie R, et al. The voltage-gated Kv1.3 K(+) channel in effector memory T cells as new target for MS. *J Clin Invest.* 2003;111(11): 1703–1713.

Xiao BG, Linington C, Link H. Antibodies to myelin-oligodendrocyte glycoprotein in cerebrospinal fluid from patients with multiple sclerosis and controls. *J Neuroimmunol.* 1991;31(2):91–96.

Zeman AZ, Kidd D, McLean BN, et al. A study of oligoclonal band negative multiple sclerosis. *J Neurol Neurosurg Psychiatry.* 1996;60(1):27–30.

Zhang J, Markovic-Plese S, Lacet B, Raus J, Weiner HL, Hafler DA. Increased frequency of interleukin 2-responsive T cells specific for myelin basic protein and proteolipid protein in peripheral blood and cerebrospinal fluid of patients with multiple sclerosis. *J Exp Med.* 1994;179(3):973–984.

5 Taking a Microscopic Look at Multiple Sclerosis

Claudia F. Lucchinetti

Multiple sclerosis (MS) is a chronic inflammatory demyelinating disease of the central nervous system (CNS) and the most common cause of non-traumatic disability in young adults (Anderson et al., 1992). Multiple sclerosis has major social and economic ramifications over the lifetime of the patient (Whetten-Goldstein et al., 1996). About 50% of MS patients become dependent on a walking aid and many need a wheelchair after 15 years of disease (Weinshenker et al., 1989). Relapses and progression are the two basic clinical phenomena in MS. Relapses are considered to be the clinical expression of acute inflammatory demyelinating focal lesions disseminated in the CNS, whereas progression is considered to reflect the occurrence of demyelination, axonal loss, gliosis, and diffuse global pathology involving the normal appearing white matter and cortex. There is considerable heterogeneity in the clinical characteristics of MS, but the disease is principally classified based on the clinical course of disease into relapsing remitting at onset and primary progressive at onset (no attacks) (Lublin and Reingold, 1996). Clinical predictors of natural history are far from perfect to be applied on an individual basis, and there are no surrogate markers that reliably predict course or outcome early in MS. Pathological features that clearly distinguish relapsing-remitting from progressive courses, or mild versus poor prognoses, need to be established. Furthermore, the biologic basis for the variable treatment response observed among MS patients is not well understood, and it may reflect clinical, genetic, and/or pathologic heterogeneity. With the advent of more sophisticated immunological and molecular tools, coupled with advances in neuroimaging, a greater appreciation for the complex and dynamic nature of MS pathology has emerged, and it has led to novel pathogenic insights into this enigmatic disorder.

THE DYNAMIC NATURE OF MULTIPLE SCLEROSIS PATHOLOGY

Over the last, decade MS pathological studies have shifted from the descriptive to the interpretive, in an attempt to draw dynamic conclusions from static pathological observations. However, it is essential to recognize that MS pathology changes over time, and the neuropathological features are influenced by numerous factors, including demyelinating activity, disease severity, and disease duration. Most pathological studies are based on archival autopsy samples from patients with longstanding chronic progressive disease, when relapses and magnetic resonance imaging (MRI) activity are no longer evident. Other pathological cohorts are largely based on biopsies or autopsies derived from MS patients in whom initially the diagnosis was in question, or who died in the midst of a fulminant attack. These samples are biased toward patients with very early disease, when relapses and MRI activity are typically prominent. From these two distant pathologic windows, investigators attempt to draw dynamic conclusions about this complex disease (Fig. 5-1). It is critical that in order to compare interpretations between different published pathological studies, it is necessary to compare similar pathological cohorts before concluding that observed differences represent contradictions or inconsistencies.

The pathological hallmarks of MS were beautifully described and illustrated in the 1800s by Carswell (1838), Cruveilhier (1841), and Charcot

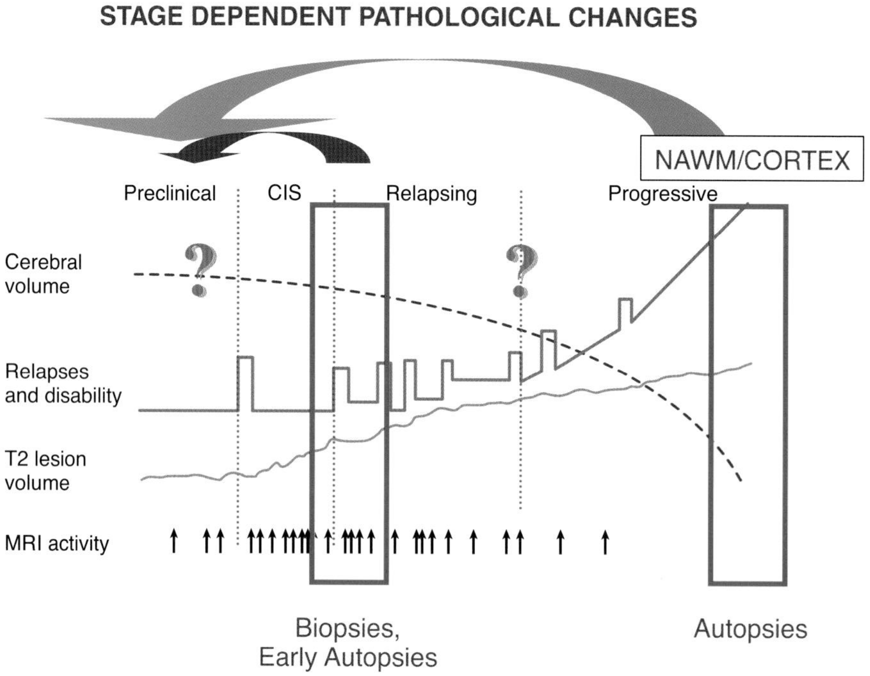

STAGE DEPENDENT PATHOLOGICAL CHANGES

Figure 5-1 Stage-dependent pathological changes in multiple sclerosis. Biopsies and early acute autopsies from fulminant disease typically capture MS during the inflammatory phase of the disease when there is evidence of ongoing relapses, and MRI activity is characterized by accumulating T2 lesion burden and gadolinium enhancement. However, most MS autopsies are derived from chronic late disease stages, when degenerative noninflammatory pathology predominates and relapses and MRI activity are less evident. CIS, clinically isolated syndrome; MRI, magnetic resonance imaging; MS, multiple sclerosis; NAWM, normal appearing white matter.

(1868, 1880). Classic MS lesions are present in all forms and stages and are characterized by areas of focal demyelination, with variable inflammation, gliosis, and relative axonal preservation. Lesions are disseminated throughout the CNS with a predilection for the optic nerves, spinal cord, brain stem, cerebellum, and periventricular white matter. Despite years of histopathological study and sophisticated magnetic resonance (MR) technology, the MS lesion is incompletely understood. How it is initiated, changes over time, correlates with clinical symptoms and other markers of disease activity, and impacted by therapeutic intervention are all largely unknown. As the site of disease pathology, the MS lesion remains the target of therapy.

Multiple sclerosis lesions evolve differently during early versus chronic *phases* of the disease, and within each phase, different *stages* and *types* of

demyelinating activity are evident. The criteria for defining an actively demyelinating MS lesion are controversial. A stringent definition of demyelinating activity within a plaque can be obtained by studying the sequence of myelin degradation products within macrophages (Bruck et al., 1995). Whenever myelin sheaths are destroyed, their remnants are phagocytosed by macrophages. Minor myelin proteins, such as myelin oligodendrocyte glycoprotein (MOG) or myelin-associated glycoprotein (MAG), are rapidly degraded in 1–4 days, whereas major myelin proteins, such as myelin basic protein (MBP) or proteolipid protein (PLP), may persist for 6–12 days. In later stages, macrophages contain sudanophilic and PAS-positive "granular lipids" that may persist for several months. Active MS lesions are characterized by an intimate admixture of macrophages and reactive astrocytes, and variable T cell (CD4+ and CD8+) and

B cell perivascular and parenchymal infiltrates. Early active lesions contain myelin–laden macrophages immunoreactive for minor myelin proteins (MOG/MAG), whereas late active lesions contain major myelin proteins (MBP/PLP). Neither minor nor major myelin proteins are present in inactive areas, although macrophages may still persist up to 6 months in the lesion. Early remyelinating lesions are notable for the presence of clusters of short, thin, irregularly organized myelin sheaths. Brains of MS patients may consist of multiple lesions, any of which may contain regions of different demyelinating stages. Stage of demyelinating activity must be differentiated from inflammatory activity, which may be present even in the absence of ongoing active demyelination.

Based on the presence and distribution of myelin-laden macrophages within MS lesions, four types of plaques can be distinguished (Figs. 5-2 and 5-3) and include the following: *(1) acute active plaque* (macrophages contain early [red] and late [green] degradation products throughout the lesion), *(2) chronic active plaque* (active macrophages [red] accumulate at plaque edge and diminish toward inactive center), *(3) smoldering plaque* (few active macrophages [red] present at plaque edge) (Prineas et al., 2001), and *(4) inactive plaque*. Acute and chronic active plaques are mainly found in acute or early MS, and in secondary progressive MS patients with ongoing relapses. Smoldering and inactive MS plaques predominate in late MS phases, in particular in PPMS or SPMS.

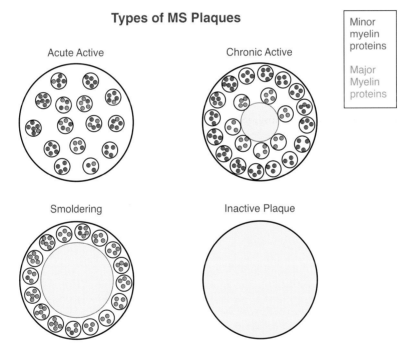

Types of MS Plaques

Acute Active   Chronic Active

Smoldering   Inactive Plaque

Minor myelin proteins

Major Myelin proteins

Figure 5-2 Multiple sclerosis plaque types. The acute active plaque is characterized by the presence of macrophages containing early (red) and late (green) myelin degradation products distributed throughout the extent of the lesion. The chronic active plaque shows the accumulation of numerous macrophages containing both early (red) and late (green) myelin degradation products clustered at the plaque edge and diminishing in number toward the plaque center (blue). The smoldering plaque is defined by the presence of very few macrophages containing early and late myelin degradation products restricted to the plaque edge, whereas the inactive plaque contains no early or late myelin degradation products within macrophages. (Reprinted with permission from Lucchinetti CF and Springer Science+Business Media. Pathological heterogeneity of idiopathic central nervous system inflammatory demyelinating disorders. *Current Topics in Microbiology and Immunology.* 2008; 318:19–43.)

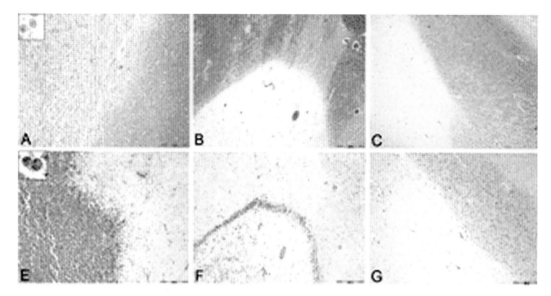

Figure 5-3 Multiple sclerosis plaque types. (A) Active lesion from a patient with acute multiple sclerosis with active demyelination. (B) Slowly expanding lesion from a patient with pathologically active progressive multiple sclerosis (SPMS), with focal demyelination. (C) Inactive lesion from a patient with pathologically active progressive multiple sclerosis (SPMS; i.e., presence of active or slowly expanding lesions at other locations). The focal demyelination is sharply demarcated from the surrounding normal-appearing white matter. (E) Profound macrophage infiltration is evident throughout the lesion. (F) A small but dense rim of CD68-positive macrophages and microglia are present at the plaque edge. Some of them contain early myelin degradation products. (G) Some CD68-positive macrophages or microglia cells are seen within the inactive lesion. (A–C) Luxol fast blue myelin staining with PAS reaction (A–D ×13). (E–G) Immunohistochemistry for CD 68 (E–G ×13). (Reprinted with permission from Frischer JM, Bramow S, Dal-Bianco A, Lucchinetti CF, Rauschka H, Schmidbauer M, et al. The relation between inflammation and neurodegeneration in multiple sclerosis brains. Brain. 2009;132:1175–1189.)

PATHOLOGIC HETEROGENEITY IN EARLY ACTIVE MULTIPLE SCLEROSIS LESIONS

Multiple sclerosis is a heterogeneous disease with respect to clinical, genetic, radiographic, and pathological features. Nevertheless, MS research has largely focused on identifying a single cause and therapy effective for all patients. The limited efficacy of T cell–directed therapies may result from a failure to abolish inflammation or intervene more specifically, since neither the trigger nor target antigen is known. In vitro and in vivo experimental data suggest multiple immune effector pathways may contribute to focal demyelination in MS. Binding of T cells to myelin epitopes can lead to macrophage activation and secondary myelin destruction. T cells and microglia/macrophages can release a toxic mediators (i.e., cytokines, proteases, reactive oxygen and nitrogen species or excitotoxins), resulting in direct tissue damage. Antibodies can mediate tissue damage via complement activation or interaction with activated macrophages. Cytotoxic T cells can directly attack oligodendrocytes and axons. Although MS pathological studies confirm the involvement of multiple immune factors are present in active MS lesions, whether there is a dominant immune effector pathway of lesion formation, or alternatively, whether multiple immune effector pathways occur in parallel or sequentially within a given patient, is controversial and has significant clinical implications. If multiple pathways within a given patient act in parallel leading to plaque formation, there would be little chance to treat or prevent lesions by blocking a single mechanism. However if focal plaque formation was the consequence of a dominant immune effector operating within a given MS patient or subgroup, specific therapy tailored towards a specific dominant immune effector mechanism might be possible.

Studies on early active MS lesions reported profound heterogeneity in immunopatterns of demyelination (Lucchinetti et al., 2000), based on loss of specific myelin proteins, extent and topography of plaques, destruction of oligodendrocytes, and evidence for complement activation (Fig. 5-4). *Pattern I* lesions were associated with T cell inflammation, and activated macrophages and microglia, suggesting demyelination was in part mediated by toxic products produced by activated monocytes. *Pattern II* lesions not only showed dense T cell and macrophage infiltration but also demonstrated evidence for immunoglobulin (Ig) deposition and complement activation on myelin and within macrophages at sites of active demyelination, suggesting a potentially important role for antibody (Ab) and complement mediated mechanisms in plaque formation. Both patterns I and II were characterized by sharp macrophage plaque borders, as well as evidence for oligodendrocytes and remyelination in the plaque center. *Pattern III* lesions also contained T cells; however, macrophage plaque borders were often ill defined, and lesions were further differentiated by a selective loss of MAG, a myelin protein located in distal oligodendrocyte processes. Based on its location, MAG loss is considered a reliable marker of a metabolically stressed oligodendrocyte, whereby the cell body is unable to support and maintain the distal axon, thereby leading to a dying back oligodendrogliopathy (Ludwin and Johnson, 1981). The finding of numerous apoptotic oligodendrocytes in pattern III lesions is compatible with this interpretation. Furthermore, MAG loss and prominent nuclear expression of hypoxia inducible factor (HIF)-1α, a specific and sensitive marker for hypoxia-like metabolic injury, was observed in both pattern III MS, as well as in acute ischemic lesions, suggesting that a hypoxia-like metabolic injury may contribute to the pathogenesis of inflammatory white matter damage in a subset of MS patients (Aboul-Enein et al., 2003; Aboul-Enein and Lassmann, 2005). *Pattern IV* lesions were exceedingly rare and associated with profound nonapoptotic oligodendrocyte death in the periplaque nondemyelinated white matter.

Analysis of a large subset of early MS lesions revealed pattern II was most frequent (~58%), followed by pattern III (~26%), I (~15%), and IV (~1%) (Lucchinetti et al., 2000, 2004; Hoftberger et al., 2004). Immunopathological patterns among early active MS lesions demonstrate high interindividual heterogeneity but intraindividual homogeneity, suggesting the dominant immune effector mechanism of tissue injury may differ among patient subgroups. Pathological heterogeneity may also reflect different host genetic factors influencing the character of immune-mediated inflammation, as well as the susceptibility of the tissue with respect glial, axonal, and neuronal injury. It is also important to emphasize that the median disease duration among patients immunopattern classified was approximately 4 years, and the majority were based on biopsies performed at the time of clinical presentation. Detailed clinical and radiographic longitudinal follow-up of this biopsied cohort confirms that although initial presentations may have been atypical, the majority of patients developed typical MS, with a disability similar to a nonbiopsied MS prevalence cohort (Pittock et al., 2005; Lucchinetti et al., 2008). Since the presence of an early active MS plaque is a prerequisite for immunopattern classification, it remains to be determined how long into chronic disease phases immunopatterns can still be differentiated. It is probable that evidence for distinct immunopatterns in late-stage established MS will be less common, given the paucity of acute and chronic active plaques available for analysis in a typical archival MS autopsy cohort. Immunopattern heterogeneity most likely is associated with focal white matter pathology typical of early disease, when relapses are still occurring. Although ongoing analysis of an expanding cohort of early active MS lesions continues to demonstrate distinct immunopatterns that are identical among all the lesion areas, or active lesions from a given patient, it is possible that with disease chronicity, heterogeneous immunopatterns ultimately converge into a more uniform homogenous pattern that contributes to disease progression in the absence of ongoing relapses.

CONTROVERSIES REGARDING IMMUNOPATTERN HETEROGENEITY

The concept of pathogenic heterogeneity has been debated. A single neuropathological series of 12 MS cases dying during or shortly after a relapse described evidence for extensive oligodendrocyte apoptosis and microglial activation, in the absence of myelin breakdown and inflammation (Barnett and Prineas,

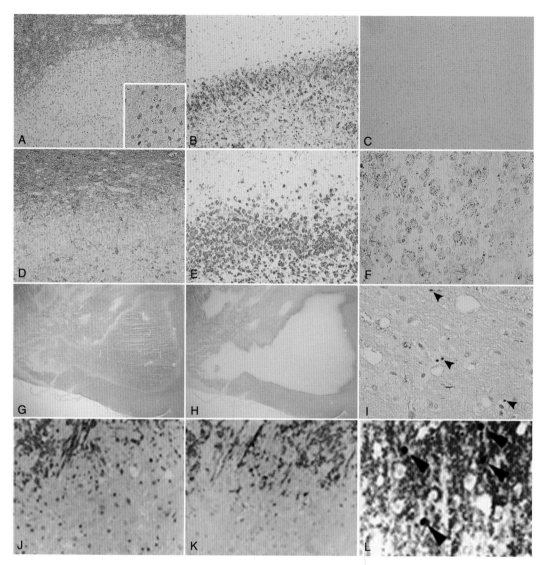

Figure 5-4 Histopathology of multiple sclerosis immunopatterns I–IV. (*A–C*) IP I. *A*: A perivenous confluent active demyelinating lesion. Macrophages contain myelin debris within their cytoplasm (insert). *B*: Macrophages accumulate in a sharp rim at the lesion border. *C*: Complement deposition is absent. (*D–F*) IP II.
D: A perivenous confluent active demyelinating lesion. Clustering of oligodendrocytes and labeling of oligodendrocyte processes is suggestive of concurrent remyelination. *E*: macrophages accumulate in a sharp rim
at the lesion border. *F*: Macrophages contain complement immunoreactive debris within their cytoplasm.
(*G–I*) IP III. *G*: MOG overexpression within active MS lesion compared to adjacent normal appearing white
matter. *H*: A striking loss of MAG is demonstrated within the lesion corresponding to the region of MOG
overexpression. *I*: Condensed oligodendrocyte nuclei suggestive of apoptosis (arrowheads). Note residual
MAG immunoreactivity in the oligodendrocyte process at upper left corner. (*J–L*) IP IV. J/K: Distribution
of myelin antigens MOG (*J*) and MAG (*K*) is similar in the lesions. *L*: DNA fragmentation of oligodendrocytes is seen in the PPWM (double staining of in-site tailing [DNA fragmentation] and CNPase [myelin and
oligodendrocytes]). ([*A–I*] Reprinted with permission from Lucchinetti CF and Springer Science+Business
Media. Pathological heterogeneity of idiopathic central nervous system inflammatory demyelinating disorders. *Current Topics in Microbiology & Immunology.* 2008; 318:19–43. [*J–K*] Reprinted with permission from
Lucchinetti et al., 2000.)

2004a, 2004b). Most of the data illustrated was based on a pediatric autopsy case of fulminant MS of short duration that died in the setting of pulmonary edema and hypoxia (Barnett and Prineas, 2004b). The presence of oligodendrocyte apoptosis in the absence of overt inflammation in some areas, as well as complement activation with evidence of remyelination in others, was interpreted as evidence of immunopattern overlap in a single patient resembling patterns III and II, respectively. This challenged the concept of pathogenic heterogeneity within MS patients and suggested immunopathological heterogeneity was stage dependent and not patient dependent (Barnett and Prineas, 2004a, 2004b). Another recent study suggested antibody and complement-mediated myelin phagocytosis was the dominant mechanism of demyelination in all lesions examined among patients with established MS (Breij et al., 2008). Although at first glance this would seemingly contradict the concept of pathogenic heterogeneity (Lucchinetti et al., 2000), it is important to recognize that this study analyzed MS lesions from late disease stages (median: 22.2 years), whereas the Lucchinetti et al. study focused on an MS cohort with early disease (median: 3.8 years) (Lucchinetti et al., 2000). It is unlikely that early active lesions (a prerequisite for immunopattern classification) were readily available for analysis in this published series, given their paucity in chronic established disease.

Published data from several independent laboratories support the concept of pathogenic heterogeneity in early MS. Distinct cellular expression patterns of chemokine receptors were observed in pattern II and pattern III MS lesions, further supporting distinct lesion microenvironments. (Mahad et al., 2004). Antigen microarrays recently identified unique serum autoantibody signatures in pattern II versus pattern I (Quintana et al., 2008). Mitochondrial defects have been described in pattern III, but not in pattern II MS lesions (Mahad et al., 2008), suggesting mitochondrial impairment may contribute to the hypoxia-like tissue injury observed in pattern III MS. Prelesional areas characterized by focal areas of white matter edema, microglial activation, and mild axonal injury in the absence of overt demyelination with minimal T cell infiltration largely restricted to the perivascular space have also been described in pattern III but not pattern II MS (Marik et al., 2007). In addition, a retrospective clinical study reported pattern II MS patients were more likely to respond favorably to plasma exchange compared to patterns I or III (Keegan et al., 2005). Similarly, a recent case report demonstrated that a patient with pattern II MS pathology experienced disease stabilization with plasma exchange (Haupts et al., 2008). These clinical and pathological observations further strengthen the concept of immunopathogenic heterogeneity in MS lesion formation.

DO IMMUNOPATTERNS CORRELATE WITH SPECIFIC CLINICAL PHENOTYPES?

To date, there is limited evidence suggesting a specific immunopattern is associated with a dominant clinical course in prototypic early MS. Although pattern IV was only seen in three cases of PPMS, these were cases of short duration, and PPMS was seen with other immunopatterns. Longer follow-up of the original cohort is needed in order to determine whether a specific immunopattern is predictive of patients who convert to secondary progression. Nevertheless, among the larger family of CNS inflammatory demyelinating disorders, several clear pathological correlations have been observed.

Baló's concentric sclerosis (BCS) is pathologically characterized by large demyelinating lesions with a peculiar pattern of alternating layers of preserved and destroyed myelin, mimicking the rings of a tree trunk. Clinically, BCS is often characterized by an acute fulminant onset followed by rapid progression to major disability or death within months. Similar to pattern III MS lesions, BCS lesions are associated with MAG loss, as well as high expression of iNOS in macrophages and microglia, and upregulated expression of proteins involved in tissue preconditioning, such as $hsp70$, HIF-1α and D-110 present at the edge of actively demyelinating Balo lesions. Due to their neuroprotective effects, the rim of peri-plaque tissue expressing these proteins may resist further hypoxia-like injury in an expanding lesion and, therefore, remain as a rim of preserved myelin (Stadelmann et al., 2005).

A distinct pattern of complement immunoreactivity has also been observed in Neuromyelitis optica, an idiopathic inflammatory CNS demyelinating disease, typically characterized by relapsing attacks of optic neuritis and myelitis. NMO lesions demonstrate extensive demyelination across multiple spinal cord levels with necrosis, cavitation, and acute axonal damage in both gray and white matter. Active NMO lesions are characterized by Ig and complement deposition in a characteristic rim and rosette vasculocentric pattern, which is distinct from the pattern of immune complex deposition along myelin sheaths and in macrophages that is observed in pattern II MS lesions (Lucchinetti et al., 2002). The specific serum autoantibody biomarker for NMO has recently been identified as NMO-IgG, which targets aquaporin 4 (AQP4) (Lennon et al., 2004, 2005), the most abundant water channel protein in the CNS, which is highly concentrated in astrocytic foot processes, with a similar rim and rosette pattern of expression in the normal human CNS (Venero et al., 1999). In contrast to MS lesions, which exhibit stage-dependent loss of AQP4, all NMO lesions show a striking loss of AQP4 regardless of the stage of demyelinating activity, extent of tissue necrosis, or site of CNS involvement and thus support a role for a complement activating AQP4-specific autoantibody as the initiator of the NMO lesion, further distinguishing NMO from MS (Roemer et al., 2007).

REMYELINATION IN MULTIPLE SCLEROSIS

Both necrosis and apoptosis of oligodendrocytes has been described in MS. Oligodendrocytes are susceptible to damage via a number of immune mediators present in the MS lesion, and they include cytokines such as TNF-α (Bitsch et al., 2000), reactive oxygen or nitrogen species, excitatory amino acids such as glutamate (Pitt et al., 2000), complement components, proteolytic and lipolytic enzymes, T cell–mediated injury via T cell products (perforin/lymphotoxin) (Selmaj et al., 1991), the interaction of Fas antigen with Fas-ligand (D'Souza et al., 1996), CD8+ class I MHC-mediated cytotoxicity (Jurewicz et al., 1998), or persistent viral infection (Merrill and Scolding, 1999). Oligodendrocyte loss is highly variable in active MS lesions. Two distinct patterns of oligodendrocyte pathology have been described in early MS lesions (Lucchinetti et al., 1999). The first pattern is characterized by oligodendrocyte survival or

progenitor recruitment, and the second is characterized by extensive oligodendrocyte destruction. The pattern of oligodendrocyte pathology reportedly remains uniform among active MS plaques examined from a single individual, further supporting the concept that the targets and mechanism of injury in MS may differ between MS patients.

Remyelination during the early stages of some MS lesions can be extensive (Prineas and Connell, 1979; Lassmann et al., 1997), however, and appears to depend on the availability of oligodendrocytes within the lesion (Raine et al., 1981; Prineas et al., 1993; Brück et al., 1994). It is not uncommon to find evidence of both active demyelination, and early remyelination, occurring simultaneously within an MS lesion examined during early disease phases, indicating the inflammatory microenvironment has both destructive and reparative capabilities. Mononuclear immune cells, like T cells, are capable of releasing anti-inflammatory cytokines including IL-4 and IL-10 and neurotrophic factors like brain-derived neurotrophic factor (BDNF) (Kerschensteiner et al., 1999), which has been found to be produced by immune cells in MS lesions (Stadelmann et al., 2002). It is probable that a delicate balance exists between the destructive and reparative inflammatory mechanisms within the MS plaque, which dictates the final outcome of the MS lesion. Conceivably, the complete blockage of all inflammatory responses in the MS lesion might be counterproductive.

The presence of oligodendrocyte progenitor cells in chronic burnt-out MS plaques lacking remyelination (Wolswijk, 1998) suggests that the failure of remyelination during these late disease phases may be less dependent on progenitor availability and more relevant to an absence of factors required for their differentiation into mature oligodendrocytes, or a defect in axons rendering progenitors less receptive to myelination signals (Chang, 2002; Charles et al., 2002). Remyelination in chronic lesions may be restricted to the plaque edge or form a completely remyelinated shadow plaque. Shadow plaques typically contain relatively few macrophages, they are associated with fibrillary gliosis. In one series, approximately 40% of chronic MS lesions demonstrated evidence for remyelination (Barkhof et al., 2003). However, profound variability in the extent of remyelination between MS patients has been reported (Patrikios et al., 2006). Patients segregated into two groups characterized either by extensive or low remyelinating capacity. This diverse capacity to form shadow plaques did not associate with clinical subtype, age of disease onset, or gender. Shadow plaques were not limited to patients with early and relapsing MS and, in fact, could be extensive even among PPMS cases. Shadow plaques were also prominent in patients with longstanding chronic disease who died at an old age. The variable and patient-dependent extent of remyelination observed in MS may need to be considered in the design of future clinical trials aimed to promote CNS repair.

PATHOLOGIC SUBSTRATE OF DISEASE PROGRESSION IN MULTIPLE SCLEROSIS

Irreversible disability in MS can occur either in a stepwise fashion due to incomplete recovery from a relapse (i.e., relapse-related disability) (Lublin et al., 2003) or as a result of gradual slow progression (i.e., progression-related disability) that occurs typically independent of clinical exacerbations or MRI evidence of lesion activity. Attack-related disability can be seen in relapsing forms of the disease (i.e., RRMS or SPMS with ongoing exacerbations), whereas progression-related disability is common in progressive forms of the disease (i.e., PPMS or SPMS with or without superimposed exacerbations). Patients with MS may experience both relapse-related and progression-related disability over the duration of their disease, and the pathogenic basis for each type of progression may differ.

Axonal Damage in Multiple Sclerosis

Axon injury and loss is a well-recognized feature of MS pathology with the last decade seeing a major emphasis on axonal damage as an important pathological correlate of disease progression. There is a high incidence of acute axonal injury in active MS lesions, and the extent of axonal transection correlates with the amount of inflammation in the lesion (Ferguson et al., 1983; Trapp et al., 1998; Kornek and Lassmann, 1999; Bitsch et al., 2000; Frischer et al., 2009). Furthermore, disability metrics (clinical/imaging) correlate with

the extent of axonal transection in MS lesions. During acute inflammatory demyelination, axons are likely damaged due to the release of toxic inflammatory mediators in the lesion, such as proteases, cytokines, excitotoxins, and free radicals (Kornek et al., 2000). A correlation between the numbers of CD8+ T cells and the extent of axonal damage further supports an important role for cytotoxic T cells in tissue damage via their production of perforin and/or granzymes (Bitsch et al., 2000). The acute axonal injury that occurs in early active MS lesions most likely contributes to the relapse-related disability predominantly seen during inflammatory phases of the disease.

However, axonal injury and loss is also evident in chronically demyelinated lesions with little or no active inflammation, and they likely contributes to gradual progression in the disease that often occurs independent of measurable clinical or radiographic inflammatory activity. In chronic MS lesions, axon loss is variable, tract specific, and size specific (DeLuca et al., 2004). Axon density is reduced by 20%–80% and can be found in the plaque, the periplaque white matter, and even in the normal appearing white matter distant from the lesion (Bitsch et al., 2000). A recent study suggested that PPMS patients show a greater reduction in axonal density in the NAWM of the cervical spinal cord compared to SPMS; however, limited sampling (1 block per case) in this series precludes any definitive conclusions regarding axonal density differences between secondary and primary progressive disease (Tallantyre et al., 2009).

Chronic inactive MS lesions may demonstrate evidence for a low-grade ongoing axonal injury, which likely accumulates over the years (Kornek et al., 2000). Several mechanisms have been proposed to account for chronic axonal damage in MS and include (1) repeated demyelination within previously remyelinated lesions (Prineas et al., 1993), (2) axonal degeneration due to the lack of trophic support from myelin and oligodendrocytes; (3) damage from soluble or cellular immune factors that may still be present in the inactive plaque; and (4) chronic mitochondrial failure in setting of increased energy demands. Demyelinated axons suffer large current leaks through newly exposed K^+ channels and the large capacitance of the naked internodal axolemma. In an attempt to restore conduction, these fibers upregulate Na^+ channels along their surface. Impulse conduction under these conditions is inefficient compared to normal saltatory conduction, and it results in increased energy demands as ion gradients are restored by ATPase consuming pumps (Stys, 2004). Mitochondria are recruited to demyelinated regions in order to meet the increased energy requirements necessary to maintain conduction and are functioning at full capacity. Although the axon may be able to support its function for several years via antioxidant defenses, free radical damage will accumulate and eventually mitochondrial function will be compromised (Andrews et al., 2005). As a result, ATP concentration in the mitochondria decreases, resulting in irreversible damage to the axon. Recent studies show reduced mitochondrial complex I and III activity in the brain and spinal cord of MS patients, raising the possibility that in addition to extrinsic inhibitors of mitochondrial respiration such as NO, there may be inherent defects in the organelles in MS that may further compromise energy-producing capacity (Lu et al., 2000). This damage could develop initially in association with inflammation, but it could also occur late in the absence of inflammation, whereby the mitochondria themselves produce excess reactive oxygen species (ROS) driving the oxidative damage that leads to eventual cell degeneration. A recent study based on global transcript profiles, biochemical analysis, and morphological studies of motor cortex samples suggested that motor neurons in chronic MS patients have significantly impaired mitochondrial function and decreased inhibitory innervations (Dutta et al., 2006). These data support increased excitability of upper motor neurons that have reduced capacity to produce ATP. This mismatch between energy demand and ATP supply could cause further degeneration of chronically demyelinated axons in MS and contribute to neurological disability.

Once axonal injury has been triggered, a cascade of downstream mechanisms leading ultimately to axonal disintegration occurs (Lassmann, 2003). Acute axonal injury leads to a disturbance in the axoplasmic membrane permeability and subsequent energy failure leading to uncontrolled Na^+ influx into the axoplasm, which reverses the Na^+/Ca^{2+} exchanger and results in excess intraxonal calcium. This activates Ca^{2+}-dependent proteases, which degrade cytoskeletal proteins, further impairing

axonal transport. Voltage-gated calcium channels (VGCCs) accumulate at sites of disturbed axonal transport, leading to further Ca^{2+} influx and eventually dissolution of the axonal cytoskeleton and axonal disintegration. Neuroprotective therapies that target different steps in this execution phase of axonal destruction such as Na^+ channel blockers, inhibitors of the Na^+/Ca^{2+} exchanger, blockade of VGCCs, or inhibition of calcium-dependent proteases, may help limit axonal destruction in MS (Dutta and Trapp, 2006).

CONTRIBUTION OF CORTICAL AND NORMAL-APPEARING WHITE MATTER PATHOLOGY TO DISEASE PROGRESSION IN MULTIPLE SCLEROSIS

Cortex

Although chronic axonal damage is a contributor to progressive disability in MS, the magnitude of axonal loss in chronic MS lesions suggests mechanisms other than inflammatory demyelination may contribute to axonal damage and disease progression at later disease phases. The focus on white matter lesions may have missed relevant pathological differences between relapsing and progressive MS. Historically MS has been considered a disease primarily affecting CNS white matter; however, recent imaging and pathological studies confirm MS is also a gray matter disease, with extensive cortical involvement (Brownwell and Hughes, 1962; Lumsden, 1970; Richert et al., 1998; Kidd et al., 1999; Peterson et al., 2001; Bo et al., 2003a; Kutzelnigg et al., 2005; Wegner et al., 2006). Multiple sclerosis may involve the cortex either as a classically demyelinated plaque or as neuronal loss and atrophy following retrograde degeneration from white matter lesions (Lumsden, 1970). Different schemes for classifying cortical plaques have been used, with three main types described (Bo et al., 2003a, 2003b). Leukocortical lesions extend from white matter into adjacent cortex; intracortical lesions are small and centered on vessels; and subpial lesions extend from pia into deeper cortex. Subpial demyelinated cortical plaques are most common in chronic MS, and they may span extended distances, penetrating variable depths, occasionally reaching white matter (Bo et al., 2003b; Kutzelnigg et al., 2005). Subpial lesions have a predilection for cortical sulci, as well as cingulate, temporal, insular, and cerebellar cortex (Kutzelnigg and Lassmann, 2006). Cortical demyelination is most prominent in SPMS and PPMS, suggesting it may be an important pathologic correlate of irreversible disability (Kutzelnigg et al., 2005). Although conventional MRI techniques are typically not sensitive enough to detect intracortical or subpial lesions, more recent imaging protocols using double inversion recovery demonstrate intracortical and subpial lesions are more frequent in SPMS, however already present in early disease (i.e., in both clinically isolated syndromes and early RRMS). Cortical atrophy is present early and becomes more prominent during progressive disease (De Stefano, 2003; Sailer et al., 2003; Amato et al., 2004; Dalton et al., 2004; Sastre-Garriga et al., 2004; Sanfilipo et al., 2005; Tiberio et al., 2005). Magnetization transfer ratios are decreased early in the cortex (Audoin et al., 2004). A longitudinal MRS study of cortex in RRMS showed periodic peaks consistent with breakdown of myelin (Sharma et al., 2001), and normal-appearing cortex shows increased apparent diffusion coefficients, both regionally and globally, likely reflecting focal and diffuse cortical damage (Vrenken et al., 2006). Diffusion-tensor MRI indicates cortical damage is more severe in disabling MS phenotypes (Bozzali et al., 2002; Rovaris et al., 2002; Dehmeshki et al., 2003; Miller et al., 2003; Rovaris et al., 2005; Vrenken et al., 2006). As cortical damage is the strongest predictor of MS disability, it is critical to better understand its pathology and pathogenic basis.

The mechanisms involved in cortical demyelination in MS are unknown, and it is uncertain whether MS therapies used to limit white matter demyelination influence cortical pathology. Emerging pathological and neuroimaging studies support the concept that cortical demyelination occurs, in part, independent of white matter lesions, and extensive subpial cortical demyelination in the near absence of white matter lesions has been described (Kutzelnigg et al., 2005). Although immunopathological heterogeneity has been described in early active white matter MS lesions (Lucchinetti et al., 2000), it remains to be determined whether the four patterns (i.e., I: T cell/macrophage; II: antibody/complement;

III: dying back oligodendrogliopathy; or IV: primary oligodendrogliopathy) segregate with specific cortical plaque types or patients. One study reported complement deposition was absent in cortical demyelination, despite its presence in active white matter plaques, suggesting a dissociation of the mechanisms mediating cortical and white matter demyelination (Brink et al., 2005). Furthermore, cortical EAE lesions in marmosets reveal Ig leakage and complement deposition in leukocortical but not subpial demyelination (Merkler et al., 2006). Recent studies suggest that subpial demyelination is specific to MS and not seen in progressive multifocal leukoencephalopathy (PML) or adrenoleukodystrophy (ALD) (Moll et al., 2008). Subpial cortical MS lesions are topographically associated with meningeal inflammation (Serafini et al., 2004; Magliozzi et al., 2007). These meningeal infiltrates reportedly resemble lymphoid follicular structures and predominate among patients with SPMS (Magliozzi et al., 2007). A recent study suggested these follicles were immunoreactive for Epstein Barr virus (Serafini et al., 2007). The damaged cortex may also differ in degree of injury and repair in comparison to white matter lesions. Cortical MS lesions are generally less destructive than white matter lesions. Light and electron microscopic studies show extensive cortical remyelination in chronic MS patients, with a higher propensity toward remyelination in cortical versus white matter lesions, suggesting a high remyelinative capacity in the cortex (Albert et al., 2007).

Despite limited inflammation in chronic cortical demyelination lesions, there is clear evidence for neural degeneration, which includes glial loss (Wegner et al., 2006), transected neurites, apoptotic neurons (Peterson et al., 2001), and reduced neuronal density (Vercellino et al., 2005). Central chromatolysis is occasionally found in cortical neurons and may reflect retrograde or anterograde degeneration. Loss of trophic support from glia within neocortical lesions could also contribute to neuronal damage and distal axonal degeneration. Discordance between neurodegeneration in the setting of minimal inflammation in chronic cortical demyelination has been interpreted by some as evidence that MS may be a primarily neurodegenerative disease. However, the presence of inflammatory cells in early cortical lesions may contribute to inflammation-dependent tissue injury possibly related to microglial activation, iNOS, complement/ antibody, cytotoxic lymphocytes, oxidative stress, and/or excitotoxic mechanisms.

Normal-Appearing White Matter

Although normal-appearing white matter (NAWM) in MS appears grossly "normal," subtle alterations in the NAWM of MS patients have been reported and include blood–brain-barrier abnormalities, mild inflammation (mainly CD8[+] T cells), microglial activation, gliosis, diffuse axonal injury, and nerve fiber degeneration (Allen et al., 1981, 2001; Fu et al., 1998; Aboul-Enein et al., 2003). Diffuse injury of the white matter is also most prominent in progressive MS patients with long-standing disease. Recent MRI data indicate the extent of tissue damage within focal plaques does not fully explain the degree of diffuse white matter changes (Filippi et al., 1995, 1998) and suggests that global permanent neurological deficits may in part be determined by global and diffuse changes in the NAWM (Rovaris et al., 2002; Dehmeshki et al., 2003). Diffuse NAWM microglial activation and axonal injury are most prominent in patients with PPMS or SPMS (Kutzelnigg et al., 2005). Interestingly, the extent of NAWM pathology in the forebrain did not correlate with the extent of white matter demyelination, suggesting that diffuse white matter changes may develop independently from focal white matter lesions (Kutzelnigg et al., 2005). Microarray analysis of NAWM in MS revealed the upregulation of a number of functionally related genes that are involved in endogenous neuroprotection, as well as pro- and anti-inflammatory mechanisms (Zeis et al., 2008). These microarray data support that a diffuse inflammatory reaction may occur throughout MS white matter, and they are consistent with findings described in neuropathological studies. These diffuse changes may be the consequence of a compartmentalized inflammatory reaction within the CNS.

CAN NEURODEGENERATION IN MULTIPLE SCLEROSIS OCCUR INDEPENDENTLY OF INFLAMMATION?

Several clinical, radiographic, and pathological observations have led some to hypothesize that MS pathogenesis is mediated by two independent events, an inflammatory reaction driving the formation of white matter lesions, and primary neurodegeneration, which drives progression. This apparent dissociation between early inflammation and subsequent disease progression is referred to as the "inflammation-neurodegeneration paradox." Clinical and radiographic evidence that highlights this paradox include the following: (1) relapse frequency early in disease influences time to onset of progression; however, once a threshold of disability is reached, rate of disability progression is not affected by relapses either before or during the progressive phase (Confavreux et al., 2000; Pittock et al., 2004); (2) MS immunomodulatory therapies reduce relapse rate along with some relapse-related disability, but their impact on disease progression remains to be proven (Coles et al., 1999); (3) brain atrophy in MS is, in part, independent of T2 lesion load (Pelletier et al., 2003); and (4) diffuse white matter damage and axonal loss can be severe despite very few white matter MRI lesions (Rocca et al., 2003). Pathological support for a primary neurodegenerative disease is circumstantial and includes the following: (1) initial oligodendrocyte injury in MS occurs in the absence of inflammation (Barnett and Prineas, 2004b); (2) evidence for ongoing axonal loss in inactive MS lesions (Kornek and Lassmann, 1999); (3) axonal loss in NAWM independent from lesions (Evangelou et al., 2000; Lovas et al., 2000; DeLuca et al., 2004); and (4) lack of inflammation in chronic cortical demyelinated lesions (Bo et al., 2003a). However, in contrast to classical neurodegenerative diseases, all MS lesions, regardless of the stage and type of the disease, are associated with inflammation. A recent large neuropathological study systematically analyzed the interdependence of inflammation, neurodegeneration, and disease progression in various MS stages in relation to lesional activity and clinical course (Frischer et al., 2009). Prominent brain inflammation was not restricted to acute and relapsing MS, but was also observed in secondary and primary progressive disease. T and B cell infiltrates correlated with demyelinating activity, whereas plasma cell infiltrates were most pronounced in patients with SPMS and PPMS. A highly significant association between inflammation and axonal injury was seen in all MS subtypes, including the progressive phenotypes.

Among older patients with longer disease duration, inflammatory infiltrates and extent of axonal injury declined to levels similar to age-matched controls. Evidence for ongoing neurodegeneration was typically attributed to confounding pathologies such as Alzheimer disease or vascular disease. These data suggest a close association between inflammation and neurodegeneration in all lesions and disease stages of MS.

CONCLUSION

Multiple sclerosis neuropathology provides important insights into the essential nature of the MS lesion, as well as tantalizing clues on disease pathogenesis. Figure 5-5 attempts to schematically consolidate current and evolving concepts of MS pathology as it relates to disease duration, clinical course, extent of inflammation/degeneration, site of pathology, stage of demyelinating activity, and heterogeneity. Early MS is typically characterized by attacks, whereas with increasing

disease duration, progression predominates. Inflammatory processes drive early disease, and degenerative processes accumulate with disease chronicity. However, there is a close interdependence between these two processes. White matter pathology dominates in early phases of MS, with more extensive cortical and NAWM pathology accumulating in chronic progressive disease. Actively demyelinating lesions can be pathologically identified in early MS; however, smoldering and inactive plaques are more prevalent in later disease stages. Finally, heterogeneous immunopatterns (I, II, III, IV) can be discerned in early active MS, but may ultimately converge into a homogenous pattern in smoldering and inactive plaques.

It is important to underscore the inherent limitations in relying on static observations to draw dynamic conclusions. The paucity of suitable MS brain tissue from different stages of lesion formation, in particular from active lesions, has resulted in much of what is known regarding MS

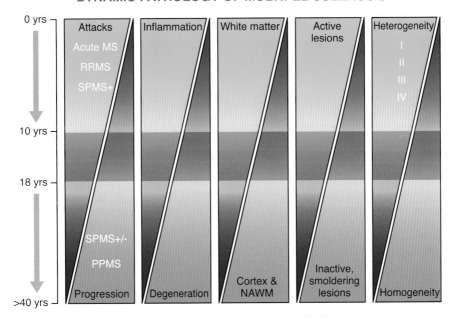

DYNAMIC PATHOLOGY OF MULTIPLE SCLEROSIS

FROM RELAPSES TO PROGRESSION

Figure 5-5 Dynamic pathology of multiple sclerosis. PPMS, primary progressive multiple sclerosis; RRMS, relapsing-remitting multiple sclerosis; SPMS, secondary progressive multiple sclerosis.

pathophysiology and immunology being based largely on experimental animal models. There remains a significant ongoing need to systematically and rigorously analyze MS lesions from different stages and phases of the disease. An appreciation for the evolving and changing aspects of MS pathology is critical as one attempts to understand and reconcile different pathogenic interpretations reported in the literature. Although qualitative observations are useful, conclusions are strengthened by the use of rigorous statistical methods. Perhaps most important is recognizing one's own limitations and biases when analyzing MS pathology. Through the lens of a microscope we see but a fraction of the global, dynamic pathology of this complex disease.

REFERENCES

Aboul-Enein F, Lassmann H. Mitochondrial damage and histiotoxic hypoxia: a pathway of tissue injury in inflammatory brain disease. *Acta Neuropathol*. 2005; 109:49–55.

Aboul-Enein F, Rauschka H, Kornek B, et al. Preferential loss of myelin-associated glycoprotein reflects hypoxia-like white matter damage in stroke and inflammatory brain diseases. *J Neuropath Exp Neurol*. 2003;62: 25–33.

Albert M, Antel J, Bruck W, Stadelmann C. Extensive cortical remyelination in patients with chronic multiple sclerosis. *Brain Pathol*. 2007;17:129–138.

Allen IV, Glover G, Anderson R. Abnormalities in the macroscopically normal white matter in cases of mild or spinal multiple sclerosis. *Acta Neuropathol (Berl)*. 1981;Suppl VII:176–181.

Allen IV, McQuaid S, Mirakhur M, Nevin G. Pathological abnormalities in the normal-appearing white matter in multiple sclerosis. *Neurol Sci*. 2001;22:141–144.

Amato MP, Bartolozzi ML, Zipoli V, et al. Neocortical volume decrease in relapsing-remitting MS patients with mild cognitive impairment. *Neurology*. 2004;63: 89–93.

Anderson DW, Ellenberg JH, Leventhal CM, Reingold SC, Rodriguez M, Silberberg DH. Revised estimate of the prevalence of multiple sclerosis in the United States. *Ann Neurol*. 1992;31:333–336.

Andrews HE, Nichols PP, Bates D, Turnbull DM. Mitochondrial dysfunction plays a key role in progressive axonal loss in multiple sclerosis. *Medical Hypotheses*. 2005;64:669–677.

Audoin B, Ranjeva JP, Au Duong MV, et al. Voxel-based analysis of MTR images: a method to locate gray matter abnormalities in patients at the earliest stage of multiple sclerosis. *J Magn Reson Imaging*. 2004;20:765–771.

Barkhof F, Bruck W, De Groot C, et al. Remyelinated lesions in multiple sclerosis: magnetic resonance image appearance. *Arch Neurology*. 2003;60:1073–1081.

Barnett MH, Parratt JD, Cho ES, Prineas JW. Immunoglobulins and complement in postmortem multiple sclerosis tissue. *Ann Neurol*. 2009;65: 32–46.

Barnett MH, Prineas JW. Pathological heterogeneity in multiple sclerosis: a reflection of lesion stage? *Ann Neurol*. 2004a;56:309.

Barnett MH, Prineas JW. Relapsing and remitting multiple sclerosis: pathology of the newly forming lesion. *Ann Neurol*. 2004b;55:458–468.

Bitsch A, Schuchardt J, Bunkowski S, Kuhlmann T, Bruck W. Acute axonal injury in multiple sclerosis. Correlation with demyelination and inflammation. *Brain*. 2000;123:1174–1183.

Bo L, Vedeler C, Nyland H, Trapp B, Mork S. Intracortical multiple sclerosis lesions are not associated with increased lymphocyte infiltration. *Mult Scler*. 2003a;9: 323–331.

Bo L, Vedeler C, Nyland H, Trapp B, Mork S. Subpial demyelination in the cerebral cortex of multiple sclerosis patients. *J Neuropathol Exp Neurol*. 2003b;62: 723–732.

Bozzali M, Cercignani M, Sormani MP, Comi G, Filippi M. Quantification of brain gray matter damage in different MS phenotypes by use of diffusion tensor MR imaging. *AJNR*. 2002;23:985–988.

Breij EC, Brink BP, Veerhuis R, et al. Homogeneity of active demyelinating lesions in established multiple sclerosis. *Ann Neurol*. 2008;63:16–25.

Brink BP, Veerhuis R, Breu ECW, et al. The pathology of multiple sclerosis is location dependent: no significant complement activation is detected in purely cortical lesions. *J Neuropathol Exp Neurol*. 2005;64:147–155.

Brownwell B, Hughes AE. The distribution of plaques in the cerebrum in multiple sclerosis. *J Neurol Neurosurg Psychiatry*. 1962;25:315–320.

Bruck W, Porada P, Poser S, et al. Monocyte-macrophage differentiation in early multiple sclerosis lesions. *Ann Neurol*. 1995;38:788–796.

Carswell R. *Pathological Anatomy: Illustrations on Elementary Forms of Disease*. London: Logman; 1838.

Chang A, Tourtellotte W, Rudick R, Trapp BD. Premyelinating oligodendrocytes in chronic lesions of multiple sclerosis. *N Engl J Med*. 2002;346:165–173.

Charcot J. *Lecons sur les Maladies du Systeme Nerveux Faites a la Salpetriere*. Paris: Cert et fils; 1880.

Charcot JM. Histologie de la sclérose en plaques. *Gaz Hop civils et militaires* 1868;140,141,143:554–555, 557–558,566.

Charles P, Reynolds R, Seilhean D, et al. Re-expression of PSA-NCAM by demyelinated axons: an inhibitor of remyelination in multiple sclerosis? *Brain*. 2002;125: 1972–1979.

Coles AJ, Wing MG, Molyneux P, et al. Monoclonal antibody treatment exposes three mechanisms underlying the clinical course of multiple sclerosis. *Ann Neurol*. 1999;46:296–304.

Confavreux C, Vukusic S, Moreau T, Adeleine P. Relapses and progression of disability in multiple sclerosis. *N Engl J Med*. 2000;343:1430–1438.

Cruveilier J. Anatomie pathologique du corps humain. 1841:1829–1842.

Dalton CM, Chard DT, Davies GR, et al. Early development of multiple sclerosis is associated with progressive grey matter atrophy in patients presenting with clinically isolated syndromes. *Brain.* 2004;127:1101–1107.

De Stefano N, Matthews PM, Filippi M, et al. Evidence of early cortical atrophy in MS: Relevance to white matter changes and disability. *Neurology.* 2003;60:1157–1162.

Dehmeshki J, Chard DT, Leary SM, et al. The normal appearing grey matter in primary progressive multiple sclerosis: a magnetisation transfer imaging study. *J Neurol.* 2003;250:67–74.

DeLuca GC, Ebers GC, Esiris MM. Axonal loss in multiple sclerosis: a pathological survey of the corticospinal and sensory tracts. *Brain.* 2004;127:1009–1018.

Dutta R, McDonough J, Yin X, et al. Mitochondrial dysfunction as a cause of axonal degeneration in multiple sclerosis patients. *Ann Neurol.* 2006;59:478–489.

Evangelou N, Esiri MM, Smith S, Palace J, Matthews PM. Quantitative pathological evidence for axonal loss in normal appearing white matter in multiple sclerosis. *Ann Neurol.* 2000;47:391–395.

Ferguson TB, Clifford DB, Montgomery EB, Bruns KA, McGregor PJ, Trotter JL. Thymectomy in multiple sclerosis. Two preliminary trials. *J Thorac Cardiovasc Surg.* 1983;85:88–93.

Filippi M, Campi A, Dousset V, et al. A magnetization transfer imaging study of normal-appearing white matter in multiple sclerosis. *Neurology.* 1995;45:478–482.

Filippi M, Rocca M, Martino G, Horsfield M, Comi G. Magnetization transfer changes in the normal appearing white matter precede the appearance of enhancing lesions in patients with multiple sclerosis. *Ann Neurol.* 1998;43:809–814.

Frischer JM, Bramow S, Dal-Bianco A, et al. The relation between inflammation and neurodegeneration in multiple sclerosis brains. *Brain.* 2009;132:1175–1189.

Fu L, Matthews PM, De Stefano N, et al. Imaging axonal damage of normal-appearing white matter in multiple sclerosis. *Brain.* 1998;121 (pt 1):103–113.

Haupts MR, Schimrigk SK, Brune N, et al. Fulminant tumefactive multiple sclerosis: therapeutic implications of histopathology. *J Neurol.* 2008;255:1272–1273.

Hoftberger R, Aboul-Enein F, Brueck W, et al. Expression of major histocompatibility complex class I molecules on the different cell types in multiple sclerosis lesions. *Brain Pathol.* 2004;14:43–50.

Keegan M, Konig F, McClelland R, et al. Relation between humoral pathological changes in multiple sclerosis and response to therapeutic plasma exchange. *Lancet.* 2005;366:579–582.

Kerschensteiner M, Gallmeier E, Behrens L, et al. Activated human T cells, B cells and monocytes produce brain-derived neurotrophic factor (BDNF) in vitro and in brain lesions: a neuroprotective role for inflammation? *J Exp Med.* 1999;189:865–870.

Kidd D, Barkhof F, McConnell R, Algra PR, Allen IV, Revesz T. Cortical lesions in multiple sclerosis. *Brain.* 1999;122:17–26.

Kornek B, Lassmann H. Axonal pathology in multiple sclerosis: a historical note. *Brain Pathol.* 1999;9:651–656.

Kornek B, Storch MK, Weissert R, et al. Multiple sclerosis and chronic autoimmune encephalomyelitis: a comparative quantitative study of axonal injury in active, inactive, and remyelinated lesions. *Am J Pathol.* 2000; 157:267–276.

Kutzelnigg A, Lassmann H. Cortical demyelination in multiple sclerosis: a substrate for cognitive deficits. *J Neurosci.* 2006;245:123–126.

Kutzelnigg A, Lucchinetti C, Stadelmann C, et al. Cortical demyelination and diffuse white matter injury in multiple sclerosis. *Brain.* 2005;128:2705–2712.

Lassmann H. Axonal injury in multiple sclerosis. *J Neurol Neurosurg Psychiatry.* 2003;74:695–697.

Lennon VA, Kryzer TJ, Pittock SJ, Verkman AS, Hinson SR. IgG marker of optic-spinal MS binds to the aquaporin-4 water channel. *J Exp Med.* 2005;202:473–477.

Lennon VA, Wingerchuk DM, Kryzer TJ, et al. A serum autoantibody marker of neuromyelitis optica: distinction from multiple sclerosis. *Lancet.* 2004;364:2106–2112.

Lovas G, Szilagyi N, Majtenyi K, Palkovits M, Komoly S. Axonal changes in chronic demyelinated cervical spinal cord plaques. *Brain.* 2000;123:308–317.

Lu F, Selak M, O'Connor J, et al. Oxidative damage to mitochondrial DNA and activity of mitochondrial enzymes in chronic active lesions of multiple sclerosis. *J Neurol Sci.* 2000;177:95–103.

Lublin FD, Baier M, Cutter G. Effect of relapses on development of residual deficit in multiple sclerosis. *Neurology.* 2003;61:1528–1532.

Lublin FD, Reingold SC. Defining the clinical course of multiple sclerosis: results of an international survey. *Neurology.* 1996;46:907–911.

Lucchinetti CF. Pathological heterogeneity of idiopathic central nervous system inflammatory demyelinating disorders. *Curr Top Microbiol Immunol.* 2008;318: 19–43.

Lucchinetti CF, Bruck W, Lassmann H. Evidence for pathogenic heterogeneity in multiple sclerosis. *Ann Neurol.* 2004;56:308.

Lucchinetti CF, Bruck W, Parisi J, Scheithauer B, Rodriguez M, Lassmann H. Heterogeneity of multiple sclerosis lesions: implications for the pathogenesis of demyelination. *Ann Neurol.* 2000;47:707–717.

Lucchinetti CF, Brueck W, Rodriguez M, Parisi J, Scheithauer B, Lassmann H. A quantitative study on the fate of the oligodendrocyte in multiple sclerosis lesions: a study of 113 cases. *Brain.* 1999;122:2279–2295.

Lucchinetti CF, Gavrilova RH, Metz I, et al. Clinical and radiographic spectrum of pathologically-confirmed tumefactive multiple sclerosis. *Brain.* 2008;137(7):1759–1775.

Lucchinetti CF, Mandler RN, McGavern D, et al. A role for humoral mechanisms in the pathogenesis of Devic's neuromyelitis optica. *Brain.* 2002;125:1450–1461.

Ludwin S, Johnson E. Evidence of a "dying back" gliopathy in demyelinating disease. *Ann Neurol.* 1981:301–305.

Lumsden C. The neuropathology of multiple sclerosis. In: Vinken P, Bruyn G, eds. *Handbook of Clinical Neurology.* Vol 9. New York: Elsevier; 1970: 217–309.

Magliozzi R, Howell O, Vora A, et al. Meningeal B-cell follicles in secondary progressive multiple sclerosis associate with early onset of disease and severe cortical pathology. *Brain.* 2007;130:1089–1104.

Mahad D, Ziabreva I, Lassmann H, Turnbull D. Mitochondrial defects in acute multiple sclerosis lesions. *Brain.* 2008;131:1722–1735.

Mahad DJ, Trebst C, Kivisakk P, et al. Expression of chemokine receptors CCR1 and CCR5 reflects differential activation of mononuclear phagocytes in pattern II and pattern III multiple sclerosis lesions. *J Neuropath Exp Neurol.* 2004;63:262–273.

Marik C, Felts PA, Bauer J, Lassmann H, Smith KJ. Lesion genesis in a subset of patients with multiple sclerosis: a role for innate immunity? *Brain.* 2007;130: 2800–2815.

Merkler D, Ernsting T, Kerschensteier M, Bruck W, Stadelmann C. A new focal EAE model of cortical demyelination multiple sclerosis lesions with rapid resolution of inflammation and extensive remyelination. *Brain.* 2006:129(pt 8):1–12.

Miller DH, Thompson AJ, Filippi M. Magnetic resonance studies of abnormalities in the normal appearing white matter and grey matter in multiple sclerosis. *J Neurol.* 2003;250:1407–1419.

Moll NM, Rietsch AM, Ransohoff AJ, et al. Cortical demyelination in PML and MS: similarities and differences. *Neurology.* 2008;70:336–343.

Patrikios P, Stadelmann C, Kutzelnigg A, et al. Remyelination is extensive in a subset of multiple sclerosis patients. *Brain.* 2006;129:3165–3172.

Pelletier D, Nelson SJ, Oh J, et al. MRI lesion volume heterogeneity in primary progressive MS in relation with axonal damage and brain atrophy. *J Neurol Neurosurg Psychiatry.* 2003;74:950–952.

Peterson JW, Bo L, Mork S, Chang A, Trapp BD. Transected neurites, apoptotic neurons, and reduced inflammation in cortical multiple sclerosis lesions. *Ann Neurol.* 2001;50:389–400.

Pittock SJ, Mayr WT, McClelland RL, et al. Change in MS-related disability in a population-based cohort - a 10-year follow-up study. *Neurology.* 2004;62:51–59.

Pittock SJ, McClelland RL, Achenbach SJ, et al. Clinical course, pathologic correlations and outcome of biopsy proven inflammatory demyelinating disease. *J Neurol Neurosurg Psychiatry.* 2005;767:1693–1697.

Prineas JW, Barnard RO, Revesz T, Kwon EE, Sharer L, Cho ES. Multiple sclerosis. Pathology of recurrent lesions. *Brain.* 1993;116(pt 3):681–693.

Prineas JW, Kwon EE, Cho ES, et al. Immunopathology of secondary-progressive multiple sclerosis. *Ann Neurol.* 2001;50:646–657.

Quintana FJ, Farez MF, Viglietta V, et al. Antigen microarrays identify unique serum autoantibody signatures in clinical and pathologic subtypes of multiple sclerosis. *Proc Natl Acad Sci USA.* 2008;105:18889–18894.

Richert ND, Ostuni JL, Bash CN, Duyn JH, McFarland HF, Frank JA. Serial whole-brain magnetization transfer imaging in patients with relapsing-remitting multiple sclerosis at baseline and during treatment with interferon beta-1b. *AJNR: Am J Neuroradiol.* 1998;19:1705–1713.

Rocca MA, Iannucci G, Rovaris M, Comi G, Filippi M. Occult tissue damage in patients with primary progressive multiple sclerosis is independent of T2-visible lesions-a diffusion tensor MR study. *J Neurology.* 2003; 250:456–460.

Roemer SF, Parisi JE, Lennon VA, et al. Pattern specific loss of aquaporin 4 immunoreactivity distinguishes neuromyelitis optica from multiple sclerosis. *Brain.* 2007;130:1194–1205.

Rovaris M, Bozzali M, Iannucci G, et al. Assessment of normal-appearing white and gray matter in patients with primary progressive multiple sclerosis: a diffusion-tensor magnetic resonance imaging study. *Arch Neurol.* 2002;59:1406–1412.

Rovaris M, Gallo A, Valsasina P, et al. Short term accrual of gray matter pathology in patients with progressive multiple sclerosis: an in vivo study using diffusion tensor MRI. *Neuroimage.* 2005;13:307–314.

Sailer M, Fischl B, Salat D, et al. Focal thinning of the cerebral cortex in multiple sclerosis. *Brain.* 2003; 126:1734–1744.

Sanfilipo MP, Benedict RH, Sharma J, Weinstock-Guttman B, Bakshi R. The relationship between whole brain volume and disability in multiple sclerosis: a comparison of normalized gray vs. white matter with misclassification correction. *Neuroimage.* 2005;26: 1068–1077.

Sastre-Garriga J, Ingle GT, Chard DT, Ramio-Torrenta L, Miller DH, Thompson AJ. Grey and white matter atrophy in early clinical stages of primary progressive multiple sclerosis. *Neuroimage.* 2004;22:353–359.

Serafini B, Rosicarelli B, Magliozzi R, Stigliano E, Aloisi F. Detection of ectopic B-cell follicles with germinal centers in the meninges of patients with secondary progressive multiple sclerosis. *Brain Pathol.* 2004; 14:164–174.

Serafini B, Rosicarelli B, Franciotta D, et al. Dysregulated Epstein-Barr virus infection in the multiple sclerosis brain. *J Exp Med.* 2007;epub Nov 5.

Sharma R, Ponnada N, Wolinsky JS. Grey matter abnormalities in multiple sclerosis: proton magnetic resonance spectroscopic imaging. *Mult Scler.* 2001;7:221–226.

Stadelmann C, Kerschensteiner M, Misgeld T, Brück W, Hohlfeld R, Lassmann H. BDNF and gp145trkB in multiple sclerosis brain lesions: neuroprotective interactions between immune cells and neuronal cells. *Brain.* 2002;125:75–85.

Stadelmann C, Ludwin SK, Tabira T, et al. Hypoxic preconditioning explains concentric lesions in Balo's type of multiple sclerosis. *Brain.* 2005;128: 979–987.

Stys PK. Axonal degeneration in multiple sclerosis: is it time for neuroprotective strategies? *Ann Neurol.* 2004; 55:601–603.

Tallantyre EC, Bo L, Al-Rawashdeh O, et al. Greater loss of axons in primary progressive multiple sclerosis plaques compared to secondary progressive disease. *Brain.* 2009;132:1190–1199.

Tiberio M, Chard DT, Altmann DR, et al. Gray and white matter volume changes in early RRMS: a 2-year longitudinal study. *Neurology*. 2005;64:1001–1007.

Trapp BD, Peterson J, Ransohoff RM, Rudick R, Mork S, Bo L. Axonal transection in the lesions of multiple sclerosis. *N Engl J Med*. 1998;338:278–285.

Venero JL, Vizuete ML, Ilundain AA, Machado A, Echevarra M, Cano J. Detailed localization of aquaporin-4 messenger RNA in the CNS; preferential expression in periventricular organs. *Neuroscience*. 1999;94:239–250.

Vercellino M, Plano F, Votta B, Mutani R, Giordana MT, Cavalla P. Grey matter pathology in multiple sclerosis. *J Neuropath Exp Neurol*. 2005;64:1101–1107.

Vrenken H, Pouwels PH, Jeroen JG, et al. Altered diffusion tensor in multiple sclerosis normal-appearing brain tissue: cortical diffusion changes seem related to clinical deterioration. *J Mag Res Imaging*. 2006;23:628–636.

Wegner C, Esiri MM, Chance SA, Palace J, Matthews PM. Neocortical neuronal, synaptic, and glial loss in multiple sclerosis. *Neurology*. 2006;67:960–967.

Weinshenker BG, Bass B, Rice GP, et al. The natural history of multiple sclerosis: a geographically based study. I. Clinical course and disability. *Brain*. 1989;112:133–146.

Whetten-Goldstein K, Sloan F, Viscusi K, Kulas B, Chesson H. The economic burden of multiple sclerosis. *MS Mgmt*. 1996;3:33–37.

Wolswijk G. Chronic stage multiple sclerosis lesions contain a relatively quiescent population of oligodendrocyte precursor cells. *J Neurosci*. 1998;18:601–609.

Zeis T, Graumann U, Reynolds R, Schaeren-Wiemers N. Normal-appearing white matter in multiple sclerosis is in a subtle balance between inflammation and neuroprotection. *Brain*. 2008;131:288–303.

Part 3 **Diagnosis and Prognosis**

Diagnosis of Multiple Sclerosis

Loren A. Rolak

There is no way to prove a person has multiple sclerosis (MS). Even a brain biopsy is subject to mistakes from sampling errors and the inability of pathologists to distinguish various causes of inflammation and demyelination. There is no laboratory test nor imaging study that is highly sensitive and highly specific, and there is thus no "gold standard" to confirm the diagnosis. Neurologists must diagnose other diseases for which there are also no definitive tests—migraine headaches, Parkinson disease, and amyotrophic lateral sclerosis are just some examples. Nevertheless, for these patients, neurologists can usually integrate features of the history, physical examination, and laboratory tests to achieve such accuracy that they rarely doubt their conclusions. Yet neurologists often find this same diagnostic process more difficult when dealing with the great variability and complexity of MS, and thus the diagnostic uncertainty is often greater.

Nevertheless, the diagnosis of MS—and its differential diagnosis—relies on the same process as for any other disease, which is to say that it relies on determining whether the patient has a presentation "typical" of the disease (Fleming, 2002, 2007). This requires a clinician who is both knowledgeable and experienced: knowledgeable enough to understand the typical symptoms, signs, and laboratory tests of MS, and experienced enough to understand the atypical features that sometimes occur as well as the atypical features ("red flags") that refute the diagnosis. For example, if a 25-year-old woman has a headache at the onset of her menses, which is preceded by 30 minutes of flashing lights, followed by a periorbital and hemicranial pulsatile pain, accompanied by photophobia and phonophobia, with nausea and vomiting, and

lasting several hours, she is probably experiencing a migraine headache. Her presentation is sufficiently typical of migraines that if her neurological examination and tests were normal, there would still be little doubt that she had a migraine headache. An experienced clinician would recognize that if some unusual features were present—such as transient tingling in her left hand—she would still have a migraine. If some typical features were absent—such as no nausea or gastrointestinal symptoms—she would still have a migraine. But if some highly atypical red flags were present—fever and obtundation—it would be less likely she was having a migraine. Similarly for MS, the diagnosis must be reached through questioning, examining, and testing to determine whether the evidence is sufficiently typical or atypical to find the patient "guilty" or "not guilty" of having MS. Even when great care is used, the diagnosis may be made in error (innocent people found guilty), or inappropriately dismissed (guilty people found innocent), and expert neurologists may disagree among themselves (hung juries). As with any endeavor dependent upon human judgment, in the end some doubt may exist as to whether justice was done (correct diagnosis achieved). The reputation of MS as a challenging disease to diagnose is well earned.

TYPICAL FEATURES OF MULTIPLE SCLEROSIS

The most common symptoms of MS are well known to neurologists, and they are summarized in Table 6-1. Visual symptoms are very common, including transient painful monocular visual loss of optic neuritis, double vision from brainstem

TABLE 6-1 Typical Features of Multiple Sclerosis

1. Optic neuritis

2. Internuclear ophthalmoplegia

3. Lhermitte's sign

4. Sensory level

5. Pyramidal tract signs: Weakness, spasticity, Babinski sign

6. Neurogenic bladder

lesions, or blurred vision from internuclear oph-thalmoplegia (INO). Myelopathic symptoms are also common, including Lhermitte sign, a sensory-level paraparesis or quadriparesis, and numbness or paresthesias of the limbs. Interestingly, hemi-paresis and hemisensory loss are unusual in MS and should be a red flag to consider vascular disease or other diagnoses. Neurogenic bladder symptoms of urgency and frequency are also typical. Cerebellar deficits of ataxic gait or tremors may be seen.

The time course is an important aspect of "typical" MS symptoms. Attacks or relapses of MS usually have a subacute onset, appearing abruptly or progressing over a few days, then reaching a plateau with stable symptoms for days or weeks, then showing partial or complete recovery over several weeks or months. Multiple sclerosis should be doubted if symptoms are transient (last-ing minutes or hours) or if they are very indolent (progressing over weeks or months). Relapses strike every 2–3 years, on average, and often repro-duce previous symptoms. Long periods without problems are characteristic. Suspicions should be aroused if complaints are constant.

Typical physical examination findings correlate with the symptoms, including monocular visual loss with optic nerve pallor and an afferent papillary defect, an internuclear ophthalmoplegia, a sensory level corresponding to a spinal cord dermatome, or upper motor neuron weakness with loss of strength in a pyramidal pattern accompanied by spasticity, hyperreflexia, and Babinski signs.

"Red flags" that are atypical of MS are listed in Table 6-2. One of the most important features of patients who do not have MS is that they do not have typical symptoms of MS (Boster et al., 2008). Therefore, one of the most important atypical fea-tures is the absence of typical features. In one pro-spective study of the misdiagnosis of MS, the most important clue that the patient actually had a different disease was that she "lacked typical fea-tures of MS" (Katzan and Rudick, 1996).

It is particularly difficult to make a diagnosis of MS in a patient who has another disease that pro-duces the same symptoms and signs. For example, a patient with diabetes might suffer a stroke, numb feet from a peripheral neuropathy, a hemisensory level from a thoracoabdominal radiculopathy, double vision from a third nerve palsy, or any

TABLE 6-2 Atypical "Red Flags" for Multiple Sclerosis

1. Normal neurologic examination

2. Lack of typical symptoms: No problems with vision, bladder, sensation, etc.

3. Abnormality in a single location: No dissemination in space

4. Persistent or slowly progressive symptoms: No dissemination in time

5. Gray matter symptoms: Dementia, seizures, aphasia

6. Peripheral symptoms: Neuropathy, fasciculations

7. Other diseases present: Psychiatric, genetic, systemic

8. Normal MRI of the brain

9. Normal spinal fluid

number of other neurologic complications which could mimic the signs and symptoms and time course of MS. Multiple sclerosis should thus be diagnosed only when there is "no better explanation" or no good alternative diagnosis to account for the symptoms.

A typical MS case is an otherwise healthy 25–40-year-old woman who had optic neuritis 3 years ago which recovered completely. She presents now with the sudden onset of double vision and Lhermitte sign. Her examination shows an internuclear ophthalmoplegia and bilateral Babinski signs. A diagnosis of MS can be confidently assumed and appropriate discussions and treatments initiated. In patients whose symptoms and signs less perfectly match this typical case, good clinical judgment should still allow for an appropriate diagnosis.

DIAGNOSTIC CRITERIA FOR MULTIPLE SCLEROSIS

The diagnosis of MS thus depends upon the judgment of an experienced clinician as to whether the various features of a patient's presentation are sufficiently typical to conclude that MS is present. This is a subjective process that relies to some degree on interpretation, experience, and opinion. In an effort to make this process more objective, over the years several physicians (and expert committees) have devised formal criteria to codify the typical features into indisputable diagnostic criteria. This has been done in part to assist physicians who are less experienced with the characteristic features of MS and with the nuances that can confuse the diagnosis. The primary driving force for these diagnostic criteria, however, has been the necessity of identifying patients for research trials. It is not possible to study the natural history of

MS, or potential new treatments, or other scientific aspects of MS, unless everyone can agree (regardless of their experience, biases, or opinions) on exactly which patients have MS. These criteria are designed to be very specific, to make sure that all patients who qualify must have MS. They are not designed to be sensitive, and there are patients with MS who do not meet these criteria. Their value to the practicing neurologist is thus limited. Confirming or refuting MS is not done by adhering to any standardized criteria for the diagnosis of MS nor by following any set algorithm on each and every patient. The adage remains true that "a patient has MS when an experienced neurologist says he or she has MS."

The first "official" criteria for the diagnosis of MS were developed in 1965 by the Schumacher Committee (Schumacher et al., 1965), and they remain the basis upon which all other criteria have been derived. These are essentially a list of the typical features of MS (Table 6-3).

The venerable Schumacher criteria solidified the concept of MS as a disease disseminated in time and in space. It forbade a diagnosis unless the patient had experienced two separate neurologic symptoms (with objective abnormalities on neurologic examination) at two separate times. This "dissemination in time and in space" has been the concept anchoring (or shackling depending upon your perspective) all future criteria. These criteria accomplished their goal of identifying patients with MS, but at a cost of excluding some genuine cases—we know the disease can begin before age 10 or after age 50, for example.

Throughout the next 20 years, evoked potentials and spinal fluid evaluations increasingly became common tests to provide objective support for the clinical impression of MS. In an effort to standardize the role of these tests, new criteria

TABLE 6-3 Schumacher Committee Criteria for the Diagnosis of MS

1. Onset of symptoms between 10 and 50 years of age

2. Objective abnormalities on the neurologic examination

3. The signs and symptoms indicate CNS white matter damage

4. The lesions are disseminated in space (two or more separate lesions)

5. The lesions are disseminated in time (two attacks at least one month apart)

6. No better explanation

were developed that incorporated these into the purely clinical guidelines of the Schumacher criteria. These new Poser Committee criteria of 1983 (Poser et al., 1983) determined whether a patient had possible, probable, or definite MS (Table 6-4). They still relied on the concept of different lesions at different times, but they now allowed for documentation of clinically occult, asymptomatic attacks—called paraclinical lesions—by using the new laboratory tests of evoked potentials and spinal fluid (Table 6-4).

Shortly afterward, in the mid 1980s, magnetic resonance imaging (MRI) became widely available and was soon almost universally performed on patients with suspected MS. Now, a diagnosis of MS is seldom made anywhere in the developed world without examining the results of an MRI scan. Areas of "abnormal" high signal are common on MRI scans of any adult brain, however, so criteria were needed to clarify precisely what constitutes MS on an MRI. For this reason, a new set of diagnostic criteria was proposed in 2001 (and modified in 2005) by the McDonald Committee (McDonald et al., 2001; Polman et al., 2005). These criteria reaffirm dissemination in time and in space (with no better explanation) and thus permit a diagnosis on clinical grounds alone.

However, if clinical data cannot fulfill these requirements, then MRI findings can supplement clinical features to establish dissemination in time and in space (Table 6-5). By incorporating MRI imaging, these criteria have supplanted the Poser criteria to become the most widely used standard. These guidelines are derived from a small number of evidence-based studies and are weighted toward high specificity so the imaging studies must conform to very exacting standards. This makes them rather cumbersome to use in routine clinical practice. Even when the multitude of complex rules are strictly adhered to, many other diseases can still produce an MRI appearance identical to typical MS (Charil et al., 2006). Nevertheless, because the MRI is a frequent source of errors in the diagnosis of MS, the McDonald Committee criteria can sometimes be of value to the discriminating clinician.

Although the various criteria for the diagnosis of MS provide a useful framework for clinicians, there is no set of guidelines that will unfailingly generate a correct diagnosis of MS. Physicians must instead consider typical signs and symptoms, the presence of other diseases, imaging features, and all other available evidence to arrive at a determination that MS is or is not present.

TABLE 6-4 Poser Committee Criteria for the Diagnosis of Multiple Sclerosis

	Attacks	Clinical Lesions		Laboratory or Paraclinical Lesions	Csf Bands or IgG
1. Clinically definite MS:	2	2			
	2	1	and	1	
2. Laboratory-supported definite MS:	2	1	or	1	+
	1	2			+
	1	1	and	1	+
3. Clinically probable MS:	2	1			
	1	2			
	1	1	and	1	
4. Laboratory-supported probable MS:	2				+

CSF, cerebrospinal fluid; IgG, xxx; MS, multiple sclerosis.

TABLE 6-5   Revised Mcdonald Committee MRI Criteria for the Diagnosis of MS

I. Dissemination in space: At least 3 of the following 4 features must be present:

   1. At least one gadolinium-enhancing lesion

               or

    Nine T2 hyperintense lesions

               or

    Eight T2 lesions plus one spinal cord lesion

   2. At least one infrat entorial (brain stem or cerebellum) lesion

               or

    One spinal cord lesion

   3. At least one juxtacortical lesion (at the gray-white junction)

   4. At least three periventricular lesions

II. Dissemination in time: Either one of the following must be present:

   1. A gadolinium-enhancing lesion at a site not corresponding to the initial clinical event, on a scan done at least three months after symptom onset

   2. If an initial scan is done at least 30 days after a clinical event, then any new T2 lesion on a second scan done any time afterwards proves dissemination in time

MAGNETIC RESONANCE IMAGING

The introduction and refinement of magnetic resonance imaging has substantially changed the diagnostic process in MS, but it has also caused more mischief than any other diagnostic study (Frohman et al., 2003). Chapter 7 in this volume will review the role of MRI in the diagnosis of MS, but it is important to mention here that the most common reason for misdiagnosing MS is faulty interpretation of the MRI (Rudick et al., 1986). Signal abnormalities of various kinds are so common on MRI scans as to be ubiquitous, and over-interpretation of such scans, erroneously assuming the signal changes to be caused by MS, is a common diagnostic error.

COMMUNICATING THE DIAGNOSIS

Patients want to know if they have a serious medical problem. They do not wish to have important information withheld in the mistaken belief that this is humane and will spare them from emotional distress. Indeed, most are relieved to find an explanation for their troubling symptoms (O'Connor et al., 1994; Papathanasopoulos et al., 2005). Nevertheless, receiving news of a chronic potentially disabling neurologic disease is very emotionally charged and conveying a diagnosis of MS should be done compassionately, considering the patient's personality, life circumstances, and medical sophistication (Isaksson and Ahlstrom, 2006). It is thus usually best to give the diagnosis in a clear and straightforward way, avoiding euphemisms such as "demyelinating disease" or "inflammation of the nervous system." Explain the nature of MS, but briefly since long or technical discussions are unlikely to be retained by the patient in the initial office setting. Dispel unrealistic pessimism that MS is an inevitably crippling or fatal disease—it is possible to be realistic and still hopeful. Then outline a management plan, emphasizing that treatments are now available for MS and many of the symptoms it produces. It is usually then helpful to schedule a follow-up visit in the immediate future to discuss the diagnosis and treatment plan further, after the patient has had time to psychologically absorb the information.

Of course, an important reason why physicians strive for an early, accurate diagnosis of any patient's symptoms is so they can begin appropriate therapy. Treating sick patients to restore their health is a fundamental goal of medicine, and this begins with the correct diagnosis. The currently available therapies for MS are only partially effective and of uncertain long-term benefit, so which drugs to choose and when to begin treatment remain controversial. Nevertheless, the discussion cannot even begin until a diagnosis is achieved.

Multiple sclerosis is a chronic disease that will require many future visits to doctors. The tact and sympathy with which physicians present the diagnosis of MS begins the long-term patient relationship so critical to managing chronic illness. It is thus a vital part of the diagnostic process.

DIFFERENTIAL DIAGNOSIS OF MULTIPLE SCLEROSIS

Multiple sclerosis is an inflammatory, autoimmune disease. But the differential diagnosis of MS is not other inflammatory, autoimmune diseases. Multiple sclerosis is a white matter disease. But the differential diagnosis of MS is not other white matter diseases. Instead, the other conditions confused with MS are those that produce fluctuating neurologic symptoms in young people. By far the most common of these is psychiatric disease. This spans a range of conditions from conversion disorder, hysteria, somatization disorder, malingering, depression, and anxiety (Crimlisk et al., 1998). Such patients usually have multiple somatic complaints that can include numbness and tingling throughout their body and limbs, vague problems with balance and dizziness, generalized weakness, fatigue, difficulty concentrating, and similar nonspecific symptoms. These frequently assume a pattern of "symptoms disseminated in time and in space" and are thus easily confused with MS. In three specialized MS clinics that have reported the diagnoses of referred patients who proved not to have MS, the most common correct diagnosis at each center was psychiatric disease (Table 6-6) (Murray and Murray, 1984; Carmosino et al., 2005; Rolak and Fleming, 2007).

The two most useful features in distinguishing psychiatric symptoms from those of MS are the anatomy and the time course. Anatomically, psychogenic symptoms tend to be diffuse such as tingling of the hands and feet simultaneously, or numbness of the entire face, or feeling "weak all over." In contrast, MS symptoms usually have a clear anatomic location such as optic nerve, spinal cord, or other focal lesion. Relapses of MS also have a distinct time course, occurring abruptly and evolving over hours to days, persisting for days to weeks, and then slowly resolving. Conversely, psychiatric symptoms tend to be very brief and last just seconds to minutes, but recur repeatedly without ever remitting. Patients are seldom free of symptoms and seldom feel well. When these nonlocalized and persistent symptoms are accompanied by nonspecific MRI signal changes, they are frequently confused with MS.

The other conditions that mimic MS are the other common conditions causing neurologic symptoms in young people. It is true that "common things are common" and the other diseases

TABLE 6-6 Differential Diagnosis of Multiple Sclerosis

	Colorado	Nova Scotia	Wisconsin
Psychiatric disease	63	14	70
Migraine	29	7	3
Stroke or TIA	7	3	2
Peripheral neuropathy	6	3	1
Cervical spondylosis	4	1	2
Benign paresthesias	0	11	10
Total	78% of 139	75% of 52	88% of 100

Of the 139 Colorado patients found not to have MS, 78% of them had one of these six diagnoses. These accounted for 75% of the 52 non-MS patients in Nova Scotia and 88% of the 100 patients in Wisconsin.

MS, multiple sclerosis; TIA, transient ischemic attack.

Source: Modified from Carmosino et al. (Colorado); Murray and Murray (Nova Scotia); and Rolak and Fleming, 2007 (Wisconsin).

in the differential diagnosis of MS are the mundane problems frequently encountered in most neurologic clinics: migraine headaches, peripheral neuropathy, cervical spondylosis, and strokes (Table 6-6). Most clinicians do not conceptualize these illnesses as usually occurring disseminated in time and in space and so they can easily be overlooked when considering the differential diagnosis of MS. But these are the most frequent other diseases that send patients to MS clinics.

FALSE POSITIVES

Equally true is that "uncommon conditions are uncommon." Other white matter diseases, inflammatory conditions, and autoimmune diseases are all uncommon. They rarely present like MS, but sometimes they may produce symptoms (and especially MRI changes) similar to MS and so by tradition they are often listed in a differential diagnosis of MS (Rolak and Fleming, 2007; Miller et al., 2008). However, most of these are exotic illnesses that are seldom encountered in a general population. Inflammatory and autoimmune diseases such as systemic lupus, vasculitis, Sjogren syndrome, sarcoid, and similar illnesses may mimic MS, but searching for such rare conditions is seldom productive on a routine basis. Another problem is the high incidence of false positives. In the Optic Neuritis Treatment Trial (Beck et al., 1992), which did screen hundreds of patients with demyelinating disease with complete blood counts, metabolic profile, chest X-ray (to exclude sarcoid), flourescent treponemal antigen (FTA) and antinuclear antibody (ANA), all of the "positive" screening tests proved to be false except for one single patient. All other screening tests—including the 31% of patients who had a spinal tap—were normal or produced distracting false positive results that actually hindered and delayed the true diagnosis (Optic Neuritis Study Group, 1991). Indeed, one later study found a "positive" but clinically unimportant ANA in 81% of MS patients (Barned et al., 1995).

The futility of screening suspected MS patients for Lyme disease or antiphospholipid syndromes has also been demonstrated (Coyle et al., 1993; Halperin et al., 1996; Quadrad et al., 2000). Checking for vitamin B12 deficiency, another white matter disease, is usually equally unproductive

(Reynolds et al., 1991). Attempts have been made to develop a consensus on the differential diagnosis of MS and to standardize the diagnostic evaluation (Miller et al., 2008), but blanket application of these guidelines to all patients is not always valuable. Clinicians must be very careful about searching for inflammatory or white matter diseases disseminated in time and in space since they are so seldom present that even when one is "found" it is probably really not there. Table 6-7 lists these diseases traditionally discussed in the differential diagnosis of MS, but diagnose them with caution.

TABLE 6-7 Rare diseases which share some features of MS

1. Inflammatory
   A. Sarcoid
   B. Sjogren's disease
   C. Systemic lupus erythematosis
   D. Systemic sclerosis (scleroderma)
   E. Acute disseminated encephalomyelitis

2. Vascular
   A. CNS vasculitis
   B. Anti-phospholipid antibody syndrome
   C. Susac's disease

3. Infectious
   A. Lyme disease
   B. Progressive multifocal leukoencephalopathy
   C. Whipple's disease
   D. Syphilis
   E. HIV
   F. HTLV-1/2

4. Degenerative/Metabolic
   A. Central pontine myelinolysis
   B. Celiac disease (sprue)
   C. Amyotrophic lateral sclerosis

5. Genetic
   A. Adrenoleukodystrophy syndromes
   B. Spinocerebellar ataxias
   C. Mitochondrial cytopathies: MELAS, MERRF
   D. Leber's hereditary optic neuropathy
   E. CADASIL

6. Other
   A. CNS lymphoma
   B. Syringomyelia
   C. Paraneoplastic syndromes

MULTIPLE SCLEROSIS VARIANTS

Neuromyelitis optica (NMO), sometimes also called Devic disease, is a relapsing inflammatory immune-mediated white matter disease often clinically indistinguishable from MS. It is very uncommon. It characteristically produces recurrent optic neuritis and transverse myelitis in a pattern of distinct relapses with variable degrees of remission. Magnetic resonance imaging scans occasionally reveal lesions outside the optic nerves and cord, but these are rarely clinically active. Evidence that this is a separate disease distinct from conventional MS came with the discovery of an autoantibody present in NMO patients that is absent in MS. This is an immunoglobulin (IgG) directed against aquaporin channels in the nervous system. This humoral attack seems to produce, by unknown mechanisms, the inflammatory demyelination responsible for the white matter lesions. Diagnostically, suspicion should be aroused in patients who present with the combination of optic neuritis and myelitis. This is especially true when the cord lesions are extensive, extending over three or more segments sagitally and affecting the entire cord transversely. Because the clinical picture may be indistinguishable from typical MS, some authorities recommend testing for the NMO antibody in all patients presenting with optic neuritis or an extensive transverse myelitis (Wingerchuck, 2007).

TABLE 6-8 McDonald Committee Criteria for Primary Progressive MS

1. Insidious neurological progression suggestive of MS

2. Abnormal CSF with oligoclonal bands or increased IgG is essential

3. Dissemination in time proven by:
   A. New MRI lesions
                or
   B. Continued progression for 1 year

4. Dissemination in space proven by:
   A. MRI showing multifocal lesions
                or
   B. Visual evoked response abnormalities

5. No better explanation

The differentiation of other MS variants is less clear. Balo's concentric sclerosis is a very rare demyelinating condition characterized by alternating bands of demyelination separated by strips of normal myelin. These produce a characteristic pattern of concentric rings of demyelination on magnetic resonance imaging. The few autopsy cases have shown findings indistinguishable from typical MS and this may not be a separate disease at all, but rather just a fortuitous juxtaposition of lesions (Korte et al., 1994). Intensely inflammatory demyelination that relapses relentlessly, sometimes leading to death within 1 or 2 years, is sometimes labeled Marburg disease. Too little data are available about this rare condition to determine whether it is a distinct demyelinating disease or simply unusually severe MS.

PRIMARY PROGRESSIVE MULTIPLE SCLEROSIS

The disease conventionally diagnosed as MS seems to involve two different processes. One is an inflammatory, immune-mediated attack on central nervous system myelin which occurs intermittently in distinct relapses followed by periods of remission. The other process is a "neurodegenerative" one characterized by slow, gradual deterioration in neurologic function, usually with diffuse and progressive brain (and possibly spinal cord) atrophy. This progression is accompanied by less (or perhaps no) inflammation, may or may not be immune mediated, and is progressive rather than relapsing-remitting. The relationship between these two processes of inflammatory relapses and degenerative atrophy is unclear. Some authorities believe that the progressive degeneration is somehow caused by the cumulative effects of the relapsing inflammation, but other authorities dispute this. In any event, approximately 15% of MS patients have only the progressive clinical course, never experiencing relapses or remissions. These patients are referred to as primary progressive MS (PPMS). They are much more likely to be male (more than 60%) and to be older (more than 40 years) than other MS patients.

The diagnosis of PPMS can be even more challenging than the relapsing-remitting form. The McDonald Committee suggested that patients should still show evidence of dissemination in time and in space, though this may require more reliance upon testing rather than clinical evidence (Table 6-8). Because the differential diagnosis of slowly progressive neurologic deficits is much more extensive and difficult to distinguish than relapsing-remitting symptoms, these diagnostic criteria are less reliable. Indeed, the authors of these guidelines noted that they "had particular difficulty in reaching a consensus on the criteria for diagnosis in this clinical group." Ideally, patients should have abnormal MRI scans, visual evoked responses, and spinal fluid. However, many of the patients diagnosed by academic MS experts as having primary progressive multiple sclerosis for inclusion in a trial of a new therapeutic agent had normal spinal fluid and did not meet the McDonald criteria (Wolinsky et al., 2004). Patients with this clinical presentation thus demand more careful follow-up and diagnostic flexibility.

REFERENCES

Barned S, Goodman AD, Mattison DH. Frequency of anti-nuclear antibodies in multiple sclerosis. *Neurol.* 1995; 45:384–389.

Beck RW, Cleary PA, Anderson MM, et al. A randomized, controlled trial of corticosteroids in the treatment of acute optic neuritis. *N Engl J Med.* 1992;236: 581–588.

Boster A, Caon C, Perumal J, et al. Failure to develop multiple sclerosis in patients with neurologic symptoms without objective evidence. *Mult Scler.* 2008;14:804–808.

Carmosino MJ, Brousseau KM, Arciniegas DB, Corboy JR. Initial evaluations for multiple sclerosis in a university multiple sclerosis center: outcomes and role of magnetic resonance imaging in referral. *Arch Neurol.* 2005;62:585–590.

Charil A, Yousry TA, Rovaris M, et al. MRI and the diagnosis of multiple sclerosis: expanding the concept of "No Better Explanation." *Lancet Neurol.* 2006;5: 841–852.

Coyle PK, Krupp LB, Doscher C. Significance of a reactive lyme serology in multiple sclerosis. *Ann Neurol.* 1993; 34:745–747.

Crimlisk HL, Bhatia K, Cope H, David A, Marsden CD, Ron MA. Slater revisited: 6-year follow-up study of patients with unexplained motor symptoms. *BMJ.* 1998;316:582–586.

Fleming JO. *Diagnosis and Management of Multiple Sclerosis.* West Islip, NY: Professional Communications; 2002.

Fleming JO. *The Diagnosis of Multiple Sclerosis. Education Program Syllabus. St Paul, MN:* American Academy of Neurology; 2007.

Frohman EM, Goodin DS, Calabresi PA, et al. The utility of MRI in suspected MS. Report of the Therapeutics and Technology Assessment Subcommittee of the American Academy of Neurology. *Neurol.* 2003;61: 602–611.

Halperin JJ, Logigian EL, Finkel MF, Pearl RA. Practice parameters for the diagnosis of patients with nervous system lyme borreliosis (Lyme disease). *Neurol.* 1996; 46:619–627.

Isaksson AK, Ahlstrom G. From symptom to diagnosis: Illness experiences of multiple sclerosis patients. *J Neurosci Nursing.* 2006;38:229–237.

Katzan I, Rudick RA. Guidelines to avoid errors in the diagnosis of multiple sclerosis. *Neurol.* 1996;40:54.

Korte JH, Bom EP, Vos LD, Breuer TJ, Wondergem JH. Balo concentric sclerosis: MR diagnosis. *Am J Neuroradiol.* 1994;15:1284–1285.

McDonald WI, Compston A, Edan G, et al. Recommend diagnostic criteria for multiple sclerosis: guidelines from the international panel on the diagnosis of multiple sclerosis. *Ann Neurol.* 2001;50:121–127.

Miller DH, Weinshenker BG, Filippi M, et al. Differential diagnosis of suspected multiple sclerosis: a consensus approach. *Mult Scler.* 2008;14:1157–1174.

Murray TJ, Murray SJ. Characteristics of patients found not to have multiple sclerosis. *Can Med Assoc J.* 1984; 131:336–337.

Optic Neuritis Study Group. The clinical profile of optic neuritis. Experience of the optic neurtis treatment trial. *Arch Ophthalmol.* 1991;109:1673–1678.

Papathanasopoulos PG, Nikolakopoulou A, Scolding NJ. Disclosing the diagnosis of multiple sclerosis. *J Neurol.* 2005;252:1307–1309.

Polman CH, Reingold SC, Edan G, et al. Diagnostic criteria for multiple sclerosis: 2005 revisions to the McDonald criteria. *Ann Neurol.* 2005;58:840–846.

Poser CM, Paty DW, Scheinberg L, et al. New diagnostic criteria for multiple sclerosis: Guidelines for research protocols. *Ann Neurol.* 1983;13:227–231.

Quadrad MJ, Khamasta MA, Ballesteros A, et al. Can neurologic manifestations of anti-phospholipid syndrome be distinguished from multiple sclerosis? *Medicine* 2000;79:57–68.

Reynolds EH, Linnell JC, Faludy JE. Multiple sclerosis associated with Vitamin B12 deficiency. *Arch Neurol.* 1991;48:808–811.

Rolak LA, Fleming JO. The differential diagnosis of multiple sclerosis. *Neurologist.* 2007;13:57–72.

Rudick RA, Schiffer R, Schwetz KM, Herndon RM. Multiple sclerosis: The problem of incorrect diagnosis. *Arch Neurol.* 1986;54:578–583.

Schumacher G, Kibler R, Kurland L, Kurtzke J, McDowell F. Problems of experimental trials in multiple sclerosis. *Ann NY Acad Sci.* 1965;122:552–568.

Wingerchuck DM. Diagnosis and treatment of neuromyelitis optica. *The Neurologist.* 2007;13:2–11.

Wolinsky J and the PROMISE trial Study Group. The promise trial. *Mult Scler.* 2004;10:565–572.

7 Neuroimaging in Multiple Sclerosis

Nancy L. Sicotte

The basis for the diagnosis of multiple sclerosis (MS) requires finding evidence of at least two central nervous system (CNS) lesions that are separated by neuroanatomy (space) and occur in distinct episodes (time). As specific diagnostic criteria have evolved, the role of magnetic resonance imaging (MRI) has increased in importance in making the diagnosis of MS; information obtained from magnetic resonance (MR) scans can now fulfill the requirements for both dissemination in time and space. These advances have led to earlier diagnosis and access to treatment, which is associated with better long-term patient outcomes.

Standard MRI measures of disease activity, including white matter lesions and gadolinium-enhancing lesions, are useful markers of inflammation, but they show only modest correlations with current and future disability (Filippi, 2001; Fisniku et al., 2008a). Nonconventional MR techniques that more fully capture the extent of MS-related disease burden in both white and gray matter CNS regions offer promise as better markers of neurodegenerative changes associated with MS. These techniques will become more important in assessing patient outcomes and putative neuroprotective therapies.

STANDARD MAGNETIC RESONANCE IMAGING ACQUISITIONS

Magnetic Resonance Imaging Technology

A detailed description of MR physics is beyond the scope of this book, but those seeking more in-depth information are directed to a very helpful Web site (http://www.cis.rit.edu/htbooks/mri/) that offers an excellent overview of MR physics, image acquisition, and pulse sequences. Magnetic resonance imaging uses strong magnetic fields with applied radiofrequency (rf) energy and gradients to create detailed soft-tissue images. This technique has several advantages over other imaging modalities, including the ability to obtain multiple studies without the risk of radiation exposure, the generation of high-resolution images in any orientation (unlike CAT scans that are limited to the axial plane), and the ability to achieve an almost endless variety of tissue contrasts by the application of ever-more sophisticated pulse sequences.

Standard MRI sequences obtain signals from protons (hydrogen) found in fat and water, the main constituents of the brain. When placed in the strong magnetic field of an MRI scanner, proton spins will align with this field also known as B0. Energy, in the form of brief rf pulses, is applied to the tissues, displacing the spins in a uniform direction. As the spins dephase and return to alignment with the B0 field, they in turn produce rf energy that is collected and reconstructed into images. The rate at which spins "relax" after rf pulses is determined by local tissue properties, and these subtle differences provide contrast between tissue types and lead to the exquisitely detailed images produced by MRI. The timing of the application (TR, repetition time) and sampling (TE, echo time) of rf energy are the critical parameters that determine the relative tissue contrast or "weighting" of the resulting images. Sequences that that are used most commonly in clinical practice are described next.

T1

T1 (longitudinal or spin-lattice relaxation) is the time for the spins to recover longitudinal magnetization after the application of the rf pulse. T1-weighted scans are short TR (~500 msec) and TE (~25 msec) scans that can be collected quickly, routinely producing 3D images with a resolution of 1 mm³. T1-weighted images provide excellent contrast between CNS white and gray matter, while the cerebrospinal fluid appears dark. The intravenous administration of gadolinium-based contrast agents causes a shortening of the T1, leading to a higher signal in the areas where contrast is present, normally within blood vessels, but leaking into the brain parenchyma in areas of inflammation associated with blood–brain barrier breakdown.

T2

T2 (transverse or spin-spin relaxation) is the time for the loss of phase coherence in the transverse plane after the application of the rf pulse. T2-weighted images have a long TR (~2500 msec) and long TE (~90 msec) with tissue contrast that is the inverse of T1-weighted scans; CSF is bright, and white matter appears darker than gray matter. This sequence is very sensitive to any pathological process associated with excess water, including edema and/or inflammation.

Proton Density Scans

Protein density (PD) scans produce images in which the signal intensity is proportional to the number of protons present. These are long TR (~2500 msec) and short TE (~30 msec) scans that are commonly obtained at the same time as the T2-weighted scan, as the first echo of a "double echo" scan. Excess water also appears bright on PD weighted scans, and prior to the use of FLAIR imaging, these scans were used preferentially to quantify white matter lesions in MS clinical trials because of the better ventricular/lesion contrast.

Fluid Attenuated Inversion Recovery

Fluid attenuated inversion recovery (FLAIR) is essentially a T2-weighted scan obtained after the application of an additional rf pulse that is timed so that the signal from spins in free fluid are nulled at the time the image is collected. This causes CSF spaces to appear black, leading to a greater conspicuity of periventricular lesions, but also accentuating areas of high T2 signal within white and gray matter regions of the brain. The FLAIR images obtained in the sagittal plane are especially useful for identifying lesions within the corpus callosum, the presence of which increases the likelihood of demyelination, in light of the low incidence of corpus callosum lesions in vascular disease.

TECHNICAL ISSUES WITH MAGNETIC RESONANCE IMAGING

Field Strength

Magnetic field strength, as measured in Tesla (T) units, refers to the strength of the B0 field. Early scanners used static, naturally occurring magnetic materials, or permanent magnets, with the major limitation being the size and weight of the magnet, and the limited field strength generated, only to about 0.4T. Modern MR scanners are electromagnets in which an electric current generates the magnetic fields using superconducting wires that operate at zero resistance in low temperatures, achieved by the use of a liquid helium core. This technology generates high field strengths that are stable over time. What constitutes "standard" field has been evolving rapidly as typical clinical scanners that operate at 1.5T are increasingly being replaced by 3.0T "high field" scanners, since recent FDA approval. Ultra high field scanners of 7.0T and above are limited to research settings and are not in use currently for routine clinical scanning.

Besides bragging rights to having the biggest scanner on the block, high field increases the amount of detectable signal, leading to a markedly improved signal to noise ratio. As a result, images of higher resolution and better tissue contrast are possible at higher field strengths. Advanced applications that yield inherently low signals, such as functional MRI, which relies on detecting subtle signal differences between oxygenated and deoxygenated hemoglobin, or spectroscopy, which detects signal from compounds at very low concentrations in the CNS, are greatly enhanced at high field. Relaxation times are affected by the strength of the B0 field and the shortening of T1 at 3.0T and above can lead to a decrease in T1 contrast while T2 processes are enhanced at higher field strengths.

The use of higher field strength does not appear to greatly affect the ability to make a diagnosis of

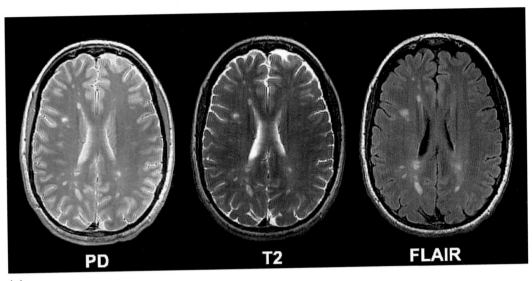

(a)

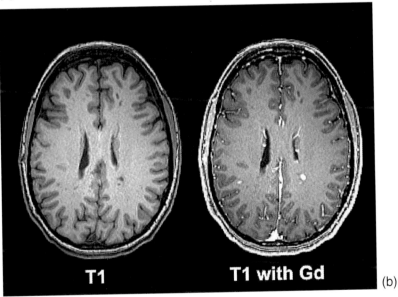

(b)

Figure 7-1 Conventional magnetic resonance imaging (MRI) in multiple sclerosis. (A) Axial slices of magnetic resonance images with typical white matter lesions seen in multiple sclerosis. FLAIR, fluid attenuated inversion recovery; PD, proton density; T2, T2-weighted scan. (B) T1-weighted images before (*left*) and after (*right*) the administration of gadolinium contrast material. Note presence of two gadolinium-enhancing lesions and T1 black holes.

MS (Lee et al., 1995; Keiper et al., 1998). However, higher numbers and volumes of both T2 and Gd+ lesions can be detected at higher field strengths (Keiper et al., 1998; Sicotte et al., 2003), and this is useful in clinical trials in which the quantification of serial scans is an important outcome measure.

Resolution

Magnetic resonance images are comprised of individual voxels, or volume elements, that have x, y, and z dimensions. The MRI scanner samples tissue within a specific field of view (FOV), typically 20–24 cm², which is then partitioned into

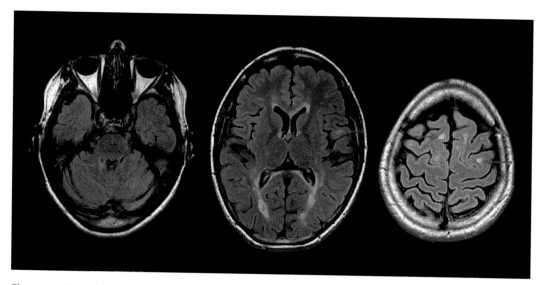

Figure 7-2 Typical demyelinating lesions as seen on fluid attenuated inversion recovery (FLAIR). Red arrows indicate infratentorial (*left*) and juxtacortical (*middle* and *right*) white matter lesions as seen on axial FLAIR magnetic resonance imaging scans of an individual diagnosed with relapsing-remitting multiple sclerosis.

individual regions specified by the matrix (typical matrix: 256 × 256). For a two-dimensional scan, dividing the FOV by the matrix yields the "in-plane" scan resolution, or x and y dimensions. In two-dimensional acquisitions, slice thickness is the z-dimension, with typical values of 3–5 mm. Of note, two-dimensional acquisitions may include a "gap" between slices, ranging from 1 to 2.5 mm; therefore, any areas of abnormality smaller than the gap will not be detected. Three-dimensional acquisitions are now increasingly used, especially with the advent of high field strengths, parallel imaging protocols, and multichannel rf coils that all increase scan speed, yielding scans with a resolution of 1 mm³ routinely.

Serial Scans

The new McDonald criteria (McDonald et al., 2001) for the diagnosis of MS includes the use of serial MRI findings to satisfy dissemination in time and the diagnosis of MS. This requires demonstrating the appearance of a new T2 or Gd+ lesion not seen on an initial scan and this emphasizes the need for accurate and reproducible scans over time. Differences in the protocols used, field strength, slice thickness, and resolution will all

affect the ability to reliably detect new lesion formation. But other subtle differences such as changes in head position across scans could lead to incorrect conclusions about disease activity. To address these concerns, the Consortium of MS Centers (CMSC) has published guidelines for the use of MRI in the diagnosis and follow-up of MS (Simon et al., 2006), described later and shown in Table 7-4.

FINDINGS ON STANDARD MAGNETIC RESONANCE IMAGING IN MULTIPLE SCLEROSIS

T1-Weighted Imaging

Gadolinium (Gd+)-enhancing lesions

Lesions that enhance after the administration of gadolinium on T1-weighted images are highly specific and sensitive for MS-related inflammation. They represent areas of acute inflammation associated with the breakdown of the blood–brain barrier (BBB). Enhancement typically resolves within 4–6 weeks; therefore, measures of Gd+ lesions are useful markers of acute inflammation.

Lesions may re-enhance later, and certain patterns of enhancement (ring-like) have been associated with more severe pathology (Masdeu et al., 1996; Morgen et al., 2001). If present at the time of a clinically isolated syndrome, a diagnosis of MS is more likely. Steroids temporarily suppress enhancing lesion activity. The number and volume of lesions are quite variable between individuals as well within a single individual; therefore, several scans done at monthly intervals are typically required in order to establish a baseline of activity for an individual patient (Stone et al., 1995).

The presence of Gd+ lesions is associated with a high risk of relapse, although new Gd+ lesions appear 7–10 times more frequently than clinical relapses (Kappos et al., 1999). Quantification of Gd+ lesion numbers and volumes are an attractive surrogate marker of disease activity in MS because of this increased sensitivity. All of the currently approved disease-modifying agents (DMAs) have been shown to reduce the number and volume of Gd+ lesions (Paty and Li, 1993; Jacobs et al., 1996; Comi and Filippi, 1999; Miller et al., 2003). In addition, Gd+ lesions are frequently used as the primary outcome measure in exploratory Phase II trials of novel MS drugs. In fact, potential therapies that cannot demonstrate an ability to suppress new Gd+ lesions are not likely to move beyond these early stages of drug development.

Of note, gadolinium-based contrast agents (GBCAs) have recently been associated with a rare but severe syndrome termed "nephrogenic systemic fibrosis" (NSF). This progressive, multisystem disorder has been reported in patients with severe renal disease either on dialysis or as part of hepato-renal syndrome who received GBCAs (Broome, 2008). This has led to a black box warning on GBCA drug inserts and recommendations for additional screening of patients for occult renal disease prior to the use of a GBCA. See FDA Web site for full details: http://www.fda.gov/Drugs/DrugSafety

T1 "black holes"

Areas of hypointensity in the white matter, termed "black holes," can be seen frequently on T1-weighted images in MS. It is important to note that all acutely Gd+-enhancing lesions will be hypointense on the noncontrast T1 scan and these "acute black holes" likely represent edema. However, while the majority of these acute black holes will resolve, serial studies show that a subset, on average 30%, will remain persistently hypointense, becoming chronic black holes (CBHs; van Waesberghe et al., 1998). Histopathological and nonconventional imaging findings show that CBHs represent areas of significant axonal loss, suggesting that CBHs may be an imaging marker of permanent damage (van Walderveen et al., 1998; Li et al., 2003). T1 black hole volumes are also better correlated with disability measures than standard T2 volumes (Truyen et al., 1996).

Difficulties with the use of this MRI marker are that T1 black holes can resolve over many months to years (Bagnato et al., 2003) and may also represent a gradient of pathological change (gray and black holes) (Bitsch et al., 2001; Riva et al., 2009). Reliable serial measures require the careful exclusion of new enhancing lesions and long-term monitoring. Some but not all disease-modifying therapies have been shown to affect black hole formation (Filippi et al., 2001; Bagnato et al., 2005), although longer studies are needed.

Atrophy

Diffuse changes occur in the brain in patients with MS even at the earliest stages of the disease. Studies have shown that compared to age-matched controls, MS patients have diffuse loss of brain tissue as measured by decreased brain volumes, ventricular enlargement, and spinal cord atrophy (Losseff et al., 1996; Stevenson et al., 1998; Rudick et al., 1999; Brex et al., 2000; Ge et al., 2000; Filippi et al., 2003) and have detectable brain volume loss before converting to clinically definite MS (Dalton et al., 2002a). The number and volume of enhancing lesions are associated with the development of subsequent atrophy, but other, as yet unidentified, factors must play a role (Fisher et al., 2002). Demyelination in subcortical and cortical regions, which is largely invisible using standard imaging techniques (Stadelmann et al., 2008), is one plausible factor. Recent pathological studies have found significant axonal loss in the spinal cord and brain of MS patients (Ganter et al., 1999; Schmierer et al., 2004), but while axonal density was severely decreased, tissue volumes were not as significantly affected, suggesting that MRI volume measures may underestimate the true extent of axonal and neuronal loss (DeLuca et al., 2004; Evangelou et al., 2005).

The loss of volume within gray matter regions is also evident on standard T1-weighted scans and can be measured using relatively simple linear techniques (Butzkueven et al., 2008). In particular, early loss is seen in thalamus, reflected in enlargement of the third ventricle and associated with cognitive impairment (Houtchens et al., 2007). Basal ganglia atrophy is reflected in part by measures such as the bicaudate ratio (Bermel et al., 2002). Other gray matter areas are involved early in MS, including the hippocampus, which is also associated with verbal memory impairment (Sicotte et al., 2008).

T2/Proton Density Imaging

T2 lesions

Areas of high signal within white matter regions, termed "T2 lesions," are a key marker of MS and are used as a measure of cumulative disease activity or "disease burden" in MS. Although T2 lesions can be useful and sensitive markers of demyelination, it is important to recognize that areas of high signal on T2 lack neuropathological specificity, can be seen in otherwise healthy individuals, and are a feature of disorders other than MS, including migraine, hypertension, and a variety of other potential MS "mimics." However, key features of T2 lesions such as size and location increase the likelihood that these represent demyelination. These characteristics have been formalized into specific criteria in order to facilitate the diagnosis of MS while preventing false diagnosis due to the presence of minor, nonspecific changes, or other disease conditions (see Table 7-2). Other characteristics of white matter lesions that suggest demyelination include ovoid shape, involvement of the corpus callosum, and orientation perpendicular to the long axis of the lateral ventricles. When viewed in the sagittal plane, these white matter lesions appear to stand on end, due to their perivenule orientation, and have been given the eponym "Dawson's fingers."

T2 hypointensity

Areas of *decreased* T2 signal are seen in deep gray matter regions of MS patients and have been

correlated with disability measures and brain atrophy (Bakshi et al., 2002). These changes, which are also found in other neurological disorders such as Parkinson disease and Alzheimer disease, appear to reflect progressive iron deposition related to neurodegeneration (Brass et al., 2006). A recent study found that worsening T2 hypointensity in the putamen and thalamus predicted clinical progression in a large cohort of MS patients (Neema et al., 2009). Iron deposition in other areas may also reflect disease activity. At ultra high field (7T), signal changes thought to represent iron-laden macrophages can be detected in rims around white matter lesions (Hammond et al., 2008). These findings have spurred the development of iron-sensitive imaging as a biomarker for neurodegeneration in MS (Schenck and Zimmerman, 2004).

Fluid Attenuated Inversion Recovery Imaging

The incorporation of FLAIR imaging to routine clinical practice has led to new, key insights into the pathophysiology of MS, as areas of high signal on FLAIR scans can be seen in juxtacortical and cortical areas, not seen well on PD/T2 scans (Bakshi et al., 2001). The number and volume of these areas increase with disease duration and severity (Geurts et al., 2005; Calabrese et al., 2008). Findings on FLAIR imaging can be especially useful in establishing the diagnosis of MS, by revealing the presence of juxtacortical lesions and involvement of the corpus callosum, both of which are more closely associated with demyelination. Of note, FLAIR may be less sensitive to lesions in the posterior fossa (Bastianello et al., 1997), requiring careful inspection of the PD/T2 scans in this region.

Spinal Cord Imaging

It is more difficult to detect lesions involving the spinal cord, due to several factors, including the small size of the cord and artifacts due to respiration and cardiac activity. However, spinal cord lesions are very common in MS, occurring in up to 83% of individuals recently diagnosed with MS with a predilection for the cervical and upper thoracic regions (Ikuta and Zimmerman, 1976; Bot et al., 2004). Sagittal T2-weighted scans are most helpful in identifying areas of high signal, which can then be further assessed on axial acquisitions, along with pre- and postcontrast T1-weighted scans. In cases of diagnostic uncertainty when brain lesions appear nonspecific, the finding of a spinal cord lesion can be very helpful in clarifying the diagnosis of MS. In the case of neuromyelitis optica (NMO), an MS variant with a distinct pathogenesis, evidence of a confluent multilevel signal abnormality on spinal cord imaging is a key diagnostic component (Wingerchuk et al., 2007).

DIAGNOSIS OF MULTIPLE SCLEROSIS: WHEN MAGNETIC RESONANCE IMAGING PLAYS A PIVOTAL ROLE

In moving from exam-based diagnosis (Schumacher et al., 1965) to the incorporation of paraclinical supportive data including MRI and evoked potentials (Poser et al., 1983), the usefulness of MRI in identifying those patients at high risk for developing clinically definite MS became evident. Furthermore, with the development of disease-modifying therapies, it became a matter of good medical practice to begin treatment as soon as a diagnosis of MS could be made. In this way, individuals with a clinically isolated syndrome (CIS)—a single episode suggestive of demyelination (e.g., optic neuritis)—could be stratified into low risk and high risk on the basis of initial MRI results.

Clinically Isolated Syndrome

Magnetic resonance imaging findings play an especially important role in establishing the risk of developing clinically definite MS. In a seminal longitudinal study of 81 patients who presented with clinically isolated syndrome of optic neuritis, transverse myelitis, or a brainstem syndrome and were subsequently followed for 10 years, O'Riordan et al. (1998) showed that the presence of an abnormal MRI (two or more T2 lesions) at presentation predicted a transition to clinically definite MS (CDMS) in 83% of patients. The number of T2 lesions at presentation was not associated with a greater risk of eventual development of clinically definite MS if there were two or more lesions. However, greater numbers of lesions at baseline predicted an earlier conversion to CDMS and a higher EDSS score at 5 and 10 years. In the group with a normal MRI at the time of clinically isolated event, 11% were eventually diagnosed with CDMS, suggesting that a negative MRI at

symptom onset does not completely rule out a subsequent diagnosis of CDMS.

Final results of the Optic Neuritis Treatment Trial, in which 389 patients who presented with isolated optic neuritis were followed prospectively, revealed that the cumulative risk of developing MS was 50% in the subsequent 15 years. However, if MR imaging was abnormal at presentation, the risk was 72%, while those with normal imaging had a 25% risk. Even a single lesion at onset more than doubled the risk of developing CDMS to 60%, while those with three or more lesions at baseline had a 78% risk of conversion to CDMS (Beck et al., 2008).

Studies have compared the relative sensitivity and specificity of the presence of MR lesions at the time of an initial clinical event in predicting the conversion to clinically definite MS within a relatively short time period of 2 years. Barkhof assessed a variety of MRI findings associated with MS, including the size, location, number, and presence of Gd+ lesions in a group 74 patients who presented with clinically isolated syndromes suggestive of MS. Using a logistic regression analysis, the strongest predictors of subsequent conversion to CDMS were in descending order: Gd+ lesions, juxtacortical lesions, infratentorial lesions, and periventricular lesions. Compared to previously reported criteria, Barkhof found that these criteria predicted conversion to CDMS with an accuracy of 80%. Paty's criteria (Paty et al., 1994), which requires four lesions or only three if one is periventricular, and Fazekas' criteria (Fazekas et al., 1998), which requires three lesions (including two with the following characteristics: infratentorial location, periventricular location, size >6 mm), both had an accuracy of 69% in predicting conversion to CDMS. A subsequent prospective study by Tintore also found that the Barkhof criteria had better specificity and accuracy in predicting the development of CDMS compared to the Paty and Fazekas criteria (Tintore et al., 2000). As described later, the Barkhof criteria, as modified by Tintore, is used in the McDonald criteria to fulfill the requirement for dissemination in space.

Nonspecific Complaints

In clinical practice, it is not uncommon for patients to present with a variety of vague and nonspecific neurologic complaints that do not fit classic CIS syndromes of optic neuritis, transverse myelitis, or a brainstem syndrome. In these cases, a normal MRI scan can be reassuring in decreasing the likelihood of a diagnosis of MS. Conversely, given the high incidence of nonspecific white matter lesions that can be detected in the general population, routine MRI scans can frequently lead to consultation requests to "rule out MS." In these cases it is important to carefully review the actual MRI scans and not rely on the radiologist's report. As described previously, careful evaluation of MRI data shows that abnormalities that are most likely to represent MS have certain characteristics that can differentiate them from other disease processes. Obtaining additional scans such as postcontrast and/or spinal cord imaging can also increase the diagnostic specificity of suspected demyelinating lesions. Finally, other paraclinical tests such as spinal fluid evaluation and evoked potential testing should be considered if the presentation or examination is questionable (Miller et al., 2008).

Multiple Sclerosis Variants

Relapsing-remitting MS (RRMS) is the initial diagnosis in 85% of MS cases. The other categories include primary progressive MS (10%) and progressive relapsing (5%). These forms of MS are defined clinically, but MR features can differ between these categories. For example, primary progressive MS is frequently associated with smaller numbers and volumes of T2 lesions and Gd+ lesions, more spinal cord atrophy, and diffuse rather than focal white matter abnormalities as compared to RRMS (Miller and Leary, 2007).

In addition there are several MS variants with distinct MRI features. Acute disseminated encephalomyletis (ADEM) is a monophasic illness that can be confused with the first attack of MS. It is more frequent in children after a viral illness or vaccination, and encephalopathy is common. Classic MRI findings are large, multifocal white matter lesions, with many or all showing Gd+ enhancement, although this is not a constant finding and in some cases it is difficult to differentiate ADEM from classic RRMS (Wingerchuk, 2006). Other rare forms of MS include Marburg disease or acute MS in which rapidly progressive, massive demyelination frequently leads to death

and MRI shows evidence of severe, confluent white matter involvement (Mendez and Pogacar, 1988). Schilder disease and Balo concentric sclerosis have also been described as separate MS entities, supported in part by findings on neuropathology (Stadelmann and Bruck, 2004) as well as imaging (Poser et al., 1992; Canellas et al., 2007; Simon and Kleinschmidt-DeMasters, 2008).

Neuromyelitis optica (NMO), also known as Devic's disease, is a devastating MS variant associated with a clinical presentation of severe optic neuritis, frequently affecting both eyes in turn, and/or an aggressive transverse myelitis involving multiple spinal levels with significant edema and enhancement. Recently, the presence of a novel antibody (NMO Ab) that binds to the Aquaporin 4 receptor found on water channels in CNS has been associated with the clinical syndrome of NMO (Wingerchuk et al., 2007). The identification of a specific biomarker for NMO has furthered our understanding of the clinical variability of this form of MS. The presence of typical white matter brain lesions does not preclude the diagnosis of NMO, and it is now clear that high signal seen on FLAIR imaging in the region of the fourth ventricle and hypothalamus are also common findings (Pittock et al., 2006). Testing for the NMO variant should be done if there is any clinical suspicion, as this variant does not respond to the typical DMAs available for RRMS and more aggressive inmmunosuppression is indicated (Cree, 2008).

Tumefactive MS can present as a single, large, Gd-enhancing lesion, sometimes confused with glioma, resulting in unnecessary biopsy (Enzinger et al., 2005; Smith et al., 2008). Initial published cohort studies suggest that tumefactive cases represented a clinically unique syndrome that was frequently monophasic (Kepes, 1993), but subsequent studies suggest that many individuals that present with tumefactive MS will show subsequent disease activity and MRI activity consistent with RRMS (Lucchinetti et al., 2008).

Multiple Sclerosis Mimics

There is a long list of potential mimics of MS, and many can present with nonspecific white matter or other MRI changes. Two recent review articles have addressed this issue (Charil et al., 2006;

Miller et al., 2008). In a consensus approach, Miller et al. (2008) identified a number of clinical and MRI red flags that should lead to consideration of alternate diagnoses in individuals presenting with syndromes suspicious for MS. Charil et al. (2006) reviewed commonly seen MR abnormalities that are sometimes confused with MS. Table 7-1 lists the major MRI variables and associated disorders.

Radiologically Isolated Syndrome

Finally, it should be reiterated that an abnormal scan, even one that fulfills dissemination in space by McDonald criteria, in the absence of a clinical event or exam abnormality, is not sufficient to make the diagnosis of MS. This radiologically isolated syndrome (RIS) (Okuda et al., 2009) or preclinical MS (Lebrun et al., 2008) is increasingly recognized, especially as routine MRI studies become more common. Serial studies of individuals with RIS suggest that at least a third will develop a clinical attack and the majority will show evidence of radiological progression in a relatively short period of time (Lebrun et al., 2008; Okuda et al., 2009). Current practice is to monitor these individuals closely, but to begin treatment only if there is clinical activity.

DEVELOPMENT OF SPECIFIC MAGNETIC RESONANCE IMAGING CRITERIA FOR MULTIPLE SCLEROSIS DIAGNOSIS

Dissemination in Space

Recognizing the high incidence of nonspecific white matter changes on MRI that could result in errors in diagnosis, along with the emotional, financial, and insurance implications of a diagnosis of MS, there has been an effort to develop more formal criteria in evaluating abnormalities on MRI that are suggestive of MS. Several MRI criteria were developed to better specify lesion characteristics most consistent with demyelinating lesions seen in MS. After testing several of these criteria, it was found that the Barkof criteria had the best sensitivity and specificity (Tintore et al., 2000) (see Table 7-2) and were subsequently incorporated into the McDonald (McDonald et al.,

2001) criteria to fulfill "dissemination in space" by MRI.

In the initial publication, dissemination in space can be satisfied if a single scan meets three of the four Barkhof criteria (McDonald et al., 2001). Note that the presence of a lesion showing enhancement after the administration of gadolinium is equivalent to the presence of nine T2 lesions, an indication of the high specificity associated with the presence of gadolinium enhancement in identifying demyelinating lesions associated with MS. Subsequent modifications to the McDonald criteria have focused on simplifying and streamlining these criteria (Polman et al., 2005; Swanton et al., 2006). The modifications in 2005 allowed for spinal cord lesions to count as an infratentorial lesion, contribute to the overall total of T2 lesions, and if enhancing, substitute for the brain-enhancing lesion (Polman et al., 2005).

Dissemination in Time

Perhaps the most important advance resulting from the McDonald criteria is the ability to demonstrate dissemination in time with MRI changes rather than clinical events. This has undoubtedly led to earlier diagnosis and earlier treatment (Dalton et al., 2002b). Evidence of disease progression on MRI is a strong patient motivator for otherwise reluctant patients to begin treatment. As initially described, the criteria to fulfill dissemination in time are complex. In order to avoid counting lesions that developed around the time of the initial clinical event, a baseline MRI was required at least 30 days after symptom onset. Dissemination in time could then be fulfilled if a subsequent MRI 3 months later showed a gadolinium-enhancing lesion. If no Gd+ lesion was seen, another MRI done at least 3 months later that demonstrated a Gd+ or new T2 lesion was required. Since its publication in 2001, the McDonald criteria have undergone several modifications, all intended to simplify the application of the criteria to real-life clinical practice. The first modification in 2005 allowed for the detection of either a Gd+ lesion or a new T2 lesion to satisfy dissemination in time (Polman et al., 2005). See Table 7-3 for a review of these changes.

Further modifications recently described allow for a single follow-up scan to satisfy dissemination

TABLE 7-1 MRI Findings Suggestive of a Non-Multiple Sclerosis Diagnosis

MRI "Red Flag"	Alternative Diagnoses
White Matter	
Hemorrhages/microhemorrhages	Amyloid angiopathy; moya moya disease; CADASIL; vasculitis
Selective anterior and temporal lobe involvement	CADASIL
Persistent gadolinium enhancement	Lymphoma; glioma; vasculitis; sarcoidosis
Simultaneous enhancement of all lesions	Vasculitis; lymphoma; sarcoidosis; ADEM
Lacunar infarcts	Hypertensive ischemic disease; CADASIL; Susac syndrome
Complete ring enhancement	Brain abscess; glioblastoma; metastatic cancer
Diffuse white matter involvement	Behcet disease; HIV; small vessel disease; CADASIL
Large lesions starting in juxtacortical location with progressive enlargement	Progressive multifocal leukoencephalopathy
Lesions in the temporal pole, U-fibers, external capsule, insula	CADASIL
Extensive and bilateral periventricular abnormalities in isolation	B12 deficiency; acquired copper deficiency
Gray Matter	
Cortical Infarcts	Embolic disease; thrombotic thrombocytopenic purpura; vasculitis
T2-hyperintensity in the dentate nucleus	Cerebrotendinous xanthomatosis
T1-hyperintensity of the pulvinar	Fabry disease; hepatic encephalopathy; manganese toxicity
Large, infiltrating brainstem lesions	Behcet disease; pontine glioma
Predominance of lesions at cortical/subcortical junction	Embolic infarction; vasculitis; progressive multifocal leukoencephalopathy
Multiple discrete lesions of the basal ganglia and thalamus	Susac syndrome
Spinal Cord	
Large lesions with mass effect	NMO; ADEM; acute transverse myelitis; Sjogren syndrome
Diffuse abnormalities in the posterior columns	Vitamin B12 deficiency; acquired copper deficiency
Other	
Cerebral venous sinus thrombosis	Behcet disease; vasculitis; chronic meningitis; hypercoagulable state
Meningeal enhancement	Chronic meningitis; sarcoidosis; lymphomatosis; Primary angiitis of the CNS; Lyme disease
Calcifications on CT scans	Neurocysticercosis; toxoplasmosis; mitochondrial disorders
Hydrocephalus	Sarcoidosis
Dilation of Virchow-Robin spaces	Hyperhomocysteinemia; Primary angiitis of the CNS
Regional atrophy of the brain stem	Behcet disease; adult-onset Alexander disease

ADEM, acute disseminated encephalomyletis; CNS, central nervous system; CT, computed tomography; NMO, neuromyelitis optica.

Source: Adapted from Charil et al., 2006 and Miller et al., 2008.

TABLE 7-2 Magnetic Resonance Imaging Criteria for Dissemination in Space

At least three out of four of the following:

1. One gadolinium-enhancing lesion or nine T2 hyperintense lesions if no gadolinium-enhancing lesion is present

2. At least one infratentorial lesion

3. At least one juxtacortical lesion

4. At least three periventricular lesions

Source: From Tintore et al., 2000.

in time (Swanton et al., 2006). And a recent study found that a single MRI with both enhancing and nonenhancing white matter lesions characteristic of MS accurately predicted conversion to CDMS, suggesting that one MRI scan might be sufficient to satisfy dissemination in time *and* space (Rovira et al., 2009). In all cases, of course, there must be the presence of a clinical episode, consistent with a demyelinating process, such as optic neuritis or partial transverse myelitis, and careful consideration of other diagnostic entities.

Guidelines for Magnetic Resonance Imaging Scans to Assess Multiple Sclerosis

Interpreting serially acquired scans to establish the diagnosis of MS or to look for evidence of disease progression can be complicated by several technical issues, touched on previously. Serial scans are rarely performed using the same scanner, slice orientation, or even slice thickness. Because the appearance of a new area of signal abnormality is key to fulfilling dissemination in time, it is

TABLE 7-3 Modifications of Magnetic Resonance Imaging Criteria for Dissemination in Time

Original McDonald Criterion	*2005 Revision*
1. If a first scan occurs 3 months or more after the onset of the clinical event, the presence of a gadolinium-enhancing lesion is sufficient to demonstrate dissemination in time, provided that it is not at the site implicated in the original clinical event. If there is no enhancing lesion at this time, a follow-up scan is required. The timing of this follow-up scan is not crucial, but 3 months is recommended. A new T2- or gadolinium-enhancing lesion at this time then fulfills the criterion for dissemination in time.	1. There are two ways to show dissemination in time using imaging: a. Detection of gadolinium enhancement at least 3 months after the onset of the initial clinical event, if not at the site corresponding to the initial event b. Detection of a *new* T2 lesion if it appears at any time compared with a reference scan done at least 30 days after the onset of the initial clinical event
2. If the first scan is performed less than 3 months after the onset of the clinical event, a second scan done 3 months or longer after the clinical event showing a new gadolinium-enhancing lesion provides sufficient evidence for dissemination in time. However, if no enhancing lesion is seen at this second scan, a further scan not less than 3 months after the first scan that shows a new T2 lesion or an enhancing lesion will suffice.	

important that serial scans are done using the same orientation, with relatively thin slices (3 mm) and no "gap" between slices. In the past, a radiology requisition with the clinical information "rule out MS" would result in the application of the "tumor protocol," a series of 5 mm slices with 2.5 mm gaps aimed at ruling out a large brain mass. Radiology practices have certainly advanced, but they are not uniform across centers. In recognition of the importance of properly collected MRI data, and the lack of commonly accepted guidelines, the Consortium of MS Centers (CMSC), in collaboration with neuroradiologists and MS researchers and clinicians, has developed guidelines for MRI acquisition at the time of MS diagnosis and follow-up. These are available in published form (Simon et al., 2006) and on their Web site (http://www.mscare.org/cmsc/images/pdf/MRIprotocol2003.pdf). Included are protocols for the initial evaluation and subsequent follow-up studies of patients with MS. Key features include archiving initial studies and the collection of 3 mm, nongapped slices obtained at the same orientation. See Table 7-4 for details.

ROLE OF MAGNETIC RESONANCE IMAGING IN DISEASE MONITORING

Prognosis

Findings on initial imaging studies are only of modest help in providing reliable prognostic information regarding disease progression. In general, higher numbers and volumes of T2 lesions, and especially the presence of gadolinium-enhancing lesions, at the time of the first demyelinating event are associated with a more rapid progression to clinically definite MS (O'Riordan et al., 1998; Gauthier et al., 2007; Rocca et al., 2008). Recently published long-term studies have shown that CIS patients who demonstrated the greatest amount of T2 lesion volume accumulation, especially during the 5 years after diagnosis, were much more likely to develop progressive disability after 20 years (Fisniku et al., 2008a), suggesting that in the early stages of RRMS, T2 lesion accumulation may be an important marker of future disability. However, in later disease stages, absolute T2 volumes may plateau,

in part due to ongoing brain atrophy (Tintore et al., 2000). At these later stages of disease, ongoing neurodegenerative changes as reflected by increasing global and gray matter atrophy may be more relevant MRI markers to monitor (Horakova et al., 2009).

Monitor Treatment Response

There is wide variability in the use of serial MRIs to monitor response to therapy among MS clinicians, due in part to the lack of validated imaging metrics that can be followed. A reasonable approach is to obtain a new set of baseline scans at the time of treatment initiation or a change to a new therapy. Determining a "suboptimal" response is a primarily a clinical assessment with imaging serving a potentially confirmatory role. Keeping in mind that all of the currently approved DMAs have been shown to decrease the rate of lesion accumulation on MRI and relapse rates tend to decrease over time without therapy, a sudden increase in relapse rate or substantial worsening of disease burden should prompt a reappraisal of the therapeutic approach (Cohen et al., 2004).

Monitoring Disease Progression

Conventional measures alone have only modest association with subsequent disease progression, but composite MRI measures may be more informative (Mainero et al., 2001; Wolinsky et al., 2001). Bakshi et al. recently described an MS disease severity scale that utilized baseline T2 volumes, the ratio of T1 black holes to T2 lesion volumes, and brain parenchymal fraction to yield a disease severity scale from 0 to 10 that was associated with disease progression over the subsequent 3 years and was able to distinguish relapsing remitting from secondary progressive MS (Bakshi et al., 2008). A large cross-sectional study of MS patients examined multiple MRI parameters, including lesion volumes and numbers and brain volumes and found that gray matter atrophy was the best predictor of disability (Tedeschi et al., 2005). Recently published longitudinal studies have also identified gray matter atrophy as the key driver of overall brain atrophy and disability progression (Fisher et al., 2008; Fisniku et al., 2008b).

TABLE 7-4 Consortium of Multiple Sclerosis Centers (CMSC) Magnetic Resonance Imaging (MRI) Guidelines

I. Clinical Guidelines for Brain and Spinal Cord MRI in MS

Clinically Isolated Syndrome (CIS) and Suspected MS
Baseline evaluation:
- Brain MRI with gadolinium recommended
- Spinal cord MRI if brain MRI is nondiagnostic
- Spinal cord MRI if presenting symptoms or signs are at the level of the spinal cord

Follow-up evaluation:
- Brain MRI with gadolinium recommended to demonstrate new disease activity

Established MS Indications
Baseline evaluation:
- Brain MRI with gadolinium recommended

Follow-up of MS:
- To evaluate an unexpected clinical worsening concerning for a secondary diagnosis.
- For the re-assessment of the original diagnosis.
- For the re-assessment before starting or modifying therapy.
- To assess subclinical disease activity should be *considered* every 1–2 years. The exact frequency may vary depending on clinical course and other clinical features.

II. MRI Protocols for Brain and Spinal Cord

Slice Thickness: ≤3 mm and no gap and in plane resolution of ≤1 mm × 1 mm for both Brain and spinal cord. (Note: ≤5 mm and no gap is acceptable for brain MRI for centers that are unable to acquire 3 mm slices in the allotted time).

Scan Orientation and Coverage
Reproducible coverage and orientation for the axial slices using the subcallosal line as a reference on an appropriate sagittal localizer is critical for longitudinal comparisons.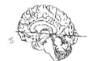

Minimum Required Brain MRI Sequences (diagnostic, baseline, and follow-up studies)
1st: Sagittal FLAIR (fluid attenuating inversion recovery).
2nd: Axial T2 weighted (axial PD optional)
3rd: Axial FLAIR
4th: Axial pre- and post-gadolinium-enhanced T1-weighted (gadolinium optional if no T2 lesions)

Cervical Cord Sequences
1st: Sagittal T2/Proton Density or STIR
2nd: Sagittal pre-Gad T1
3rd: Axial T2
4th: Sagittal post-Gad T1 (optional)
5th: Axial post-Gad T1 (optional).Slice thickness ≤3 mm (sagittal) or ≤4mm (axial), no gap. In plane resolution ≤1 mm × 1 mm

OTHER IMAGING MODALITIES

Advancements in MRI technology have led to the development of several novel techniques, many of which are not used routinely for clinical purposes but have been studied extensively in research settings. Given the limitations of conventional techniques to fully capture the extent of disease burden in MS, these new approaches may provide better, more sensitive measures of inflammatory and degenerative changes. Magnetic resonance techniques are continually evolving and applications are limited only by the imagination and perhaps hardware capabilities. A few of the techniques most commonly used in the study of MS are reviewed briefly in the next section.

Nonconventional Magnetic Resonance Imaging Techniques

Magnetization transfer imaging

Magnetization transfer imaging (MTI) exploits a principle that protons bound to macromolecules (like myelin) behave differently than protons that are freely moving. An extra rf pulse is applied that is preferentially absorbed by bound protons. These protons will then "transfer" the absorbed rf energy to nearby tissues, leading to a decrease in the MR signal. A second set of images is collected without the MT pulse and a ratio image is then created. The magnetization transfer ratio (MTR) image is calculated using the formula:

$$MTR = \frac{Mo - Ms}{Mo} \times 100$$

Mo = signal without MT pulse

Ms = signal with MT pulse

In areas with intact myelin, Ms will be smaller (greater signal loss due to the transfer of energy from bound protons) and therefore will have a larger MTR value. Whereas in areas that are devoid of intact structural elements, Ms will not decrease as much, resulting in a lower MTR value. The values from the MTR image can be quantified using a histogram approach to identify a variety of parameters, including peak height, mean MTR, and so on (Horsfield, 2005). These quantitative approaches have shown that both lesion areas and NAWM regions show decreases in MTR compared to healthy controls (Traboulsee et al., 2003). Gray matter regions also show decreased MTR (Ge et al., 2001; Sharma et al., 2006). Histopathology suggests that MTR measures are closely related to myelin content in the brain (Brochet and Dousset, 1999; Schmierer et al., 2004) and spinal cord (Mottershead et al., 2003). In some studies, low MTR measures at baseline predicted future disease progression better than conventional MR markers (Filippi et al., 2000b; Fernando et al., 2005; De Stefano et al., 2006). To date, MTI has not been used as an outcome measure in clinical trials in part due to technical constraints that limit the comparison of data obtained across multiple sites. However, recent approaches suggest that these limitations may not be insurmountable (Dwyer et al., 2009).

Diffusion tensor imaging

Diffusion tensor imaging (DTI) is an application of diffusion-weighted imaging (used routinely for stroke imaging) in which images are collected after the application of diffusion gradients in multiple directions (at least six) in order to calculate the tensor, a mathematical construct that specifies direction and magnitude (Pierpaoli et al., 1996). This technique exploits the physiological principle that more diffusion will occur in the direction of the axon, and less will occur across intact myelin. Color-coded maps created from these data make it possible to identify specific white matter tracts on the basis of their location and projection pathways as seen in Fig. 7-3. Diffusion tensor imaging data also yield specific diffusion parameters that quantify the directional specific flow; these include mean diffusivity (MD), an average of overall diffusion, and fractional anisotropy (fA), a dimensionless number that reflects the degree of anisotropy or preferential flow (Pierpaoli and Basser, 1996). Values of fA can range from 0 (purely isotropic or nonpreferential flow) to 1 (anistropic flow in a single direction). In practice, highly oriented white matter bundles such as the corpus callosum can have fA values over 0.6, while gray matter areas are lower at 0.3–0.4, for example. The application of DTI to the study of MS has revealed diffuse abnormalities along white matter pathways distal to T2 lesion areas as reflected by decreased fA and increased diffusion parameters (Roosendaal et al., 2009). Increases in radial diffusivity (perpendicular to the axon) are detectable early and may be a more specific measure of demyelination (Song et al., 2005), while changes in axial diffusivity (parallel to the axon) may reflect axonal loss (Budde et al., 2009). Finally, this approach allows for the identification and monitoring of specific pathways within the brain (Salamon et al., 2005, 2007) and may be useful in monitoring disease progression and the effects of neuroprotective therapies (Fox, 2008).

Spectroscopy

Proton magnetic resonance spectroscopy (1H-MRS) is another MR imaging approach that has been applied to the study of MS. Rather than image the protons associated with fat and water,

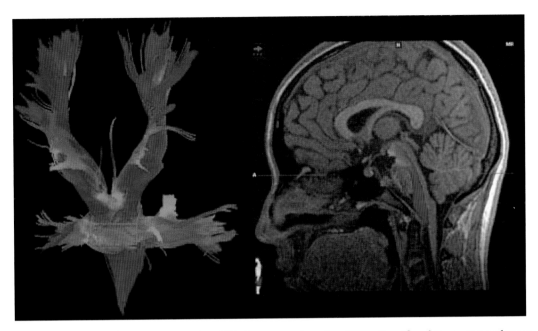

Figure 7-3 Example of tract tracing using diffusion tensor imaging (DTI). Specific white matter pathways traveling through the brain stem can be identified and tracked as seen on the left image. Image on the right shows sagittal T1-weighted image with overlaid color-coded DTI. Color coding is based on the fiber direction with blue indicating rostral-caudal; green, anterior posterior; red, right to left.

this technique is used to obtain an NMR spectrum of metabolites present within nervous system tissue. The concentrations of these metabolites are orders of magnitude lower than fat and water; therefore, in order to obtain interpretable spectra, signals from water and fat must be suppressed. In addition, because the signal is small, the technique is limited in resolution, with typical imaging protocols producing voxel sizes of 1 cm³. Metabolites of interest include N-acetylaspartate (NAA), choline, creatine, inositol, and glutamine (Sajja et al., 2009). The use of higher field strengths (3.0T and above) has resulted in better defined spectra; for example, Pelletier and colleagues have been able to identify a separate peak for glutamate at 3.0T using advanced techniques (Srinivasan et al., 2005). NAA is localized within neurons and has been most extensively studied as a marker of neuronal integrity (Rigotti et al., 2007). Many studies have shown that NAA concentrations are decreased in both the white and gray matter of MS patients and may offer prognostic information for future disability (Chard et al., 2002). Interestingly, some groups suggest

that NAA levels may reflect *functional* integrity of axons, in part because serial studies have shown dramatic recovery of NAA levels in lesion areas over time as inflammation resolves and axonal transport resumes in intact axons (De Stefano et al., 1997; Narayanan et al., 2001). Part of the recovery could also be due to a relative increase in NAA concentration with decreased edema.

Absolute quantification of metabolite concentrations requires sophisticated pre- and postscanning processing, and these challenges have limited the use of MRS across sites as an outcome measure in clinical trials. However, the European MRI consortium recently published guidelines for the use of MRS in multicenter trials of MS, suggesting that this will be possible in the near future (De Stefano et al., 2007).

Functional magnetic resonance imaging

Functional MRI (fMRI) is possible because the rate of MR signal decay, or T2*, is slightly faster for deoxygenated hemoglobin than for oxygenated hemoglobin. Functional MRI (fMRI) uses imaging parameters that are optimized to detect these slight differences. When the brain is active, neuronal activity increases, metabolic demands increase, and blood flow increases, delivering increased amounts of oxygenated blood. This causes a relative decrease in deoxygenated hemoglobin concentrations, resulting in a slightly slower rate of signal loss, so that relative to the preactivation state, the MR signal detected is increased. This technique, known as blood oxygen level-dependent (BOLD) fMRI is used extensively in cognitive neuroscience applications and has been used to study MS (Filippi et al., 2002).

Functional imaging studies in MS have demonstrated aberrant activation patterns during both motor and cognitive tasks when compared to healthy controls (Reddy et al., 2002; Mainero et al., 2004). Differences detected include more extensive areas of activation and the engagement of the opposite hemisphere. These patterns have also been seen in other neurological conditions, including stroke and early Alzheimer disease, and have been characterized as evidence of "compensation" for ongoing tissue damage (Bookheimer et al., 2000; Cramer and Bastings, 2000). Other possibilities include the loss of inhibitory input that could lead to the "uncovering" of previously nonactivated regions (Lenzi et al., 2007), but other evidence supports the idea that the brain can engage new areas in order to maintain performance (Staffen et al., 2002). This ability may contribute to the "MRI-disability" paradox by limiting clinical manifestations of ongoing disease activity.

Emerging nonconventional techniques

There are several promising MR-based techniques that are being applied to the study of MS and hold promise as potentially more sensitive markers to tissue-specific disease manifestations. These include quantitative measures of T_1 and T_2 relaxation (Deoni et al., 2008) that may be useful in detecting the early changes in myelin (Laule et al., 2008), perfusion measures using arterial spin labeling techniques (Inglese et al., 2008), and ultrahigh field imaging to visualize cortical plaques (Mainero et al., 2009), susceptibility weighted imaging to detected iron deposition (Haacke et al., 2009), and multimodal techniques that monitor the relationship between structural and functional

changes (Kern et al., 2009). Look for these and other, yet-to-be-developed techniques to be applied to the study of disease progression and treatment effects in persons with MS in the future.

LIMITATIONS OF STANDARD TECHNIQUES

Missed Lesions

As mentioned previously, the addition of FLAIR imaging to standard clinical MRI studies led to the recognition of large numbers of cortical and juxtacortical lesions that were previously missed on PD/T2 scans (Bakshi et al., 2001). Newer approaches, including double inversion recovery (DIR) and ultrahigh field imaging are even better at revealing these areas of abnormal cortex (Bagnato et al., 2006; Calabrese et al., 2008). However, detailed neuropathological correlations show that even these techniques miss a majority of the demyelinating lesions that are present in cortical regions (Geurts et al., 2005; Stadelmann et al., 2008).

Normal-Appearing White Matter Is Not Normal

The normal-appearing white matter (NAWM) shows abnormalities on pathological examination, including severe axonal loss (Evangelou et al., 2000), ubiquitination of axons (Bo et al., 2003), and the presence of activated microglia (Allen et al., 2001; Giordana et al., 2002). Nonconventional imaging approaches using magnetization transfer imaging, spectroscopy, and diffusion-weighted imaging have detected abnormalities in the NAWM (Narayanan et al., 1997; Richert et al., 1998; Gonen et al., 2000, 2002; Tortorella et al., 2000), including decreases in the magnetization transfer ratio (MTR), lower levels of NAA, and increased diffusion indicating that axonal damage extends along the white matter pathways distant from the site of the demyelinating plaque (Gasperini et al., 1996; De Stefano et al., 1999; Filippi et al., 2000a; Simon et al., 2000; Allen et al., 2001; Bjartmar et al., 2001; Giordana et al., 2002). Furthermore, the degree of change in the NAWM as determined by magnetization transfer imaging was a strong predictor of future clinical progression (Santos et al., 2002).

Gray Matter Involvement

Only recently have studies focused on gray matter involvement in MS (Catalaa et al., 1999; Peterson et al., 2001; Bo et al., 2003). Pathological findings have shown large areas of demyelination in the cortical rim, hippocampus, and thalamus (Peterson et al., 2001; Cifelli et al., 2002; Geurts et al., 2005; Kutzelnigg and Lassmann, 2005; Geurts et al., 2007). In addition, there is evidence of neuronal death with the presence of activated microglia-engulfing neurons (Bo et al., 2003). Volumetric MRI measures reveal that the cortical ribbon is atrophied, and there is some preliminary evidence that this cortical atrophy may follow a specific pattern as the disease progresses (De Stefano et al., 2003). A sophisticated analysis reveals focal atrophy of the frontal and temporal cortices early in the course of MS with eventual involvement of the primary motor cortex as the disease progresses, as measured by the EDSS and by the time from diagnosis (Sailer et al., 2003). In addition to the cortical gray matter, there is ample evidence that the deep gray matter structures are abnormal in MS patients with tissue loss demonstrated by volumetric MRI analysis and increased diffusion as measured by diffusion-weighted imaging in the hippocampus, thalamus, and basal ganglia (Cifelli et al., 2002; Wylezinska et al., 2003; Sicotte et al., 2008). There is evidence that gray matter atrophy occurs early in the course of MS and precedes white matter volume changes (Dalton et al., 2004).

Functional Compensation

Conventional imaging approaches provide only structural information about the brain, but fMRI studies have demonstrated significant changes in cortical activation patterns in MS patients even at the earliest stages of the disease (Pantano et al., 2002; Rocca et al., 2003c). Early on, when behavioral measures are still normal, the brain may compensate for subtle, diffuse, pathological processes by increasing the magnitude and extent of functional activity (Rocca et al., 2003b; Filippi et al., 2004), and this may contribute to the poor correlation of conventional measures with overt disability. In cases of acute loss of function such a MS relapse, compensatory activity in "latent" pathways may become evident. In the case of

motor function, this usually involves the ipsilateral sensorimotor cortex (SMC) (Lee et al., 2000; Reddy et al., 2000a; Pantano et al., 2002) perhaps utilizing the uncrossed motor fibers that make up 10% of the corticospinal tracts. In a serial study of recovery after a relapse, Reddy showed that as hand function recovered, activity shifted from the ipsilateral SMC to the more normal contralateral > ipsilateral SMC pattern (Reddy et al., 2000a). The degree to which activity patterns differ from normal has also been correlated with global measures of tissue loss such as decreased NAA or MTR histogram values (Reddy et al., 2000b; Rocca et al., 2003a). Taken together, the results seen to date suggest that the brain shows functional adaptation early in the course of MS and that the pattern of changes may progress from a strategy of initially enlisting more local tissue, to the "uncovering" of latent pathways such as uncrossed corticospinal tracts.

CONCLUDING REMARKS

As discussed earlier, information gleaned from standard MRI sequences obtained in routine clinical practice can yield important information supporting the diagnosis of MS, but they have limited value in predicting future disability, response to therapy, and for monitoring disease progression. Cross-sectional studies show that T2 volumes are only modestly correlated with disability measures. This MRI-clinical paradox has been discussed extensively in the literature. Areas of high signal detectable on T2-weighted images lack pathological specificity, representing anything from reversible edema to permanent axonal loss. Standard scans are not sensitive to cortical demyelination, and these lesions seem more likely to have a significant clinical impact. The brain's ability to compensate functionally for ongoing damage will limit the ability to measure a direct imaging/disability connection, especially in cross-sectional studies. Findings on spinal cord imaging are only rarely included in these analyses, but studies show a better correlation of spinal cord atrophy with disability as measured by the EDSS, which preferentially reflects clinical changes in mobility. Finally, classic disability measures such as the EDSS are relatively insensitive to many important MS disease manifestations such as cognitive impairment. Recent studies show better MRI/disability correlations using elements of the MSFC (Rudick et al., 2008). Therefore, it is probably not surprising that nonspecific measures of tissue damage show only a modest correlation with insensitive measures of disability. In the future, newer, nonconventional techniques, obtained at higher field strengths will be increasing applied to the study of MS and the effectiveness of treatments for this complex disease.

REFERENCES

Allen IV, McQuaid S, Mirakhur M, Nevin G. Pathological abnormalities in the normal-appearing white matter in multiple sclerosis. *Neurol Sci*. 2001;22:141–144.

Bagnato F, Butman JA, Gupta S, et al. In vivo detection of cortical plaques by MR imaging in patients with multiple sclerosis. *AJNR Am J Neuroradiol*. 2006;27: 2161–2167.

Bagnato F, Gupta S, Richert ND, et al. Effects of interferon beta-1b on black holes in multiple sclerosis over a 6-year period with monthly evaluations. *Arch Neurol*. 2005;62:1684–1688.

Bagnato F, Jeffries N, Richert ND, et al. Evolution of T1 black holes in patients with multiple sclerosis imaged monthly for 4 years. *Brain*. 2003;126:1782–1789.

Bakshi R, Ariyaratana S, Benedict RH, Jacobs L. Fluid-attenuated inversion recovery magnetic resonance imaging detects cortical and juxtacortical multiple sclerosis lesions. *Arch Neurol*. 2001;58:742–748.

Bakshi R, Benedict RH, Bermel RA, et al. T2 hypointensity in the deep gray matter of patients with multiple sclerosis: a quantitative magnetic resonance imaging study. *Arch Neurol*. 2002;59:62–68.

Bakshi R, Neema M, Healy BC, et al. Predicting clinical progression in multiple sclerosis with the magnetic resonance disease severity scale. *Arch Neurol*. 2008; 65:1449–1453.

Bastianello S, Bozzao A, Paolillo A, et al. Fast spin-echo and fast fluid-attenuated inversion-recovery versus conventional spin-echo sequences for MR quantification of multiple sclerosis lesions. *AJNR Am J Neuroradiol*. 1997;18:699–704.

Bermel RA, Bakshi R, Tjoa C, Puli SR, Jacobs L. Bicaudate ratio as a magnetic resonance imaging marker of brain atrophy in multiple sclerosis. *Arch Neurol*. 2002; 59:275–280.

Bitsch A, Kuhlmann T, Stadelmann C, Lassmann H, Lucchinetti C, Bruck W. A longitudinal MRI study of histopathologically defined hypointense multiple sclerosis lesions. *Ann Neurol*. 2001;49:793–796.

Bjartmar C, Kinkel RP, Kidd G, Rudick RA, Trapp BD. Axonal loss in normal-appearing white matter in a patient with acute MS. *Neurology*. 2001;57:1248–1252.

Bo L, Vedeler CA, Nyland HI, Trapp BD, Mork SJ. Subpial demyelination in the cerebral cortex of multiple sclerosis patients. *J Neuropathol Exp Neurol*. 2003; 62:723–732.

Bookheimer SY, Strojwas MH, Cohen MS, et al. Patterns of brain activation in people at risk for Alzheimer's disease. *N Engl J Med*. 2000;343:450–456.

Bot JC, Barkhof F, Polman CH, et al. Spinal cord abnormalities in recently diagnosed MS patients: added value of spinal MRI examination. *Neurology*. 2004;62: 226–233.

Brass SD, Chen NK, Mulkern RV, Bakshi R. Magnetic resonance imaging of iron deposition in neurological disorders. *Top Magn Reson Imaging*. 2006;17:31–40.

Brex PA, Jenkins R, Fox NC, et al. Detection of ventricular enlargement in patients at the earliest clinical stage of MS. *Neurology*. 2000;54:1689–1691.

Brochet B, Dousset V. Pathological correlates of magnetization transfer imaging abnormalities in animal models and humans with multiple sclerosis. *Neurology*. 1999; 53:S12–S17.

Broome DR. Nephrogenic systemic fibrosis associated with gadolinium based contrast agents: a summary of the medical literature reporting. *Eur J Radiol*. 2008; 66:230–234.

Budde MD, Xie M, Cross AH, Song SK. Axial diffusivity is the primary correlate of axonal injury in the experimental autoimmune encephalomyelitis spinal cord: a quantitative pixelwise analysis. *J Neurosci*. 2009; 29:2805–2813.

Butzkueven H, Kolbe SC, Jolley DJ, et al. Validation of linear cerebral atrophy markers in multiple sclerosis. *J Clin Neurosci*. 2008;15:130–137.

Calabrese M, Filippi M, Rovaris M, et al. Morphology and evolution of cortical lesions in multiple sclerosis. A longitudinal MRI study. *Neuroimage*. 2008;42: 1324–1328.

Canellas AR, Gols AR, Izquierdo JR, Subirana MT, Gairin XM. Idiopathic inflammatory-demyelinating diseases of the central nervous system. *Neuroradiology*. 2007; 49:393–409.

Catalaa I, Fulton JC, Zhang X, et al. MR imaging quantitation of gray matter involvement in multiple sclerosis and its correlation with disability measures and neurocognitive testing. *AJNR Am J Neuroradiol*. 1999;20: 1613–1618.

Chard DT, Griffin CM, McLean MA, et al. Brain metabolite changes in cortical grey and normal-appearing white matter in clinically early relapsing-remitting multiple sclerosis. *Brain*. 2002;125:2342–2352.

Charil A, Yousry TA, Rovaris M, et al. MRI and the diagnosis of multiple sclerosis: expanding the concept of "no better explanation". *Lancet Neurol*. 2006;5:841–852.

Cifelli A, Arridge M, Jezzard P, Esiri MM, Palace J, Matthews PM. Thalamic neurodegeneration in multiple sclerosis. *Ann Neurol*. 2002;52:650–653.

Cohen BA, Khan O, Jeffery DR, et al. Identifying and treating patients with suboptimal responses. *Neurology*. 2004;63:S33–S40.

Comi G, Filippi M. The effect of glatiramer acetate (Copaxone(R)) on disease activity as measured by cerebral MRI in patients with relapsing-remitting multiple sclerosis (RRMS): a multi-center, randomized, double-blind, placebo-controlled study extended by open-label treatment. *Neurology*. 1999;52:A289.

Cramer SC, Bastings EP. Mapping clinically relevant plasticity after stroke. *Neuropharmacology*. 2000;39: 842–851.

Cree B. Neuromyelitis optica: diagnosis, pathogenesis, and treatment. *Curr Neurol Neurosci Rep*. 2008;8: 427–433.

Dalton CM, Brex PA, Jenkins R, et al. Progressive ventricular enlargement in patients with clinically isolated syndromes is associated with the early development of multiple sclerosis. *J Neurol Neurosurg Psychiatry*. 2002a;73:141–147.

Dalton CM, Brex PA, Miszkiel KA, et al. Application of the new McDonald criteria to patients with clinically isolated syndromes suggestive of multiple sclerosis. *Ann Neurol*. 2002b;52:47–53.

Dalton CM, Chard DT, Davies GR, et al. Early development of multiple sclerosis is associated with progressive grey matter atrophy in patients presenting with clinically isolated syndromes. *Brain*. 2004;127:1101–1107.

DeLuca GC, Ebers GC, Esiri MM. Axonal loss in multiple sclerosis: a pathological survey of the corticospinal and sensory tracts. *Brain*. 2004;127:1009–1018.

Deoni SC, Rutt BK, Arun T, Pierpaoli C, Jones DK. Gleaning multicomponent T1 and T2 information from steady-state imaging data. *Magn Reson Med*. 2008;60:1372–1387.

De Stefano N, Battaglini M, Stromillo ML, et al. Brain damage as detected by magnetization transfer imaging is less pronounced in benign than in early relapsing multiple sclerosis. *Brain*. 2006;129:2008–2016.

De Stefano N, Filippi M, Miller D, et al. Guidelines for using proton MR spectroscopy in multicenter clinical MS studies. *Neurology*. 2007;69:1942–1952.

De Stefano N, Matthews PM, Filippi M, et al. Evidence of early cortical atrophy in MS: relevance to white matter changes and disability. *Neurology*. 2003;60:1157–1162.

De Stefano N, Matthews PM, Narayanan S, Francis GS, Antel JP, Arnold DL. Axonal dysfunction and disability in a relapse of multiple sclerosis: longitudinal study of a patient. *Neurology*. 1997;49:1138–1141.

De Stefano N, Narayanan S, Matthews PM, Francis GS, Antel JP, Arnold DL. In vivo evidence for axonal dysfunction remote from focal cerebral demyelination of the type seen in multiple sclerosis. *Brain*. 1999;122: 1933–1939.

Dwyer M, Bergsland N, Hussein S, Durfee J, Wack D, Zivadinov R. A sensitive, noise-resistant method for identifying focal demyelination and remyelination in patients with multiple sclerosis via voxel-wise changes in magnetization transfer ratio. *J Neurol Sci*. 2009; 282:86–95.

Enzinger C, Strasser-Fuchs S, Ropele S, Kapeller P, Kleinert R, Fazekas F. Tumefactive demyelinating lesions: conventional and advanced magnetic resonance imaging. *Mult Scler*. 2005;11:135–139.

Evangelou N, DeLuca GC, Owens T, Esiri MM. Pathological study of spinal cord atrophy in multiple sclerosis suggests limited role of local lesions. *Brain*. 2005;128: 29–34.

Evangelou N, Esiri MM, Smith S, Palace J, Matthews PM. Quantitative pathological evidence for axonal loss in normal appearing white matter in multiple sclerosis. *Ann Neurol*. 2000;47:391–395.

Fazekas F, Barkhof F, Filippi M. Unenhanced and enhanced magnetic resonance imaging in the diagnosis of multiple sclerosis. *J Neurol Neurosurg Psychiatry*. 1998:S2–S5.

Fernando KT, Tozer DJ, Miszkiel KA, et al. Magnetization transfer histograms in clinically isolated syndromes suggestive of multiple sclerosis. *Brain*. 2005;128: 2911–2925.

Filippi M. Magnetic resonance imaging findings predicting subsequent disease course in patients at presentation with clinically isolated syndromes suggestive of multiple sclerosis. *Neurol Sci*. 2001;22(suppl 2): S49–S51.

Filippi M, Bozzali M, Rovaris M, et al. Evidence for widespread axonal damage at the earliest clinical stage of multiple sclerosis. *Brain*. 2003;126:433–437.

Filippi M, Iannucci G, Cercignani M, Assunta RM, Pratesi A, Comi G. A quantitative study of water diffusion in multiple sclerosis lesions and normal-appearing white matter using echo-planar imaging. *Arch Neurol*. 2000a;57:1017–1021.

Filippi M, Inglese M, Rovaris M, et al. Magnetization transfer imaging to monitor the evolution of MS: a 1-year follow-up study. *Neurology*. 2000b;55:940–946.

Filippi M, Rocca MA, Colombo B, et al. Functional magnetic resonance imaging correlates of fatigue in multiple sclerosis. *NeuroImage*. 2002;15(3):559–567.

Filippi M, Rocca MA, Mezzapesa DM, et al. Simple and complex movement-associated functional MRI changes in patients at presentation with clinically isolated syndromes suggestive of multiple sclerosis. *Hum Brain Mapp*. 2004;21:108–117.

Filippi M, Rovaris M, Rocca MA, Sormani MP, Wolinsky JS, Comi G. Glatiramer acetate reduces the proportion of new MS lesions evolving into "black holes". *Neurology*. 2001;57:731–733.

Fisher E, Lee JC, Nakamura K, Rudick RA. Gray matter atrophy in multiple sclerosis: a longitudinal study. *Ann Neurol*. 2008;64:255–265.

Fisher E, Rudick RA, Simon JH, et al. Eight-year follow-up study of brain atrophy in patients with MS. *Neurology*. 2002;59:1412–1420.

Fisniku LK, Brex PA, Altmann DR, et al. Disability and T2 MRI lesions: a 20-year follow-up of patients with relapse onset of multiple sclerosis. *Brain*. 2008a; 131:808–817.

Fisniku LK, Chard DT, Jackson JS, et al. Gray matter atrophy is related to long-term disability in multiple sclerosis. *Ann Neurol*. 2008b;64:247–254.

Fox RJ. Picturing multiple sclerosis: conventional and diffusion tensor imaging. *Semin Neurol*. 2008;28: 453–466.

Ganter P, Prince C, Esiri MM. Spinal cord axonal loss in multiple sclerosis: a post-mortem study. *Neuropathol Appl Neurobiol*. 1999;25:459–467.

Gasperini C, Horsfield MA, Thorpe JW, et al. Macroscopic and microscopic assessments of disease burden by MRI in multiple sclerosis: relationship to clinical parameters. *J Magn Reson Imaging*. 1996;6:580–584.

Gauthier SA, Mandel M, Guttmann CR, et al. Predicting short-term disability in multiple sclerosis. *Neurology*. 2007;68:2059–2065.

Ge Y, Grossman RI, Udupa JK, et al. Brain atrophy in relapsing-remitting multiple sclerosis and secondary progressive multiple sclerosis: longitudinal quantitative analysis. *Radiology*. 2000;214:665–670.

Ge Y, Grossman RI, Udupa JK, Babb JS, Kolson DL, McGowan JC. Magnetization transfer ratio histogram analysis of gray matter in relapsing-remitting multiple sclerosis. *AJNR Am J Neuroradiol*. 2001;22:470–475.

Geurts JJ, Bo L, Pouwels PJ, Castelijns JA, Polman CH, Barkhof F. Cortical lesions in multiple sclerosis: combined postmortem MR imaging and histopathology. *AJNR Am J Neuroradiol*. 2005;26:572–577.

Geurts JJ, Bo L, Roosendaal SD, et al. Extensive hippocampal demyelination in multiple sclerosis. *J Neuropathol Exp Neurol*. 2007;66:819–827.

Giordana MT, Richiardi P, Trevisan E, Boghi A, Palmucci L. Abnormal ubiquitination of axons in normally myelinated white matter in multiple sclerosis brain. *Neuropathol Appl Neurobiol*. 2002;28:35–41.

Gonen O, Catalaa I, Babb JS, et al. Total brain N-acetylaspartate: a new measure of disease load in MS. *Neurology*. 2000;54:15–19.

Gonen O, Moriarty DM, Li BS, et al. Relapsing-remitting multiple sclerosis and whole-brain N-acetylaspartate measurement: evidence for different clinical cohorts initial observations. *Radiology*. 2002;225:261–268.

Haacke EM, Makki M, Ge Y, et al. Characterizing iron deposition in multiple sclerosis lesions using susceptibility weighted imaging. *J Magn Reson Imaging*. 2009; 29:537–544.

Hammond KE, Metcalf M, Carvajal L, et al. Quantitative in vivo magnetic resonance imaging of multiple sclerosis at 7 Tesla with sensitivity to iron. *Ann Neurol*. 2008;64:707–713.

Horakova D, Dwyer MG, Havrdova E, et al. Gray matter atrophy and disability progression in patients with early relapsing-remitting multiple sclerosis: a 5-year longitudinal study. *J Neurol Sci*. 2009;282:112–119.

Horsfield MA. Magnetization transfer imaging in multiple sclerosis. *J Neuroimaging*. 2005;15:58S–67S.

Houtchens MK, Benedict RH, Killiany R, et al. Thalamic atrophy and cognition in multiple sclerosis. *Neurology*. 2007;69:1213–1223.

Ikuta F, Zimmerman HM. Distribution of plaques in seventy autopsy cases of multiple sclerosis in the United States. *Neurology*. 1976;26:26–28.

Inglese M, Adhya S, Johnson G, et al. Perfusion magnetic resonance imaging correlates of neuropsychological impairment in multiple sclerosis. *J Cereb Blood Flow Metab*. 2008;28:164–171.

Jacobs LD, Cookfair DL, Rudick RA, et al. Intramuscular interferon beta-1a for disease progression in relapsing multiple sclerosis. The Multiple Sclerosis Collaborative Research Group (MSCRG). *Ann Neurol*. 1996;39:285–294.

Kappos L, Moeri D, Radue EW, et al. Predictive value of gadolinium-enhanced magnetic resonance imaging for relapse rate and changes in disability or impairment in multiple sclerosis: a meta-analysis. Gadolinium MRI Meta-analysis Group. *Lancet*. 1999;353:964–969.

Keiper MD, Grossman RI, Hirsch JA, et al. MR identification of white matter abnormalities in multiple sclerosis: a comparison between 1.5 T and 4 T. *AJNR Am J Neuroradiol*. 1998;19:1489–1493.

Kepes JJ. Large focal tumor-like demyelinating lesions of the brain: intermediate entity between multiple sclerosis and acute disseminated encephalomyelitis? A study of 31 patients. *Ann Neurol*. 1993;33:18–27.

Kern KC, Ekstrom A, Giesser BS, Montag M, Sicotte NL. Role of hippocampal connectivity in functional verbal memory compensation in multiple sclerosis. *Mult Scler*. 2009.

Kutzelnigg A, Lassmann H. Cortical lesions and brain atrophy in MS. *J Neurol Sci*. 2005;233:55–59.

Laule C, Kozlowski P, Leung E, Li DK, Mackay AL, Moore GR. Myelin water imaging of multiple sclerosis at 7 T: correlations with histopathology. *Neuroimage*. 2008; 40:1575–1580.

Lebrun C, Bensa C, Debouverie M, et al. Unexpected multiple sclerosis: follow-up of 30 patients with magnetic resonance imaging and clinical conversion profile. *J Neurol Neurosurg Psychiatry*. 2008;79:195–198.

Lee DH, Vellet AD, Eliasziw M, et al. MR imaging field strength: prospective evaluation of the diagnostic accuracy of MR for diagnosis of multiple sclerosis at 0.5 and 1.5 T. *Radiology*. 1995;194:257–262.

Lee M, Reddy H, Johansen BH, et al. The motor cortex shows adaptive functional changes to brain injury from multiple sclerosis. *Ann Neurol*. 2000;47:606–613.

Lenzi D, Conte A, Mainero C, et al. Effect of corpus callosum damage on ipsilateral motor activation in patients with multiple sclerosis: a functional and anatomical study. *Hum Brain Mapp*. 2007;28:636–644.

Li BS, Regal J, Soher BJ, Mannon LJ, Grossman RI, Gonen O. Brain metabolite profiles of t1-hypointense lesions in relapsing-remitting multiple sclerosis. *AJNR Am J Neuroradiol*. 2003;24:68–74.

Losseff NA, Kingsley DP, McDonald WI, Miller DH, Thompson AJ. Clinical and magnetic resonance imaging predictors of disability in primary and secondary progressive multiple sclerosis. *Mult Scler*. 1996;1: 218–222.

Lucchinetti CF, Gavrilova RH, Metz I, et al. Clinical and radiographic spectrum of pathologically confirmed tumefactive multiple sclerosis. *Brain*. 2008;131: 1759–1775.

Mainero C, Benner T, Radding A, et al. In vivo imaging of cortical pathology in multiple sclerosis using ultra-high field MRI. *Neurology*. 2009;73:941–948.

Mainero C, Caramia F, Pozzilli C, et al. fMRI evidence of brain reorganization during attention and memory tasks in multiple sclerosis. *Neuroimage*. 2004;21: 858–867.

Mainero C, De Stefano N, Iannucci G, et al. Correlates of MS disability assessed in vivo using aggregates of MR quantities. *Neurology.* 2001;56:1331–1334.

Masdeu JC, Moreira J, Trasi S, Visintainer P, Cavaliere R, Grundman M. The open ring. A new imaging sign in demyelinating disease. *J Neuroimaging.* 1996;6: 104–107.

McDonald WI, Compston A, Edan G, et al. Recommended diagnostic criteria for multiple sclerosis: guidelines from the International Panel on the Diagnosis of Multiple Sclerosis. *Ann Neurol.* 2001;50:121–127.

Mendez MF, Pogacar S. Malignant monophasic multiple sclerosis or "Marburg's disease". *Neurology.* 1988; 38:1153–1155.

Miller DH, Khan OA, Sheremata WA, et al. A controlled trial of natalizumab for relapsing multiple sclerosis. *N Engl J Med.* 2003;348:15–23.

Miller DH, Leary SM. Primary-progressive multiple sclerosis. *Lancet Neurol.* 2007;6:903–912.

Miller DH, Weinshenker BG, Filippi M, et al. Differential diagnosis of suspected multiple sclerosis: a consensus approach. *Mult Scler.* 2008;14:1157–1174.

Morgen K, Jeffries NO, Stone R, et al. Ring-enhancement in multiple sclerosis: marker of disease severity. *Mult Scler.* 2001;7:167–171.

Mottershead JP, Schmierer K, Clemence M, et al. High field MRI correlates of myelin content and axonal density in multiple sclerosis–a post-mortem study of the spinal cord. *J Neurol.* 2003;250:1293–1301.

Narayanan S, De Stefano N, Francis GS, et al. Axonal metabolic recovery in multiple sclerosis patients treated with interferon beta-1b. *J Neurol.* 2001;248: 979–986.

Narayanan S, Fu L, Pioro E, et al. Imaging of axonal damage in multiple sclerosis: spatial distribution of magnetic resonance imaging lesions. *Ann Neurol.* 1997; 41:385–391.

Neema M, Arora A, Healy BC, et al. Deep gray matter involvement on brain MRI scans is associated with clinical progression in multiple sclerosis. *J Neuroimaging.* 2009;19:3–8.

O'Riordan JI, Thompson AJ, Kingsley DP, et al. The prognostic value of brain MRI in clinically isolated syndromes of the CNS. A 10-year follow-up. *Brain.* 1998; 121(pt 3):495–503.

Okuda DT, Mowry EM, Beheshtian A, et al. Incidental MRI anomalies suggestive of multiple sclerosis. The radiologically isolated syndrome. *Neurology.* 2009; 72(9):800–805.

Optic Neuritis Study Group. Multiple sclerosis risk after optic neuritis: final optic neuritis treatment trial follow-up. *Arch Neurol.* 2008;65:727–732.

Pantano P, Iannetti GD, Caramia F, et al. Cortical motor reorganization after a single clinical attack of multiple sclerosis. *Brain.* 2002;125:1607–1615.

Paty DW, Li DK. Interferon beta-1b is effective in relapsing-remitting multiple sclerosis. II. MRI analysis results of a multicenter, randomized, double-blind, placebo-controlled trial. UBC MS/MRI Study Group and the IFNB Multiple Sclerosis Study Group. *Neurology.* 1993;43:662–667.

Paty DW, Li DK, Oger JJ, et al. Magnetic resonance imaging in the evaluation of clinical trials in multiple sclerosis. *Ann Neurol.* 1994;36:S95–S96.

Peterson JW, Bo L, Mork S, Chang A, Trapp BD. Transected neurites, apoptotic neurons, and reduced inflammation in cortical multiple sclerosis lesions. *Ann Neurol.* 2001;50:389–400.

Pierpaoli C, Basser PJ. Toward a quantitative assessment of diffusion anisotropy. *Magn Reson Med.* 1996;36: 893–906.

Pierpaoli C, Jezzard P, Basser PJ, Barnett A, Di CG. Diffusion tensor MR imaging of the human brain. *Radiology.* 1996;201:637–648.

Pittock SJ, Weinshenker BG, Lucchinetti CF, Wingerchuk DM, Corboy JR, Lennon VA. Neuromyelitis optica brain lesions localized at sites of high aquaporin 4 expression. *Arch Neurol.* 2006;63:964–968.

Polman CH, Reingold SC, Edan G, et al. Diagnostic criteria for multiple sclerosis: 2005 revisions to the "McDonald Criteria". *Ann Neurol.* 2005;58:840–846.

Poser CM, Paty DW, Scheinberg L, et al. New diagnostic criteria for multiple sclerosis: guidelines for research protocols. *Ann Neurol.* 1983;13:227–231.

Poser S, Luer W, Bruhn H, Frahm J, Bruck Y, Felgenhauer K. Acute demyelinating disease. Classification and non-invasive diagnosis. *Acta Neurol Scand.* 1992; 86:579–585.

Reddy H, Narayanan S, Arnoutelis R, et al. Evidence for adaptive functional changes in the cerebral cortex with axonal injury from multiple sclerosis. *Brain.* 2000a;123:2314–2320.

Reddy H, Narayanan S, Matthews PM, et al. Relating axonal injury to functional recovery in MS. *Neurology.* 2000b;54:236–239.

Reddy H, Narayanan S, Woolrich M, et al. Functional brain reorganization for hand movement in patients with multiple sclerosis: defining distinct effects of injury and disability. *Brain.* 2002;125:2646–2657.

Richert ND, Ostuni JL, Bash CN, Duyn JH, McFarland HF, Frank JA. Serial whole-brain magnetization transfer imaging in patients with relapsing-remitting multiple sclerosis at baseline and during treatment with interferon beta-1b. *AJNR Am J Neuroradiol.* 1998; 19:1705–1713.

Rigotti DJ, Inglese M, Gonen O. Whole-brain N-acetylaspartate as a surrogate marker of neuronal damage in diffuse neurologic disorders. *AJNR Am J Neuroradiol.* 2007;28:1843–1849.

Riva M, Ikonomidou VN, Ostuni JJ, et al. Tissue-specific imaging is a robust methodology to differentiate in vivo T1 black holes with advanced multiple sclerosis-induced damage. *AJNR Am J Neuroradiol.* 2009;30:1394–1401.

Rocca MA, Agosta F, Sormani MP, et al. A three-year, multi-parametric MRI study in patients at presentation with CIS. *J Neurol.* 2008;255:683–691.

Rocca MA, Iannucci G, Rovaris M, Comi G, Filippi M. Occult tissue damage in patients with primary progressive multiple sclerosis is independent of T2-visible lesions–a diffusion tensor MR study. *J Neurol.* 2003a; 250:456–460.

Rocca MA, Mezzapesa DM, Falini A, et al. Evidence for axonal pathology and adaptive cortical reorganization in patients at presentation with clinically isolated syndromes suggestive of multiple sclerosis. *Neuroimage.* 2003b;18:847–855.

Rocca MA, Pagani E, Ghezzi A, et al. Functional cortical changes in patients with multiple sclerosis and nonspecific findings on conventional magnetic resonance imaging scans of the brain. *Neuroimage.* 2003c;19: 826–836.

Roosendaal SD, Geurts JJ, Vrenken H, et al. Regional DTI differences in multiple sclerosis patients. *Neuroimage.* 2009;44:1397–1403.

Rovira A, Swanton J, Tintore M, et al. A single, early magnetic resonance imaging study in the diagnosis of multiple sclerosis. *Arch Neurol.* 2009;66:587–592.

Rudick RA, Fisher E, Lee JC, Simon J, Jacobs L. Use of the brain parenchymal fraction to measure whole brain atrophy in relapsing-remitting MS. Multiple Sclerosis Collaborative Research Group. *Neurology.* 1999;53: 1698–1704.

Rudick RA, Lee JC, Nakamura K, Fisher E. Gray matter atrophy correlates with MS disability progression measured with MSFC but not EDSS. *J Neurol Sci.* 2008;284:223.

Sailer M, Fischl B, Salat D, et al. Focal thinning of the cerebral cortex in multiple sclerosis. *Brain.* 2003;126: 1734–1744.

Sajja BR, Wolinsky JS, Narayana PA. Proton magnetic resonance spectroscopy in multiple sclerosis. *Neuroimaging Clin N Am.* 2009;19:45–58.

Salamon N, Sicotte N, Alger J, et al. Analysis of the brainstem white-matter tracts with diffusion tensor imaging. *Neuroradiology.* 2005;47:895–902.

Salamon N, Sicotte N, Drain A, et al. White matter fiber tractography and color mapping of the normal human cerebellum with diffusion tensor imaging. *J Neuroradiol.* 2007;34:115–128.

Santos AC, Narayanan S, de Stefano N, et al. Magnetization transfer can predict clinical evolution in patients with multiple sclerosis. *J Neurol.* 2002;249:662–668.

Schenck JF, Zimmerman EA. High-field magnetic resonance imaging of brain iron: birth of a biomarker? *NMR Biomed.* 2004;17:433–445.

Schmierer K, Scaravilli F, Altmann DR, Barker GJ, Miller DH. Magnetization transfer ratio and myelin in postmortem multiple sclerosis brain. *Ann Neurol.* 2004; 56:407–415.

Schumacher F, Beeve G, Kibler F, et al. Problems of experimental trials of therapy in multiple sclerosis. *Ann N Y Acad Sci.* 1965;122:552–568.

Sharma J, Zivadinov R, Jaisani Z, et al. A magnetization transfer MRI study of deep gray matter involvement in multiple sclerosis. *J Neuroimaging.* 2006;16: 302–310.

Sicotte NL, Kern KC, Giesser BS, et al. Regional hippocampal atrophy in multiple sclerosis. *Brain.* 2008; 131:1134–1141.

Sicotte NL, Voskuhl RR, Bouvier S, Klutch R, Cohen MS, Mazziotta JC. Comparison of multiple sclerosis lesions at 1.5 and 3.0 Tesla. *Invest Radiol.* 2003;38:423–427.

Simon JH, Kinkel RP, Jacobs L, Bub L, Simonian N. A Wallerian degeneration pattern in patients at risk for MS. *Neurology.* 2000;54:1155–1160.

Simon JH, Kleinschmidt-DeMasters BK. Variants of multiple sclerosis. *Neuroimaging Clin N Am.* 2008;18: 703–16, xi.

Simon JH, Li D, Traboulsee A, et al. Standardized MR imaging protocol for multiple sclerosis: Consortium of MS Centers consensus guidelines. *AJNR Am J Neuroradiol.* 2006;27:455–461.

Smith PD, Cook MJ, Trost NM, Murphy MA. Teaching NeuroImage: open-ring imaging sign in a case of tumefactive cerebral demyelination. *Neurology.* 2008; 71:e73.

Song SK, Yoshino J, Le TQ, et al. Demyelination increases radial diffusivity in corpus callosum of mouse brain. *Neuroimage.* 2005;26:132–140.

Srinivasan R, Sailasuta N, Hurd R, Nelson S, Pelletier D. Evidence of elevated glutamate in multiple sclerosis using magnetic resonance spectroscopy at 3 T. *Brain.* 2005;128:1016–1025.

Stadelmann C, Albert M, Wegner C, Bruck W. Cortical pathology in multiple sclerosis. *Curr Opin Neurol.* 2008;21:229–234.

Stadelmann C, Bruck W. Lessons from the neuropathology of atypical forms of multiple sclerosis. *Neurol Sci.* 2004;25(suppl 4):S319–S322.

Staffen W, Mair A, Zauner H, et al. Cognitive function and fMRI in patients with multiple sclerosis: evidence for compensatory cortical activation during an attention task. *Brain.* 2002;125:1275–1282.

Stevenson VL, Leary SM, Losseff NA, et al. Spinal cord atrophy and disability in MS: a longitudinal study. *Neurology.* 1998;51:234–238.

Stone LA, Frank JA, Albert PS, et al. The effect of interferon-beta on blood-brain barrier disruptions demonstrated by contrast-enhanced magnetic resonance imaging in relapsing-remitting multiple sclerosis. *Ann Neurol.* 1995;37:611–619.

Swanton JK, Fernando K, Dalton CM, et al. Modification of MRI criteria for multiple sclerosis in patients with clinically isolated syndromes. *J Neurol Neurosurg Psychiatry.* 2006;77:830–833.

Tedeschi G, Lavorgna L, Russo P, et al. Brain atrophy and lesion load in a large population of patients with multiple sclerosis. *Neurology.* 2005;65:280–285.

Tintore M, Rovira A, Martinez MJ, et al. Isolated demyelinating syndromes: comparison of different MR imaging criteria to predict conversion to clinically definite multiple sclerosis. *AJNR Am J Neuroradiol.* 2000; 21:702–706.

Tortorella C, Viti B, Bozzali M, et al. A magnetization transfer histogram study of normal-appearing brain tissue in MS. *Neurology.* 2000;54:186–193.

Traboulsee A, Dehmeshki J, Peters KR, et al. Disability in multiple sclerosis is related to normal appearing brain tissue MTR histogram abnormalities. *Mult Scler.* 2003;9:566–573.

Truyen L, van Waesberghe JH, van Walderveen MA, et al. Accumulation of hypointense lesions ("black holes") on T1 spin-echo MRI correlates with disease progression in multiple sclerosis. *Neurology.* 1996;47: 1469–1476.

van Waesberghe JH, van Walderveen MA, Castelijns JA, et al. Patterns of lesion development in multiple sclerosis: longitudinal observations with T1-weighted spin-echo and magnetization transfer MR. *AJNR Am J Neuroradiol.* 1998;19:675–683.

van Walderveen MA, Kamphorst W, Scheltens P, et al. Histopathologic correlate of hypointense lesions on T1-weighted spin-echo MRI in multiple sclerosis. *Neurology.* 1998;50:1282–1288.

Wingerchuk DM. The clinical course of acute disseminated encephalomyelitis. *Neurol Res.* 2006;28:341–347.

Wingerchuk DM, Lennon VA, Lucchinetti CF, Pittock SJ, Weinshenker BG. The spectrum of neuromyelitis optica. *Lancet Neurol.* 2007;6:805–815.

Wolinsky JS, Narayana PA, Johnson KP. United States open-label glatiramer acetate extension trial for relapsing multiple sclerosis: MRI and clinical correlates. Multiple Sclerosis Study Group and the MRI Analysis Center. *Mult Scler.* 2001;7:33–41.

Wylezinska M, Cifelli A, Jezzard P, Palace J, Alecci M, Matthews PM. Thalamic neurodegeneration in relapsing-remitting multiple sclerosis. *Neurology.* 2003;60: 1949–1954.

8 Cerebrospinal Fluid Profile

Wallace W. Tourtellotte

The cerebrospinal fluid (CSF) profile has been determined by including multiple sclerosis (MS) patients with relapsing-remitting MS with Kurtzke disability scores less than 6 (no aids of ambulation are necessary). Patients were included based on Schumacher et al. (1965) and Poser et al. (1983) criteria. The CSF and matched blood were obtained at the onset of a trial. Each component is based on more than 500 patients (Tourtellotte and Tumani, 1997).

APPEARANCE

Multiple sclerosis CSF is crystal clear except in some cases of transverse myelitis. The edematous spinal cord might produce a block or partial block of the subarachnoid space and hence CSF flow is impaired. In some cases the CSF obtained below the block or partial block can appear yellow and clot (Froin syndrome).

CEREBROSPINAL FLUID DYNAMICS

The pressure is normal (200 mm of water) except when transverse myelitis has resulted in a block of CSF flow: At first CSF flows into the lumbar puncture needle and then suddenly ceases when the fluid below the block is drained and pressure falls to zero. This is referred to as a dry tap.

It has been reported that draining fluid below a spinal subarachnoid block can produce a worsening of symptoms and signs. Accordingly, it is recommended that a spinal cord magnetic resonance image (MRI) be performed prior to a lumbar puncture in cases suspected of being clinically afflicted with transverse myelitis. If the MRI shows a block or partial block, a lumbar puncture should not be performed. If it is necessary to check the MS CSF profile or to check for other reasons, fluid can be obtained by tapping the cisterna magna.

CYTOLOGY

A total leukocyte count of 5 cells or less per microliter (mean + 2 standard deviations [M + 2 SD]) is normal. Sixty-six percent of cases were normal and cell counts more than 50 are very rare ($p = 0.001$) and make MS unlikely. In such cases, other diseases should be considered, or rarely a patient has a comorbidity.

The differential count (Wright stain) is normal and all are mononuclear cells (no polymorphonuclear cells and no erythrocytes).

Total CSF leukocyte and differential cells counts showed no relationship to relapses, but the total cell count is modestly proportional to elevated intrathecal IgG synthesis rate or IgG index. There is a tendency that cases with the lowest synthesis rates and the lowest cell counts have had MS the longest.

GLUCOSE

Cerebrospinal fluid and matched blood should be obtained in the fasting state at least 3 hours after eating. The normal ratio of CSF to plasma glucose concentration is 0.6. In all cases CSF/plasma glucose ratio was normal. If the CSF glucose is high or low because of hyperglycemia or hypoglycemia caused by diabetes mellitus, the ratio is still normal. High CSF ratio in the fasting state has been reported in viral encephalitis. A low ratio is an expected result with bacterial meningitis and meningeal carcinomatosis.

CEREBROSPINAL FLUID ALBUMIN/SERUM ALBUMIN(Q_{ALB})

Dynamic studies with intravenously injected radio-labeled albumin have shown that albumin in CSF is exclusively derived from blood, and blood albumin is derived from liver synthesis. Further, albumin is not synthesized or catabolized within the central nervous system (CNS). The absolute concentration of CSF albumin, the major CSF protein, depends on many factors, including its blood concentration, integrity of blood–brain-CSF barrier (BBCB), rate of CSF flow, age of the patient, and the volume of CSF sample taken for analysis because of the gradient in the CSF space (highest in the lumbar CSF space to lowest in the ventricles).

The normal albumin concentration in the CSF is equal to or less than 34 mg/dl (M + 2 SD) in 77% of the cases. An albumin concentration in the CSF of more than 65 mg/dl is very rare ($p = 0.001$) and makes MS unlikely. In such cases, other diseases should be considered, or rarely a patient has MS with a comorbidity.

Albumin quotient is calculated by dividing the albumin concentration in the CSF by the concentration in the serum. It is a quantitative method to assess the overall integrity of the BBCB to mid-sized proteins such as albumin and IgG. The Q_{ALB} is age dependent. For the first 10 ml of lumbar fluid Q_{ALB} is 6.5–8.0 for individuals 16–40 years old; if an individual is 40–60 years old, 8–9; if an individual is more than 60 years old, the ratio is >9. Values higher than 14 in MS are very rare ($p = 0.001$) and make MS unlikely. In such cases, other diseases should be considered, or rarely a MS patient has a comorbidity.

TOTAL PROTEIN

Multiple sclerosis CSF total protein concentration is normal, 54 mg/dl or less (M + 2 SD) in 77% of cases. A value of more than 110 mg/dl is very rare in MS ($p = 0.001$). The significance of an elevated CSF total protein is similar to an elevated albumin. Albumin determination is the preferred method in a modern clinical laboratory.

INTRATHECAL IgG SYNTHESIS RATE PER DAY

The intrathecal IgG rate per day is more than 6 in 92% of cases. It is rarely more than 130 ($p = 0.001$). In such cases other diseases should be considered, or rarely a patient has a comorbidity.

In MS, CSF IgG is elevated by synthesis of IgG by plasma cells inside the BBCB. It is proposed that B-lymphocytes are recruited from the blood across the blood–brain barrier (BBB) to the CNS for an unknown reason in MS. Some of the B-lymphocytes mature to plasma cells, which synthesize IgG. Increased intrathecal IgG synthesis rate is temporally and clonally stable (Walsh and Tourtellotte, 1986). This information has led to the proposal that the MS CNS has been turned into a type of immune organ.

The empirical formula to calculate intrathecal IgG sythesis rate per day requires total CSF IgG concentration be corrected for leaks across the BBB into the CSF. The formula is given in detail in the CSF chapter in our MS textbook (Tourtellotte & Tumani, 1997).

IgG INDEX

Our empirical formula is the basis of the IgG index, which is used by all CSF laboratories and clinicians. Further, the correlation coefficient between our formula and IgG index is $r = 0.96$. The MS plaque load in a case correlates with the formula and IgG index and even better with the circumference of the plaque load. It is our observation that active demyelination is primarily located at plaque edges.

Here is the IgG index formula:

$$IgG\,index = \frac{CSF\,IgG}{serum\,IgG} \div \frac{CSF\,albumin}{serum\,albumin}$$

A value of more than 0.73 (M+ 2 SD) is abnormal and is present in 92% of clinical definite MS cases. Index more than 4 is very rare ($p = 0.001$). In such cases, other diseases should be considered, or rarely a MS patient has a comorbidity.

UNIQUE CEREBROSPINAL FLUID OLIGOCLONDAL IgG BANDS

This is a very different way to detect intrathecal IgG synthesis by plasma cells. In our MS patients' data set 97% of cases had 1 or more bands. It has been proposed that bands are specific for an antigen. This proposal is based on subacute sclerosis panencephalitis (SSPE) studies (Conrad, et al., 1994). SSPE has many CSF oligoclonal IgG bands similar to MS, and when absorbed with measles antigen all the bands are removed.

SUMMARY OF CEREBROSPINAL FLUID PROFILE SUPPORTING A CLINICAL DEFINITE DIAGNOSIS OF MULTIPLE SCLEROSIS

The following conditions support a clinical definite MS diagnosis:

- Crystal-clear CSF under normal pressure and normal fasting CSF-plasma glucose ratio
- The CSF cell count is less than 50 cells/cmm
- The differential cell count shows only mononuclear cells (no neutrophils and no erythrocytes).
- The Q_{ALB} is less than 14.
- Intrathecal IgG synthesis rate per day shows an abnormal synthesis rate more than 6 mg/day in 92% of cases, but it is less than 130 mg/day ($p = 0.001$).
- The IgG index: a value more than 0.73 is present in 92% of cases and is less than 4.
- The unique CSF oligoclonal IgG bands are found in 97% of MS cases.
- Furthermore, if there is an elevated intrathecal IgG synthesis rate per day, an elevated IgG index, and the presence of unique CSF oligoclonal IgG bands is found, then a patient has a 99% chance of having MS.
- Clinical isolated syndrome: CSF oligoclonal IgG bands are more sensitive than MRI; see data presented under "Issues."

RED FLAG: LABORATORY TESTS TO RULE OUT OTHER DISEASES THAT CAN MIMIC MULTIPLE SCLEROSIS

Since there is no proven etiology of MS, there is no specific diagnostic test. Many diseases/syndromes can mimic symptoms/signs and course of MS (see Table 6-7 in Chapter 6). Various laboratory tests need to be done to rule out mimicker diagnoses when clinically indicated. It is also important to perform an extremely detailed history and a detailed neurological/physical exam. Brain and spinal cord MRI should also be included in the final decision; only then does the MS CSF profile becomes more valid to support the clinical diagnosis of MS.

Tests that may indicate the presence of vasculitis (ESR, ANA, ACE), infections (Lyme, HIV, HTLV-1, HHV-6, RPR), metabolic derangements (thyroid dysfunction, B12 deficiency), or other uncommon conditions that may produce clinical, radiologic, and spinal fluid profile similar to that seen in persons with MS, should be run if there is clinical suspicion of these conditions. However, false positives are not uncommon with some of these assays. For example antinuclear antibodies (ANA) and ANA titers up to 1:200 have been found in persons with MS.

Cerebrospinal fluid findings in Neuromyelitis Optica (NMO) (Devic's Disease)

Often neutrophils are present and albumin is elevated indicating fulminant demyelination with necrosis in the central nervous system. In contrast to MS the oligoclonal bands frequently may be absent or may be present and then disappear (Zaffaroni 2004).

Aquoporin-4 (AQP4) is the most abundant water channel in the central nervous system. It has been shown that AQP4-antibodies are related to the clinical activities of NMO (Jarius et al, 2008), and the presence of AQP4 antibodies in the serum is 73% sensitive and 91% specific in individuals with a clinical diagnosis of NMO (Lennon et al 2004). These antibodies have not been seen in MS. However cases have been described in a few patients with clinical NMO who were seronegative for AQP4 antibodies, but in whom AQP4 antibodies were detected in CSF.(Klawiter et al 2009). The authors suggest that testing for CSF AQP4 antibodies is warranted in AQP4 seronegative patients in whom the dx. of NMO is "strongly suspected".

MULTIPLE SCLEROSIS CEREBROSPINAL FLUID TASK FORCE

The proposal by McDonald et al. (2001) stated that CSF testing was an integral part of making the diagnosis of MS, but the proposal did not present enough detail to be useful for MS specialists and clinical laboratories. Accordingly, a MS CSF Task Force (Freedman et al., 2005) composed of international MS CSF experts recommended laboratory methods and a CSF profile that supports the clinical definite multiple sclerosis diagnosis.

The MS CSF Task Force presented the following conclusions:

1. Oligoclonal IgG bands in the CSF and not in serum or more intense in the CSF than serum is "the gold standard" of the MS CSF profile. Proteins in CSF and serum should be separated by isoelectric focusing in agarose gel.

2. After electrophoresis the gel should be immunofixed with an antibody reagent to human IgG. After washing the gels to remove the nonreactive proteins, an antibody reagent is added to react with the immunofixed complex, which has attached peroxidase molecules. When hydrogen peroxidase is added to the gel, the oligoconal bands turn brownish pink. Bands are counted by inspection (Thompson, 2005).

3. In addition to CSF IgG oligoclonal bands, neurologists must consider results only from crystal-clear fluid removed under normal pressure with less than 50 mononuclear cells, no neutrophils or erthyrocytes, Q_{ALB} less than 14, daily intrathecal IgG synthesis rate less than 130 mg/day, and an IgG index less than 4.

4. The Task Force members concurred that in certain cases the evaluation of light chains can help resolve equivocal IgG oligoclonal patterns, but this did not rise to the level that it should be a routine determination.

5. The neurologist should consider repeating a lumbar puncture and CSF analysis in 6 months if clinical suspicion is high but CSF is equivocally negative or shows only one band.

6. Neurologists must use clinical judgment and laboratory tests to rule out patients whose symptoms and signs mimic MS.

BUNDLED RECOMMENDATIONS BASED ON OUR CEREBROSPINAL FLUID LABORATORY RESULTS AND THE CEREBROSPINAL FLUID TASK FORCE CONCLUSIONS

Neurologists must consider appearance, CSF pressure, cell counts and differential counts, glucose, Q_{ALB}, intrathecal IgG synthesis rate per day, and IgG index when evaluating significance of unique CSF oligoclonal IgG bands. It is necessary that components which make up the MS CSF profile are normal, or elevated and fall below cut-off points. It is only then that CSF oligoclonal IgG bands are unique for MS and become the gold standard of the MS CSF examination.

There is a red flag reminder in evaluating the validity of the specificity and sensitivity of the CSF profile to support a clinical definite MS diagnosis: specific tests for other diseases should be performed and results should be normal.

ISSUES

Clinically Isolated Syndrome and Multiple Sclerosis Cerebrospinal Fluid Profile

Is the profile present in clinically isolated syndrome (CIS) patients? Masjuan et al. (2006) concluded that the presence of oligoclonal IgG bands is highly specific and sensitive for early prediction of conversion to MS. They found head MRI images have a high specificity but less sensitivity. They finally concluded the simultaneous use of both tests showed highest sensitivity and specificity in predicting CIS conversion to MS.

In a much earlier study, Tumani et al. (1998) studied CSF/blood obtained from patients in the Acute Optic Neuritis Treatment Trial (ONTT). Optic neuritis is a type of CIS. Twelve of 28 patients with acute optic neuritis had abnormal head MRI images, but all had a MS CSF profile. Accordingly, 6 of 16 patients with optic neuritis had a positive MS CSF profile but a normal head MRI. It was concluded that the CSF profile was a more sensitive marker than head MRI to predict conversion to MS in optic neuritis.

FUTURE APPLICATIONS

Recent reports suggest that CSF levels of neurofilament proteins, which are markers of axonal injury, could be used as a biomarker to monitor disease activity in persons with MS and may predict future disability(Salzer et al 2010, Giovannoni, 2010). Larger studies are needed to confirm these associations.

REFERENCES

Conrad AJ, Chiang EY, Andeen LE, et al. Quantitation of intrathecal measles virus IgG synthesis rate: subacute sclerosing panencephalitis and multiple sclerosis. *J Neuroimmunol.* 1994;54:99–108.

Freedman MS, Thompson EJ, Deisnhammer F, et al. Recommended standard of cerebrospinal fluid analysis in the diagnosis of multiple sclerosis. A consensus statement. *Arch Neurol.* 2005;62:8865–8870.

Giovannoni G. Cerebrospinal fluid neurofilament: the biomarker that will resuscitate the "Spinal Tap". *Mult. Sclerosis.* 2010;16(3):285–286.

Masjuan J, Alvarez-Cermeno JC, Garcia-Barragan N, et al. Clinically isolated syndromes. A new oligoclonal band test accurately predicts conversion to MS. *Neurology.* 2006;66:576–578.

Jarius S, Aboul-Enein F, Waters P, et al. Antibody to aquoporin-4 in the long-term course of neuromyelitis optica. *Brain.* 2008;131:3072–3080.

Klawiter E, Alvarez E, Xu J et al. NMO-IgG detected in seronegative neuromyelitis optica. *Neurology.* 2009; 72(12):1101–1103.

Lennon V, Wingerchuk D, Kryzer T et al. A serum antibody marker of neuromyelitis optica: distinction from multiple sclerosis. *Lancet.* 2004;364: 2106–2112.

McDonald WI, Compston A, Edan G, et al. Recommended diagnostic criteria for multiple sclerosis. Guidelines from the International Panel on the Diagnosis of Multiple Sclerosis. *Ann Neurol.* 2001;50:121–127.

Poser CM, Paty DW, Scheinberg L, et al. New diagnostic criteria for multiple sclerosis: guidelines for research protocols. *Ann Neurol.* 1983;13(3):227–231.

Salzer J, Svenningsson A, Sundstrom P. Neurofilament light as a prognostic marker in MS. *Mult. Sclerosis.* 2010;16(3):287–292.

Schumacher GA, Beebe G, Kibler RF, et al. Problems of experimental trials of therapy in multiple sclerosis: report by the panel on the evaluation of experimental trials of therapy in multiple sclerosis. *NY Acad Sci.* 1965;122:552–568.

Thompson EJ. Proteins of the Cerebrospinal Fluid: Analysis and Interpretation in the Diagnosis and Treatment of Neurological Disease. 2nd ed. Amsterdam, Netherlands: Elsevier Academic Press; 2005.

Tourtellotte WW, Tumani H. Multiple Sclerosis Cerebrospinal Fluid. In: Raine CS, McFarland HF, Tourtellotte WW, eds. *Multiple Sclerosis. Clinical and Pathogenetic Basis.* New York: Chapman & Hall Medical;1997:57–79.

Tumani H, Tourtellotte WW, Peter JB, Felgenhauer K, The Optic Study Group. Acute optic neuritis: combined immunological markers and magnetic resonance imaging predict subsequent development of multiple sclerosis. *J Neurol Sci.* 1998;155(1):44–49.

Walsh MJ, Tourtellotte WW. Temporal invariance and clonal uniformity of brain and cerebrospinal IgG, IgA, and IgM in multiple sclerosis. *J Exp Med.* 1986;163:41–53.

Zaffaroni M. Cerebrospinal fluid findings in Devic's neuromyelitis optica. *Neurol. Sci.* 2004;25(Suppl.4) S368–70.

SUGGESTED READING

Fleming JO. *Diagnosis and Management of Multiple Sclerosis.* 1st ed. Caddo, OK: Professional Communications Inc; 2002.

Jarius S, Aboul-Enein F, Waters P, et al. Antibody to aquaporin-4 in the long-term course of neuromyelitis optica. *Brain.* 2008;131:3072–3080.

Tourtellotte WW. What every physician should know about multiple sclerosis (MS) diagnosis and primary treatment. *NNI Journal.* 2007;3(3):126–131.

9 Evoked Potentials

Marc R. Nuwer

Evoked potentials (EPs) are nervous system electrical potentials evoked by certain brief stimuli. For 35 years EP tests have helped clinically to diagnose multiple sclerosis (MS) (Comi et al., 1998, 1999; Leocani et al., 2000; Leocani and Comi, 2000; Fuhr and Kappos, 2001). They are a research tool to explore the pathophysiology of demyelination as well as an adjunct useful for MS therapeutic trials (Nuwer et al., 1987; Emerson, 1998).

Evoked potentials are sensitive, objective, and reproducible. They easily are quantified to 2–3 significant figures. Evoked potentials can detect "silent lesions," physiologic impairment without accompanying signs or symptoms that can provide evidence of an additional lesion. The tests are objective because they require only that the patient lie quietly or watch a video screen. The patient's cooperation does not alter EP results. Test scoring is standardized. Evoked potentials are reproducible in that they yield the same values when tested again. The standard scoring is quantified to 2–3 significant figures for comparison to normal values. These precisely quantified measurements facilitate their use with parametric statistics, a substantially more powerful research tool than categorical variables.

Evoked potentials are electrical potentials (voltages) evoked by brief stimuli. After each stimulus, nerve volleys travel along the peripheral and central nervous system pathways of the stimulated sensory or motor modality. These axon volleys are delayed or blocked by regions of demyelination (Raminsky, 1981; Sears and Bostock, 1981; Waxman, 1981; Waxman and Ritchie, 1981; Sedgwick, 1983). Beyond the region of demyelination, the EP signals are delayed, attenuated, or absent. Because the peaks' generator sites are known, the EP reader can determine the level of impairment. Several modalities of EPs can assess several specific nervous system pathways: central visual, brainstem auditory, lemniscal sensory, and corticospinal motor pathways (Cowan et al., 1984; Mills and Murray, 1985; Hess et al., 1987). Event-related potentials measure cognitive processing speed.

Evoked potentials are used also in other neurologic disorders. Brainstem auditory EPs can screen infants for hearing impairment (Starr et al., 1977). In comatose patients, EPs assess degree and location of impairment (Karnaze et al., 1982; Cant et al., 1986). They can help distinguish among some hereditary-degenerative neurologic conditions that have specific patterns of EP changes (Nuwer et al., 1983). In the operating room, EPs can monitor the nervous system, allowing early identification of complications and allowing for early intervention (Nuwer, 2008). They can help separate peripheral from central levels of impairment, analogous to the clinical use of deep tendon reflexes to separate central from peripheral motor pathway impairment.

VISUAL EVOKED POTENTIALS

Visual evoked potentials (VEPs) are triggered by a strobe flash or a checkerboard visual pattern. Flash was described first (Richey et al., 1971), but the pattern reversal checkerboard VEP technique is more sensitive for detecting optic neuritis (Halliday et al., 1972). In the pattern reversal checkerboard techniques, each black and each white checkerboard square reverses color twice each second. This is displayed on a television screen or by a slide projector projected through a galvinometer-mounted mirror. The patient is tested one eye at a time in a darkened room. The test times the interval from the moment of each checkerboard reversal to an occipital positive electrical polarity peak, named P100, seen at around 100 milliseconds. Results from 100 separate stimulus presentations are averaged together before making measurements. The P100 event is preceded with axon volleys from the eye, along the optic nerve, across the chiasm, and up the optic tract to the lateral geniculate body. From that point the axon volley travels up the optic radiations, directly through the periventricular white matter for rather long distances, eventually reaching occipital cortex. Substantial processing occurs at the occipital cortex for up to 50 msec after the volley arrives. Finally an electrically positive P100 peak is seen at the occipital scalp, a potential generated from striate cortex (see Fig. 9-1).

Delayed conduction may occur at several points along this pathway in MS patients (Fig. 9-2). Delays at the optic nerve are well known. Less appreciated are the VEP delays that may occur along the optic tract and especially in the periventricular white matter. Prechiasmatic optic neuritis can be separated from the postchiasmatic lesions by comparing results from each eye. Interocular P100 latency differences are attributed to optic neuritis.

For detecting demyelination, VEPs are more sensitive than even a careful clinical visual function examination (Brooks and Chiappa, 1982; Kupersmith et al., 1983; Chiappa, 1990). Neuro-ophthalmologic examinations always were normal when the VEP was normal (Brooks and Chiappa, 1982). Even when the VEP was abnormal, various clinical examinations were often normal for visual fields by confrontation or formal testing, normal pupillary reflexes, and many had normal optic fundi and no red desaturation.

The checkerboard VEP technique is abnormal in almost all patients with a history of optic neuritis. In a summary of the literature (Halliday et al., 1973a, 1973b; Asselman et al., 1975; Hume and Cant, 1976; Lowitzsch et al., 1976; Mastaglia et al., 1976; Celesia and Daly, 1977; Hennerici et al., 1977; Matthews et al., 1977; Cant et al., 1978; Collins et al., 1978; Duwaer and Spekreijse, 1978; Nillson, 1978; Shahrokhi et al., 1978; Wist et al., 1978; Rigolet et al., 1979; Tackmann et al., 1979; Trojaborg and Petersen, 1979; Chiappa, 1980; Diener and Scheibler, 1980; Kjaer, 1980a; Wilson and Keyser, 1980; Purves et al., 1981; van Buggenhout et al., 1982; Walsh et al., 1982). Chiappa (1990) found that 90% of optic neuritis patients had abnormal VEPs, and close to 100% in many published series. When there was no clinical evidence for optic neuritis, the VEPs still were abnormal in 51% of 715 MS patients.

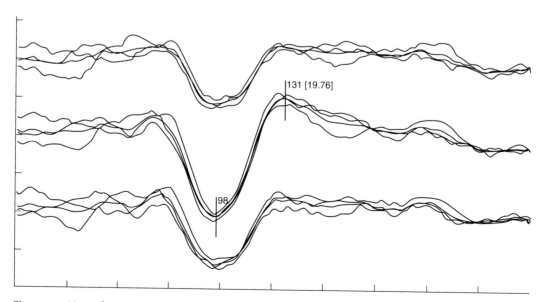

131 [19.76]

98

Figure 9-1 Normal pattern-reversal checkerboard visual evoked potentials. The P100 peak occurred at 98 msec. The three channels are from the right, midline, and left occipital regions.

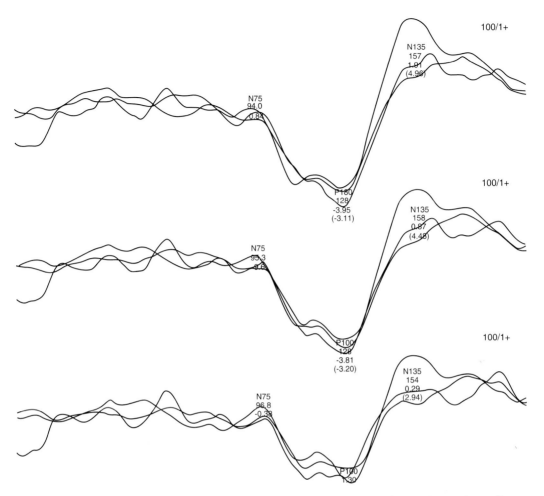

Figure 9-2 Abnormal visual evoked potentials with a delayed P100 seen as a down-going peak at 128 msec. The three channels are from the right, midline, and left occipital channels.

Visual EPs improve partially after an optic neuritis or postchiasmatic demyelination episode, but they do not return to normal (Matthews and Small, 1979; Jones and Brusa, 2003). An initial delay of 30 msec improves gradually over months to a 16 msec delay (Brusa et al., 2001; Jones and Brusa, 2003), improved but still remaining in the abnormal range. Visual EPs help the clinician to decide whether a history of visual changes years ago was from optic neuritis; if the VEP is normal, the episode was not optic neuritis.

For patients presenting with an isolated spinal or brainstem lesion, VEP can determine whether optic neuritis occurred in the past. This search for

a silent second lesion is an established use of VEPs (Polman et al., 2005).

Other disorders can affect VEPs. Some hereditary-degenerative neurologic disorders, for example, Friedreich ataxia (Nuwer et al., 1983) and adrenoleukodystrophy (Mamoli et al., 1979), as well as B12 deficiency (Krumholz et al., 1981), neurosyphillis (Lowitzsch and Westhoff, 1980), and other disorders (Streletz et al., 1981), can slow VEP latencies. These changes usually are mild or moderate bilateral delays. Severe delay or interocular latency difference is usually from demyelination. Mild to moderate symmetrical delays could be bilaterally demyelination, or they might be from another disorder, confirming an abnormality but nonspecific for the pathology.

Several useful MS VEP facts are notable:

- Idiopathic optic neuritis (ON) patients often develop MS (Rodriguez et al., 1995; Ghezzi et al., 2000).
- Initial VEPs are abnormal in nearly all (Frederiksen et al., 1996; Frederiksen and Petrera, 1999; Bee et al., 2003; Jones and Brusa, 2003) eyes affected with ON.
- Visual EP is abnormal in the clinically unaffected eye in 25% to 35% of ON patients (Frederiksen et al., 1996; Frederiksen and Petrera, 1999; Bee et al., 2003; Jones and Brusa, 2003; Simó et al., 2008), greatly increasing the likelihood that those patients will progress from idiopathic ON to MS.
- Visual EP is twice as sensitive as MRI to confirm optic nerve, chasm, and optic tract symptomatic demyelination (Farlow et al., 1986; Paty et al., 1988; Martinelli et al., 1991; Frederiksen et al., 1996).
- Magnetic resonance imaging (MRI) is more sensitive than VEP (Farlow et al., 1986; Paty et al., 1988; Frederiksen et al., 1990, 1996; Martinelli et al., 1991) to find a second lesion in the asymptomatic eye in ON patients.
- Brain MRI has a high yield of abnormalities in other brain areas (Giesser et al., 1987; Paty et al., 1988; Lee et al., 1991), whereas VEP is sensitive only along visual axis.
- The length of the MRI-detected demyelination correlated with the severity of VEP delay (Davies et al., 1998).
- The amount of VEP delay does not predict the amount of MRI-detected long-term atrophy (Hickman et al., 2003).
- Time needed for resolution of optic nerve gadolinium enhancement correlates with time for VEP latency improvement (Youl et al., 1991).

The American Academy of Neurology evidence-based assessment of VEPs recommends the technique as useful to identify patients at increased risk for developing clinically defined MS (Gronseth and Ashman, 2000). Visual EP has been adopted into the MacDonald criteria for diagnosis of MS (Polman et al., 2005).

When evaluating for possible MS those patients presenting with acute or chronic spinal cord lesions, multimodality EPs have a high yield of abnormalities (69% sensitivity) and fewer false positives than MRI (5% false positives for EPs, 9% for MRI). Abnormal VEPs clarify that demyelination is the likely cause of enhancing spinal MRI lesions (McDonald, 1988). The diagnostic yield for VEP in that circumstance was moderately low (7%–28%), so it is often normal and not specifically helpful for predicting which spinal lesions patients will progress to MS (Miller et al., 1987; Cordonnier et al., 2003).

Visual EPs help understand the physiology of demyelination. Analogous to the Uhthoff phenomenon, heat alters VEPs (Regan et al., 1977; Bajada et al., 1980; Persson and Sachs, 1980) in ways that can be studied precisely. Hyperventilation can increase VEP amplitudes (Davies et al., 1986), corresponding to clinical observations that hyperventilation, alkalosis, and hypocalcemia can transiently improve clinical deficits. The calcium channel blocker verapamil (Gilmore et al., 1985) and the potassium channel blocker 4-aminopyridine (Jones et al., 1983) can improve VEPs transiently.

An investigational VEP technique is to test each portion of the visual field, a kind of visual field testing using VEPs. Known as multifocal VEPs (Fraser et al., 2006a, 2006b; Grover et al., 2008; Hood et al., 2004a, 2004b), these can better define the central scotomas that may be seen in some optic neuritis. Routine VEPs also can show evidence of a central scotoma, which presents with a bifid (doubled) P100 peak (Rousseff et al., 2005).

Visual EPs can help study genetic predisposition to MS (Nuwer et al., 1985). Some asymptomatic first-degree relatives of MS patients have mild VEP abnormalities. A genetic predisposition toward subclinical pathology may underlie this (e.g., subclinical optic nerve edema without demyelination). Epidemiology of MS tells us that most such abnormalities are unlikely to develop into frank clinical MS. Some additional factors must be needed to convert such subtle processes into clinical MS.

Overall, checkerboard reversal pattern VEP helps the clinical evaluation of patients with possible MS. Abnormalities commonly occur in these visual pathways even in patients with no visual signs or symptoms. Visual EPs are more sensitive than MRI to detect optic neuritis. A VEP clarifies whether history of a previous visual event was optic neuritis. They can also identify a silent second lesion in the visual pathway in patients with isolated brainstem or spinal cord lesions.

BRAINSTEM AUDITORY EVOKED POTENTIALS

Brainstem auditory evoked potentials (BAEPs) record at the scalp signals generated in the brainstem. These signals are evoked by 100-microsecond clicks delivered by earphones. The sources of the signals are nuclei and tracks associated with auditory localization, not speech discrimination, in the pons and midbrain.

The proximal eighth cranial nerve is the source of wave I. That wave I assesses the peripheral portions of the auditory pathway. Wave I is normal in MS patients who have no hearing problem. The BAEP has four central waves labeled II–V (see Fig. 9-3). Wave II is generated by the cochlear nucleus. Wave III is generated around the superior olive and trapezoid body in the central pons. Waves IV and V arise from lateral lemniscus bilaterally in the upper pons to lower midbrain. Internuclear ophthalmoplegia is the most common clinical sign corresponding to BAEP abnormalities.

Table 9-1 shows the correlation between BAEP and signs and symptoms.

Typical BAEP abnormalities in MS patients are delayed waves II–V and wave V amplitude decrease or absence. Figure 9-4 shows examples of BAEP abnormalities in MS of progressively worsening degrees.

Other neurologic disorders also affect BAEPs, for example, tumors (House and Brackmann, 1979; Brown et al., 1981), ischemia (Brown et al., 1981), and some hereditary-degenerative neurological disorders (Nuwer et al., 1983). Therefore, BAEP abnormalities are not pathognomonic of MS. Abnormalities just indicate impairment at the pons or lower midbrain.

In Chiappa's (1990) aggregate results from many published reports (Robinson and Rudge, 1977a, 1977b; Stockard and Rossiter, 1977; Lacquanti et al., 1979; Mogensen and Kristensen, 1979; Chiappa et al., 1980a; Green et al., 1980; Hausler and Levine, 1980; Robinson and Rudge, 1980; Stockard and Sharbrough, 1980; Tackman et al., 1980; Fischer et al., 1981; Khoshbin and Hallett, 1981; Parving et al., 1981; Purves et al., 1981; Shanon et al., 1981; Barajas, 1982; Elidan et al., 1982; Green et al., 1982; Prasher et al., 1982;

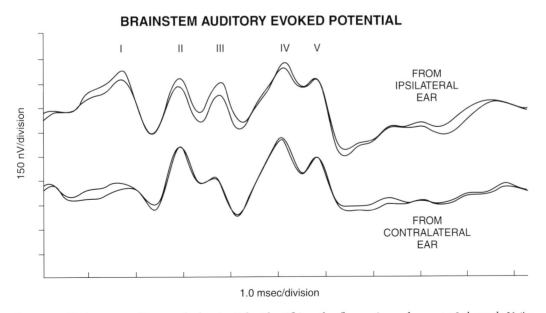

Figure 9-3 Brainstem auditory evoked potentials, identifying the five main peaks waves I through V (in Roman numerals). (From Nuwer et al. 1994b.)

TABLE 9-1 Correlation between Degree of BAEP Abnormality and Multiple Sclerosis Patient Signs and Symptoms

Correlation with Change	
In BAEPs	History
0.41	Diplopia
0.23	Dysphagia
0.16	Vertigo
0.12	Hearing Impairment
0.10	Dysarthria
0.03	Facial Sensory Impairment
	Physical Signs
0.39	Ocular Dysmetria or Gaze Paresis
0.32	Nystagmus
0.29	Facial Weakness
0.25	Dysarthria
0.23	Facial Sensory Loss
0.21	Slow Tongue Movements
0.09	Other Brainstem Signs
0.04	Subjective Hearing Threshold

BAEP, brainstem auditory evoked potential.

Source: From Nuwer et al., 1988.

BRAINSTEM AUDITORY EVOKED POTENTIALS WITH VARIOUS DEGREES OF CHANGE IN WAVES IV &V

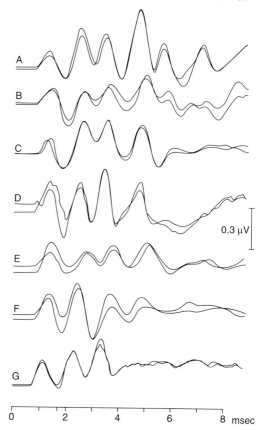

Figure 9-4 Examples of various degrees of abnormality in the brainstem auditory evoked potential test in multiple sclerosis. The upper evoked potential traces are less affected, and the lower traces are more affected. Demyelination causes some prolongation of latencies, with loss of amplitude and eventual absence of peaks II–V. (From Nuwer et al., 1988.)

Tackmann and Ettlin, 1982; Hutchinson et al., 1984; Kayamori et al., 1984; Koffler et al., 1984), 46% of approximately 1000 MS patients had abnormal BAEPs (Table 9-2). Among patients without brainstem symptoms or signs, 38% had clinically silent BAEP abnormalities.

Brainstem auditory evoked potentials are more sensitive for pontine lesions than MRI (Cutler et al., 1986; Comi et al., 1987, 1989; Baum et al., 1988). Brain MRI advantage is in finding lesions in many places, whereas BAEP is specific to a limited part of the brain stem. Among studies directly comparing the two tests, brain MRI was abnormal among 68%–83% of patients, whereas BAEP was abnormal among 41%–50% (Giesser et al., 1987; Comi et al., 1989; Gilmore et al., 1989).

Overall, BAEP can confirm that cranial nerve signs or symptoms are due to central brainstem impairment, as opposed to impairment along the peripheral pathways. The test is sensitive to pons and lower midbrain impairment.

SOMATOSENSORY EVOKED POTENTIALS

Somatosensory testing begins with a brief electrical stimulus to the median nerve at the wrist or posterior tibial nerve at the ankle. Recordings are made using electrodes over the brachial plexus or lumbar spine, cervical spine, and scalp. The somatosensory evoked potentials (SEPs) travel along the posterior columns, medial lemniscus, and internal capsule.

TABLE 9-2 Rates of Abnormalities for Evoked Potentials in Multiple Sclerosis: Aggregate Results of 26–31 Separate Research Series

	VEP	BAEP	SEP
No. of patients	1950	1006	1006
No. of research series	26	26	31
Rates of EP abnormality			
Definite MS	85%	67%	77%
Probable MS	58%	41%	67%
Possible MS	37%	30%	49%
Asymptomatic patients	51%	38%	42%
All patients	63%	46%	58% (upper extremity) 76% (lower extremity)

BAEP, brainstem auditory evoked potential; EP, evoked potential; MS, multiple sclerosis; SEP, somatosensory evoked potential; VEP, visual evoked potential.

Source: From Chiappa, 1990.

Median nerve SEP peaks are generated at brachial plexus, mid-cervical cord, cervicomedullary junction, upper midbrain or thalamus, and Rolandic fissure (see Fig. 9-5). Posterior tibial nerve SEPs' main potentials are from lumbar spinal cord and Rolandic fissure. Comparison among these peaks reveals the anatomic level of lemniscal pathway disruption. This is useful when approximate anatomic localization is valuable.

In Chiappa's (1990) summary of results among clinical studies in MS (Namerrow, 1968, 1970; Anziska et al., 1978; Dorfman et al., 1978; Mastaglia et al., 1978; Small et al., 1978; Eisen et al., 1979; Eisen and Nudleman, 1979; Matthews and Esiri, 1979; Matthews and Small, 1979; Trojaborg and Petersen, 1979; Abbruzzese et al., 1980; Chiappa, 1980; Chiappa et al., 1980b; Dau et al., 1980; Diener and Scheibler, 1980; Eisen and Odusote, 1980; Ganes, 1980; Green et al., 1980; Hausler and Levine, 1980; Kjaer, 1980a, 1980b; Noel and Desmedt, 1980; Stockard and Sharbrough, 1980; Tackmann et al., 1980; Weiner and Dawson, 1980; Eisen et al., 1981, 1982; Purves et al., 1981; Trojaborg et al., 1981; Kazis et al., 1982; van Buggenhout et al., 1982; Walsh et al., 1982; Larrea and Mauguiere, 1988), median nerve SEP was abnormal in 42% of MS patients without sensory signs or symptoms; and abnormal in 75% of patients who *did* have sensory signs or

symptoms. Posterior tibial SEPs had somewhat higher rates of clinically silent abnormalities (see Table 9-3). Delays in SEP correlated with the expanded disability status scale (EDSS) findings (Koehler et al., 2000). Abnormalities in SEP parallel clinical measures of limb impairment in MS patients (Nociti et al., 2008).

Various neurologic disorders can affect SEPs. Peripheral effects can be identified by measuring central conduction separately from peripheral conduction, which is checked at the brachial plexus or lumbar spinal cord. Some hereditary-degenerative neurologic conditions can impair central sensory conduction (Nuwer et al., 1983). So can B12 deficiency (Fine and Hallet, 1980; Misra et al., 2003). Focal ischemia, tumors, and cervical myelopathy can disrupt central lemniscal conduction. Central delay of SEP is not specific to MS (Cruccu et al., 2008).

Brain MRI tests a much wider area of brain and spinal anatomy, so that the MRI is more sensitive than either median or posterior tibial nerve SEP in MS. In two direct comparisons, 48%–54% of early MS patients had an abnormal median nerve SEP and 61%–72% had abnormal posterior tibial nerve SEPs, whereas brain MRI more often had abnormalities among the same patients (Comi et al., 1989; Gilmore et al., 1989). In a series of patients with spinal cord symptoms being

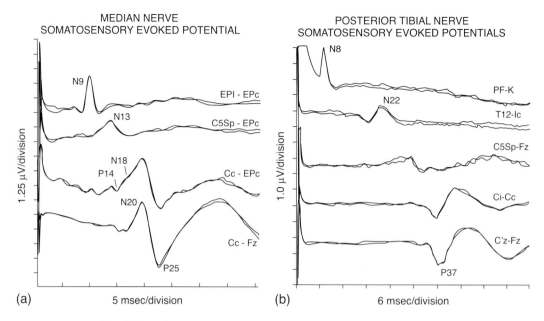

Figure 9-5 Examples of the peaks seen in normal short latency (*A*) median nerve and (*B*) posterior tibial nerve, somatosensory evoked potential testing. Negative potentials are upward deflections here. Recording sites EPi and EPc are at shoulders; C5Sp and T12 over the spine; PF, K, and IC at popliteal fossa, knee, and iliac crest; Ci, Cc, C'z, and Fz on scalp. The several standard peaks are identified here. (From Nuwer et al., 1994a.)

evaluated for MS, 67% (31/46) had an abnormal cervical MRI, whereas 57% (26/46) had abnormal SEPs (Miller et al., 1987).

The American Academy of Neurology evidence-based assessment of SEPs recommends the technique as possibly useful to identify patients at increased risk for developing clinically definite MS (Gronseth and Ashman, 2000).

Overall, SEPs are a useful tool for detecting clinically silent lesions, and they can contribute to the diagnosis of MS. They provide a sensitive way to assess the lemniscal spinal and intracranial pathways.

MOTOR EVOKED POTENTIALS

Cerebral neurons can be discharged by a brief electrical stimulus. This can be delivered through the intact skull. Considerable voltage is needed to drive transcranial electrical currents from the scalp through the skull to the cortex. In awake patients such electrical stimulation is painful.

An ingenious painless solution is to use a powerful magnetic device held above the scalp. Each stimulus is a brief, extremely intense magnetic field. The skull is a resistor for electrical currents, but magnetic fields pass unimpeded through the intact skull. Faraday's law of electromagnetic induction describes that a change in a magnetic field creates an electrical potential. The brief intense magnetic field above the scalp evokes an electric current in the cerebral cortex strong enough to discharge neurons (Barker et al., 1985, 1986). This can be focused in a particular small region under the magnetic stimulator. The specific cortical region stimulated is chosen by locating the magnetic coil over the corresponding scalp.

Clinicians studying motor pathways now use the magnetically stimulated motor evoked potentials (MEPs). These have been evaluated in MS and other neurological disorders (Merton and Morton, 1980; Merton et al., 1982). Motor EPs are sensitive to corticospinal impairment early in the course of MS (Rico et al., 2009). Markedly prolonged central

TABLE 9-3 Evoked Potential Findings among 101 Patients with Chronic Progressive Multiple Sclerosis (Left and Right Sides Scored Separately)

Pattern Visual EPs	
Median P100 latency	119 msec (normal < 105)
Number normal	50/202 (25%)
present but abnormal	132/202 (65%)
absent	20/202 (10%)
Median P100 amplitude	4.0 microV
Brainstem Auditory EPs	
Median I–V interpeak latency	4.4 msec (normal < 4.6)
Median V/I amplitude ratio	64% (normal > 50%)
Number normal	105/202 (52%)
wave V present but abnormal	24/202 (12%)
wave V absent	63/202 (32%)
all peaks absent	2/202 (1%)
Median Nerve Somatosensory EPs	
Number normal	15/202 (7%)
Number N9 absent	0/202
N13 absent	70/202 (35%)
N20 absent	115/202 (57%)
N20 latency	26 msec
N20 amplitude	0.8 microV

Source: From Nuwer et al., 1987.

Note. Small adjustments to normal limits for individual patients were made for age, gender, and height (details not shown here). Absent peaks were excluded from median latency determination here. Somatosensory normal limits were N20-N9 <10.5 msec, N20-N13 <7.0 msec plus N13-N9 < 4.3 msec; absolute latencies of N20 were not used when assessing normality.

EPs, evoked potentials.

motor conduction times are seen in most MS patients tested (Cowan et al., 1984; Mills and Murray, 1985; Hess et al., 1986, 1987; Ingram et al., 1988; Jones et al., 1991; Mayr et al., 1991; Ravnborg et al., 1992; Segura et al., 1994; Di Lazzaro et al., 1999; Cruz-Martinez et al., 2000; Dan et al., 2000). In MS, lower-extremity MEPs are abnormal more often than upper-extremity MEPs. Exercise increases the abnormality rate (Nielsen and Norgaard, 2002; Perretti et al., 2004). Motor EPs are well suited for identifying silent lesions in MS patients. They are an objective measure for MS therapeutic trials (Kandler et al., 1991a, 1991b; Andersson et al., 1995). Motor EP correlates well with MRI lesions in cervical corticospinal tracks (Cruz-Martinez et al., 2000). They correspond less well with physical signs of weakness (Segura et al., 1994; Humm et al., 2003).

Ongoing muscle activity is disrupted by some MEPs. The duration of this disruption is known as the silent period. Ongoing investigations suggest that this is dependent on spinocerebellar pathways. A prolonged silent period may be a sign of cerebellar involvement in MS patients (Tataroglu et al., 2003).

Other versions of MEPs have looked at the science of fatigue with repetitive stimulation (Brasil-Neto et al., 1994; Liepert et al., 1996; Schubert et al., 1998; Petajan and White, 2000). Further studies note relationships between MS symptoms and variations on MEP techniques (Fuhr and Kappos, 2001).

Central motor conduction tests can be abnormal in other neurological disorders. Slowed MEPs were found in 85% of amyotrophic lateral sclerosis patients (Berardelli et al., 1987; Hugon et al., 1987), whereas SEPs were normal. Patients with hereditary motor and sensory neuropathy (HMSN) patients had delayed central conduction when they had clinical signs of corticospinal disease (Claus et al., 1990).

Motor EP is used more widely outside the United States. It is used less in the United States partly because the Food and Drug Administration (FDA) has not given full approval for magnet use for clinical brain stimulation. It is approved for peripheral nerve stimulation. Central use is off label. Motor EPs should be considered as a diagnostic test for MS, as well as in the diagnosis evaluation of other possible central motor disorders.

EVENT-RELATED POTENTIALS

Cognitive processes can be measured by special EPs known as event-related potentials (ERPs). These mark certain internal recognition events and decision-making processes. P300, the most common ERP, uses the auditory oddball paradigm (Goodin et al., 1994). A series of brief tones is presented, most at one pitch intermixed with occasional (rare) tones at a different pitch. The patient is asked to count silently the rare tones. An extra positive polarity potential occurs around 300 msec after each rare tone. That peak, measured over the scalp vertex, is referred to as the P300. It corresponds to the brain recognizing the rare tone, "Oh, that's it! Count it!"

The P300 ERP peak latency is delayed in dementia but not in depression. In MS patients, P300 often is delayed (Aminoff and Goodin, 2001) as are earlier primary auditory cortical peaks. The results may be a combination of primary sensory system and cognitive processing speed delays. P300 delay in MS is worse among patients with secondary progressive MS (Ellger et al., 2002). Visual P300 also is often abnormal (Sailer et al., 2001).

Serial ERP studies in MS measured progression of the P300 cognitive processing delays over time (Gerschlager et al., 2000), which did not correspond to EDSS changes.

MULTIMODALITY EVOKED POTENTIAL TESTING

It is worthwhile to compare EP modalities with each other, and to compare EPs with MRI and cerebral spinal fluid (CSF) findings. Chiappa (1990) summarized results from several thousand patients among 26–31 published reports of VEP, BAEP, and SEP in MS patients (Namerow, 1968, 1970; Halliday et al., 1973a, 1973b; Asselman et al., 1975; Hume and Cant, 1976; Lowitzsch et al., 1976; Mastaglia et al., 1976; Celesia and Daly, 1977; Hennerici et al., 1977; Matthews et al., 1977; Robinson and Rudge, 1977a, 1977b; Stockard and Rossiter, 1977; Anziska et al., 1978; Cant et al., 1978; Collins et al., 1978; Dorfman et al., 1978; Duwaer and Spekreijse, 1978; Mastaglia et al., 1978; Nillson, 1978; Shahrokhi et al., 1978; Small et al., 1978; Wist et al., 1978; Eisen et al., 1979; Eisen and Nudleman, 1979; Lacquanti et al., 1979; Matthews and Esiri, 1979; Matthews and Small, 1979; Mogensen and Kristensen, 1979; Rigolet et al., 1979; Tackmann et al., 1979; Trojaborg and Petersen, 1979; Abbruzzese et al., 1980; Chiappa, 1980, Chiappa et al., 1980a, 1980b; Dau et al., 1980; Diener and Scheibler, 1980; Eisen and Odusote, 1980; Ganes, 1980; Green et al., 1980; Hausler and Levine, 1980; Kjaer, 1980a, 1980b; Noel and Desmedt, 1980; Robinson and Rudge, 1980; Stockard and Sharbrough, 1980; Tackman et al., 1980; Weiner and Dawson, 1980; Wilson and Keyser, 1980; Eisen et al., 1981; Fischer et al., 1981; Khoshbin and Hallett, 1981; Parving et al., 1981; Purves et al., 1981; Shanon et al., 1981; Trojaborg et al., 1981; Barajas, 1982; Eisen et al., 1982; Elidan et al., 1982; Green et al., 1982; Kazis et al., 1982; Prasher et al., 1982; Tackmann and Ettlin, 1982; van Buggenhout et al., 1982; Walsh et al., 1982; Hutchinson et al., 1984; Kayamori et al., 1984; Koffler et al., 1984; Larrea and Mauguiere, 1988). See Table 9-2. Visual EP had the highest overall rate of abnormality and BAEPs the lowest. Abnormality rates of SEPs were similar to VEPs, even higher in the possible and probable MS categories. Lower extremity SEPs from nerves are abnormal more often than median nerve SEPs. Silent lesions, that is, EP abnormalities despite no signs or symptoms in that sensory modality, are seen in a third to a half of the MS patients.

Among patients with a more severe degree of MS, SEPs are more likely to be abnormal compared to VEP or BAEP. In one study (Nuwer et al., 1987) of the three sensory EP modalities in 101 patients with chronic progressive MS, median nerve SEPs were abnormal in EPs in 93%, VEPs in 75%, and BAEPs in 48%. Table 9-3 compares sensory EPs. Similar results have been reported in children with MS (Brass et al., 2003; Pohl et al., 2006).

Comparing MEPs to sensory EPs in MS, one study found that lower extremity SEPs were abnormal most often (75% of patients), followed by lower-extremity MEPs (65%), VEPs (64%), upper-extremity MEPs and SEPs (56% and 52%), and finally BAEPs (39%) (Filippi et al., 1995). In another study of early relapsing-remittting MS (Jung et al., 2008), the lower-extremity MEPs were most sensitive (68%), followed by VEP (62%) and then lower-extremity SEPs (57%). Patients with chronic progressive MS had the highest rate and greatest degrees of EP abnormalities. Other reports noted worse MEPs among secondary progressive than relapsing-remitting MS (Facchetti et al., 1997), and that MEPs were abnormal more often than SEPs (Andersson et al., 1995).

Motor EPs have been compared to multimodality sensory EPs (VEP, BAEP, SEP) and MRI in patients clinically suspected of MS. In one study of patients who eventually were diagnosed with MS (Ravnborg et al., 1992), the MRI was positive in 88%; MEP, 83%; VEP, 67%; SEP, 63%; and BAEP, 42%. For some patients eventually diagnosed with MS, the MRI initially was normal but the EPs were abnormal.

How useful are EPs for patients being evaluated for possible MS? For 2 1/2 years, Hume and Waxman (1988) followed 222 patients suspected of having MS. Among those patients, 48 eventually developed clinically definite MS. Among those 48 patients, 90% had abnormal sensory EPs during their initial clinical workup, providing positive diagnostic evidence of a silent lesion previously unsuspected. Abnormal EPs were occasionally seen in other disorders (De Seze et al., 2001).

Hume and Waxman (1988) assessed also the likelihood of MS progression in patients with possible MS. They found a 71% chance of clinical deterioration over 2 1/2 years if the patient had abnormal EPs, but only a 16% chance if the EPs were normal. Several CSF measures were not so accurate in predicting disease progression. Kallman et al. (2006) assessed 94 MS patients from first presentation until 10 years later. They found that SEP and MEP at first presentation predicted EDSS at 5 and 10 years: the worse the initial EPs, the worse the disability years later. Similarly, Leocani et al. (2006) found that among 84 MS patients, those with worse sensory and motor EPs had twice the chance of EDSS progression over 2 ½ years compared to those with fewer EP abnormalities. Changes in VEP and MRI also measured and predicted changes in EDSS and clinical progression over several years (Fuhr et al., 2001, Jung et al., 2008).

Magnetic resonance imaging has been considered more reliable for predicting a future diagnosis of MS (Polman et al., 2005) compared to CSF or EPs, although the EPs do provide helpful information (Filippini et al., 1994; Ghezzi et al., 1996, 2000). Magnetic resonance imaging has been compared directly to EPs in several studies. Both MRI and sensory EP testing are abnormal in at least 70% patients with definite or probable MS (Cutler et al., 1986; Farlow et al., 1986; Comi et al., 1987; Giesser et al., 1987; Baum et al., 1988; Guerit and Argile, 1988; Hume and Waxman, 1988; Comi et al., 1989; Gilmore et al., 1989; Rodriguez et al., 1995). Brainstem auditory EPs are more sensitive than MRI for detecting lesions in the pons (Cutler et al., 1986; Baum et al., 1988). Visual EPs are better than MRI at detecting optic nerve lesions. Magnetic resonance imaging can show multiplicity of lesions or classical MS distribution of lesions more effectively than multimodal EPs (Cutler et al., 1986; Farlow et al., 1986). Magnetic resonance imaging and sensory EPs were similarly effective in predicting an MS diagnosis, its course, or severity (Guerit and Argile, 1988; Hume and Waxman, 1988; Lee et al., 1991; O'Connor et al., 1998). Magnetic resonance imaging and MEP taken together were more effective at predicting disability than either alone (Kalkers et al., 2007). In the recent review by Leocani and Comi (2008), EPs were considered more useful for the assessment of disease progression, since EP abnormalities are more strictly related to disability than MRI lesion burden. Evoked potentials were considered useful to identify therapeutic nonresponders, to assess patients with ambiguous new symptoms, to confirm a dubious relapse, and to measure disease progression.

Compared to oligoclonal banding and similar CSF abnormalities, multimodal sensory EPs were slightly more likely to be abnormal in early or possible MS (Trojaborg et al., 1981; Bartel et al., 1983; Miller et al., 1983; Ganes et al., 1986; Cosi et al., 1987; Hume and Waxman, 1988; Lee et al., 1991; Irkec et al., 2001). Evoked potential abnormality is more accurate for predicting MS progression than are CSF changes. Patients with normal results on both EP and CSF studies are most likely to remain stable over time.

In a formal technology assessment, the American Academy of Neurology (AAN) looked at EPs in MS (Gronseth and Ashman, 2000). They used a structured literature review to assess the usefulness of evoked potentials in identifying clinically silent lesions in patients with suspected multiple sclerosis. The reports recommend using VEPs and SEPs to search for clinically silent lesions. Visual EPs were scored as probably useful and SEPs as possibly useful in predicting progression from initial evaluation to clinically definite MS within a few years. For BAEPs, there is a trend toward usefulness to search for silent lesions, but the magnitude of an effect is much less than for VEPs and SEPs. The reports note that there are other reasons for using EPs in MS beyond just searching for silent lesions. They may aid in localizing lesions, confirm clinically ambiguous lesions or the organic basis of symptoms, and suggest demyelination as the cause of a suspicious lesion.

In these days of limited health-care resources, it is appropriate to compare resource utilization. In the United States, the Medicare Fee Schedule allows 9.58 relative value units (RVUs) for brain, 8.64 for cervical, and 8.66 for thoracic MRIs. In contrast, each sensory EP test is valued at an average of 2.83 RVUs, far less cost than for MRI testing.

The different types of tests are complementary to each other, MRI assessing anatomy and EPs assessing physiology (Cruccu et al., 2008). Evoked potentials, MRI, and CSF studies have their own niches in the diagnostic evaluation paradigm.

USE OF EVOKED POTENTIALS IN MULTIPLE SCLEROSIS THERAPEUTIC TRIALS

Evoked potentials are useful as a measuring tool in MS therapeutic trials (Nuwer et al., 1987). Evoked potential testing is easily repeated at modest costs. Grouped EP data track the accumulating disease burden (Hennerici et al., 1977; Nuwer et al., 1987; Brigell et al., 1994). Evoked potentials tend to worsen progressively in MS. They can detect the physiologic remnants of previous demyelination that may have become inapparent on MRIs. The gradual progression of EPs provides an objective, quantified measure that parallels progression in EDSS (O'Connor et al., 1998; Koehler et al., 2000; Niklas et al., 2009). Because the EPs detect clinically silent lesions, they are not redundant with any signs or symptoms detectable by physical examination or history.

In therapeutic trials EPs ought to be scored in terms of the actual latency values. Test-retest differences ought to be measured by direct, careful comparison of EP traces themselves, not by completely separate scoring of the individual traces. This substantially reduces the trial-to-trial interpretation variability. Year-to-year comparisons can be carried out using parametric statistics. This is far superior to the better/worse/unchanged, changed/unchanged, or normal/abnormal scoring that is used in some MS trials.

Evoked potentials can reliably measure and predict the courses in groups in MS patients (Fuhr et al., 2001). They were valuable in several therapeutic trials. In a trial of azathioprine and steroids, VEP and SEP predicted 3-year study outcome at year one (Nuwer et al., 1987). In a trial of azathioprine, antilymphocyte globulin, and steroid (Mertin et al., 1982), VEPs deteriorated in the control group but were stable in the immunosuppressed group. In a study of steroid treatment, EPs correlated with clinical disability scores (La Mantia et al., 1994). In interferon studies, VEPs were reliable indices to follow clinical progress (Sipe et al., 1984; Anlar et al., 2003; Weinstock-Guttman et al., 2003). Similar improvements were seen for MEPs in a steroid and cyclophosphamide study (Manova et al., 2001), where it paralleled the EDSS. P300 steroid therapy showed P300 (Filipovic et al., 1997) and MEP (Fierro et al., 2002) improvement.

Other studies found change neither in clinical scores nor in EPs. Those drugs may be ineffective in MS, for example, hyperbaric oxygen (Neiman et al., 1985; Harpur et al., 1986) and acyclovir (Lycke et al., 1996). In studies of plasmapheresis, EPs paralleled clinical findings (Dau et al., 1980; Weiner and Dawson, 1980; Gordon et al., 1985; Khatrie et al., 1985; Sorensen et al., 1996).

Overall, EPs are cost-effective tools that can add easily measured and quantified statistical significance to the results of an MS therapeutic trial.

REFERENCES

Abbruzzese G, Abbruzzese M, Favale E, Ivaldi M, Leandri M, Ratto S. The effect of hand muscle vibration on the somatosensory evoked potential in man: an interaction between lemniscal and spinocerebellar inputs? *J Neurol Neurosurg Psychiat.* 1980;43:433–437.

Aminoff JC, Goodin DS. Long-latency cerebral event-related potentials in multiple sclerosis. *J Clin Neurophysiol.* 2001;18:372–377.

Andersson T, Siden A, Persson A. A comparison of motor evoked potentials and somatosensory evoked potentials in patients with multiple sclerosis and potentially related conditions. *Electromyogr Clin Neurophysiol.* 1995;35:17–24.

Anlar O, Kisli M, Tombul T. Visual evoked potentials in multiple sclerosis before and after two years of interferon therapy. *Intern J Neurosci.* 2003;113:483–489.

Anziska B, Cracco RQ, Cook AW, Feld EW. Somatosensory far field potentials: studies in normal subjects and patients with multiple sclerosis. *Electroencephalogr clin Neurophysiol.* 1978;45:602–610.

Asselman P, Chadwick DW, Marsden CD. Visual evoked responses in the diagnosis and management of patients suspected of multiple sclerosis. *Brain.* 1975; 98:261–282.

Bajada S, Mastaglia FL, Black JL, Collins DWK. Effects of induced hyperthermia on visual evoked potentials and saccade parameters in normal subjects and multiple sclerosis patients. *J Neurol Neurosurg Psychiat.* 1980; 43:849–852.

Barajas JJ. Evaluation of ipsilateral and contralateral brainstem auditory evoked potentials in multiple sclerosis patients. *J Neurol Sci.* 1982;54:69–78.

Barker AT, Freeston IL, Jalinous R, Jarratt JA. Clinical evaluation of conduction time measurements in central motor pathways using magnetic stimulation of the human brain. *Lancet.* 1986;1:1325–1326.

Barker AT, Jalinous R, Freeston IL. Non–invasive magnetic stimulation of human motor cortex. *Lancet.* 1985; 2:1106–1107.

Bartel DR, Markand ON, Kolar OJ. The diagnosis and classification of multiple sclerosis: evoked responses and spinal fluid electrophoresis. *Neurology.* 1983; 33:611–617.

Baum K, Scheuler W, Hegerl U, Girke W, Schörner W. Detection of brainstem lesions in multiple sclerosis: comparison of brainstem auditory evoked potentials with nuclear magnetic resonance imaging. *Acta Neurol Scand.* 1988;77:283–288.

Bee YS, Lin MC, Wang CC, Sheu SJ. Optic neuritis: clinical analysis of 27 cases. *Kaohsiung J Med Sci.* 2003;19: 105–112.

Berardelli A, Inghilleri M, Formisano R, Accornero N, Manfredi M. Stimulation of motor tracts in motor neuron disease. *J Neurol Neurosurg Psychiat.* 1987; 50:732–737.

Brasil-Neto JP, Cohen LG, Hallett M. Central fatigue as revealed by postexercise decrement of motor evoked potentials. *Muscle Nerve.* 1994;17:713–719.

Brass SD, Caramanos Z, Santos C, Dilenge ME, Lapierre Y, Rosenblatt B. Multiple sclerosis vs acute disseminated encephalomyelitis in childhood. *Pediatr Neurol.* 2003;29:227–231.

Brigell M, Kaufman DI, Bobak P, Beydoun A. The pattern visual evoked potential: a multicenter study using standardized techniques. *Doc Ophthalmol.* 1994;86:65–79.

Brooks EB, Chiappa KH. A comparison of clinical neuro-ophthalmological findings and pattern shift visual evoked potentials in multiple sclerosis. In: Courjan JJ, Mauguiere F, Revol M, eds. *Clinical Applications of Evoked Potentials in Neurology.* New York: Raven Press; 1982:453–457.

Brown RH, Chiappa KH, Brooks EG. Brainstem auditory evoked responses in 22 patients with intrinsic brainstem lesions: implications for clinical interpretations. *Electroencephalogr Clin Neurophysiol.* 1981;51:38P.

Brusa A, Jones SJ, Plant GT. Long-term remyelination after optic neuritis. *Brain.* 2001;124:468–479.

Cant BR, Hume AL, Judson JA, Shaw NA. The assessment of severe head injury by short-latency somatosensory and brain-stem auditory evoked potentials. *Electroencephalogr Clin Neurophysiol.* 1986;65:188–195.

Cant BR, Hume AL, Shaw NA. Effects of luminance on the pattern visual evoked potential in multiple sclerosis. *Electroencephalogr Clin Neurophysiol.* 1978;45:496–504.

Celesia GG, Daly RF. Visual electroencephalographic computer analysis (VECA). *Neurology.* 1977;27:637–641.

Chiappa KH. Pattern shift visual, brainstem auditory, and short-latency somatosensory evoked potentials in multiple sclerosis. *Neurology.* 1980;30(7 pt 2):110–123.

Chiappa KH. *Evoked Potentials in Clinical Medicine.* 2nd ed. New York: Raven Press; 1990.

Chiappa KH, Choi S, Young RR. Short latency somatosensory evoked potentials following median nerve stimulation in patients with neurological lesions. *Progr Clin Neurolphysiol.* 1980b;7:264–281.

Chiappa KH, Harrison JL, Brooks EB, Young RR. Brainstem auditory evoked responses in 200 patients with multiple sclerosis. *Ann Neurol.* 1980a;7:135–143.

Claus D, Waddy HM, Harding AE, Murray NMF, Thomas PK. Hereditary motor and sensory neuropathies and hereditary spastic paraplegia: a magnetic stimulation study. *Ann Neurol.* 1990;28:43–49.

Collins DWK, Black JL, Mastaglia FL. Pattern reversal visual evoked potential. *J Neurol Sci.* 1978;36:83–95.

Comi G, Canal N, Martinelli V, et al. Comparison between magnetic resonance imaging and other techniques in 39 multiple sclerosis patients. *Rivista de Neurologia.* 1987;57:44–47.

Comi G, Filippi M, Rovaris M, Leocani L, Medaglini S, Locatelli T. Clinical, neurophysiological, and magnetic resonance imaging correlations in multiple sclerosis. *J Neurol Neurosurg Psychiat.* 1998;64(suppl 1):S21–S25.

Comi G, Locatelli T, Leocani L, Medaglini S, Rossi P, Martinelli V. Can evoked potentials be useful in monitoring multiple sclerosis evolution? *Clin Neurophysiol.* 1999;40:349–357.

Comi G, Martinelli V, Medaglini S, et al. Correlation between multimodal evoked potentials and magnetic resonance imaging in multiple sclerosis. *Neurology.* 1989;39:4–8.

Cordonnier C, de Seze J, Breteau G, et al. Prospective study of patients presenting with acute partial transverse myelopathy. *J Neurol.* 2003;250:1447–1452.

Cosi V, Citterio A, Battelli G, Bergamaschi R, Grampa G, Callieco R. Multimodal evoked potentials in multiple sclerosis: a contribution to diagnosis and classification. *Ital J Neurol Sci.* 1987;8(suppl 6):109–112.

Cowan JMA, Rothwell JC, Dick JPR, Thompson PD, Day BL, Marsden CD. Abnormalities in central motor pathway conduction in multiple sclerosis. *Lancet.* 1984; 2:304–307.

Cruccu G, Aminoff MJ, Curio G, et al. Recommendations for the clinical use of somatosensory-evoked potentials. *Clin Neurophysiol.* 2008;119(8):1705–1719.

Cruz-Martinez A, Gonzalez-Orodea JI, Lopez Pajares R, Arpa J. Disability in multiple sclerosis: the role of transcranial magnetic stimulation. *Electromyogr Clin Neurophysiol.* 2000;40:441–447.

Culter JR, Aminoff MJ and Brant-Zawadzki M. Evaluation of patients with multiple sclerosis by evoked potentials and magnetic resonance imaging: a comparative study. *Ann Neurol.* 1986;20:645–648.

Dan B, Christiaens F, Christophe C, Dachy B. Transcranial magnetic stimulaton and other evoked potentials in pediatric multiple sclerosis. *Pediatr Neurol.* 2000;22: 136–138.

Dau PC, Petajan JH, Johnson KP, Panitch HS, Borenstein MB. Plasmapheresis in multiple sclerosis: preliminary findings. *Neurology.* 1980;30:1023–1028.

Davies HD, Carroll WM, Mastaglia FL. Effects of hyperventilation on pattern-reversal visual evoked potentials in patients with demyelination. *J Neurol Neurosurg Psychiat.* 1986;49:1392–1396.

Davies MB, Williams R, Haq N, Pelosi L, Hawkins CP. MRI of optic nerve and postchiasmal visual pathways and visual evoked potentials in secondary progressive multiple sclerosis. *Neuroradiology.* 1998;40:765–770.

De Seze J, Stojkovic T, Breteau G, et al. Acute myelopathies: clinical, laboratory and outcome profiles in 79 cases. *Brain.* 2001;124:1509–1521.

Diener HC, Scheibler H. Follow-up studies of visual potentials in multiple sclerosis evoked by checkerboard and foveal stimulation. *Electroencephalogr Clin Neurophysiol.* 1980;49:490–496.

Di Lazzaro V, Oliviero A, Profice P. The dignostic value of motor evoked potentials *Clin Neurophysiol.* 1999;110: 1297–1307.

Dorfman LJ, Bosley TM, Cummins KL. Electrophysiological localization of central somatosensory lesions in patients with multiple sclerosis. *Electroencephalogr Clin Neurophysiol.* 1978;44:742–753.

Duwaer AL, Spekreijse H. Latency of luminance and contrast evoked potentials in multiple sclerosis patients. *Electroencephalogr Clin Neurophysiol.* 1978;45:244–258.

Eisen A, Nudleman K. Cord to cortex conduction in multiple sclerosis. *Neurology.* 1979;29:189–193.

Eisen A, Odusote K. Central and peripheral conduction times in multiple sclerosis. *Electroencephalogr Clin Neurophysiol.* 1980;48:253–265.

Eisen A, Paty D, Purves S, Hoirch M. Occult fifth nerve dysfunction in multiple sclerosis. *Can J Neurol Sci.* 1981;8:221–225.

Eisen A, Purves S, Hoirch M. Central nervous system amplification: its potential in the diagnosis of early multiple sclerosis. *Neurology.* 1982;32:359–364.

Eisen A, Stewart J, Nudleman K, Cosgrove JBR. Short-latency somatosensory reponses in multiple sclerosis. *Neurology.* 1979;29:827–834.

Elidan J, Sohmer H, Gafni M, Kahana E. Contribution of changes in click rate and intensity on diagnosis of multiple sclerosis by brainstem auditory evoked potentials. *Acta Naurol Scand.* 1982;65:570–585.

Ellger T, Bethke F, Frese A, et al. Event-related potentials in different subtypes of multiple sclerosis: a cross-sectional study. *J Neurol Sci.* 2002;205:35–40.

Emerson R. Evoked potentials in clinical trials for multiple sclerosis. *J Clin Neurophysiol.* 1998;15:109–116.

Facchetti D, Mai R, Micheli A, et al. Motor evoked potentials and disability in secondary progressive multiple sclerosis. *Can J Neurol Sci.* 1997;24:332–337.

Farlow MR, Markand ON, Edwards MK, Stevens JC, Kolar OJ. Multiple sclerosis: magnetic resonance imaging, evoked responses, and spinal fluid electrophoresis. *Neurology.* 1986;36:828–831.

Fierro B, Salemi G, Brighina F, et al. A transcranial magnetic stimulation study evaluating methylprednisolone treatment in multiple sclerosis. *Acta Neurol Scand.* 2002;105:152–157.

Filipovic SR, Drulovic J, Stojsavljevic N, Levic Z. The effects of high-dose intravenous methylprednisolone on event-related potentials in patients with multiple sclerosis. *J Neurol Sci.* 1997;152:147–153.

Filippi M, Campi A, Mammi S, et al. Brain magnetic resonance imaging and multimodal evoked potentials in benign and secondary progressive multiple sclerosis. *J Neurol Neurosurg Psychiat.* 1995;58:31–37.

Filippini G, Comi GC, Cosi V, et al. Sensitivities and predictive values of paraclinical tests for diagnosing multiple sclerosis. *J Neurol.* 1994;241:132–137.

Fine EJ, Hallet M. Neurophysiological study of subacute combined degeneration. *J Neurol Sci.* 1980;45: 331–336.

Fischer C, Blanc A, Mauguiere F, Courjon J. Apport des potentiels evoqués auditifs précoces au diagnostic neurologique. *Rev Neurol.* 1981;137:229–240.

Fraser C, Klistorner A, Graham S, Garrick R, Billson F, Grigg J. Multifocal visual evoked potential latency analysis: predicting progression to multiple sclerosis. *Arch Neurol.* 2006b;63:847–850.

Fraser CL, Klistorner A, Graham SL, Garrick R, Billson FA, Grigg JR. Multifocal visual evoked potential analysis of inflammatory or demyelinating optic neuritis. *Ophthalmology.* 2006a;113: 315–323.

Frederiksen JL, Larsson HBW, Olesen J. Stigsby G. MRI, VEP, SEP, and biothesiometry suggest monosymptomatic acute optic neuritis to be a first manifestation of multiple sclerosis. *Acta Neurol Scand.* 1990;83: 343–350.

Frederiksen JL, Petrera J. Serial visual evoked potentials in 90 untreated patients with acute optic neuritis. *Surv Ophthalmol.* 1999;44:S54–S62.

Frederiksen JL, Petrera J, Larsson HBW, Stigsby B, Olesen J. Serial MRI, VEP, SEP and biotesiometry in acute optic neuritis: value of baseline results to predict the development of new lesions at one year follow up. *Acta Neurol Scand.* 1996;93:246–252.

Fuhr P, Borggrefe-Chappuis A, Schindler C, Kappos L. Visual and motor evoked potentials in the course of multiple sclerosis. *Brain.* 2001;124:2162–2168.

Fuhr P, Kappos L. Evoked potentials for evaluation of multiple sclerosis. *Clin Neurophysiol.* 2001;112: 2185–2189.

Ganes T. Somatosensory evoked response and central afferent conduction times in patients with multiple sclerosis. *J Neurol Neurosurg Psychiat.* 1980;43:948–953.

Ganes T, Brautaset NJ, Nyberg-Hansen, Vandvik B. Multimodal evoked response and cerebrospinal fluid oligoclonal immunoglobulins in patients with multiple sclerosis. *Acta Neurol Scand.* 1986;73:472–476.

Gerschlager W, Beisteiner R, Deecke L, et al. Electrophysiological, neuropsychological and clinical findings in multiple sclerosis patients receiving interferon B-1b: a 1-year follow-up. *Eur Neurol.* 2000;44:205–209.

Ghezzi A, Martinelli V, Rodegher M, Zaffaroni M, Comi G. The prognosis of idiopathic optic neuritis. *Neurol Sci.* 2000;21:S865–S869.

Ghezzi A, Torri V, Zaffaroni M. Isolated optic neuritis and its prognosis for multiple sclerosis: a clinical and paraclinical study with evoked potentials, CSF examination and brain MRI. *Ital J Neurol Sci.* 1996;17:325–332.

Giesser BS, Kurtzberg D, Vaughan HG, et al. Trimodal evoked potentials compared with magnetic resonance imaging in the diagnosis of multiple sclerosis. *Arch Neurol.* 1987;44:281–284.

Gilmore RL, Kasarskis EJ, Carr WA, Norvell E. Comparative impact of paraclinical studies in establishing the diagnosis of multiple sclerosis. *Electroencephalogr Clin Neurophysiol.* 1989;73:433–442.

Gilmore RL, Kasarskis EJ, McAllister RG. Verapamil-induced changes in central conduction in patients with multiple sclerosis. *J Neurol Neurosurg Psychiat.* 1985;48:1140–1146.

Goodin D, Desmedt J, Maurer K, Nuwer MR. IFCN recommended standards for long-latency auditory event-related potentials. *Electroencephalogr Clin Neurophysiol.* 1994;91:18–20.

Gordon PA, Carroll DJ, Etches WS, et al. A double-blind controlled pilot study of plasma exchange versus sham apheresis in chronic progressive multiple sclerosis. *Can J Neurol Sci.* 1985;12:39–44.

Green JB, Price R. Woodbury SG. Short-latency somatosensory evoked potentials in multiple sclerosis: comparison with auditory and visual evoked potentials. *Arch Neurol.* 1980;37:630–633.

Green JB, Walcoff M, Lucke JF. Phenytoin prolongs far-field somatosensory and auditory evoked potentials interpeak latencies. *Neurology.* 1982;32:85–88.

Gronseth GS, Ashman EJ. Practice parameter: the usefulness of evoked potentials in identifying clinically silent lesions in patients with suspected multiple sclerosis (an evidence-based review) Report of the Quality Standards Subcommittee of the American Academy of Neurology. *Neurology.* 2000;54:1720–1725.

Grover LK, Hood DC, Ghadiali Q, et al. A comparison of multifocal and conventional visual evoked potential techniques in patients with optic neuritis/multiple sclerosis. *Doc Ophthalmol.* 2008;117:121–128.

Guerit JM, Argile AM. The sensitivity of multimodal evoked potentials in multiple sclerosis: a comparison with magnetic resonance imaging and cerebrospinal fluid analysis. *Electroencephalogr Clin Neurophysiol.* 1988;70:230–238.

Halliday AM, McDonald WI, Mushin J. Delayed visual evoked response in optic neuritis. *Lancet.* 1972;1: 982–985.

Halliday AM, McDonald WI, Mushin J. Delayed pattern evoked responses in optic neuritis in relation to visual acuity. *Trans Ophthalmol Soc UK.* 1973a;93: 314–324.

Halliday AM, McDonald, WI, Mushin J. Visual evoked response in the diagnosis of multiple sclerosis. *Br Med J.* 1973b;4:661–664.

Harpur GD, Suke R, Bass BH, et al. Hyperbaric oxygen therapy in chronic stable multiple sclerosis: double-blind study. *Neurology.* 1986;36:988–991.

Hausler R, Levine RA. Brain stem auditory evoked potentials are related to interaural time discrimination in patients with multiple sclerosis. *Brain Res.* 1980;191: 589–594.

Hennerici M, Wenzel D, Freund HJ. The comparison of small-size rectangle and checkerboard stimulation for the evaluation of delayed visual evoked response in patients suspected of multiple sclerosis. *Brain.* 1977;100:119–136.

Hess CW, Mills KR, Murray NMF. Measurement of central motor conduction in multiple sclerosis by magnetic brain stimulation. *Lancet.* 1986;2:596–600.

Hess CW, Mills KR, Murray NMF, Schriefer TN. Magnetic brain stimulation: central motor conduction studies in multiple sclerosis. *Ann Neurol.* 1987;22:744–752.

Hickman SJ, Kapoor R, Jones SJ, Altmann DR, Plant GT, Miller DH. Corticosteroids do not prevent optic nerve atrophy following optic neuritis. *J Neurol Neurosurg Psychiat.* 2003;74:1139–1141.

Hood DC, Ohri N, Yang EB, et al. Determining abnormal latencies of multifocal visual evoked potentials: a monocular analysis. *Doc Ophthalmol.* 2004b;109:189–199.

Hood DC, Zhang X, Rodarte C, et al. Determining abnormal interocular latencies of multifocal visual evoked potentials. *Doc Ophthalmol.* 2004a;109:177–187.

House JW, Brackmann DE. Brainstem audiometry in neurotologic diagnosis. *Arch Otolaryngol.* 1979;105:305–309.

Hugon J, Lubeau M, Tabaraud F, Chazot F, Vallat JM, Dumas M. Central motor conduction in motor neuron disease. *Ann Neurol.* 1987;22:544–546.

Hume AL, Cant BR. Pattern visual evoked potentials in the diagnosis of multiple sclerosis and other disorders. *Proc Austr Assoc Neurol.* 1976;13:7–13.

Hume AL, Waxman SG. Evoked potentials in suspected multiple sclerosis: diagnostic value and prediction of clinical course. *J Neurol Sci.* 1988;83:191–210.

Humm AM, Magistris MR, Truffert A, Hess CW, Rosler KM. Central motor conduction differs between acute relapsing-remitting and chronic progressive multiple sclerosis. *Clin Neurophysiol.* 2003;114:2196–2203.

Hutchinson M, Blandford S, Glynn D, Martin EA. Clinical correlates of abnormal brainstem auditory evoked responses in multiple sclerosis. *Acta Neurol Scand.* 1984;69:90–95.

Ingram, DA, Thompson AJ, Swash M. Central motor conduction in multiple sclerosis: evaluation of abnormalities revealed by transcutaneous magnetic stimulation of the brain. *J Neurol Neurosurg Psychiat.* 1988;51:487–494.

Irkec C, Nazhel B, Kocer B. The correlation between cerebrospinal fluid findings and evoked potentials during an acute MS attack. *Electromyogr Clin Neurophysiol.* 2001;41:117–122.

Jones RE, Heron JR, Foster DH, Snelgar RS, Mason RJ. Effects of 4-aminopyridine in patients with multiple sclerosis. *J Neurol Sci.* 1983;60:353–362.

Jones SJ, Brusa A. Neurophysiological evidence for long-term repair of MS lesions: implications for axon protection. *J Neurol Sci.* 2003;206:193–198.

Jones SMJ, Streletz LJ, Raab VE, Knobler RL, Lublin FD. Lower extremity motor evoked potentials in multiple sclerosis. *Arch Neurol.* 1991;48:944–948.

Jung P, Beyerle A, Ziemann U. Multimodal evoked potentials measure and predict disability progression in early relapsing-remitting multiple sclerosis. *Mult Scler.* 2008;14(4):553–556.

Kalkers NF, Strijers RL, Jasperse MM, et al. Motor evoked potential: a reliable and objective measure to document the functional consequences of multiple sclerosis? Relation to disability and MRI. *Clin Neurophysiol.* 2007;118(6):1332–1340.

Kallmann BA, Fackelmann S, Toyka KV, Rieckmann P, Reiners K. Early abnormalities of evoked potentials and future disability in patients with multiple sclerosis. *Mult Scler.* 2006;12(1):58–65.

Kandler RH, Jarratt JA, Gumpert EJ, et al. Magnetic stimulation in the diagnosis of multiple sclerosis. *J Neurol Neurol Sci.* 1991a;106:25–30.

Kandler RH, Jarratt JA, Davis-Jones GA, et al. The role of magnetic stimulation as a quantifier of motor disability in patients with multiple sclerosis. *J Neurol Sci.* 1991b;106:31–34.

Karnaze DS, Marshall LF, McCarthy CS, Klauber MR, Bickford RG. Localizing and prognostic value of auditory evoked responses in coma after closed head injury. *Neurology.* 1982;32:299–302.

Kayamori R, Dickins S, Yamada T, Kimura J. Brainstem auditory evoked potential and blink reflex in multiple sclerosis. *Neurology.* 1984;34:1318–1323.

Kazis A, Vlaikidis N, Xafenias D, Papanastasiou J, Pappa P. Fever and evoked potentials in multiple sclerosis. *J Neurol.* 1982;227:1–10.

Khatri BO, McQuillen MP, Harrington GJ, Schmoll D, Hoffmann RG. Chronic progressive multiple sclerosis: double-blind controlled study of plasmapheresis in patients taking immunosuppressive drugs. *Neurology.* 1985;35:312–319.

Khoshbin S, Hallett M. Multimodality evoked potentials and blink reflex in multiple sclerosis. *Neurology.* 1981;31:138–144.

Kjaer M. Visual evoked potentials in normal subjects and patients with multiple sclerosis. *Acta Neurol Scand.* 1980a;62:1–13.

Kjaer M. The value of brainstem auditory, visual and somatosensory evoked potentials and blink reflexes in the diagnosis of multiple sclerosis. *Acta Neurol Scand.* 1980b;62:220–236.

Koehler J, Faldum A, Hopf HC. EDSS correlated analysis of median nerve somatosensory evoked potentials in multiple sclerosis. *Neurol Sci.* 2000;21:217–221.

Koffler B, Oberascher G, Pommer B. Brain-stem involvement in multiple sclerosis: a comparison between brain-stem auditory evoked potentials and the acoustic stapedius reflex. *Neurology.* 1984;34:145–147.

Krumholz A, Weiss HD, Goldstein PJ, Harris KC. Evoked responses in vitamin B-12 deficiency. *Ann Neurol.* 1981;9:407–409.

Kupersmith MJ, Nelson JI, Seiple WH, Carr RE, Weiss PA. The 20/20 eye in multiple sclerosis. *Neurology.* 1983;33:1015–1020.

La Mantia L, Riti F, Salmaggi MC, Eoli M, Ciano C, Avanzini G. Serial evoked potentials in multiple sclerosis bouts: relation to steroid treatment. *Ital J Neurol Sci.* 1994;15:333–340.

Lacquaniti F, Benna P, Gilli M, Troni W, Bergamasco B. Brain stem auditory evoked potentials and blink reflex in quiescent multiple sclerosis. *Electroencephalogr Clin Neurophysiol.* 1979;47:607–610.

Larrea LG, Mauguiere F. Latency and amplitude abnormalities of the scale far-field P14 to median nerve stimulation in multiple sclerosis. A SEP study of 122 patients recorded with a non-cephalic reference montage. *Electroencephalogr Clin Neurophysiol.* 1988;71:180–186.

Lee KH, Hashimoto SA, Hooge JP, et al. Magnetic resonance imaging of the head in the diagnosis of multiple sclerosis: a prospective 2-year follow-up with comparison of clinical evaluation, evoked potentials, oligoclonal banding, and CT. *Neurology.* 1991;41:657–660.

Leocani L, Comi G. Neurophysiological investigations in multiple sclerosis. *Curr Opin Neurol.* 2000;13(3): 255–61.

Leocani L, Comi G. Neurophysiological markers. *Neurol Sci.* 2008;29(suppl 2):S218–S221.

Leocani L, Medaglini S, Comi G. Evoked potentials in monitoring multiple sclerosis. *Neurol Sci.* 2000;21: S889–S891.

Leocani L, Rovaris M, Boneschi FM, et al. Multimodal evoked potentials to assess the evolution of multiple sclerosis: a longitudinal study. *J Neurol Neurosurg Psychiat.* 2006;77(9):1030–1035.

Liepert J, Kotterba S, Tegenthoff M, Malin JP. Central fatigue assessed by transcranial magnetic stimulation. *Muscle Nerve.* 1996;19:1429–1434.

Lowitzsch K, Kuhnt U, Sakmann Ch, et al. Visual pattern evoked responses and blink reflexes in assessment of MS diagnosis. *J Neurol.* 1976;213:17–32.

Lowitzsch K, Westhoff M. Optic nerve involvement in neurosyphillis: diagnostic evaluation by pattern-reversal visual evoked potentials (VEP). *EEG EMG.* 1980;11: 77–80.

Lycke J, Svennerholm B, Hjelmquist E, et al. Acyclovir treatment of relapsing-remitting multiple sclerosis. A randomized, placebo-controlled, double-blind study. *J Neurol.* 1996;243:214–24.

Mamoli B, Graf M, Toifl K. EEG, pattern-evoked potentials and nerve conduction velocity in a family with adrenoleukodystrophy. *Electroencephalogr Clin Neurophysiol.* 1979;47:411–419.

Manova MG, Kostadinova II, Chalakova-Atanasova NT, Temenlieva VK, Petrova NS. Clinico-electrophyisiological correlates in patients with relapsing-remitting multiple sclerosis. *Folia Medica.* 2001;23:5–9.

Martinelli V, Comi G, Filippi M, et al. Paraclinical tests in acute-onset optic neuritis: basal data and results of a short follow-up. *Acta Neurol Scand.* 1991;84:231–236.

Mastaglia FL, Black JL, Collins DWK. Visual and spinal evoked potentials in the diagnosis of multiple sclerosis. *Br Med J.* 1976;2:732.

Mastaglia FL, Black JL, Edis R, Collins DWK. The contribution of evoked potentials in the functional assessment of the somatosensory pathway. *Clin Exp Neurol.* 1978; 15:279–298.

Matthews WB, Esiri M. Multiple sclerosis plaque related to abnormal somatosensory evoked potentials. *J Neurol Neurosurg Psychiat.* 1979;42:940–942.

Matthews WB, Small DG. Serial recording of visual and somatosensory evoked potentials in multiple sclerosis. *J Neurol Sci.* 1979;40:11–21.

Matthews WB, Small DG, Small M, Pountney E. Pattern reversal evoked visual potential in the diagnosis of multiple sclerosis. *J Neurol Neurosurg Psychiat.* 1977; 40:1009–1014.

Mayr N, Baumgartner C, Zeitlhofer J, Deecke L. The sensitivity of transcranial cortical magnetic stimulation in detecting pyramidal tract lesions in clinically definite multiple sclerosis. *Neurology.* 1991;41:566–569.

Mertin J, Rudge P, Kremer M, et al. Double-blind controlled trial of immunosuppression in the treatment of multiple sclerosis: final report. *Lancet.* 1982;2: 351–354.

Merton PA, Morton HB. Stimulation of the cerebral cortex in the intact human subjects. *Nature.* 1980;285:227.

Merton PA, Morton HB, Hill DK, Marsden CD. Scope of a technique for electrical stimulation of human brain, spinal cord and muscle. *Lancet.* 1982;2:596–600.

McDonald WI. The role of NMR imaging in the assessment of multiple sclerosis. *Clin Neurol Neurosurg.* 1988;90:3–9.

Miller DH, McDonald WI, Blumhardt LD, et al. Magnetic resonance imaging in isolated noncompressive spinal cord syndromes. *Ann Neurol.* 1987;22:714–723.

Miller JR, Burke AM, Bever CT. Occurrence of oligoclonal bands in multiple sclerosis and other CNS diseases. *Ann Neurol.* 1983;13:53–58.

Mills KR, Murray NMF. Corticospinal tract conduction time in multiple sclerosis. *Ann Neurol.* 1985;18: 601–605.

Misra UK, Kalita J, Das A. Vitamin B12 deficiency neurological syndromes: a clinical, MRI and electrodiagnostic study. *Electromyogr Clin Neurophysiol.* 2003;43:57–64.

Mogensen F, Kristensen O. Auditory double click evoked potentials in multiple sclerosis. *Acta Neurol Scand.* 1979;59:96–107.

Namerow NS. Somatosensory evoked response in multiple sclerosis patients with varying sensory loss. *Neurology.* 1968;18:1197–1204.

Namerow NS. Somatosensory recovery functions in multiple sclerosis patients. *Neurology.* 1970;20:813–817.

Neiman J, Nilsson BY, Barr PO, Perkins DJD. Hyperbaric oxygen in chronic progressive multiple sclerosis: visual evoked potentials and clinical effects. *J Neurol Neurosurg Psychiat.* 1985;48:497–500.

Nielsen JF, Norgaard P. Increased post-exercise facilitation of motor evoked potentials in multiple sclerosis. *Clin Neurophysiol.* 2002;113:1295–1300.

Niklas A, Sebraoui H, Hess E, Wagner A, Then Bergh F. Outcome measures for trials of remyelinating agents in multiple sclerosis: retrospective longitudinal analysis of visual evoked potential latency. *Mult Scler.* 2009; 15(1):68–74.

Nilsson BY. Visual evoked responses in multiple sclerosis: comparison of two methods for pattern reversal. *J Neurol Neurosurg Psychiat.* 1978;41:499–504.

Nociti V, Batocchi AP, Bartalini S, et al. Somatosensory evoked potentials reflect the upper limb motor performance in multiple sclerosis. *J Neurol Sci.* 2008;273: 99–102.

Noel P, Desmedt JE. Cerebral and far-field somatosensory evoked potentials in neurological disorders involving the cervical spinal cord, brainstem, thalamus and cortex. *Prog Clin Neurophysiol.* 1980;7:205–230.

Nuwer MR. *Intraoperative Monitoring of Neural Function.* Amsterdam, Netherlands: Elsevier; 2008.

Nuwer MR, Aminoff M, Desmedt J, et al. IFCN recommended standards for short latency somatosensory evoked potentials. *Electroencephalogr Clin Neurophysiol.* 1994a;91:6–11.

Nuwer MR, Aminoff M, Goodin D, et al. IFCN recommended standards for brain-stem auditory evoked potentials. *Electroencephalogr Clin Neurophysiol.* 1994b; 91:12–17.

Nuwer MR, Packwood JW, Ellison GW, Meyers LW. A parametric scale for BAEP latencies in multiple sclerosis. *Electroencephalogr Clin Neurophysiol.* 1988; 71:33–39.

Nuwer MR, Packwood JW, Myers LW, Ellison GW. Evoked potentials predict the clinical changes in multiple sclerosis drug study. *Neurology.* 1987;37:1754–1761.

Nuwer MR, Perlman SL, Packwood JW, Kark RAP. Evoked potential abnormalities in the various inherited ataxias. *Ann Neurol.* 1983;13:20–27.

Nuwer MR, Visscher BR, Packwood JW, Namerow NS. Evoked potential testing in relatives of multiple sclerosis patients. *Ann Neurol.* 1985;18:30–34.

O'Connor P, Marchetti P, Lee L, Perera M. Evoked potential abnormality scores are a useful measure of disease burden in relapsing-remitting multiple sclerosis. *Ann Neurol.* 1998;44:404–407.

Parving A, Elbering C, Smith T. Auditory electrophysiology: findings in multiple sclerosis. *Audiology.* 1981;20: 123–142.

Paty DW, Oger JJF, Kastrukoff LF, et al. MRI in the diagnosis of MS: a prospective study with comparison of clinical evaluation, evoked potentials, oligoclonal banding and CT. *Neurology.* 1988;38:180–185.

Perretti A, Balbi P, Orefice G, et al. Post-exercise facilitation and depression of motor evoked potentials to transcranial magnetic stimulation: a study in multiple sclerosis. *Clin Neurophysiol.* 2004;115(9):2128–2133.

Persson HE, Sachs C. VEPs during provoked visual impairment in multiple sclerosis. In: Barber C, ed. *Evoked Potentials.* Baltimore: University Park Press; 1980: 575–579.

Petajan JH, White AT. Motor-evoked potentials in response to fatiguing grip exercise in multiple sclerosis patients. *Clin Neurophysiol.* 2000;111:2188–2195.

Pohl D, Rostasy K, Treiber-Held S, Brockmann K, Gärtner J, Hanefeld F. Pediatric multiple sclerosis: detection of clinically silent lesions by multimodal evoked potentials. *J Pediatr.* 2006;149(1):125–127.

Polman CH, Reingold SC, Edan G, et al. Diagnostic criteria for multiple sclerosis: 2005 revisions to the "McDonald Criteria". *Ann Neurol.* 2005;58:840–846.

Prasher DK, Sainz M, Gibson WPR, Findley LJ. Binaural voltage summation of brain stem auditory evoked potentials: an adjunct to the diagnostic criteria for multiple sclerosis. *Ann Neurol.* 1982;11:86–91.

Purves SJ, Low MD, Galloway J, Reeves B. A comparison of visual brainstem auditory, and somatosensory evoked potentials in multiple sclerosis. *Can J Neurol Sci.* 1981;8:15–19.

Raminsky M. Hyperexcitability of pathologically myelinated axons and positive symptoms in multiple sclerosis. In: Waxman SG, Ritchie JM, eds. *Demyelinating Disease: Basic and Clinical Electrophysiology.* New York: Raven Press; 1981: 289–298.

Ravnborg M, Liguori R, Christiansen P, Larsson H, Sørenson PS. The diagnostic reliability of magnetically evoked motor potentials in multiple sclerosis. *Neurology.* 1992;42:1296–1301.

Regan D, Murray TJ, Silver R. Effect of body temperature on visual evoked potential delay and visual perception in multiple sclerosis. *J Neurol Neurosurg Psychiat.* 1977;40:1083–1091.

Richey ET, Kooi KA, Tourtellotte WW. Visually evoked responses in multiple sclerosis. *J Neurol Neurosurg Psychiat.* 1971;34:275–280.

Rico A, Audoin B, Franques J, et al. Motor evoked potentials in clinically isolated syndrome suggestive of multiple sclerosis. *Mult Scler.* 2009;15(3):355–362.

Rigolet MH, Mallecourt J, LeBlanc M, Chain F. Etude de la vision des couleurs et des potentiels evoqués dans diagnostic de la sclérose en plaques. *J Fr Ophthalmol.* 1979;2:553–560.

Robinson K, Rudge P. Abnormalities of the auditory evoked potentials in patients with multiple sclerosis. *Brain.* 1977a;100:19–40.

Robinson K, Rudge P. The early components of the auditory evoked potential in multiple sclerosis. *Prog Clin Neurophysiol.* 1977b;2:58–67.

Robinson K, Rudge P. The use of the auditory evoked potential in the diagnosis of multiple sclerosis. *J Neurol Sci.* 1980;45:235–244.

Rodriguez M, Siva A, Cross SA, O'Brien PC, Kurland LT. Optic neuritis: a population-based study in Olmsted County, Minnesota. *Neurology.* 1995;45:244–250.

Rousseff RT, Tzvetanov P, Rousseva MA. The bifid visual evoked potential—normal variant or a sign of demyelination? *Clin Neurol Neurosurg.* 2005;107:113–116.

Sailer M, Heinze HJ, Tendolkar I, et al. Influence of cerebral lesion volume and lesion distribution on event-related brain potentials in multiple sclerosis. *J Neurol.* 2001;248:1049–1055.

Schubert M, Wohlfahrt K, Rollnik JD, Dengler R. Walking and fatigue in multiple sclerosis: the role of the corticospinal system. *Muscle Nerve.* 1998;21:1068–1070.

Sears TA, Bostock H. Conduction failure in demyelination: is it inevitable? In: Waxman SG, Ritchie JM, eds. *Demyelinating Disease: Basic and Clinical Electrophysiology.* New York: Raven Press; 1981: 357–376.

Sedgwick EM. Pathophysiology and evoked potentials in multiple sclerosis. In: Hallpike JF, Adams CWM, Tourtellotte WW, eds. *Multiple Sclerosis: Pathology, Diagnosis and Management.* Baltimore: Williams and Wilkins; 1983: 177–201.

Segura MJ, Garcea O, Gandolfo CN. Multiple sclerosis: assessment of lesional levels by means of transcranial stimulation. *Electromyogr Clin Neurophysiol.* 1994;34: 249–255.

Shahrokhi F, Chiappa KH, Young RR. Pattern shift visual evoked responses: Two hundred patients with optic neuritis and/or multiple sclerosis. *Arch Neurol.* 1978;35: 65–71.

Shanon E, Himmelfarb MZ, Gold S. Pontomedullary vs pontomesencephalic transmission time: a diagnostic aid in multiple sclerosis. *Arch Otolaryngol.* 1981;107: 474–475.

Simó M, Barsi P, Arányi Z. Predictive role of evoked potential examinations in patients with clinically isolated optic neuritis in light of the revised McDonald criteria. *Mult Scler.* 2008;14:472–478.

Sipe JC, Knobler RL, Braheny SL, Rice GPA, Panitch HS, Oldstone MBA. A neurologic rating scale (NRS) for use in multiple sclerosis. *Neurology.* 1984;34:1368–1372.

Small DG, Matthews WB, Small M. The cervical somatosensory evoked potential (SEP) in the diagnosis of multiple sclerosis. *J Neurol Sci.* 1978;35:211–224.

Sorensen PS, Wanscher B, Szpirt W, et al. Plasma exchange combined with azathioprine in multiple sclerosis using serial gadolinium-enhanced MRI to monitor disease activity: a randomized single-masked cross-over pilot study. *Neurology.* 1996;46:1620–1625.

Starr A, Amlie RN, Martin WH, Sanders S. Development of auditory function in newborn infants revealed by auditory brainstem potentials. *Pediatrics.* 1977;60: 831–839.

Stockard JJ, Rossiter VS. Clinical and pathologic correlates of brain stem auditory response abnormalities. *Neurology.* 1977;27:316–325.

Stockard JJ, Sharbrough FW. Unique contributions of short-latency somatosensory evoked potentials in patients with neurological lesions. *Prog Clin Neurophysiol.* 1980; 7:231–263.

Streletz LJ, Chambers RA, Bae SH, Israel HL. Visual evoked potentials in sarcoidosis. *Neurology.* 1981;31: 1545–1549.

Tackmann W, Ettlin T. Blink reflexes elicited by electrical, acoustic and visual stimuli. II: their relation to visual-evoked potentials and auditory brain stem evoked potentials in the diagnosis of multiple sclerosis. *Eur Neurol.* 1982;21:264–269.

Tackmann W, Strenge H, Barth R, Sojka-Raytscheff A. Diagnostic validity for different components of pattern shift visual evoked potentials in multiple sclerosis. *Eur Neurol.* 1979;18:243–248.

Tackmann W, Strenge H, Barth R, Sojka-Raytscheff A. Evaluation of various brain structures in multiple

sclerosis with multimodality evoked potentials, blink reflex and nystagmography. *J Neurol.* 1980;224: 33–46.

Tataroglu C, Genc A, Idiman E, et al. Cortical silent period and motor evoked potentials in patients with multiple sclerosis. *Clin Neurol Neurosurg.* 2003;105:105–10.

Trojaborg W, Bottcher J, Saxtrup O. Evoked potentials and immunoglobulin abnormalities in multiple sclerosis. *Neurology.* 1981;31:866–871.

Trojaborg W, Petersen E. Visual and somatosensory evoked cortical potentials in multiple sclerosis. *J Neurol Neurosurg Psychiat.* 1979;42:323–330.

van Buggenhout E, Ketelaer P, Carton H. Success and failure of evoked potentials in detecting clinical and subclinical lesions in multiple sclerosis patients. *Clin Neurol Neurosurg.* 1982;84:3–14.

Walsh JC, Garrick R, Cameron J, McLeod JG. Evoked potential changes in clinically definite multiple sclerosis: a two year follow up study. *J Neurol Neurosurg Psychiat.* 1982;45:494–500.

Waxman SG. Clinicopathological correlations in multiple sclerosis and related diseases. In: Waxman SG, Ritchie JM, eds. *Demyelinating Disease: Basic and Clinical Electrophysiology.* New York: Raven Press; 1981: 169–182.

Waxman SG, Ritchie JM. Electrophysiology of demyelinating disease: future directions and questions. In: Waxman SG, Ritchie JM, eds. *Demyelinating Disease: Basic and Clinical Electrophysiology.* New York: Raven Press; 1981:511–514.

Weiner HL, Dawson DM. Plasmapheresis in multiple sclerosis: preliminary study. *Neurology.* 1980;30:1029–1033.

Weinstock-Guttman B, Baier M, Stockton R,. Pattern reversal visual evoked potentials as a measure of visual pathway pathology in multiple sclerosis. *Mult Scler.* 2003;9(5):529–534.

Wilson WB, Keyser RB. Comparison of the pattern and diffuse-light visual evoked responses in definite multiple sclerosis. *Arch Neurol.* 1980;37:30–34.

Wist ER, Hennerici M, Dichgans J. The Pulfrich spatial frequency phenomenon: a psycholophysical method competitive to visual evoked potentials in the diagnosis of multiple sclerosis. *J Neurol Neurosurg Psychiat.* 1978;41:1069–1077.

Youl BD, Turano G, Miller DH, et al. The pathophysiology of acute optic neuritis. *Brain.* 1991;114:2437–2450.

10 Temporal and Clinical Course of Multiple Sclerosis

Erica Grazioli, Cornelia Mihai, and Bianca Weinstock-Guttman

Multiple sclerosis (MS), similar to other chronic autoimmune diseases, has a heterogeneous disease course that is often unpredictable (Compston et al., 2006;). Natural history data collected over the years from different geographical regions apply in general to groups of MS patients rather than to individuals, and therefore it is essential for the clinician and researcher to acknowledge the value but also the limitation of this information. Nevertheless, identifying sensitive predictors associated with a milder versus a more aggressive disease is critical. Entering into a new era of beneficial therapeutic interventions available for MS is raising anticipation for a significant positive impact on the natural history of disease.

DIFFERENT TEMPORAL AND CLINICAL COURSES

Multiple sclerosis clinical course can vary between patients, but it also can change over time within the same individual. Nonetheless, the majority of patients experience acute neurologic events (relapses, attacks, or exacerbations), disease progression, or a combination of both patterns. In 1996, the results of an international survey of clinicians involved in MS care and revised by the NMSS (USA) Advisory Committee on Clinical Trials of New Agents in Multiple Sclerosis was published. This report attempted to clarify the terminology used to describe the disease course patterns in patients with MS, based on either clinical or severity criteria (Lublin and Reingold, 1996).

Based on specific clinical characteristics, four MS disease courses were determined to be representative and fully accepted by clinicians and researchers:

1. Relapsing-remitting MS (RRMS) characterized by "clearly defined relapses with full recovery or with sequelae and residual deficits upon recovery; the periods between disease relapses are characterized by a lack of disease progression"
2. Secondary progressive MS (SPMS): "initial RR disease course followed by progression with or without occasional relapses, minor remissions, and plateaus"
3. Primary-progressive MS (PPMS): "disease progression from onset with occasional plateaus and temporary minor improvements allowed"
4. Progressive-relapsing MS (PRMS): "progressive disease from the onset, with clear acute relapses, with or without full recovery; periods between relapses characterized by continuing progression"

There are also two consensus definitions based on clinical severity:

1. Benign MS: "disease in which the patient remains fully functional in all neurologic systems 15 years after disease onset." This entity remains a challenging diagnosis taking in consideration that in general the diagnosis is based on a retrospective analysis. A continuous search is carried on for identifying sensitive predictive markers of MS early on its disease course.
2. Malignant MS: "disease with a rapid progressive course, leading to significant disability in multiple neurologic systems or death in a relatively short time after disease onset"

Clinically isolated syndrome (CIS) has been defined as the first attack of neurologic deficit associated with MRI findings suggestive of demyelinating disease. It may present as a spinal cord syndrome (incomplete transverse myelitis), optic neuritis, or brainstem dysfunction as the most common clinical pictures (Frohman, 2003). Because most of such patients will develop a second event over months or years, more specific criteria became necessary in order to identify the highest patient at risk to become MS. Clinically isolated syndrome can also be classified as based on the initial clinical and MRI findings as monofocal (no dissemination in space) or multifocal (dissemination in space), with (multilesional) or without (monolesional) MRI abnormalities additional to the lesion responsible for the clinical presentation. Based on these several combinations (clinical and MRI) identified at the first event, a more specific classification was recommended including five CIS types (CIS 1–5) (Miller et al., 2008). This recent classification based on U.S. National MS Society task force recommendations remains an operational classification with further value to be proven. One of the more challenging presentations is the CIS type 5 characterized by incidental MRI findings suggestive for MS but with no clinical support. This entity recently became referred to as the radiologically isolated syndrome (RIS) (Okuda et al., 2009). Future prospective studies are necessary to define the risk of these patients to progress/convert to MS.

The second neurologic event usually marks the clinically definite (CD) MS and also a RR course. The T2-weighted MRI lesion load is the best predictor for conversion to CDMS, with an 85% conversion rate if the initial MRI shows two or more lesions (Comi et al., 2001). New diagnostic principles, the McDonald Criteria, endorse new MRI parameters as surrogate markers to support the diagnosis of MS providing the potential for an earlier diagnosis (McDonald et al., 2001; Polman et al., 2005; see more on Chapter 4).

In most instances, up to 80%, MS begins as a relapsing-remitting disease (RRMS), while 15%–20% present with a primary progressive course (PPMS) (Lublin and Reingold, 1996). In a clinic-based cross-sectional study of 1100 MS patients from London, Ontario, Weinshenker found 60% had RRMS and 15% PPMS. Depending of the duration of the disease, RRMS can convert to a secondary progressive MS course (SPMS) (Weinshenker, 1994). At 11–15 years disease duration, 58% had progressive MS and at 16–25 years duration, 66% had progressive MS (Weinshenker et al., 1989). Similar data were reported by Runmarker and Andersen who followed a cohort of 308 patients for 25 years, 80% of their MS cohort becoming progressive at the 25-year follow-up assessment (Runmarker and Anderson, 1993). The relapsing stage of the disease is assumed to be associated with an inflammatory underlying pathobiology, while during the progressive stage a neurodegenerative process dominates. However, a coexistence of the two processes from the early stages is increasingly accepted (Lassmann, 2007). As previously mentioned, during the initial phase of secondary progressive disease, patients may still experience relapses; this stage was previously classified as relapsing–progressive disease. This early transition stage is often difficult to differentiate on clinical grounds from a relapsing remitting stage with incomplete recovery, supporting the statement that RRMS and SPMS represent a continuum within the same disease process. Often these two entities are combined within the term of *relapsing MS*.

Central nervous system (CNS) inflammation is considered the primary cause of the nervous tissue injury in MS in which the adaptive immune system including T cells (CD4+ and CD8+) but also B cells and NK cells being shown to be involved in MS pathology and certainly contributing to the MS disease heterogeneity (McFarland and Martin, 2007; Lunemann and Munz, 2008). The innate immune system comprised from monocytes, dendritic cells, and microglia is becoming increasingly recognized to play also an important role in immunopathogenesis of MS.

However, there are no proven surrogate or biological markers that can differentiate between the various clinical courses of MS. Recent throughput arrays methodology data suggest that during the relapsing stage a pro-inflammatory milieu that combines both the innate and adaptive immune system predominates, whereas in the progressive stage abnormalities of the innate immune system outweigh (Weiner, 2009). Quintana et al. found unique autoantibody patterns that distinguished RRMS, SPMS, and PPMS from healthy controls and other neurological and autoimmune diseases, using antigen microarray analysis. RRMS patients have autoantibodies to heat shock proteins that were not observed in SPMS or PPMS. Also, RRMS, SPMS, and PPMS were found to have unique patterns of reactivity to CNS antigens, and these findings were also linked to each type of pathology as determined by brain biopsy (Quintana et al., 2008). These findings may help monitor the disease course and guide therapy in the near future.

GUIDELINES FOR DEFINING PROGNOSIS

The outcome and prognosis of MS is quite variable among those affected. In an individual, it is difficult to reliably predict the disease course and ultimate disability. Identifying clinical predictors early in the disease course that may foretell long-term outcome becomes important. In the overall MS population, several demographic and clinical features have been identified as predictors of disability in both the short and long term.

Weinshenker et al. (1996) prospectively studied a sample population of both relapsing and progressive MS patients with average disease duration of 13.5 years for predictors of short-term outcome (3 years). Baseline EDSS scores and disease duration were significant predictors (Weinshenker et al., 1996).

Scott et al. (2000) examined a cohort of patients from the onset of diagnosis of clinically definite RRMS as defined by Poser's criteria (Poser et al., 1983). This population overall was earlier in their disease course than that studied by Weinshenker et al. The average follow-up was 37 months from the time of diagnosis. Six prognostic factors were found to influence the progression of short-term disability:

1. Age at onset; less than 40 or greater than 40
2. Symptoms at onset; isolated sensory or cranial nerve versus motor or sensory plus motor
3. MRI status at onset of first attack and time of onset of CDMS;"negative" versus "suspicious" versus "suggestive." Patients who had ≥4 white matter lesions measuring ≥3 mm on T2-weighted imaging were considered suggestive and those who had 1–3 white matter lesions ≥3 mm were considered suspicious.
4. Interval between the first and second attack, >2.5 years or <2.5 years
5. Attack frequency in the first 2 years, ≤ 2 versus > 2
6. Completeness of recovery from initial attacks, good versus poor. Patients who had

a postattack EDSS of ≤1.5 were considered to have a good recovery and ≥2 were considered to have a poor recovery.

Of the above, the risk factors for a poor prognosis were older age at disease onset, motor symptoms, presence of suggestive white matter lesions on MRI, a shorter attack interval or greater attack frequency, and poor recovery from attacks. Patients were grouped according to the number of these risk factors present. Low risk was considered 0–1 risk factor, medium risk 2–3 risk factors, or high more than 3 risk factors. The high risk factor group had the highest final EDSS as well as the greatest change in EDSS over the course of the study. There was no difference in progression seen between the low- and medium-risk factor groups. Of the individual risk factors, the strongest correlation was seen in those having a second attack in less than 2.5 years and more than 2 attacks in the first 2 years. Status of MRI alone did not predict final EDSS (Scott et al., 2000).

Age at onset may also influence the disease course and progression as shown, suggesting an increased risk of progression with age of onset after age 40. Pediatric-onset patients (onset before age of 18, present in 4%–5% of MS cases), on the other hand, tend to take longer to reach disability landmarks than adult-onset patients, but tend to do so at a younger age (Renoux et al., 2007). Delayed disability progression in children could result from more robust or efficient neuronal repair mechanisms than those of adults.

Gender may also interfere with the disease severity. Although MS affects more often women than men (ratio 2–3:1), men appear to be more severely affected than women, often presenting with a later disease onset and a progressive disease course (Wynn et al., 1990; Kantarci et al., 1998; Schwendimann and Alekseeva, 2007).

Relapses early in the disease course have been shown to influence the time to reach certain disability levels using the well-accepted disability status scale (DSS) and the corresponding Kurtzke extended disability status scale (EDSS); a higher first 2-year attack rate correlated with a shorter time to early disability (DSS 3) and need for an assistive device (DSS of 6) as seen in Table 10-1 (Weinshenker et al., 1989). A 25-year observational study (Ebers, 2001) found that relative risk

Table 10-1 First 2-Year Attack Rate

	Years to DSS 3	Years to DSS 6
One attack	13	20
Two attacks	8	17
Three attacks	9	18
Four attacks	8	14
Five or more attacks	3	7

of progression to long-term disability with an EDSS of 6 (corresponding to the need of a unilateral assistance for ambulation) was influenced by the following:

1. Progressive course from onset
2. Relapse rate
3. First inter-attack interval
4. Polysymptomatic onset
5. Time to early disability, defined as time from onset to EDSS of 3

Of these factors, the greatest predictor of development of disability was a progressive disease course (Ebers, 2001).

Mechanisms for clinical worsening in MS include both stepwise worsening secondary to incomplete recovery from relapses as well as gradual progressive worsening independent of relapses. Lublin (2007) analyzed EDSS scores before, during, and after relapses of 224 patients who had been randomized to the placebo group of clinical trials. The "after" time period was at least 30 days from the "during" acute period evaluation. A residual disability of ≥ 0.5 EDSS point was seen in 42% of patients and ≤ 1.0 EDSS point in 28% (Lublin, 2007).

Once a certain disability phase of the disease is reached, it has been suggested that the rate of disease progression is no longer influenced by either prior or subsequent relapses (Confavreux et al., 2000; Ebers, 2001; Confavreux, 2003). Confavreux studied 1844 relapsing and progressive MS patients from the Lyons, France database. Overall, the median time from disease onset to an EDSS of 4 was 8.4 years, to an EDSS of 6 was 20.1 years, and an EDSS of 7 was 29.9 years. The times to reach these markers of disability from time of

disease onset were significantly longer in those with relapsing as compared to progressive disease at disease onset ($p < 0.001$). The median time from an EDSS of 4 to an EDSS of 6 was 5.7 years, from an EDSS of 6 to an EDSS of 7 was 3.4 years, and from an EDSS of 4 to an EDSS of 7 was 12.1 years. Once an EDSS of 4 was reached, the median time to reach an EDSS of 6 or 7 was similar regardless of whether the patients had an initially relapsing remitting or progressive course (Confavreux et al., 2000). These results were mirrored in the London, Ontario natural history cohort (Ebers, 2001). These data suggest that the inflammatory and neurodegenerative components of MS may be both interdependent and independent. Remarkably, the finding that the time of reaching progressive disability milestones is similar between patients after reaching an EDSS of 4 suggests a certain threshold of accumulated damage beyond which the repair and plasticity mechanisms may not be able to compensate.

A subgroup of MS patients is known retrospectively to have a benign course with minimal accumulation of disability. Clinical features early in the MS disease course predictive of a benign course are similar to those portending a good prognosis as discussed previously. Prognostic factors for a benign MS course include onset age less than 40 years, optic neuritis as the presenting symptom, absence of pyramidal signs at onset, duration of the first remission of more than 1 year, and only one exacerbation in the first 5 years (Ramsaransing, 2001). Additional MRI characteristics may be helpful to distinguish patients with this benign course as described later.

Racial and ethnic factors also contribute to MS prognosis. African Americans (AAs) develop MS less frequently than White Americans (WAs) (Alter, 1962; Kurtzke et al., 1979) but have an earlier diagnosis following the initial symptom and more aggressive disease (Weinstock-Guttman et al., 2003; Cree et al., 2004). African Americans have increased occurrence of multifocal signs and symptoms (Cree et al., 2004) and greater disability over time (Weinstock-Guttman et al., 2003; Cree et al., 2004). A shorter time from symptom onset to gait impairment and greater degrees of cognitive decline have also been reported (Weinstock-Guttman et al., 2003; Cree et al., 2004). Additionally, studies suggest that AAs are also at greater risk for earlier development of severe disability requiring wheelchair dependency (Cree et al., 2004; Naismith et al., 2006). These findings have been explained by severe attacks followed by incomplete recovery even following the first episode including optic neuritis (Phillips et al., 1998) as well as more frequent pyramidal system involvement (Kaufmann et al., 2003), greater cerebellar dysfunction (Naismith et al., 2006), and often a higher number of relapses in AAs compared to WAs (Debouverie et al., 2007).

ROLE OF MAGNETIC RESONANCE IMAGING IN FORMULATING PROGOSIS AND MONITORING DISEASE ACTIVITY

Today MRI is considered the best surrogate marker for providing an earlier MS diagnosis as well as for predicting the conversion of CIS to MS. However, there are no established MRI markers for disease progression and disability. Lesions identified on T2-weighted images (WI) are nonspecific and cannot adequately distinguish between inflammation, edema, and axonal loss (Zivadinov and Bakshi, 2004). A "clinical-MRI paradaox" exists in MS in that conventional MRI imaging has only a modest association with clinical disability and disease progression.

The Optic Neuritis Treatment trial followed a cohort of patients with an initial presentation of optic neuritis. The presence of MRI lesions at baseline predicted future development of CDMS such that the 15-year cumulative probability of developing CDMS was 25% with no lesions and 72% for patients with one or more MRI lesions (Optic Neuritis Study Group, 2008). The Queens Square Group also followed a cohort of patients with CIS (Brex et al., 2002; Fishniku et al., 2008). These data demonstrate an association with the number of T2 WI lesions on MRI at presentation and the subsequent chance of conversion to CDMS over 20 years with a 21% risk with 0 lesions, 82% risk with 1–3 lesions, 85% risk with 4–9 lesions, and an 81% risk with greater than 10 lesions. Disability as measured by EDSS at 20 years was also influenced by the number of T2 lesions at baseline as shown in Table 10-2.

Magnetic resonance imaging data may also predict in a limited fashion a benign course for MS. O'Riordan reported that for patients with greater than or equal to 10 demyelinating lesions at presentation, three-quarters had an EDSS of greater than 3 after 10 years. However, with less that 10 MRI lesions at baseline, three-quarters had an EDSS less than or equal to 3 after 10 years (O' Riordan et al., 1998).

Nevertheless, as MS disease course progresses, there is a decreased association between T2 lesion volume and clinical outcomes. It cannot be assumed therefore that stabilization of T2 lesions equals stabilization of disease or that increase in T2 lesions is associated with increased disease duration. For example, T2 lesion volume may be artificially lowered as brain volume is lost to atrophy (Li et al., 2006; Dwyer et al., 2007).

A number of nonconventional MRI modalities have been developed during the past decade (Zivadinov, 2007). These newer techniques appear to be more sensitive biomarkers for measuring the pathogenic processes associated with disease activity and progression, including the presence of occult pathology in gray matter (GM) and white matter (WM). These MRI techniques are able to reveal a range of pathological substrates of MS lesions which include edema, inflammation, demyelination, and axonal loss (Lucchinetti et al., 1996). These techniques include measurement of T1-WI hypointense lesions ("black holes"), assessment of different metrics on magnetization transfer imaging (MTI), diffusion-weighted and tensor imaging (DWI and DTI), magnetic resonance spectroscopy (MRS), functional MRI (fMRI), and

TABLE 10-2 Risk of Disability at 20 Years

	T2 Lesions			
	0 Lesions	1–3 Lesions	4–9 Lesions	10+ Lesions
EDSS > 3	26%	36%	50%	65%
EDSS > 6	6%	18%	35%	45%

high- and ultrahigh-field MRI. These are emerging as useful tools for identifying more exactly the underlying pathologic processes within lesions and in normal-appearing brain tissue (NABT).

Gadolinium-contrast (Gd) on T1 WI, usually indicating blood–brain-barrier disruption secondary to inflammation is considered a predictor of moderate ability for the occurrence of relapses, but it is not predictive of cumulative impairment or disability (Kappos et al., 1999; Zivadinov and Leist, 2005). Only about a third of these acute black holes (initially enhancing after Gd) persist on T1-WI as hypointense areas. These persistent T1 lesions are called T1 chronic black holes and are characterized histopathologically by extensive axonal loss and gliosis. Their density is associated with the degree of chronic neurologic impairment, and postmortem analysis of MS lesions demonstrated that chronic T1 hypointensities correlate with axonal density, a marker of the irreversible accumulation of disability in MS (van Walderveen et al., 1998, 1999; Paolillo et al., 2000; Bitsch et al., 2000). Correlation between T1 hypointense lesion volume and clinical disability suggests that these may be clinically relevant for measuring disease progression (van Waesberghe et al., 1999; Paolillo et al., 2000; Zivadinov and Leist, 2005).

The measurement of brain atrophy seems to be of growing clinical relevance as a biomarker of the disease process (Miller et al., 2002; Anderson et al., 2006; Bermel and Bakshi, 2006). There is mounting evidence that the assessment of brain atrophy represents a potentially powerful tool for monitoring disease progression and therapeutic efficacy in MS (Zivadinov et al., 2001; Fisher et al., 2002; Miller et al., 2002; Bermel et al., 2003; Benedict et al., 2004). Brain atrophy is a predictor of clinical impairments such as physical disability (Miller et al., 2002), cognitive dysfunction (Zivadinov et al., 2001), depression (Bakshi et al., 2000), and quality of life (Janardhan and Bakshi, 2000), and is independent of the effect of conventional MRI lesions.

CONCLUSIONS

Multiple sclerosis is a heterogeneous disease with a chronic progressive course. Specific and sensitive surrogate markers able to predict future course as well as response to therapy for individual patients are still limited. Nonconventional MRI techniques have become the most promising tools for monitoring the destructive pathophysiology of MS as translated on clinical impairment, disease progression, and the accumulation of long-term physical and neuropsychological disability. Developing disease prognostic sensitive markers at the initial presentation or early on the disease course will help in individualizing the therapeutic intervention especially in the light of new MS therapies with increased efficacy but also with a considerably higher estimated side-effect profile.

REFERENCES

Alter M. Multiple sclerosis in the Negro. *Arch Neurol.* 1962;7:83–91.

Anderson V, Fox N, Miller D. Magnetic resonance imaging measures of brain atrophy in multiple sclerosis. *J Magn Reson Imaging.* 2006;23(5):605–618.

Bakshi R, Czarnecki D, Shaikh Z, et al. Brain MRI lesions and atrophy are related to depression in multiple sclerosis. *Neuroreport.* 2000;11(6):1153–1158.

Benedict RH, Weinstock-Guttman B, Fishman I, et al. Prediction of neuropsychological impairment in multiple sclerosis: comparison of conventional magnetic resonance imaging measures of atrophy and lesion burden. *Arch Neurol.* 2004;61(2):226–230.

Bermel R, Bakshi R. The measurement and clinical relevance of brain atrophy in multiple sclerosis. *Lancet Neurol.* 2006;5(2):158–170.

Bermel R, Sharma J, Tjoa C, Puli S, Bakshi R. A semiautomated measure of whole-brain atrophy in multiple sclerosis. *J Neurol Sci.* 2003;208:57–65.

Bitsch A, Schuchardt J, Bunkowski S, Kuhlmann T, Bruck W. Acute axonal injury in multiple sclerosis. Correlation with demyelination and inflammation. *Brain.* 2000;123:1174–1183.

Brex PA, Ciccarelli O, O'Riordan JI, Sailer M, Thompson AJ, Miller, DH. A longitudinal study of abnormalities on MRI and disability from multiple sclerosis. *N Engl J Med.* 2002;346:158–164.

Lassmann H, Bruck W, Lucchinetti C. The immunopathology of multiple sclerosis: an overview. *Brain Pathol.* 2007;17(2):210–218.

Comi G, Filippi M, Barkhof F, et al. Effect of early interferon treatment on conversion to definite multiple sclerosis: a randomized study. *Lancet.* 2001;357(9268): 1576–1582.

Compston A, Mcdonald I, Noseworthy J, et al. *McAlpine's Multiple Sclerosis.* 4th ed. New York: Elsevier; 2006: 69–284.

Confavreux C, Vukusic S, Adeleine P. Early clinical predictors and progression of irreversible disability in multiple sclerosis: an amnesic process. *Brain.* 2003;126:770–782.

Confavreux C, Vukusic M, Monreau T, Adeleine P. Relapses and progression of disability in multiple sclerosis. *N Engl J Med.* 2000; 343(20):1430–1438.

Cree B, Kahn O, Bourdette D, et al. Clinical characteristics of African Americans versus Caucasian Americans with multiple sclerosis. *Neurology.* 2004;63:2039–2045.

Debouverie M, Lebrun C, Jeannin S, et al. More severe disability of North Africans vs. Europeans with multiple sclerosis in France. *Neurology.* 2007;68: 29–32.

Dwyer M, Dolezal O, Hussein S, et al. Development of central atrophy may lead to underestimation of lesion accrual in patients with multiple sclerosis. *Proc Soc Magn Reson Med.* 2007;P2198:2432.

Ebers G. Natural history of multiple sclerosis. *J Neurol Neurosurg Psychiatry.* 2001;71:16–19.

Fisher E, Rudick R, Simon J, et al. Eight year follow-up study of brain atrophy in patients with MS. *Neurology.* 2002;59(9):1412–1420.

Fishniku LK, Brex PA, Altmann DR, et al. Disability and T2 MRI lesions: a 20 year follow-up of patients with relapse onset of multiple sclerosis. *Brain.* 2008;131: 808–817.

Frohman EM. Multiple sclerosis. *Med Clin North Am.* 2003;87(4):867–897.

Janardhan V, Bakshi R. Quality of life and its relationship to brain lesions and atrophy on magnetic resonance images in 60 patients with multiple sclerosis. *Arch Neurol.* 2000;57(10):1485–1491.

Kantarci O, Siva A, Eraksoy M, et al. Survival and predictors of disability in Turkish MS patients. *Neurology.* 1998;51:765–772.

Kappos L, Moeri D, Radue E, et al. Predictive value of gadolinium enhanced magnetic resonance imaging for relapse rate and changes in disability or impairment in multiple sclerosis: a meta-analysis. Gadolinium MRI Meta-analysis Group. *Lancet.* 1999;353:964–969.

Kaufman M, Johnson S, Moyer D, Birens J, Norton H. Multiple sclerosis: severity and progression rate in African Americans compared with whites. *Am J Phys Med Rehabil.* 2003;82:582–590.

Kurtzke JF, Beebe GW, Norman JE, Jr. Epidemiology of multiple sclerosis in U.S. veterans: 1. Race, sex, and geographic distribution. *Neurology.* 1979;29:1228–1235.

Li DK, Held U, Petkau J, et al. MRI T2 lesion burden in multiple sclerosis: a plateauing relationship with clinical disability. *Neurology.* 2006;66(9):1384–1389.

Lublin F. The incomplete nature of multiple sclerosis relapse resolution. *J Neurol Sci.* 2007;256:S14–S18.

Lublin FD, Reingold SC. Defining the clinical course of multiple sclerosis: results of an international survey. National Multiple Sclerosis Society (USA) Advisory Committee on Clinical Trials of New Agents in Multiple Sclerosis. *Neurology.* 1996;46:907–911.

Luccinetti C, Bruck W, Rodriguez M, Lassmann H. Distinct patterns of multiple sclerosis pathology indicate heterogeneity on pathogenesis. *Brain Pathol.* 1996;6(3):259–274.

Lunemann J, Munz C. Do natural killer cells accelerate or prevent autoimmunity in multiple sclerosis? *Brain.* 2008;131:1681–1683.

McDonald W, Compston A, Edan G, et al. Recommended diagnostic criteria for multiple sclerosis: guidelines from the International Panel on the Diagnosis of Multiple Sclerosis. *Ann Neurol.* 2001;50:121–127.

McFarland H, Martin R. Multiple sclerosis: a complicated picture of autoimmunity. *Nature Immunol.* 2007;8: 913–919.

Miller D, Barkhof F, Frank J, Parker G, Thompson A. Measurement of atrophy in multiple sclerosis: pathological basis, methodological aspects and clinical relevance. *Brain.* 2002;125:1676–1695.

Miller DH, Weinshenker BG, Filippi M, et al. Differential diagnosis of suspected multiple sclerosis: a consensus approach. *Mult Scler.* 2008;14(9):1157–1174.

Naismith R, Trinkaus K, Cross A. Phenotype and prognosis in African-Americans with multiple sclerosis: a retrospective chart review. *Mult Scler.* 2006;12:775–781.

Okuda D, Mowry E, Beheshtian A, et al. Incidental MRI findings suggestive of multiple sclerosis: the radiologically isolated syndrome. *Neurology.* 2009;27: 800–805.

O'Riordan JI, Thompson AJ, Kingsley DP, et al. The prognostic value of brain MRI in clinically isolated syndromes of the CNS: a 10 year follow-up. *Brain.* 1998; 121:495–503.

Optic Neuritis Study Group. Multiple sclerosis risk after optic neuritis. *Arch Neurol.* 2008;65:727–732.

Paolillo A, Pozzilli C, Gasperini C, et al. Brain atrophy in relapsing-remitting multiple sclerosis: relationship with 'black holes', disease duration and clinical disability. *J Neurol Sci.* 2000;174(2):85–91.

Phillips P, Newman N, Lynn M. Optic neuritis in African Americans. *Arch Neurol.* 1998;55:186–192.

Polman C, Reingold S, Edan G, et al. Diagnostic criteria for multiple sclerosis: 2005 revisions to the McDonald Criteria. *Ann Neurol.* 2005;58(6):840–846.

Poser C, Paty D, Scheinberg L, et al. New diagnostic criteria for multiple sclerosis: guidelines for research protocols. *Ann Neurol.* 1983;13:227–231.

Quintana F, Farez M, Viglietta V, et al. Antigen microarrays identify unique serum autoantibody signatures in clinical and pathologic subtypes of multiple sclerosis. *Proc Nat Acad Sci.* 2008;105(48):18889–18894.

Ramsaransing G, Maurits N, Zwanikken C, De Keyser J. Early prediction of a benign course of multiple sclerosis on clinical grounds: a systematic review. *Mult Scler.* 2001;7:345–347.

Renoux C, Vukusic S, Mikaeloff Y, et al. Natural history of multiple sclerosis with childhood onset. *N Engl J Med.* 2007;356:2603–2613.

Runmarker B, Anderson O. Prognostic factors in a multiple sclerosis incidence cohort with twenty-five years of follow-up. *Brain.* 1993;116(pt 1):117–134.

Schwendimann R, Alekseeva N. Gender issues in multiple sclerosis. *Int Rev Neurobiol.* 2007;79:377–392.

Scott T, Schramke C, Novero J, Chiefee C. Short term prognosis in early relapsing-remitting multiple sclerosis. *Neurology.* 2000;55:689–693.

Van Waesberghe J, Kamphorst W, De Groot C, et al. Axonal loss in multiple sclerosis lesions: magnetic resonance imaging insights into substrates of disability. *Ann Neurol.* 1999;46(5):747–754.

Van Walderveen M, Kamphorst W, Scheltens P, et al. Histopathologic correlate of hypointense lesions on T1-weighted spin-echo MRI in multiple sclerosis. *Neurology.* 1998;50(5):1282–1288.

Weiner H. The challenge of multiple sclerosis: how do we cure a chronic heterogeneous disease? *Ann Neurol.* 2009;65(3):239–248.

Weinshenker B. Natural history of multiple sclerosis. *Ann Neurol.* 1994;36(suppl 1): S6.

Weinshenker B, Bass B, Rice G et al. The natural history of multiple sclerosis: a geographically based study. *Brain.* 1989;112:1419–1428.

Weinshenker B, Issa M, Baskerville J. Long-term and short-term outcome of multiple sclerosis. A 3 year follow-up study. *Arch Neurol.* 1996;53:353–358.

Weinstock-Guttman B, Jacobs LD, et al. Multiple sclerosis characteristics in African American patients in the New York State Multiple Sclerosis Consortium. *Mult Scler.* 2003;9:293–298.

Wynn D, Rodriguez M, O'Fallon M, Kurland L. A reappraisal of the epidemiology of multiple sclerosis in Olmsted County, Minnesota. *Neurology.* 1990;40:780.

Zivadinov R. Can imaging techniques measure neuroprotection and remyelination in multiple sclerosis? *Neurology.* 2007;68(suppl 3):S72–S82.

Zivadinov R, Leist TP. Clinical-magnetic resonance imaging correlations in multiple sclerosis. *J Neuroimaging.* 2005;15(suppl 4):10S–21S.

Zivadinov R, Bakshi R. Role of MRI in multiple sclerosis I: inflammation and lesions. *Front Biosci.* 2004;9:665–683.

Zivadinov R, Sepcic J, Nasuelli D, et al. A longitudinal study of brain atrophy and cognitive disturbances in the early phase of relapsing-remitting multiple sclerosis. *J Neurol Neurosurg Psychiatry.* 2001;70(6):773–780.

11 | Outcome Measures in Multiple Sclerosis

Robert M. Herndon

One's knowledge of science begins when he can measure what he is speaking about and express it in numbers.

—*Lord Nelson*

Reliable measurement of neurologic changes in individuals with multiple sclerosis (MS) has proven to be extremely challenging. Multiple sclerosis has so many incommensurable signs and symptoms such that development of even an ordinal scale (a scale with an ordered sequence) is all but impossible. For example, how would you order the following impairments: a central scotoma, an internuclear ophthalmoplegia, and hand incoordination? John Kurtzke did a remarkably good job with development of the Disability Status Scale (DSS) (Kurtzke, 1955, 1961) and the subsequent Expanded Disability Status Scale (EDSS) (Kurtzke, 1983), but the problem remains, how do you quantify the extent of the disease? There is a great deal of subjectivity and significant intraobserver and inter-observer variability in use of the EDSS even with training. On the other hand, quantitative measures such as the Multiple Sclerosis Functional Composite (MSFC) (Rudick et al., 1997), which are highly reproducible with minimal intra- and inter-observer variability, cannot cover the whole range of the disease and do not include many relevant areas (e.g., oculomotor and visual function). The EDSS remains, despite its drawbacks, the gold standard.

There are certain characteristics that are desirable in useful clinical scales, and these features should be considered in selecting or evaluating a scale though few scales in neurology will have all of these characteristics (Herndon and Cutter, 2006). Scales useful in MS, when possible, should be:

- Appropriate to the task
- Valid—that is, it should measure what you want to measure (for a more extensive discussion of validity, see Herndon and Cutter, 2006)
- Accurate—it should consistently measure what it purports to measure
- Precise—it should give the same result every time if the patient has not changed
- Efficient and easy to use with little, if any, special training
- Sensitive to change in the disease without being overly sensitive to symptom fluctuation
- Cover the whole range of the disease

To be appropriate to the task, a scale must be able to measure that which you wish to measure with enough precision for the task at hand, and it must be efficient enough to be done in the time available.

The concept of validity is surprisingly complex. There are many types of validity (Herndon and Cutter, 2006). Types of validity include face validity, construct validity, criterion-related validity, content validity, predictive validity, and ecological validity. Face validity is the apparent sensibleness of the scale. For example, while leg strength might correlate fairly well with ability to ambulate, most of us would not consider it a very sensible measure because there are patients with good lower-extremity strength who are unable to ambulate because of spasticity or ataxia.

Construct validity relates to how well results of the measure concur with results predicted from the theoretical model of how things should behave. Criterion-related validity is the extent to which the results agree with another widely accepted measure. In the case of MS, most new measures are compared to the Kurtzke EDSS, which is widely considered the standard measure of impairment in MS.

Content validity is the extent to which a measure with multiple items includes all aspects of the disease and avoids irrelevancies. For example, the Hauser ambulation index is a good measure of mobility in MS, but it would not be valid as an overall measure of the disease.

Predictive validity is how well the measurement at a prior point in time can predict future change. For example, the MS Functional Composite actually predicts future EDSS better than the EDSS itself (Rudick et al., 2009).

Ecological validity is the validity of the measure in the context in which it is to be used. For example, wheelchair independence in an adapted house is not real wheelchair independence for someone whose house has doors too narrow to accommodate a wheelchair or has steps without a ramp.

There have been numerous attempts to develop and to improve scales for MS, but they all suffer from significant problems and none really rank well on these criteria. The extremely wide range of signs and symptoms characteristic of the disease and the amount of subjective judgment involved in the application of the available scales in comparing changes in different systems results in high inter-rater and even intra-rater variability. On the other hand, scales with more quantitative testing such as the Multiple Sclerosis Functional Composite (MSFC) are highly reproducible but do not cover the full variety of signs and symptoms, ignore important functions, and are unable to cover the full range of the disease. Interpretation in terms of the overall level of function of a patient

with such scales is at best difficult when it is at all possible.

Accuracy relates to how closely results center on the objective. Precision relates to how closely repeat testing mirrors the previous result if the patient has not changed (Fig. 11-1).

Most people working in MS know that an EDSS of 1 or 2 means no significant impairment, a level of 6 means the individual requires a cane or crutch for support when walking, 7.5 means wheelchair reliant but still able to self-transfer, with 10 being death from MS. No such conclusions can be drawn with the MSFC. In fact, the MSFC cannot really be used in individuals who are unable to ambulate 25 ft. In this chapter, we will present some of the measures and scales commonly used in MS and discuss their advantages and disadvantages. For additional scales and subscales the National Multiple Sclerosis Web site at http://www.nationalmssociety.org is an excellent resource. Look under the section for professionals and "research tools." The following is a list of scales available on the Web site:

9-Hole Peg Test (9-HPT)

Ambulation Index (AI)

Bladder Control Scale (BLCS)

Bowel Control Scale (BWCS)

Disease Steps (DS)

Functional Systems Scores (FSS) and Expanded Disability Status Scale (EDSS)

Health Status Questionnaire (SF-36)

Impact of Visual Impairment Scale (IVIS)

Mental Health Inventory (MHI)

Modified Fatigue Impact Scale (MFIS)

MOS Modified Social Support Survey (MSSS)

MOS Pain Effects Scale (PES)

Multiple Sclerosis Functional Composite (MSFC)

Multiple Sclerosis Quality of Life-54 (MSQOL-54)

Multiple Sclerosis Quality of Life Inventory (MSQLI)

Paced Auditory Serial Addition Test (PASAT)

Perceived Deficits Questionnaire (PDQ)

Sexual Satisfaction Scale (SSS)

Timed 25-Foot Walk (T25-FW)

Precise, Not Accurate

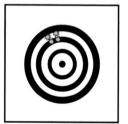

Accurate, Not Precise

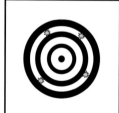

Accurate and Precise

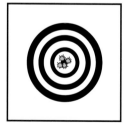

Figure 11-1 Accuracy and precision.

Since the Web site is updated regularly, additional scales are likely to be added from time to time.

In the next section of this chapter, we will present a few of the more widely used measures in MS.

COUNTING ATTACKS

This is the most common measure used in MS clinical trials and is based on exacerbations. This is used in several different forms, including time to first attack, annual attack rate, or simply number of attacks during the trial period. While simple and widely used, it regularly suffers from unrecognized bias. In order to be counted, the attack must be reported by the patient and is then typically followed by confirmation by a blinded examining physician, which gives it an air of objectivity. The problem with this measure is unreported attacks. If the patient does not report an attack, it is missed and not counted. Patients may differentially report attacks. A patient who believes he/she is on an effective drug may not report minor attacks for fear (regardless of what they have been told) that they may lose access to the drug if they report an attack. On the other hand, patients who believe they are on a placebo may report every minor new symptom. Thus, counting attacks is unbiased only when patients are blind to treatment and, given the side effects of most of the drugs used in MS, unblinding regularly occurs. Indeed, some unblinding has occurred in most of the MS clinical trials done to date. Thus, counting attacks is a poor measure unless the drug is without side effects that could reveal to the patient what treatment is being received.

THE KURTZKE EXPANDED DISABILITY STATUS SCALE

The Kurtzke Expanded Disability Status Scale (EDSS) is, by current terminology, an impairment scale. It was developed by John Kurtzke as a tool to assess the response of MS patients in a clinical trial of isoniazid (Kurtzke, 1955). He subsequently expanded the scale adding half points in an attempt to make it more sensitive (Kurtzke, 1983). It is the most widely used scale in MS trials, and its use is essential if a trial is to be compared to other MS trials. It consists of eight subscales covering pyramidal, cerebellar, brainstem, sensory,

bladder and bowel, visual, cognitive, and "other" impairments.

Strengths: The EDSS covers the whole range of the disease and is easily understood in terms of the extent of impairment by both professionals and lay persons.

Weaknesses: Intra-observer variability, even with training and examination of the same patient on the same day with other patients examined in between is one point. Inter-observer variability is even higher, around two points at the lower end of the scale but a bit less above EDSS 6. Since, despite Dr. Kurtzke's efforts to make it into a linear measure, in most neurologists' hands it acts as an ordinal scale, nonparametric statistics should be used.

The Expanded Disability Status Scale

0.0 Normal neurologic examination (all grade 0 in functional systems [FS])

0.1 No disability, minimal signs in one FS

1.5 No disability, minimal signs in more than one FS (more than one grade 1)

2.0 Minimal disability in one FS (one grade 2, others 0 or 1)

2.5 Minimal disability in two FS (two grade 2, others 0 or 1)

3.0 Moderate disability in one FS (one FS grade 3, others 0 or 1) or mild disability in (three or four FS grade 2, others 0 or 1) although fully ambulatory

3.5 Fully ambulatory but with moderate disability in one FS (one grade 3) and one or two FS grade 2; or two grade 3 (others 0 or 1) or five grade 2 (others 0 or 1)'

4.0 Fully ambulatory without aid, self-sufficient, up and about some 12 hr/day despite relatively severe disability consisting of one FS grade 4 (others 0 or 1), or combination of lesser grades exceeding limits of previous steps, and the patient should be able to walk >500 m without assistance or rest.

4.5 Fully ambulatory without aid, up and about much of the day, may otherwise require minimal assistance; characterized by relatively severe disability usually consisting of one FS grade 4 (others 1 or 0) or combination of lesser grades exceeding limits of previous steps and walks >300 m without assistance or rest.

5.0 Ambulatory without aid for at least 50 m; disability severe enough to impair full daily activities (e.g., to work a full day without special provision). (Usual FS equivalents are one grade 5 alone, other 0 or 1; combinations of lesser grade.) Patient walks >200 m without aid or rest.

5.5 Ambulatory without aid for at least 50 m; disability severe enough to preclude full daily activities. (Usual FS equivalents are one grade 5 alone, others 0 or 1; or combinations of lesser grades.) Enough to preclude full daily activities. Patient walks >100 m without aid or rest.

6.0 Intermittent or unilateral constant assistance (cane, crutch, or brace) required to walk at least 100 m. (Usual FS equivalents are combinations with more than one FS grade 3.)

6.5 Constant bilateral assistance (canes, crutches, braces) required to walk at least 20 m. (Usual FS equivalents are combinations with more than one FS grade 3.)

7.0 Unable to walk at least 5 m even with aid, essentially restricted to wheelchair; wheels self and transfers alone; up and about in wheelchair some 12 hr/day. (Usual FS equivalents are combinations with more than one FS grade 4+; very rarely pyramidal grade 5 alone.)

7.5 Unable to take more than a few steps; restricted to wheelchair; may need aid in transfer; wheels self but cannot carry on in wheelchair a full day. (Usual FS equivalents are combinations with more than one FS grade 4+; very rarely pyramidal grade 5 alone.)

8.0 Essentially restricted to chair or perambulated in a wheelchair but out of bed most of the day; retains many self-care functions; generally has effective use of arms. (Usual FS equivalents are combinations, generally grade 4+ in several systems.)

8.5 Essentially restricted to bed most of day; has some effective use of arm(s); retains some self-care functions. (Usual FS equivalents are combinations, generally grade 4 in several systems.)

9.0 Helpless bed patient; can communicate and eat. (Usual FS equivalents are combinations, mostly grade 4+.)

9.5 Totally helpless bed patient; unable to communicate effectively, eat, or swallow. (Usual FS equivalents are combinations, mostly grade 4+.)

10.0 Death due to multiple sclerosis

FUNCTIONAL SCALES

FS1-Pyramidal Functions

0. Normal

1. Abnormal signs without weakness

2. Mild weakness (4+/5)

3. Mild or moderate paraparesis or hemiparesis or severe monoparesis

4. Marked paraparesis or hemiparesis; moderate qudadriparesis; or monoplegia

5. Paraplegiak hemiplegia or marked quadriparesis

6. Quadriplegia

V. Unknown

Cerebellar Functions

0. Normal

1. Abnormal signs without disability

2. Mild ataxia

3. Moderate truncal or limb ataxia

4. Severe ataxia, all limbs

5. Unable to perform coordinated movements due to ataxia

V. Unknown

X. is used throughout after each number when weakness (grade 3 or worse on pyramidal) interferes with testing.

Brainstem Functions

0. Normal

1. Signs only

2. Moderate nystagmus or other mild disability

3. Severe nystagmus, marked extraocular weakness, or moderate disability of other cranial nerves

4. Marked dysarthria or other marked disability

5. Inability to swallow or speak

V. Unknown

Sensory Functions

0. Normal

1. Vibration or figure-writing decrease only in one or two limbs

2. Mild decrease in touch or pain or position sense, and/or moderate decrease in vibration in one or two limbs; or vibratory (c/s figure writing) decrease alone in three or four limbs

3. Moderate decrease in touch or pain or position sense and/or essentially lost vibration in one or two limbs; or mild decrease in touch or pain and/or moderate decrease in all proprioceptive tests in three or four limbs

4. Marked decrease in touch or pain or loss of proprioception, alone or combined, in one or two limbs; or moderate decrease in touch or pain and/or severe proprioceptive decrease in more than two limbs

5. Loss (essentially) of sensation in one or two limbs; or moderate decrease in touch or pain and/or loss of proprioception for most of the body below the head

V. Unknown

Bowel and Bladder Functions

0. Normal

1. Mild urinary hesitancy, urgency, or retention

2. Moderate hesitancy, urgency, retention of bowel or bladder, or rare urinary incontinence

3. Frequent urinary incontinence

4. In need of almost constant catheterization

5. Loss of bladder function

6. Loss of bowel and bladder function

V. Unknown

Visual (or Optic) Functions

0. Normal

1. Scotoma with visual acuity (corrected) better than 20/30

2. Worse eye with scotoma with maximal visual acuity (corrected) of 20/30 to 20/59

3. Worse eye with large scotoma, or moderate decrease in fields, but with maximal visual acuity (corrected) of 20/60 to 20/99

4. Worse eye with marked decrease of fields and maximal visual acuity (corrected) of 20/100 to 20/200; grade 3 plus maximal acuity of better eye of 20/60 or less

5. Worse eye with maximal visual acuity (corrected) less than 20/200; grade 4 plus maximal acuity of better eye of 20/60 or less

6. Grade 5 plus maximal visual acuity of better eye of 20/60 or less

V. Unknown

X. is added to grades 0 to 6 for presence of temporal pallor.

Cerebral (or Mental) Functions

0. Normal

1. Mood alteration only (does not affect DSS score)

2. Mild decrease in mentation

3. Moderate decrease in mentation

4. Marked decrease in mentation (chronic brain syndrome—moderate)

5. Dementia or chronic brain syndrome—severe or incompetent

V. Unknown

Other Functions

0. None

1. Any other neurologic findings attributed to MS (specify)

V. Unknown

Overall, while it requires a neurologist to administer the EDSS, it provides a reasonable scale for clinical trials and is essential if you wish to compare a current trial with results of previous MS trials.

THE MULTIPLE SCLEROSIS FUNCTIONAL COMPOSITE SCALE

The Multiple Sclerosis Functional Composite Scale is currently composed of three tests: a timed 8-meter (25 ft.) walk, 9-hole peg test done with each hand, and paced serial auditory addition test (PASAT). It was developed by a committee led by Dr. Richard Rudick supported by the National MS Society to provide a more precise measure of impairment in MS patients (Cutter et al., 1999).

Strengths: The scale is very precise and highly reproducible. It is sensitive to change and relatively insensitive to symptom fluctuation. There is very little intra- or inter-observer variability. It has excellent predictive validity and can predict future changes on the EDSS better than the EDSS itself. With regard to statistics, the results can be tested using parametric statistical methods.

Weaknesses: It does not cover the full range of the disease. Timed gait becomes uninformative when the individual can no longer walk 25 feet, and the 9-hole peg test becomes uninformative when the patient can no longer put the pegs in the holes with each hand independently. Thus, it is generally not useful beyond EDSS 6.5. It also suffers from the complexity of the statistical efforts required to establish the control baseline. Because of the complexity of calculating the Z-scores necessary for its use, we have not included it in this chapter; however, the scale and the handbook on how to use it are available on the U.S. National Multiple Sclerosis Society Web site, which was cited earlier.

QUALITY-OF-LIFE SCALES

Quality-of-life scales are now included in most clinical trials and are required by the Food and Drug Administration (FDA) for most trials. There are a number of quality-of-life scales for MS. We recommend those that are built on the Health Status Questionnaire SF-36, since this allows easy comparison with other diseases but provides additional information using disease-specific measures. The MSQOL-54 (Vickery et al., 1995) and the MSQLI (Ritvo et al., 1997) consist of disease-specific items in addition to the SF-36.

The SF-36 covers eight areas: physical functioning, role limitation due to physical problems, social functioning, bodily pain, general mental health, role limitation due to emotional problems, vitality, and general health perceptions. Because it is a generic health questionnaire, it can be used to compare the overall quality-of-life effects of different diseases. It has been used as a base to which disease-specific items can be added to create disease-specific quality of life scales.

The MSQOL-54 is a 54-item scale based on the SF-36 developed by Vickrey and colleagues. They added 18 disease-specific items based on the opinions of MS experts. They include overall quality of life (two items), health distress (four items), sexual function (five items), cognitive function (four items), and energy (one item). The scale was validated on 179 clinic cases. It is shorter than the MSQLI but does not have subscales that can be used separately.

The MS Quality of Life Inventory (MSQLI) was developed by a research group under the auspices of the Consortium of Multiple Sclerosis Clinics. They started with the SF-36 and added a number of established scales along with a few new scales. It covers some areas in more detail than the MSQOL-54 and the subscales are useful for studies of particular aspects of the disease. The following subscales are part of the MSQLI:

Modified Fatigue Impact Scale (MFIS)

MOS Pain Effects Scale (PES)

Sexual Satisfaction Scale (SSS)

Bladder Control Scale (BLCS)

Bowel Control Scale (BWCS)

Impact of Visual Impairment Scale (IVIS)

Perceived Deficits Questionnaire (PDQ)

Mental Health Inventory (MHI)

MOS Modified Social Support Survey (MSSS)

These scales cover most of the areas of concern for MS patients that relate to their quality of life. The subscales frequently prove useful in assessing the effect of particular interventions.

CONCLUSIONS

Disease measurement is important for clinical trials, for assessing the effects of various focused interventions, and for assessing disability. Selection of an appropriate scale or measurement is one of the most important steps in preparing to study any intervention in MS whether directed at the disease process or at a symptom or group of symptoms. We have presented some of the better-known, well-validated scales that we hope will be helpful in patient management and in the interpretation of reports of clinical trials.

REFERENCES

Cutter GR, Baier ML, Rudick RA, et al. Development of a multiple sclerosis functional composite as a clinical trial outcome measure. *Brain.* 1999;122:871–872.

Goodkin DE, Cookfair D, Wende K, et al. Inter- and intra-rater scoring agreement using grades 1.0-3.5 of the Kurtzke Expanded Disability Status Scale (EDSS). *Neurology.* 1992;42:859–863.

Herndon RM, Cutter G. In: eds. *Handbook of Neurologic Rating Scales.* 2nd ed. New York: Demos Medical Pub; 2006:5–6.

Kurtzke J. Rating neurologic impairment in multiple sclerosis: an Expanded Disability Status Scale (EDSS). *Neurology.* 1983;33:1444–1452.

Kurtzke JF. A new scale for evaluating disability in multiple sclerosls. *Neurology.* 1955;5:580–583.

Kurtzke JF. On the evaluation of disability in multiple sclerosis. *Neurology.* 1961;11:686–694.

Kurtzke JF, Berlin L. Isoniazid in treatment of multiple sclerosis. *JAMA.* 1957;163:172–174.

Ritvo, PG, Fischer JS, Miller DM, et al. *Multiple Sclerosis Quality of Life Inventory: A User's Manual.* New York: National Multiple Sclerosis Society; 1997.

Rudick R, Antel J, Confavreux C, et al. Recommendations from the National Multiple Sclerosis Society Clinical Outcomes Assessment Task Force. *Neurology.* 1997; 42:379–382.

Rudick RA, Polman CH, Cohen JA, et al. Assessing disease progression with the Multiple Sclerosis Functional Composite. *Mult Scler.* 2009;8:984–987.

Vickrey BG, Hays RD, Harooni R, et al. A health related quality of life measure for multiple sclerosis. *QOL Res.* 1995;4:187–206.

Part 4 Clinical Manifestations

12 Neuro-Ophthalmologic Manifestations of Multiple Sclerosis

Erik V. Burton and Elliot M. Frohman

Multiple sclerosis (MS) is one of the most common causes of neurologic and visual disability in young and middle-aged adults. Although the specific cause is unknown, the pathophysiology of MS is one of inflammatory demyelination and astrogliosis in the central nervous system (CNS) that culminates in axonal dysfunction and neuronal and axonal loss, which ultimately leads to permanent neurologic impairment. The majority of MS patients will have optic nerve and/or retinal dysfunction, and eye movement disturbances (e.g., nystagmus) at some point during the disease process. Axonal loss in the visual sensory pathways of MS patients has been documented at autopsy with 30%–45% fewer axons within the retinal nerve fiber layer (RNFL). Due to its disseminated nature, MS can produce several distinct neuro-ophthalmological syndromes that involve the anterior visual and ocular motor systems (Frohman et al., 2005).

NEURO-OPHTHALMOLOGY OF THE ANTERIOR VISUAL SYSTEM IN MS

Visual disturbances due to disease of the afferent visual system in MS may be related to pathologic changes in the uvea, retina, optic nerve, optic chiasm, and postchiasmal pathways. Changes affecting these locations may occur at any time point and may be the most significant manifestation of neurologic dysfunction in some patients. Afferent visual impairments may be the presenting feature in up to 40% of persons with MS and occur in at least 80% at some point during the disease course of those with MS (Leibowitz and Alter, 1968; Kuroiwa and Shibasaki, 1973). Additionally, visual disturbances may be subclinical and thereby go unnoticed by patients, but they may still be important in rendering the diagnosis.

The most commonly reported visual disturbances, even among those with visual acuity of 20/20 or better, are blurring and visual distortions, while visual field loss, flashes of light (phosphenes), and pain are also commonly reported (Nordmann et al., 1987). Additionally, Uhthoff first reported transient visual blurring with exercise or thermal stress—later termed *Uhthoff phenomena*—now used to describe any transient neurologic deterioration during exercise, overheating, fatigue, or emotional stress (Lepore, 1994; Selhorst and Saul, 1995). Uhthoff phenomena may be a significant source of disability and can affect any tract system that has sustained disease-related tissue injury (typically demyelination).

Optic Neuritis

Acute idiopathic demyelinating optic neuritis (ON) is frequently the initial clinical manifestation of MS and is one of the most common clinical events during the course of the disease. There is a gender difference, with women three times as likely as men to develop ON. The incidence of acute demyelinating optic neuritis in persons at high risk of developing MS is approximately 3–5/100,000 per year. In lower-risk regions the incidence approaches 1 per 100,000 per year (Wakakura et al., 1999; Kaufman et al., 2000). While the acute form of ON is the most commonly recognized by the clinician, ON may present in chronic and subclinical forms.

Clinical characteristics

The Optic Neuritis Treatment Trial (ONTT) assessed the benefits of corticosteroid treatment on visual recovery in ON and the relationship between this clinical syndrome and MS. Data on 457 patients, aged 18–46 years, with acute ON were collected in the ONTT. Patients typically experienced a decline in vision over a 7–10 day period with high variability in the degree of visual acuity loss (Optic Neuritis Study Group, 1991). Some patients experienced little change in central vision and retained a visual acuity of 20/20 or better, while no light perception vision was present in only 3% of participants initially. A progression of visual loss beyond 2 weeks was found to be distinctly unusual in this study. Typical cases exhibited some recovery of vision within 30 days of symptom onset (Beck et al., 1992).

In the ONTT, 92% of patients had pain, particularly with eye movements (Optic Neuritis Study Group, 1991). In addition to vision loss, flashes of light may be associated with ON and may be induced by eye movement (a phenomenon referred to as Moore lightning streaks) (Moore, 1935; Davis et al., 1976; McDonald and Barnes, 1992). A relative afferent papillary defect (RAPD) is often present in the affected eye unless the contralateral optic nerve is affected pathologically such that light transmission is slowed (as with demyelination). A central visual field defect is common in patients with ON, but a variety of patterns of visual field loss may be present as well (Keltner et al., 1993) (Fig. 12-1).

On funduscopic evaluation the optic disc was normal in approximately two-thirds of patients in the ONTT with classic ON (Optic Neuritis Study Group, 1991). In the remainder the optic disc is abnormal and appears swollen, as in anterior ON (also referred to as papillitis), or pale. Pallor of the optic disc is not present acutely after ON, but instead takes weeks to months in order to become manifest and is at least partially explained by astrogliosis within the optic nerve head. Retinal features that suggested nontypical ON included the presence of retinal hemorrhages, marked swelling of the optic nerve head, and retinal exudates. Additional clinical features of nontypical ON include the absence of pain and the presence of no light perception at onset (Optic Neuritis Study Group, 2003). Patients with atypical presentation had a lower risk of developing MS, particularly when a baseline magnetic resonance imaging (MRI) scan was normal (Optic Neuritis Study Group, 1997a; Optic Neuritis Study Group, 2003).

Visual recovery occured fairly rapidly but continued for up to a year in the ONTT (Beck et al., 1993b). The mean visual acuity in the affected eye at 1 year following onset of ON was 20/15 with 90% of patients having visual acuity better than 20/40 (Beck et al., 1992). Even with severe visual loss (no light perception or finger counting only), 49% of such patients regained visual acuity of 20/20 or better. Despite marked improvement in high contrast visual acuity abnormalities, abnormalities on low-contrast sensitivity, color perception, and visual field analysis persisted in approximately 30% of affected eyes and within 14%–19% of contralateral eyes (suggesting occult involvement) (Celesia et al., 1990; Ménage et al., 1993; Keltner et al., 1994; Optic Neuritis Study Group, 2004).

Demyelinating ON can occasionally be difficult to distinguish from anterior ischemic optic neuropathy (AION). The two entities have overlapping clinical features, including the rate and range of visual deterioration,11 JF Rizzo and S Lessell, Optic neuritis and ischemic optic neuropathy. Overlapping clinical profiles, Arch Ophthalmol 109 (1991), pp. 1668–1672. View Record in Scopus Cited By in Scopus (83) and up to 10%–15% of patients with ON may have an altitudinal visual field defect (a characteristic feature of AION) (Rizzo and Lessell, 1988; Rizzo and Lessell, 1991; Keltner et al., 1993) (Table 12-1). Additional evaluation may aid in distinguishing the two when appropriate.

Chronic optic neuropathy associated with MS (either following ON or in the absence of a history of ON) should be considered as a diagnosis of exclusion to avoid overlooking other, potentially treatable causes of progressive optic neuropathy. Clinical dysfunction in such chronic cases may be reported as an insidious onset or as a stepwise loss in vision over time. Fortunately most patients with chronic forms of optic neuropathy develop visual disturbance after the presentation of other characteristic features of MS, facilitating the identification of the underlying etiology in most. Evidence for subclinical or asymptomatic optic neuropathy was found in a significant proportion of fellow eyes at the time of enrollement in the ONTT and at 10 years follow-up. In particular, abnormalities in the contralateral eye included reduced visual acuity (19%), contrast sensitivity

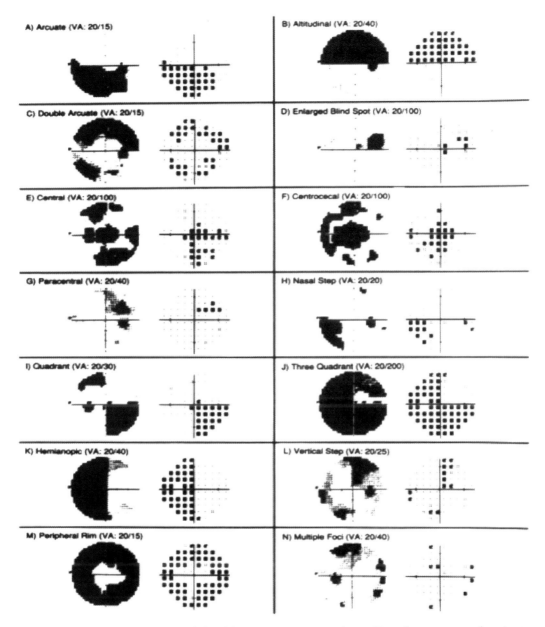

A) Arcuate (VA: 20/15)

B) Altitudinal (VA: 20/40)

C) Double Arcuate (VA: 20/15)

D) Enlarged Blind Spot (VA: 20/100)

E) Central (VA: 20/100)

F) Centrocecal (VA: 20/100)

G) Paracentral (VA: 20/40)

H) Nasal Step (VA: 20/20)

I) Quadrant (VA: 20/30)

J) Three Quadrant (VA: 20/200)

K) Hemianopic (VA: 20/40)

L) Vertical Step (VA: 20/25)

M) Peripheral Rim (VA: 20/15)

N) Multiple Foci (VA: 20/40)

Figure 12-1 Visual field defects as defined by static perimetry using a Humphrey automated perimeter and visual acuity (VA) in acute optic neuritis. (From Beck RW, Cleary PA. Optic neuritis treatment trial. One year follow-up results. *Arch Ophthalmol.* 1993;111:773–775.)

(14%), and visual fields (17%) (Optic Neuritis Study Group, 2004).

Vision testing

There are numerous bedside assessment strategies used to identify dysfunction in the afferent visual system. General routine assessment should include Snellen acuity, confrontational fields, pupillary light reflexes, and ophthalmoscopy (Table 12-2). Visual field (Humphrey 30-2, contrast sensitivity [Pelli-Robson]), visual acuity (Early Treatment Diabetic Research Study charts), and color vision testing (Ishihara pseudoisochromatic

TABLE 12-1 Clinical Characteristics of Typical Demyelinating Optic Neuritis and Anterior Ischemic Optic Neuropathy

	Demyelinating Optic Neuritis	*Anterior Ischemic Optic Neuropathy*
Age (years)	20–50	>50
Disc edema	Present in one-third typically without hemorrhage or exudates	Present, often sectoral, hemorrhage may be present
Pain	Present (>90%)	Absent (<10%)
Field defect	Central but variable	Altitudinal

plates and Farnsworth-Munsell 100-hue test) were the main visual outcome measures used in the ONTT (Beck et al., 1992). Visual acuity abnormalities were reported in 89.5% of patients at baseline (Optic Neuritis Study Group, 1991). Visual field defects (97.5%), color vision abnormalities (88%), and contrast-sensitivity abnormalities (98.2%) were present in almost all patients, with significant abnormalities present even at 5 and 10 years' follow-up (Optic Neuritis Study Group, 1997b; Optic Neuritis Study Group, 2004).

Diagnostic assessment

The risk of developing MS following an event of ON can be estimated reliably, with MRI having

TABLE 12-2 The Afferent Bedside Neuro-Ophthalmologic Exam

Visual acuity	Corrective lenses
	Pinhole
	Near or distance
Visual fields	Monocular testing
	Static and dynamic
Color	Color plates
	Red-green desaturation
Pupil	Shape and position
	Anisocoria
	Reactivity
	Relative afferent pupillary defect
Funduscopic	Edema
	Hemorrhage
	Disc pallor
	Occult nystagmus
	Perivenular phlebitis

been established as the most important predictor of this risk. Approximately 50%–70% of patients with ON will have periventricular white matter abnormalities consistent with demyelination on an initial MRI scan (Beck et al., 1993a; Morrissey et al., 1993; Dalton et al., 2003). In a report of 115 patients with clinically isolated ON, 70% of the patients had abnormal brain lesions shown by MRI scan and 27% had spinal cord lesions (Dalton et al., 2003).According to the ONTT, the cumulative risk of developing MS following optic neuritis by 15 years was 50%. In patients with no white matter lesions the risk of developing MS was approximately 25%. Nevertheless, the presence of even one white matter lesion escalates the risk of developing clinically definite MS to 72%. Of those with lesions on an initial MRI, male sex, optic disc swelling, poor vision, and no pain were associated with a lower risk for conversion to MS (Frohman et al., 2003a; Optic Neuritis Study Group, 2008).

The percentage of patients with optic nerve enhancement in the acute stage of ON may approach 90% (Rizzo et al., 2002). Newer MRI techniques—such as diffusion tensor imaging (DTI), magnetic transfer imaging, and spectroscopy—may improve our ability to detect demyelinating abnormalities in the brain and optic nerve (Filippi et al., 2003; Ge et al., 2003). Diffusion tensor imaging has demonstrated dynamic changes in acute isolated ON and, in remote disease, parameters correlate with functional, structural, and physiologic tests of vision (Naismith et al., 2009) (Fig. 12-2).

When the clinical course is typical, other diagnostic studies such as fluorescence treponemal antigen antibodies, antinuclear antibodies, angiotensin converting enzyme, Lyme titer, chest radiograph, and lumbar puncture are of limited use in

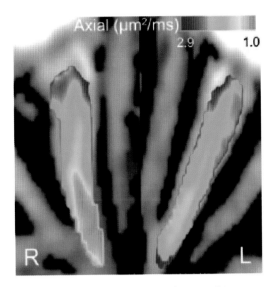

Figure 12-2 Axial diffusivety is decreased in acute optic neuritis (ON). This optic nerve was imaged 11 days after clinical onset of ON. Vision was motion perception only. Decreased axial diffusivity was manifested by a warmer color. Although this eye had a severe onset, it made a good recovery. (From Naismith RT, Xu J, Tutlam NT, et al. Disability in optic neuritis correlates with diffusion tensor-derived directional diffusivities. *Neurology.* 2009;72(7):589–594.)

eliminating other causes of optic neuropathy (Optic Neuritis Study Group, 1991). To determine risk of progression to MS oligoclonal banding in the cerebrospinal fluid (CSF) was strongly predictive but not independent of MRI and is of limited clinical utility in assessment when there is a typical course (Rolak et al., 1996). A more aggressive assessment should be considered when nontypical features of ON are present and should include tests for Lupus, Lyme disease, sarcoid, syphilis, West Nile virus, human immunodeficiency virus, ehrlichiosis, Leber optic neuropathy, and neuromyelitis optica in the appropriate clinical setting.

Electrophysiologic testing, such as visual evoked potentials, is of limited clinical utility and may be considered when there is paucity of data to confirm a clinical diagnosis of MS (Gronseth and Ashman, 2000). Multifocal visual evoked testing may be useful in select patients, particularly when the distinction between optic nerve and retinal

disease is in question, or when evidence of subclinical optic nerve dysfunction is sought (Hood et al., 2003). In routine clinical practice, computerized fields, such as Humphrey automated perimetry (using 24-2 or 30-2 test paradigms), using sita fast or full-threshold algorithms, may be used to document the visual field defect in patients with ON.

Advancements in the application of optical coherence tomography (OCT) has allowed for objective analysis of neurodegeneration and its implications within the retina (Frohman et al., 2006). The retina is unique in that the most superficial layer, the retinal nerve fiber layer (RNFL), contains axons and glia in the absence of myelin. The fibers do not become myelinated until they pass posteriorly through the lamina cribrosa. With OCT, high-resolution images of the internal retinal structures are generated by an optical beam scanned across the retina (Fig. 12-3). Measurements from these images have been correlated and validated with high-contrast and low-contrast visual acuity, visual field changes, brain atrophy, and subtype of MS (Fisher et al., 2006). The RNFL thickness is about 110–120 µm by 15 years of age. Following acute ON, about 75% of patients sustain a 10–40 µm loss of RNFL thickness that appears to be unaffected by corticosteroid or disease-modifying therapy (Costello et al., 2006). Optical coherence tomography is noninvasive and can sensitively and rapidly measure changes in the retina that are a consequence of MS and may provide an additional means of monitoring therapeutic response to neuroprotective agents (Sergott et al., 2007; Frohman et al., 2008a).

Treatment

The ONTT is the largest randomized study to examine the impact of corticosteroid treatment for inflammatory demyelinating ON. The trial used three treatment groups: *(1)* intravenous methylprednisolone (250 mg every 6 hours for 3 days) followed by an oral prednisone (1 mg/kg/day) for 12 days with 2-day taper, *(2)* oral prednisone (1 mg/kg/day) for 12 days followed by a 2-day taper, and *(3)* oral placebo for 14 days (Beck et al., 1992). Among the treatment groups there was no difference at 6 months in visual acuity ($p = 0.09$), although there were significant differences favoring the intravenous group for contrast sensitivity

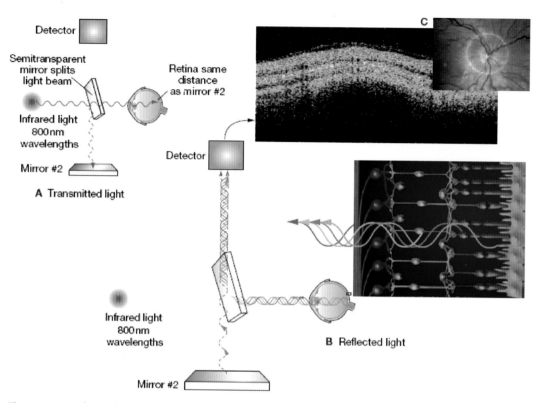

Figure 12-3 High-resolution images of the internal retinal structure taken with optical coherence tomography (OCT), demonstrating the processes involved in using this technology. (A) Low-coherence infrared light is transmitted into the eye through use of an interoferometer. (B) The infrared light is transmitted through the pupil and then penetrates through the transparent nine layers of the retina. Subsequently, the light backscatters and returns through the pupil, where detectors can analyze the interference of light returning from the layers of the retina compared with light traveling a reference path (mirror #2). An algorithm mathematically uses this information to construct a grayscale or false-color image representing the anatomy of the retina (shown in the upper right portion of the figure). (C) A fundus image from the OCT device, showing the optic disc appropriately centered and surrounded by the target image circumference marker for analysis of the retinal nerve fiber layer. (From Frohman EM, Fujimoto LG, Frohman TC, Calabresi PA, et al. Optical coherence tomography: a window into the mechanisms of multiple sclerosis. *Nat Clin Pract Neurol.* 2008b;4(12):664–675.)

($p = 0.026$) and color vision ($p = 0.033$) (Beck et al., 1992). At 1 year, however, there were no statistical differences in any of the four measures of visual function, including visual acuity, visual field, color vision, and contrast testing (Beck et al., 1993b). The ONTT therefore suggested that visual recovery may be hastened by intravenous high-dose steroids as determined by visual field and contrast sensitivity measurements, but long-term visual outcomes are not affected (Beck et al., 1992). Furthermore a meta-analysis of 12 randomized

controlled clinical trials of steroid treatment in MS and ON likewise found that corticosteroids were potentially useful in improving short-term visual recovery, but had no long-term benefit on vision (Brusaferri and Candelise, 2000). Of significance, those who received high-dose IV corticosteroids in the ONTT had a delay in the development of clinically definite MS over the following 2 years (Beck et al., 1993c).

In the ONTT the use of oral corticosteroids was associated with an increased risk of recurrent ON in the affected eye and new attacks of ON in the contralateral eye (Optic Neuritis Study Group, 1997b). Five years after an initial bout of ON, patients who received oral prednisone (1 mg/kg) had the highest rate of recurrence (41%) compared with those who received methylprednisolone or placebo (25% for both groups). This association was no longer significant at 10 years ($p = 0.07$) (Optic Neuritis Study Group, 2004). A small prospective controlled clinical trial of oral methylprednisolone (500 mg every day for 5 days) did not indicate an increased rate of demyelinating attacks, suggesting that dose as opposed to the route of administration determined response (Sellebjerg et al., 1999).

Based on findings from the ONTT, in patients with acute ON and an abnormal baseline brain MRI scan, it is recommended that treatment with a 3-day course of high-dose (1 g/day) intravenous corticosteroids followed by an oral prednisone taper be initiated given the noted delay in development of clinically definite MS and more rapid improvements in vision (Beck et al., 1993a). However, many patients with isolated ON and a normal baseline MRI scan will have spontaneous and excellent recovery of vision without the use of corticosteroids. Oral steroids in standard 1mg/kg/day doses are not to be used to treat isolated ON. In patients with severe unilateral visual loss high-dose IV corticosteroids is recommended because corticosteroids may hasten visual recovery by several weeks and have been shown to be safe with minimal adverse effects.

Other treatments such as intravenous immunoglobulin (IVIg) and plasma exchange have been reported to improve visual acuity in patients with optic neuritis (Ruprecht et al., 2004), though no effect on chronic visual loss has been reported in patients with ON treated with IVIg.

Other Afferent Manifestations

Optic chiasmal and retrochiasmal demyelinating lesions

In addition to the optic nerve, the optic chiasm, tracts, radiations, and striate cortex may be affected in MS. Any type of field defect may then occur, depending on the location of the demyelinating lesion (Plant et al., 1992; Newman, 1998).

Defects due to optic radiation and cortex involvement are uncommon in MS because of the large lesions required to produce them and the tendency for inflammation to be localized to postcapillary venules and not necessarily axonal tracts. In the ONTT, 13% of patients had evidence of a chiasmal or retrochiasmal field defect when serially screened at nine visits over 1 year (Keltner et al., 1994). Fewer than 10% of patients develop homonymous visual field defects from postchiasmal lesions in MS and symptomatic homonymous field defects are infrequent in MS, occurring in fewer than 1% of patients (Kurtzke et al., 1968; Hawkins and Behrens, 1975; Plant et al., 1992; Keltner et al., 1994). When found, defects may be quadrantic or hemianopic, complete or incomplete, and congruous or incongruous.

Chiasmal neuritis may result in typical or atypical chiasmal syndromes characterized by bitemporal visual field deficits associated with change in visual acuity and color vision (Bell et al., 1975; Sacks and Melen, 1975; Spector et al., 1980). Patients may have enlarged optic chiasms with enhancement or focal leptomeningeal enhancement along the chiasm on MRI (Kerty et al., 1991; Newman et al., 1991; Demaerel et al., 1995). These syndromes may occur like others anytime during the course of MS or as an initial manifestation of MS.

Uveitis

Ocular inflammation may be seen in patients with MS and may manifest as anterior uveitis, posterior uveitis, pars planitis, and periphlebitis. Uveitis is 10 times more common in patients with MS than in the general population and may manifest before other clinical evidence of MS exists (Ganley, 1984; Newman, 1998). Anterior uveitis, as a complication in MS, is typically granulomatous in nature and less common than posterior uveitis, which is associated with periphlebitis (Bamford et al., 1978; Arnold et al., 1984; Newman, 1998). Disease such as syphilis, sarcoidosis, Lyme disease, tuberculosis, rheumatological disorders, and Bechet disease are far more likely to produce this condition and should be excluded upon presentation. Pars planitis is an intraocular inflammation of unknown cause that occurs along the pars plana of the eye and may also be associated with periphlebitis. Although it generally has no symptoms, this type of ocular inflammation may have numerous sequelae resulting in vision loss due to cataract formation, epiretinal membrane formation, and cystoid macular edema (Malinowski et al., 1993a, 1993b). There is a strong association between pars planitis and MS, with 48% of patients with pars planitis having demyelinating lesions in the CNS in one study (Hughes and Dick, 2003).

Periphlebitis is characterized by sheathing or cuffing of the retinal veins by lymphocytes and plasma cells (Rucker, 1944; Hornsten, 1971; Arnold et al., 1984). The prevalence of periphlebitis in MS has been estimated to be in the range of 10%–36% (Adams et al., 1985; Tola et al., 1993). Generally this is asymptomatic in patients with MS and is most often identified incidentally. More aggressive forms of retinal periphlebitis may be seen, but it is more often associated with other disorders such as Eale disease, sarcoid, idiopathic uveitis, toxoplasmosis, and syphilis, all of which should be excluded (Hornsten, 1971).

NEURO-OPHTHALMOLOGY OF THE OCULAR MOTOR SYSTEM IN MULTIPLE SCLEROSIS

Patients with MS may develop disorders of ocular fixation, motility, and alignment, which may be the result of supranuclear, internuclear, nuclear, or fascicular lesions (Table 12-3). When done carefully, the bedside neuro-ophthalmological examination can detect most abnormalities within both the visual sensory and ocular motor systems of patients with MS. Examination of the ocular motor system should include testing of alignment, motility, saccades, smooth pursuit, vergence, vestibular function, and optical kinetic nystagmus (Table 12-4). Most lesions corresponding to the eye movement disorders recognized in MS are visible on MRI. Proton density and T2-weighted sequences (with thin 3 mm cuts) have been seen to be superior to fluid attenuation inversion recovery studies in detecting these lesions (Gass et al., 1998; Frohman et al., 2001).

TABLE 12-3 Ocular Motor Manifestations of Multiple Sclerosis

Disorder	Characteristics	Localization	Treatment
Saccadic intrusions	Square wave jerks Macro square waves Macro saccadic oscillations Ocular flutter Opsoclonus Microsaccadic flutter	Cerebellum Brain stem Pause cells?	Anticonvulsants Baclofen
INO	Adduction slowing Abduction nystagmus	MLF	Steroids acutely
WEBINO	Wall-eyed and bilateral Loss of convergence	Rostral midbrain involving bilateral MLF and vergence pathways or CN III pathways to medial rectus muscles	Steroids acutely
Saccadic dysmetria	Overshoots and undershoots Ipsipulsion Contrapulsion	Cerebellum Brain stem	Steroids acutely
VOR suppression	Cannot suppress VOR during head/eye tracking	Cerebellar flocculus	None
Saccadic slowing	Reduced velocity	PPRF	None

TABLE 12-3 (continued)

Disorder	Characteristics	Localization	Treatment
Cranial nerve palsies	Complete or partial Isolated In conjunction with other features	VI > III > IV	Prisms
Gaze palsies (unilateral or bilateral)	Decreased velocity and or amplitude of gaze to left, right, or both	PPRF Abducens (VI) nucleus VI + INO	Steroids acutely
One-and-a-half Syndrome	Gaze palsy to one side INO to the other Paralytic pontine exotropia	PPRF and/or VI nucleus and MLF on same side	Steroids acutely
Horizontal monocular failure	Absent or diminished adduction and abduction	VI fascicle + MLF on same side	Steroids acutely
Pursuit abnormalities	Low gain or saccadic High gain	Pursuit circuitry Attention/concentration	None
Skew deviation	Vertical misalignment Vertical diplopia Often with INO Head tilt-away from hyper Subjective vertical deviation Ocular counter-roll	Anywhere in vestibular system that can affect the linear otoliths Hyper on side of pontine lesion in most Hyper on side opposite of a medullary lesion in most	Steroids acutely
Nystagmus	Gaze evoked Multidirectional Upbeat and downbeat Vestibular Dysconjugate Rebound Pendular types Occult (with ophthalmoscopy) Periodic alternating	Cerebellum Brain stem Vesitibular apparatus either central or peripheral	Gabapentin Memantine Baclofen 3,4-diaminopyridine 4-aminopyridine Benzodiazepine Anticonvulsants Prisms Botox Particle repositioning manoeuvres for BPPV

Disorders of Fixation

Nystagmus

Nystagmus is the most common disorder of fixation in MS and may be observed in primary position or upon eccentric gaze and is often associated with the visual illusion of environmental movement (oscillopsia). The classification of nystagmus is perhaps best approached by considering the disorders of the gaze-holding networks themselves in the brain stem and cerebellum, and their inputs such as the vestibular system. The critical structures for gaze-holding—which act as a neural integrator—are located in the medulla for horizontal gaze and in the midbrain for vertical gaze. Neural integrators in the medulla include the medial vestibular nuclei and the adjacent nucleus

TABLE 12-4 Components of the Bedside Ocular Motor Exam

Ocular alignment and inspection	Tropia
	Crosscover for phoria
	Skew deviation
	Ptosis
	Head tilt
Motility	Ductions (monocular)
	Versions (binocular)
	Maddox rod/red glass testing
Smooth pursuit	High gain
	Low gain
Saccades	Latency
	Velocity
	Accuracy
	Internuclear ophthalmoplegia
	Gaze palsy
Vestibular	Vestibulo-ocular reflex (VOR)
	Head thrust for VOR gain
	VOR suppression
	Vestibular nystagmus
	Positional nystagmus
OKN	OKN strip
Intrusions	Square wave jerks
	Oscillations
	Flutter
	Opsoclonus
Nystagmus	Direction
	Primary position
	Gaze evoked
	Monocular movements
	Rebound
	Periodic alternating
	Pendular positional

prepositus hypoglossus and in the midbrain include the interstitial nucleus of Cajal (Keane, 1990; Bhidayasiri et al., 2000). The superior vestibular nuclei probably also influence vertical gaze-holding through their connection, via the medial longitudinal fasciculus (MLF), to the interstitial nucleus of Cajal. The paramedian tracts of the midline pons also contain neurons that are important for ocular motor integration. These brainstem integrators are connected to the cerebellar flocculus and paraflocculus (tonsils), which are key structures for fine tuning of the brainstem integrators.

Pathological gaze-evoked nystagmus occurs frequently in MS due to disturbances in the neural integrators and refers to a "jerk" nystagmus with a slow drift in one direction and a resetting saccade in the other. Horizontal gaze-evoked nystagmus as well as primary position downbeat nystagmus may be the result of floccular and parafloccular lesions. Often gaze-evoked nystagmus is not visually disabling and no treatment is required.

TABLE 12-5 Treatment Options for Nystagmus

Acquired pendular nystagmus	Clonazepam
	Gabapentin
	Memantine
	Scopolamine
Downbeating nystagmus	Clonazepam
	Gabapentin
	Baclofen
	3,4 diaminopyridine
	Scopolamine
Upbeating nystagmus	Baclofen
	Clonazepam
Periodic alternating nystagmus	Baclofen
	Phenothiazine
	Barbiturates
See-saw nystagmus	Clonazepam
	Baclofen

Recent studies suggest that downbeat nystagmus can be decreased using 4-aminopyridine (Kalla et al., 2004; Strupp et al., 2004). Clonazepam as well may be useful for diminishing downbeat nystagmus (Young and Huang, 2001).

Pendular nystagmus is common in MS, and it may be particularly distressing due to severe oscillopsia and decreased central acuity secondary to retinal slip (Averbuch-Heller et al., 1995; Lopez et al., 1996). Pendular nystagmus may also arise, in part, from visual loss. It is characterized by back-and-forth slow-phase oscillation with no fast phase and arises from disturbances in the neural integrators and their interconnections within the cerebellum and brainstem tegmentum (Averbuch-Heller et al., 1995; Arnold and Robinson, 1997). These movements may be horizontal, vertical, oblique, or elliptical. Examples include elliptical nystagmus and the pendullar nystagmus associated with palatal myoclonus (ocular palatal tremor) due to lesions involving Mollaret triangle (connecting the red nucleus and inferior olive ipsilaterally via the central tegmental tract to the contralateral cerebellar dentate nucleus through inferior and superior cerebellar peduncles) (Revol et al., 1990). Several drugs, including gabapentin and memantine, may improve pendular nystagmus through GABA–like effects or through NMDA-blocking, AMPA-receptor-modulating, and dopaminergic

action (Todman, 1988; Ashe et al., 1991; Starck et al., 1997; Averbuch-Heller, 1999; see Table 12-5).

Numerous other forms of nystagmus may be present in patients with MS and may result in visual dysfunction. Upbeating and downbeating forms of nystagmus may respond to clonazepam (Young and Huang, 2001; Leigh and Tomsak, 2003). Periodic alternating nystagmus, believed to be due to dysfunction of the γ-aminobutyric acid (GABA)-ergic velocity storage mechanism, may be responsive to the GABA agonist baclofen (Leigh and Tomsak, 2003). Seesaw nystagmus, characterized by a conjugate torsional component and a dysconjugate vertical component, may respond to clonazepam or baclofen (Strupp and Brandt, 2006; Table 12-5). Carbamazepine or acetazolamide may be used to suppress paroxysmal forms of nystagmus (Averbuch-Heller, 1999).

Saccadic intrusions

Various saccadic intrusions that impair fixation may occur in patients with MS and are associated with lesions in the cerebellum and caudal brain stem. These include ocular flutter, opsoclonus, square-wave jerks, microsaccadic flutter, and macrosquare-wave jerks. Disorders of pause-cell neurons, which are located in the pontine raphe between the abducens nuclei and tonicall inhibit burst neurons in the paramedian reticular formation of the pons and midbrain, may produce impaired fixation due to extraneous saccades.

The most common of these intrusions are square-wave jerks, which are 1–5 degree eye movements away and back from the primary position. Larger movements of 10–40 degrees are referred to as macrosquare-wave jerks. Large to-and-fro eccentric movements across the midline represent macrosaccadic oscillations. These movements distinguish themselves from ocular flutter, microsaccadic flutter, and opsoclonus in part by the presence of an intrasaccadic latency.

As mentioned, ocular flutter is a saccadic intrusion characterized by horizontal back-to-back saccades without an intersaccadic latency (in contrast to square-wave jerks, which have a intersaccadic interval). Similarly, opsoclonus is also characterised by back-to-back saccades without an intrasaccadic latency, but the movements are in both the horizontal and vertical planes. Finally, microsaccadic flutter is a binocular condition with similar back-to-back saccades that are generally seen only on ophthalmoscopy or on eye movement recordings (Ashe et al., 1991). Microsaccadic flutter may result in shimmering, jiggling, or wavy vision (i.e., oscillopsia). This disorder should be differentiated from superior oblique myokymia, which is strictly monocular and characterized by a strong torsional component. Spontaneous remissions, which can last for days or up to years, are typical, but there have been several reports that anticonvulsants, especially carbamazepine, have a therapeutic effect (Rosenberg and Glaser, 1983).

In addition to superior oblique myokymia, a number of other disturbances may affect fixation and are separate from nystagmus and saccadic intrusions, including ocular bobbing and oculopalatal myoclonus, which have been reported as presenting signs in MS (Revol et al., 1990). Patients with MS can also experience steady fixation interrupted by paroxysmal episodes of diplopia (Twomey and Espir, 1980; Todman, 1988).

Disorders of Cerebellar Regulation

The dorsal vermis and the posterior fastigial nuclei are cerebellar structures important in controlling saccadic. Demyelinating lesions within these structures can result in hypermetric (if the deep nuclei are involved) or hypometric (if the vermis alone is involved) saccades. Macrosaccadic oscillations are an extreme example of saccadic hypermetria. Ipsipulsion describes a hypermetric saccade toward the side of a lateral medullary lesion, while contrapulsion describes a hypermetric saccade away from a lesion of the Hook Bundle region near the superior cerebellar peduncle (Solomon et al., 1995; Frohman et al., 2001; Fig. 12-4). Floccular and parafloccular lesions, in addition to horizontal gaze-evoked nystagmus and primary-position downbeat nystagmus, may result in impaired (low-gain) smooth pursuit eye movements requiring corrective saccades, rebound nystagmus (e.g., a transient jerk nystagmus that occurs on returning the eyes to straight ahead after sustained attempted eccentric gaze-holding with the slow phase of rebound nystagmus is in the direction of prior attempted lateral gaze-holding), postsaccadic drift (glissades), and a loss of vestibulo-ocular reflex cancellation, which are commonly seen in patients with MS (Averbuch-Heller, 1999).

Disorders of Motility and Alignment

Disturbances in ocular motility and alignment are quite common in MS and often result from

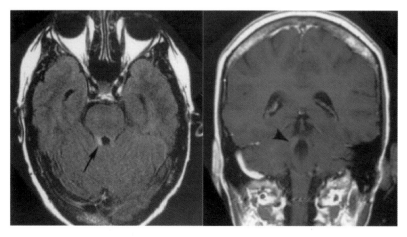

Figure 12-4 A patient with hypermetric saccades to the left has lesion within the right superior cerebellar peduncle on fluid attenuated inversion recovery (FLAIR) weighted images (*left*) with corresponding gadolinium enhancement (*right*). (From Frohman EM, Frohman TC, Fleckenstein J, et al. Ocular contrapulsion in multiple sclerosis: clinical features and pathophysiological mechanisms. *J Neurol Neurosurg Psychiatry.* 2001;70:688–692.)

demyelinating lesions of the brain stem affecting supranuclear, internuclear, nuclear, or fascicular pathways. Supranuclear lesions are characterized by saccadic and smooth pursuit dysfunction with preservation of vestibular-mediated eye movements (e.g., oculocephalic movements). Supranuclear impairment in vertical gaze is often related to dysfunction in the mesencephalon affecting the mesencephalic reticular formation or posterior commissure. Pontine dysfunction particularly affecting the paramedian pontine reticular formation results in horizontal gaze impairment.

Nuclear and fascicular lesions

Nuclear and fascicular cranial nerve syndromes have been described in MS with sixth nerve paresis being the most common (Keane, 1976; Rush and Younge, 1981). Involvement of the abducens nucleus produces a gaze palsy to the side of the lesion due to involvement of the ipsilateral projections to the lateral rectus and the internuclear neurons that connect the abducens nucleus to the contralateral third nerve nucleus through the MLF. Involvement of the abducens fascicle produces only an ipsilateral lateral rectus palsy. Bilateral horizontal gaze palsy secondary to a midline pontine lesion has been reported in MS (Joseph et al., 1985).

Isolated oculomotor (third cranial nerve) palsies can occur in MS, and partial fascicular (upper and lower division) and nuclear lesions have also been reported (Ksiazek et al., 1989; Miller, 1995). Trochlear nucleus and fascicle lesions are rare and result in an ipsilateral hypertropia that worsens on contralateral gaze and ipsilateral head tilt. A unique syndrome combining an internuclear ophthalmoplegia (INO) with a contralateral hyperdeviation secondary to superior oblique weakness has been reported. This lesion is localized to the caudal midbrain involving the MLF and trochlear nucleus and may also be associated with Horner syndrome (Vanooteghem et al., 1992).

Ptosis from a brainstem lesion can be unilateral or bilateral. When caused by oculomotor dysfunction, fascicular lesions give rise to unilateral ptosis, whereas nuclear lesions produce bilateral ptosis owing to involvement of the central caudal subnucleus of the third cranial nerve. This nucleus is unpaired and contains cells that project to both levator palpebre superioris muscles. Additional eyelid abnormalities have been reported in MS, including blepharoclonus and eyelid myokymia. Rare patients develop blepharoclonus in association with other signs of brainstem dysfunction. Blepharoclonus is characterised by paroxysms of forced eye closure that can be triggered by eccentric eye movements or occur spontaneously while looking straight ahead (Keane, 1978). Eyelid myokymia, characterized by undulating, wave-like twitching, is often self-limited but has been reported to progress to facial myokymia and hemifacial spasm.

Internuclear ophthalmoplegia

Internuclear ophthalmoplegia is a hallmark lesion of MS characterized by impairment of the adducting eye during horizontal saccades and is the result of damage to the MLF connecting the abducens nucleus to the contralateral medial rectus subnucleus within the dorsomedial pontine or midbrain tegmentum, adjacent to the fourth ventricle and cerebral aqueduct, respectively. During horizontal saccades, the burst cells in the paramedian pontine reticular formation (PPRF) innervate the abducens nucleus, which contains two distinctive sets of neurons—one to the ipsilateral lateral rectus and the other to the contralateral medial rectus subnucleus. Unilateral INO is characterized by ipsilateral impairment in the adducting eye and contralateral nystagmus in abducting eye on horizontal gaze. The discrepant movement of the two eyes in INO during saccades results in a break in binocular fusion that can lead to visual confusion, transient oscillopsia, diplopia, reading fatigue, and loss of stereopsis. The adduction impairment may be of three forms: paralysis of adduction, limitation in range of adduction with reduced velocity, and in the most subtle form range of adduction is normal with reduced velocity only (Fig. 12-5). Despite adduction weakness, convergence is generally intact; however, if the lesion is sufficiently rostral in the mesencephalon to generate generalized weakness of adduction, then convergence is compromised, potentially producing divergence of the eyes and bilateral internuclear ophthalmoplegia (WEBINO syndrome) (Frohman et al., 2000b).

When adduction limitation is present, it may not be overcome by vestibular stimulation because

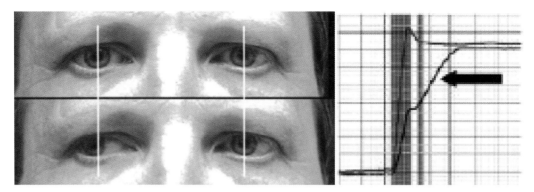

Figure 12-5 A patients with multiple sclerosis with confirmed internuclear ophthalmoparesis (INO). The vertical white bars (initially on the midpupillary line) are used to show the displacement of the eyes from the midline position. In patients with INO, the position of the adducing eye lags behind the abducting eye, with less displacement away from the midline position. During a 20° saccade to the right severe dyscon-jugacy is shown. The photographs show the position of the adducing eye at the point in time when the abducting eye has first achieved the +20° target. To the right is a corresponding infrared oculogram show-ing the divergence of the right and left eye movement tracings (arrow). (From Frohman TC, Frohman EM, O'Suilleabhain P, et al. Accuracy of clinical detection of INO in MS: corroboration with quantitative infrared oculography. *Neurology*. 2003c;61(6):848–850.)

Combined lesions of the medial longitudinal fasciculus

A lesion damaging either the PPRF or abducens nucleus (or both) together with the MLF ipsilater-ally results in a gaze palsy in one direction and INO on attempted gaze contralaterally. This is called the one-and-a-half syndrome and results in preservation of only contralateral abduction (Wall and Wray, 1983; Fig. 12-7). Patients with a one-and-a-half syndrome who have exotropia in primary position are said to have a paralytic pontine exotropia. An ipsilateral INO and sixth cranial nerve fascicle lesion can produce paralysis of both adduction and abduction in one eye (monocular horizontal gaze paralysis) (Frohman et al., 2003c).

Skew deviation and vestibular abnormalities

Skew deviation is a supranuclear vertical ocular misalignment with the higher eye most commonly on the side of the lesion in midpontine and midbrain lesions, and the lower eye on the side of the lesion in medullary lesions. It may occur in isolation or in conjunction with an INO. In addition to a change in alignment, the higher eye is usually intorted while the lower eye extorted though not necessarily concomitantly. Many patients have a head tilt away from the high eye and may also per-ceive a deviation in the vertical visual axis. Taken together, skew deviation, ocular torsion, and head tilt are referred to as the ocular tilt reaction, and this results from asymmetric disruption of oto-lithic vestibular pathways occurring peripherally or centrally (Fig. 12-8).

On occasion, MS patients will present with positional vertigo. The most common cause of vertigo in MS is benign paroxysmal positioning vertigo (BPPV) (Frohman et al., 2000a, 2003b). Demyelinating plaques within the eighth cranial nerve entry zone at the pontomedullary junction and in the medullary tegmentum are the most common MS-related lesions producing vertigo (Frohman et al., 2000b).

Vertical saccadic abnormalities

When demyelinating lesions occur in the dorsal midbrain affecting the mesencephalic reticular

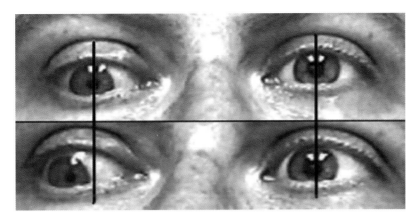

Figure 12-6 A patient with multiple sclerosis had a dorsal midbrain syndrome that included a left hyper-tropia consistent with skew deviation and a left internuclear ophthalmoparesis (on attempted right gaze as seen in the lower figure). The lesion was at the level of the left midbrain (after the decussation of the right-ward originating otolith pathways) and involved the medial longitudinal fasciculus. Also note the enlarged left pupil, which exhibited the characteristics of near-light dissociation. (From Frohman TC, Galetta S, Fox R, et al. Pearls and oy-sters: The medial longitudinal fasciculus in ocular motor physiology. *Neurology*. 2008c;70(17):e57–e67.)

the MLF contains connections from the vestibular nuclei to the ocular motor nuclei. Additionally, the pathways involved in the regulation of vertical pursuit, vertical vestibular, and otolithic mediated eye movements or vertical alignment are contained within the MLF (Frohman et al., 2008c).

Many patients with bilateral INO consequently show characteristic patterns of impaired vertical eye movements (Evinger et al., 1977; Ranalli and Sharpe, 1988), and many patients with unilateral INOs also develop a skew deviation given interruption of vestibular connections (Fig. 12-6).

Figure 12-7 A patient with multiple sclerosis has a one-and-a-half syndrome. The patient was unable to elicit saccades to the right (i.e., a right-gaze palsy) and had evidence of a right internuclear ophthalmo-paresis (INO) upon attempted gaze to the left. In this photograph, the patient is looking straight ahead. There is an exotropia, the so-called paralytic pontine exotropia with the left eye in exo (the only remaining movement possible). In this circumstance, there is an attempted leftward preference. However, only left eye abduction is possible given the right INO (with slowing and significant ocular limitation). Below is the T 2-weighted axial magnetic resonance image showing the responsible lesion involving the right pontine tegmentum (arrow). (From Frohman TC, Galetta S, Fox R, et al. Pearls and oysters: the medial longitudinal fasciculus in ocular motor physiology. *Neurology*. 2008c;70(17):e57–e67.)

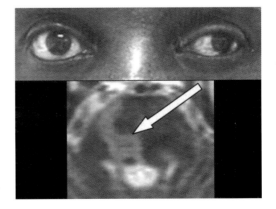

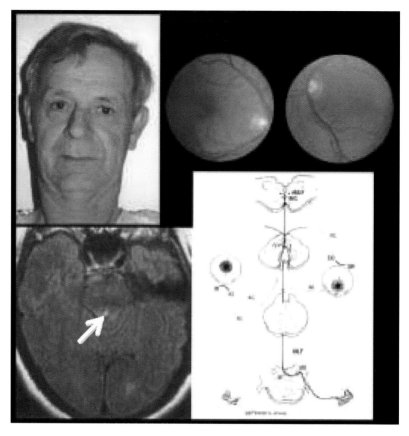

Figure 12-8 The ocular tilt reaction. (*Top left*) A mild left head tilt and right hypertropia. (*Top right*) Intorsion of the right eye and extorsion of the left eye. (*Bottom left*) Magnetic resonance imaging demonstrating lesion involving the right medial longitudinal fasciculus. (*Bottom right*) Diagram depicting causative lesion. (From Vaphiades M. The ocular tilt reaction. *Am Orthopt J.* 2003;53:127–132.)

formation or posterior commissure (or both), Parinaud syndrome may occur; it is characterized by impaired upgaze, convergent retraction nystagmus on attempted upward saccades (often best elicited when viewing a downward-moving optokinetic-nystagmus tape), and near-light dissociation (Frohman et al., 2004) (Fig. 12-9). Other concomitant features may include a skew deviation, fixation instability (square-wave jerks), convergence spasm or divergence paralysis, irregular pupils (correctopia), pseudoabducens palsy (a slower moving abducting eye during horizontal saccades perhaps related to convergence excess), downward gaze preference (setting sun sign), downbeat nystagmus, and abnormalities of vertical smooth pursuit and the vertical vestibul-ocular reflex.

Therapeutics

Other treatment modalities are targeted at improving visual function and include treatments for Uhthoff phenomena, nystagmus, superior oblique myokymia, INO, and others. Treatment for nystagmus largely depends on the type, though response to treatment varies. Visual dysfunction due to INO may respond to 4-aminopyridine (4-AP), a potassium channel antagonist, at doses up to 30 mg/day. Additionally many visual disturbances due to motility and afferent system dysfunction are

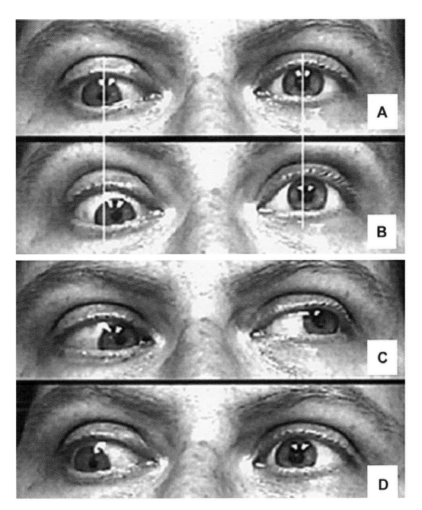

Figure 12-9 The dorsal midbrain syndrome. (*A*) In the primary position, there is a left hypertropia consistent with skew deviation in addition to anisocoria (left > right). (*B*) On attempted upgaze there is rapid convergence of the right eye and a corresponding mild divergence of the left eye (note the displacement of the pupils away from the white marker). (*C*) Attempted left gaze is relatively preserved. (*D*) During attempted right gaze there is severe limitation of the left eye and slowing of the abducting right eye was observed clinically (pseudoabducens palsy). (From Frohman EM, Dewey RB, Frohman TC. An unusual variant of the dorsal midbrain syndrome in MS: clinical characteristics and pathophysiologic mechanisms. *Mult Scler.* 2004;10(3):322–325.)

worsened by exercise, environmental heat exposure, or emotional stress (Uhthoff phenomena) (Davis et al., 2008). Attempts may be made to decrease core body temperature by the use of cooling devices or to improve neuronal function with 4-AP, which has been shown to improve heat-sensitive motor conduction and motor task performance and may be effective for temporary visual loss or degradation of eye movements as in INO.

CONCLUDING COMMENTS

The neuro-ophthalmologic manifestations of MS are broad and varied. They span the anterior visual and ocular motor systems and are some of the most common neurologic manifestations and causes of disability in MS. Indeed, the commonness of neuro-ophthalmologic abnormalities highlights the importance of recognition and appropriate treatment.

REFERENCES

Adams CWM, Poston RN, Buk SJ, Sidhu YS, Vipond H. Inflammatory vasculitis in multiple sclerosis. *J Neurol Sci.* 1985;69:269–283.

Arnold AC, Pepose JS, Hepler RS, Foos RY. Retinal periphlebitis and retinitis in multiple sclerosis, I: pathologic characteristics. *Ophthalmology.* 1984;91: 255–262.

Arnold DB, Robinson DA. The oculomotor integrator: testing of a neural network model. *Exp Brain Res.* 1997; 113:57–74.

Ashe J, Hain TC, Zee DS, Schatz NJ. Microsaccadic flutter. *Brain.* 1991;114:461–472.

Averbuch-Heller L. Acquired nystagmus. *Curr Treat Options Neurol.* 1999;1:68–73.

Averbuch-Heller L, Zivotofsky AZ, Das VE, DiScenna AO, Leigh RJ. Investigations of the pathogenesis of acquired pendular nystagmus. *Brain.* 1995;118(pt 2): 369–378.

Bamford CR, Ganley JP, Sibley WA, Laguna JF. Uveitis, perivenous sheathing and multiple sclerosis. *Neurology.* 1978;28(9 pt 2):119–124.

Beck RW, Cleary PA, Anderson MM, Jr., et al. A randomized, controlled trial of corticosteroids in the treatment of acute optic neuritis. *N Engl J Med.* 1992;326:581.

Beck RW, Arrington J, Murtagh FR, Cleary PA, Kaufman DI. Brain magnetic resonance imaging in acute optic neuritis: experience of the Optic Neuritis Study Group. *Arch Neurol.* 1993a;8:841–846.

Beck RW, Cleary PA, Optic Neuritis Study Group. Optic neuritis treatment trial. One-year follow-up results. *Arch Ophthalmol.* 1993b;11:773–775.

Beck RW, Cleary PA, Trobe JD, et al. The effect of corticosteroids for acute optic neuritis on the subsequent development of multiple sclerosis. *N Engl J Med.* 1993c; 329:1764–1769.

Beck RW, Kupersmith MJ, Cleary PA, Katz B. Fellow eye abnormalities in acute unilateral optic neuritis: experience of the Optic Neuritis Treatment Trial. *Ophthalmology.* 1993d;100:691–698.

Beck RW, Savino PJ, Schatz NJ, Smith CH, Sergott RC. Plaque causing homonymous hemianopsia in multiple sclerosis identified by computed tomography. *Am J Ophthalmol.* 1982;94(2):229–234.

Bell RA, Robertson DM, Rosen DA, Kerr AW. Optochiasmatic arachnoiditis in multiple sclerosis. *Arch Ophthalmol.* 1975;93:191–193.

Bhidayasiri R, Plant GT, Leigh J. A hypothetical scheme for the brainstem control of vertical gaze. *Neurology.* 2000;54:1985–1993.

Brusaferri F, Candelise L. Steroids for multiple sclerosis and optic neuritis: a metanalysis of randomized controlled clinical trials. *J Neurol.* 2000;247:435–442.

Celesia GG, Kaufman DI, Brigell M, et al. Optic neuritis: a prospective study. *Neurology.* 1990;40(6): 919–923.

Costello F, Coupland S, Hodge W, et al. Quantifying axonal loss after optic neuritis with optical coherence tomography. *Ann Neurol.* 2006;59:963–969.

Dalton CM, Brex PA, Miszkeil KA, et al. Spinal cord MRI in clinically isolated optic neuritis. *J Neurol Neurosurg Psychiatry.* 2003;74:1577–1580.

Davis FA, Bergen D, Schauf C, McDonald I, Deutsch W. Movement phosphenes in optic neuritis: a new clinical sign. *Neurology.* 1976;26(11):1100–1104.

Davis SL, Frohman TC, Crandall CG, et al. Modeling Uhthoff's phenomenon in MS patients with internuclear ophthalmoparesis. *Neurology.* 2008;70:1098–1106.

Demaerel P, Robberecht W, Casteels I, et al. Focal leptomeningeal MR enhancement along the chiasm as a presenting sign of multiple sclerosis. *J Comput Assist Tomogr.* 1995;19(2):297–298.

Evinger LC, Fuchs AF, Baker R. Bilateral lesions of the medial longitudinal fasciculus in monkeys: effects on the horizontal and vertical components of voluntary and vestibular induced eye movements. *Exp Brain Res.* 1977;28:1–20.

Filippi M, Bozzali M, Rovaris M, et al. Evidence for widespread axonal damage at the earliest clinical stage of multiple sclerosis. *Brain.* 2003;126:433–437.

Fisher JB, Jacobs DA, Markowitz CE, et al. Relation of visual function to retinal nerve fiber layer thickness in multiple sclerosis. *Ophthalmology.* 2006;113: 324–334.

Frohman EM, Costello F, Stuve O, et al. Modeling axonal degeneration within the anterior visual system: Implications for demonstrating neuroprotection in MS. *Arch Neurol.* 2008a;65:26–35.

Frohman EM, Costello O, Zivadinov R, et al. Optical coherence tomography in multiple sclerosis. *Lancet Neurol.* 2006;5:853–863.

Frohman EM, Dewey RB, Frohman TC. An unusual variant of the dorsal midbrain syndrome in MS: clinical characteristics and pathophysiologic mechanisms. *Mult Scler.* 2004;10:322–325.

Frohman EM, Frohman TC, Fleckenstein J, Racke MK, Hawker K, Kramer PD. Ocular contrapulsion in multiple sclerosis: clinical features and patho-physiological mechanisms. *J Neurol Neurosurg Psychiatry.* 2001;70: 688–692.

Frohman EM, Fujimoto LG, Frohman TC, Calabresi PA, Cutter G, Balcer LJ. Optical coherence tomography: a window into the mechanisms of multiple sclerosis. *Nat Clin Pract Neurol.* 2008b;4(12):664–675.

Frohman EM, Goodin D, Calabresi P, et al. The utility of MRI in suspected MS. *Neurology.* 2003a;61: 602–611.

Frohman EM, Kramer PD, Dewey RB, Kramer L, Frohman TC. Benign paroxysmal positioning vertigo in multiple sclerosis: diagnosis, pathophysiology, and therapeutic techniques. *Mult Scler.* 2003b;9:250–255.

Frohman EM, Zhang H, Dewey R, et al. Vertigo in multiple sclerosis: utility of diagnostic and particle repositioning maneuvers. *Neurology.* 2000a;55:1566–1568.

Frohman EM, Zhang H, Kramer PD, et al. MRI characteristics of the MLF in MS patients with chronic internuclear ophthalmoparesis. *Neurology.* 2001;57:762–768.

Frohman EM, Zimmerman C, Frohman TC. Neuro-ophthalmic signs and symptoms in MS. In: Burks J,

Johnson K, eds. *Multiple Sclerosis: Diagnosis, Medical Management, and Rehabilitation. Signs in Multiple Sclerosis.* New York: Demos; 2000b: 341–375.

Frohman TC, Frohman EM, O'Suilleabhain P, et al. Accuracy of clinical detection of INO in MS: corroboration with quantitative infrared oculography. *Neurology.* 2003c;61(6):848–850.

Frohman TC, Galetta S, Fox R, et al. Pearls and oysters: The medial longitudinal fasciculus in ocular motor physiology. *Neurology.* 2008c;70(17):e57–e67.

Frohman TC, Zee DS, McColl R, Galetta S. Neuroophthalmology of multiple sclerosis. *Lancet Neurol.* 2005;4:111–121.

Ganley JP. Uveitis and multiple sclerosis: an overview. In: Saari KM, ed. *Uveitis Update.* Amsterdam, Netherlands: Excerpta Medica; 1984: 345–349.

Gass A, Filippi M, Rodegher ME, Schwartz A, Comi G, Hennerici MG. Characteristics of chronic MS lesions in the cerebrum, brainstem, spinal cord, and optic nerve on T1-weighted MRI. *Neurology.* 1998;50:548–550.

Ge Y, Grossman RI, Babb JS, He J, Mannon LJ. Dirtyappearing white matter in multiple sclerosis; volumetric MR imaging and magnetization transfer ratio histogram analysis. *Am J Neuroradiol.* 2003;24:1935–1940.

Gronseth GS, Ashman EJ. Practice parameter: the usefulness of evoked potentials in identifying clinically silent lesions in patients with suspected multiple sclerosis (an evidence-based review): Report of the Quality Standards Subcommittee of the American Academy of Neurology. *Neurology.* 2000;54(9):1720–1725.

Hawkins K, Behrens MM. Homonymous hemianopia in multiple sclerosis. With report of bilateral case. *Br J Ophthalmol.* 1975;59(6):334–337.

Hood DC, Odel JG, Winn BJ. The multifocal visual evoked potential. *J Neuro Ophthalmol.* 2003;23:279–289.

Hornsten G. The relation of retinal periphlebitis to multiple sclerosis and other neurological disorders. *Acta Neurol Scand.* 1971;47:413–425.

Hughes EH, Dick AD. The pathology and pathogenesis of retinal vasculitis. *Neuropathol Appl Neurobiol.* 2003; 29:325–340.

Joseph R, Pullicino P, Goldberg CD, Rose FC. Bilateral pontine gaze palsy: nuclear magnetic resonance findings in presumed multiple sclerosis. *Arch Neurol.* 1985;42:93–94.

Kalla R, Glasauer S, Schautzer F, et al. 4-aminopyridine improves downbeat nystagmus, smooth pursuit, and VOR gain. *Neurology.* 2004;62:1228–1229.

Kaufman DI, Trobe JD, Eggenberger ER, Whitaker JN. Practice parameter: the role of corticosteroids in the management of acute monosymptomatic optic neuritis. *Neurology.* 2000;54:2039–2044.

Keane JR. Bilateral sixth nerve palsy: analysis of 125 cases. *Arch Neurol.* 1976;33:681–683.

Keane JR. Gaze evoked blepharoclonus. *Ann Neurol.* 1978; 3:243–245.

Keane JR. The pretectal syndrome: 206 patients. *Neurology.* 1990;40:684–690.

Keltner JL, Johnson CA, Spurr JO, Beck RW. Baseline visual field profile of optic neuritis. The experience of the optic neuritis treatment trial. Optic Neuritis Study Group. *Arch Ophthalmol.* 1993;111(2):231–234.

Keltner JL, Johnson CA, Spurr JO, Beck RW. Visual field profile of optic neuritis: one year follow-up in the optic neuritis treatment trial. *Arch Ophthalmol.* 1994; 112:946–953.

Kerty E, Eide N, Nakstad P, Nyberg-Hansen R. (1991). Chiasmal optic neuritis. *Acta Ophthalmol (Copenh).* 1991;69(1):135–139.

Ksiazek SM, Repka MX, Maguire A, et al. Divisional oculomotor nerve paresis caused by intrinsic brainstem disease. *Ann Neurol.* 1989;26:714–718.

Kuroiwa Y, Shibasaki H. Clinical studies of multiple sclerosis in Japan. I. A current appraisal of 83 cases. *Neurology.* 1973;23:609–617.

Kurtzke JF, Beebe GW, Nagler B, Auth TL, Kurkland LT, Nefzger MD. Studies on natural history of multiple sclerosis. 4. Clinical features of the onset bout. *Acta Neurol Scand.* 1968;44(4):467–494.

Leibowitz U, Alter M. Optic nerve involvement and diplopia as initial manifestations of multiple sclerosis. *Acta Neurol Scand.* 1968;44:70–80.

Leigh RJ, Tomsak RL. Drug treatments for eye movement disorders. *J Neurol Neurosurg Psychiatry.* 2003;74:1–4.

Lepore FE. Uhthoff's symptom in disorders of the anterior visual pathways. *Neurology.* 1994;44(6):1036–1038.

Lopez LI, Bronstein AM, Greasty MA, Du Boulay ER, Rudge P. Clinical and MRI correlates in 27 patients with acquired pendular nystagmus. *Brain.* 1996;119: 465–472.

Malinowski SM, Pulido JS, Folk JC. Long-term visual outcome and complications associated with pars planitis. *Ophthalmology.* 1993a;100(6):818–825.

Malinowski SM, Pulido JS, Goeken NE, Brown CK, Folk JC. The association of HLA-B8, B51, DR2, and multiple sclerosis in pars planitis. *Ophthalmology.* 1993b; 100(8):1199–1205.

McDonald WI, Barnes D. The ocular manifestations of multiple sclerosis. Abnormalities of the afferent visual system. *J Neurol Neurosurg Psychiatry.* 1992;55: 747–752.

Menage MJ, Papakostopoulos D, Dean Hart JC, et al. The Farnsworth-Munsell 100 hue test in the first episode of demyelinating optic neuritis. *Br J Ophthalmol.* 1993;77:68–74.

Miller N. Multiple sclerosis and related demyelinating diseases. In: 4th ed, *Clinical Neuro-Ophthalmology.* Baltimore: Williams and Wilkins; 1995: 4324.

Moore RF. Subjective "lightning streaks". *Br J Ophthalmol.* 1935;19(10):545–547.

Morrissey SP, Miller DH, Kendall BE, et al. The significance of brain magnetic resonance imaging abnormalities at presentation with clinically isolated syndromes suggestive of multiple sclerosis. A 5-year follow-up study. *Brain.* 1993;116:135–146.

Naismith RT, Xu J, Tutlam NT, et al. Disability in optic neuritis correlates with diffusion tensor-derived directional diffusivities. *Neurology.* 2009;72(7):584–585.

Newman NJ. Multiple sclerosis and related demyelinating diseases. In: Miller NR, Newman NJ, eds. *Walsh and*

Hoyt's Clinical Neuro-Ophthalmology. 5th ed. Baltimore: Williams and Wilkins; 1998: 5539–5576.

Newman NJ, Lessell S, Winterkorn JM. Optic chiasmal neuritis. *Neurology*. 1991;41(8):1203–1210.

Nordmann JP, Saraux H, Roullet E. Contrast sensitivity in multiple sclerosis: a study in 35 patients with and without optic neuritis. *Opthalmologica*. 1987;195:199–204.

Optic Neuritis Study Group. The clinical profile of optic neuritis. Experience of the Optic Neuritis Treatment Trial. *Arch Ophthalmol*. 1991;109:1673.

Optic Neuritis Study GroupOptic Neuritis Study Group. The 5 year risk of MS after optic neuritis. Experience of the optic neuritis treatment trial. Neurology. 1997a; 49:1404–1413.

Optic Neuritis Study Group. Visual function 5 years after optic neuritis: experience of the optic neuritis treatment trial. *Arch Ophthalmol*. 1997b;115:1545–1552.

Optic Neuritis Study Group. High risk and low risk profiles for the development of multiple sclerosis within 10 years after optic neuritis. Experience of the Optic Neuritis Treatment Trial. *Arch Ophthalmol*. 2003;121: 944–949.

Optic Neuritis Study Group. Visual function more than 10 years after optic neuritis: experience of the optic neuritis treatment trial. *Am J Ophthalmol*. 2004;137: 77–83.

Optic Neuritis Study Group. Multiple Sclerosis risk after optic neuritis. Final Optic Neuritis Treatment Trial Follow-up. Arch Neurol. 2008;65(6):727–732.

Plant GT, Kermode AG, Turano G, et al. Symptomatic retrochiasmal lesions in multiple sclerosis: clinical features, visual evoked potentials, and magnetic resonance imaging. *Neurology*. 1992;42:68–76.

Ranalli PJ, Sharpe JA. Vertical vestibulo-ocular reflex, smooth pursuit and eye-head tracking dysfunction in internuclear ophthalmoplegia. *Brain*. 1988;111:1299–1317.

Revol A, Vighetto A, Confavreux C, Trillet M, Aimard G. Oculo-palatal myoclonus and multiple sclerosis. *Rev Neurol (Paris)*. 1990;146:518–521.

Rizzo JF, Andreoli CM, Rabinov JD. Use of magenetic resonance imaging to differentiate optic neuritis and nonarteritic anterior ischemic optic neuropathy. *Ophthalmology*. 2002;109:1679–1684.

Rizzo JF, Lessell S. Risk of multiple sclerosis after uncomplicated optic neuritis: A long-term prospective study. *Neurology*. 1988;38(2):185–190.

Rizzo JF, Lessell S. Optic neuritis and ischemic optic neuropathy. Overlapping clinical profiles. *Arch Ophthalmol*. 1991;109:1668–1672.

Rolak LA, Beck RW, Paty DW, Tourtellotte WW, Whitaker JN, Rudick RA. Cerebrospinal fluid in acute optic neuritis: experience of the optic neuritis treatment trial. *Neurology*. 1996;46(2):368–372.

Rosenberg MI, Glaser JS. Superior oblique myokymia. *Ann Neurol*. 1983;13:667–669.

Rucker CW. Sheathing of the retinal veins in multiple sclerosis. Mayo Clinic Proc. 1944;19:176–178.

Ruprecht K, Klinker E, Dintelmann T, Rieckmann P, Gold R. Plasma exchange for severe optic neuritis: treatment of 10 patients. *Neurology*. 2004;63(6): 1081–1083.

Rush JA, Younge BR. Paralysis of cranial nerves III, IV, and VI. *Arch Ophthalmol*. 1981;99:76–79.

Sacks JG, Melen O. Bitemporal visual field defects in presumed multiple sclerosis. *JAMA*. 1975;234(1):69–72.

Selhorst JB, Saul RF. Uhthoff and his symptom. *J Neuroophthalmol*. 1995;15(2):63–69.

Sellebjerg F, Nielsen HS, Frederiksen JL, Olesen J. A randomized controlled trial of high dose methylprednisolone in acute optic neuritis. *Neurology*. 1999; 52:1474–1484.

Sergott RC, Frohman E, Glanzman R, Al-Sabbagh A, OCT in MS Expert Panel. The role of optical coherence tomography (OCT) in multiple sclerosis: expert panel consensus. *J Neurol Sci*. 2007;263:3–14.

Solomon D, Galetta SL, Liu GT. Possible mechanisms for horizontal gaze deviation and lateropulsion in the lateral medullary syndrome. *J Neuro-ophthalmol*. 1995;15: 26–30.

Spector RH, Glaser JS, Schatz NJ. Demyelinative chiamal lesions. *Arch Neurol*. 1980;37(12):757–762.

Starck M, Albrecht H, Pöllmann W, Straube A, Dieterich M. Drug therapy for acquired pendular nystagmus in multiple sclerosis. *J Neurol*. 1997;244(1):9–16.

Strupp M, Brandt T. Pharmacological advances in the treatment of neuro-otological and eye movement disorders. *Curr Opin Neurol*. 2006;19(1):33–40.

Strupp M, Schuler O, Krafczyk S, et al. Treatment of downbeat nystagmus with 3,4-diaminopyridine: a placebo-controlled study. *Neurology*. 2004;61:165–170.

Todman DH. A paroxysmal ocular motility disorder in multiple sclerosis. *Aust NZ J Med*. 1988;18:785–787.

Tola MR, Granieri E, Casetta I, et al. Retinal periphlebitis in multiple sclerosis: a marker of disease activity? *Eur Neurol*. 1993;33:93–96.

Twomey JA, Espir MLE. Paroxysmal symptoms as the first manifestations of multiple sclerosis. *J Neurol Neurosurg Psychiatry*. 1980;43:296–304.

Vanooteghem P, Dehaene I, Van Zandycke M, Casselman J. Combined trochlear nerve palsy and internuclear ophthalmoplegia. *Arch Neurol*. 1992;49:108–109.

Vaphiades M. The ocular tilt reaction. *Am Orthopt J*. 2003; 53:127–132.

Wakakura M, Minei-Higa R, Oono S, et al. Baseline features of idiopathic optic neuritis as determined by a multicenter treatment trial in Japan. *Jpn J Ophthalmol*. 1999;43:127–132.

Wall M, Wray SH. The one-and-a-half syndrome: a unilateral disorder of the pontine tegmentum: a study of 20 cases and review of the literature. *Neurology*. 1983; 33:971–980.

Young YH, Huang TW. Role of clonazepam in the treatment of idiopathic downbeat nystagmus. *Laryngoscope*. 2001;111:1490–1493.

13 Cerebellar and Brainstem Dysfunction in Multiple Sclerosis

Angeli S. Mayadev and George H. Kraft

Multiple sclerosis (MS) can affect the brain stem and cerebellum by the presence of plaques in critical structures or by disruption of connections between such structures. The resulting signs and symptoms are often among the most disabling for persons with MS. This chapter outlines the anatomical origin of dysfunction, clinical findings, and treatment options available to patients and providers.

ANATOMY OF THE BRAIN STEM AND CEREBELLUM

Anatomy

The brain stem consists of the midbrain, pons, and medulla oblongata. The midbrain connects the pons and cerebellum with the thalamencephalon and cerebral hemispheres. Functions of the midbrain include controlling responses to sight, eye movement, pupil dilation, body movement, and hearing. The midbrain contains the cell bodies of cranial nerves three and four. It consists of the tectum, which controls auditory and visual responses, and the tegmentum, which controls motor functions and regulates awareness, attention, and autonomic functions. The tegmentum consists of the cerebral aqueduct, periaqueductal gray, reticular formation, substantia nigra, and the red nucleus.

The reticular formation receives input from most of the sensory systems of the body and also from cerebral motor regions. The upper part of the formation plus the pathways to the thalamus and cortex are called the reticular activating system, which aids in maintaining the conscious state. The substania nigra contains the neurons that produce dopamine and thus is important in controlling voluntary movement and mood. The red nucleus receives many inputs from the contralateral cerebellum (interpositus nucleus and lateral cerebellar nucleus) and an input from the ipsilateral motor cortex. It sends efferent axons (the rubrospinal projection) to the contralateral half of the rhombencephalic reticular formation and spinal cord. These efferent axons cross just ventral to the nucleus and descend through the midbrain to the spinal cord. These axons make up the rubrospinal tract, which runs ventral to the lateral corticospinal tract in the lateral funiculus. The red nucleus coordinates upper-extremity movements, but in humans, these movements are dominated by the corticospinal tract.

The pons lies between the midbrain and medulla and is anterior to the cerebellum. It functions to relay sensory information between the cerebellum and cerebrum, aids in relaying other messages in the brain, controls arousal, and regulates respiration via respiratory domains. It contains the cell bodies of the cranial nerve nuclei five, six, seven, and eight.

The medulla lies below the pons and above the spinal cord. It contains pyramids that contain the corticospinal tracts from the cerebral cortex to the spinal cord. The medulla is responsible for the automatic control of heartbeat and respiration.

The cerebellum lies dorsal to the pons and posterior to the occipital lobes. It has gray and white matter, similar to the cerebral cortex. The white matter contains the four deep cerebellar nuclei which receive excitatory and inhibitory input from parts of the brain. The cerebellar peduncles process afferents and efferent signals. The superior cerebellar peduncle houses the dentate nucleus, which is where efferent fibers connect to the mid-brain, medulla, and thalamus to facilitate motor planning. The middle cerebellar peduncle receives afferent fibers from the cortex via the pons. The inferior cerebellar peduncle is concerned with motor functions that coordinate muscle tone, posture, and movement. Normally, the cerebellum is responsible for the smooth, accurate coordinated execution of movements. This portion of the brain receives information from the periphery regarding the actual position and rate of movement of the limbs, plus visual and auditory cues. It also samples information from the motor cortex regarding motor commands. Lesions of the cerebellum result in the loss of the ability to move in a smooth and coordinated manner.

Cranial Nerves

Because MS lesions in the brain stem and cervical spinal cord can affect the cell bodies of the 12 cranial nerves, it is important to review the rather complex anatomy in this small region of the central nervous system (CNS). The cranial nerves that are most often impaired by MS will be reviewed (see Table 13-1). Often, only by careful physical examination can the site of the neurologic lesion(s) be determined, and clinical signs be correlated with magnetic resonance imaging (MRI) lesions. Complementary—and sometimes supplementary information—can also be obtained from selected neurophysiologic testing (see Chapters 3 and 9 for details).

DIAGNOSIS AND CHARACTERISTICS OF BRAINSTEM AND CEREBELLAR DYSFUNCTION

Tremor

In MS, the disruption of the vestibular connections of the cerebellum and olive contribute to dysfunction. Also, the rubral pathways are commonly involved. This means that much of the apparent "cerebellar" symptoms are actually vestibular nuclei symptoms (pseudocerebellar symptoms), which in turn drive the motor symptoms of decreased ipsilateral tone, dysmetria, overshooting, hypometric saccades, lateral gaze nystagmus,

and vertigo. This leads to an organization of these cerebellar-like symptoms around the pathology, with vestibular nuclei symptoms being preeminent, followed by motor symptoms from the rubral system (e.g., dysmetria, rubral tremor, and bulbar symptoms).

In addition, the cerebellum is a major predilection site for cortical demyelination in MS. Although cerebellar cortical demyelination sometimes occurs together with demyelination in the adjacent white matter (leukocortical lesions), in most instances, the cortex is affected independently from white matter lesions. Thus, involvement of the cerebellum itself could contribute to dysfunction in MS (Kutzelnigg et al., 2007).

Disabling tremor is reported in nearly 30% of all patients with MS. In one MS population study, the median latency of tremor was 11 years from disease onset, with arms more often involved than head, trunk, or legs. *Resting tremors* are not voluntarily activated and occur in body parts with complete support. *Action tremors* occur with voluntary movements and include postural, kinetic, isometric, and *intention tremors*. Multiple sclerosis most commonly produces an intention tremor due to disruption of cerebellar outflow projection from the dentate nucleus of the cerebellum to the motor division of the thalamus. Intention tremors are large in amplitude and increase in severity with action as the limb gets closer to the target point and as the movement slows. Such a tremor typically involves the upper limbs, although the legs, head, and trunk may also be affected (Alusi et al., 2001). Some degree of tremor is found in 25%–50% of MS patients and it is often associated with severe disability and increased frequency of wheelchair use. This is mostly likely because tremor in MS is an indicator of more severe involvement of the nervous system by MS.

Tremors can be quite debilitating for patients because they interfere with the ability to perform basic activities of daily living (ADLs) such as feeding and grooming. Alusi and colleagues studied the type and severity of tremor in MS patients (Alusi et al., 2001). They evaluated 100 patients and measured the severity of tremor using finger tapping and nine-hole peg tests, and the subject's ability to draw an Archimedes spiral. Fifty-eight patients had a tremor with 20 subjects reporting asymptomatic tremors. Affected regions were

TABLE 13-1 Review of Cranial Nerves

Cranial Nerve	Anatomy: Location of Cell Bodies	Primary Function/Innervation	Clinical Correlation
II: **Optic**	Retina	Vision	Hemianopsia Scotoma
III: **Oculomotor**	Midbrain	Eyelid elevator, superior, inferior and medial rectus and inferior oblique extrinsic eye muscles; parasympathetic to papillary sphincter and ciliary muscles	Ptosis; papillary dilatation; iridoplegia; cystoplegia; rotation of the eye outward and downward; abnormal pupils
IV: **Trochlear**	Midbrain	Superior oblique muscle	Upward-outward gaze deviation
V: **Trigeminal**	Pons	Sensation via three branches to the face. Innervates muscles of mastication	Trigeminal neuralgia
VI: **Abducens**	Pons	Lateral rectus muscle	Disruption of abduction of the eye
VII: **Facial**	Ponto-medullary junction	Taste buds of anterior 2/3 of tongue; muscles of facial expression; parasympathetics	Weakness of muscles of facial expression
VIII: **Acoustic**	Medulla	Hearing; connections with the vestibulospinal tracts, medial longitudinal fasciculus, and cerebellum	Hearing loss; Tinnitus; vertigo
IX: **Glossopharyngeal**	Medulla	Taste from the posterior 1/3 of the tongue; sensation from the middle ear, Eustachian tube, and posterior wall of the pharynx; motor to stylopharyngeus and middle constrictor muscles; parasympathetics	Dysphagia; dysarthria
X: **Vagus**	Medulla	Receives visceral sensation; motor to the soft plate, pharynx and larynx	Decreased sound of voice; dysfunction of vocal cords and soft palate; diminished gag reflex
XII: **Spinal accessory**	Nucleus ambiguous at levels of C1 to C5	Trapezius and sternocleidomastoid muscles	Weakness of shoulder shrug and turning of the head
XII: **Hypoglossal**	Floor of the fourth ventricle	Extrinsic and intrinsic muscles of the tongue	Tongue weakness and atrophy

arms (56) (Alusi et al., 1999), legs (10), head (9), and trunk (7). Each case of tremor reported was of an action type (postural, kinetic, or both). The authors did not observe any true rest tremors. Exacerbating factors included anxiety, hot baths, and excessive physical exertion. While various combinations of body parts were involved, the most common included bilateral arm involvement. The most common type of tremor was a coarse distal tremor of the arms.

When comparing the tremulous and nontremulous patient groups, some significant differences between the groups were high EDSS scores and wheelchair reliance[1]; the tremulous group had higher EDSS scores (6.0 in the tremulous group vs. 5.5 in the nontremulous group) and were more likely to be wheelchair reliant. Twenty-seven percent of the subjects had a tremor-induced disability and 10% had an incapacitating tremor. The authors found no correlation between MS disease duration and tremor severity. They commented on an interesting correlation between MS patients with or without tremor and the presence of a family history of tremor. Seven percent of the MS patients reported a positive family history of tremor. This raises questions as to whether some tremor seen in an MS population may be a result of the disease, a genetic predisposition to tremor, or to some interaction of both.

Ataxia and Other Movement Disorders in Multiple Sclerosis

Movement disorders, other than tremor secondary to cerebellar or brainstem lesions, are uncommon clinical manifestations of MS. In a recent study, other movement disorders were present in only 12 of 733 patients with MS (1.6%) (Nociti et al., 2008). The authors noted that a causal correlation between movement disorders in MS is probable secondary to three reasons: (1) MS plaques can involve any part of the CNS, and therefore, the extrapyramidal pathway could be impaired at multiple levels, not only at the basal ganglia regions; (2) much of the diffuse tissue damage in MS, not detectable with standard MRI, can impair nervous fibers involved in specific motor pattern that is able to induce a movement disorder; (3) aberrant neuronal plasticity could involve

a specific motor pattern that is able to induce a movement disorder as a consequence of the demyelinating plaques (probably the least likely possibility, as CNS neuroplasticity is by nature restorative, and not disruptive).

Vertigo

Vertigo is not an uncommon complaint in patients with MS. In some cases, the disorder is caused by MS lesions (either typical MS plaques as seen on MRI or by axonal disruptions not evident on standard MRI scans) in critical areas of the brain stem in the middle region of the medulla oblongata. (See discussion in previous section on cranial nerves, especially the eighth cranial nerve.) When assessing patients with MS for this symptom, the caveat must be remembered—as it should with assessment of all other neurologic symptoms—that patients with MS are *persons* with MS. There may be some more common and treatable explanation for their symptoms; examples include carpal tunnel syndrome for hand numbness and cervical stenosis for long signs of cervical myelopathy.

With regard to vertigo, the MS specialist should not assume it is always due to the MS. Often, the history will be informative. If the vertigo is constant, and not altered by head position or movement, MS may be the cause. If the patient feels it is substantially influenced by head position or movement, it may represent benign paroxysmal positional vertigo (BPPV). Further information can be obtained by a simple office maneuver of asking the patient to rapidly rotate the head from one extreme side to the other, or rapidly tilt the head. If such maneuvers appear to precipitate the symptoms, then further assessment is in order. It is important to distinguish BPPV from MS-caused vertigo, as the Epley maneuver can typically reposition the troublesome otoconia and relieve symptoms in BPPV.

Vertigo can be a symptomatic finding in up to 20% of patients with MS. Demyelination in the medial vestibular nucleus (MVN) and the root entry zone of the eighth cranial nerve represent the most common neuroanatomical localizations that can cause vertigo. When vertigo is on the basis of demyelination, the episodes tend to be sustained for a minimum of 24 hours and are characterized by horizontal-rotary nystagmus. Although a demyelinating lesion is a suspicion in MS patients, the most common cause of vertigo in this population is BPPV. Thus, it is important to elicit history regarding whether the vertigo is induced by change in position and duration of symptoms as well as a focused exam with pro-vocative maneuvers such as the Dix- Hallpike and neuro-otologic assessment (Frohman et al., 2003). Information from the vestibular labyrinth is relayed via the vestibular portion of the eighth cranial nerve to the brainstem vestibular nuclei and from there to the cerebellum, ocular motor nuclei, and spinal cord and cerebrum. Vesti-buloocular connections are responsible for coor-dinated eye movements during head motion, while vestibulospinal pathways help maintain upright posture.

Dysphagia and Dysarthria and Dysphonia

Dysphagia, difficulty swallowing, can be a life-threatening condition, as a result of choking and aspiration. Dysarthria, the inability to enunciate clearly, is also troublesome for the individual; s/he finds that s/he cannot be easily understood. Dysphonia refers to disordered sound production at the level of the larynx, classically seen as hoarse-ness. Dysarthria is caused by neurologic damage to the motor components of speech, which may involve any or all of the speech processes, including respiration, phonation, articulation, resonance, and prosody. It may have a neurologic, structural, or functional etiology. These conditions are a result of brainstem lesions (see previous section on cranial nerves, especially the ninth and tenth cranial nerves). These conditions are caused by MS lesions in the lower medulla oblongata. The quality of voice and pitch can vary in patients with MS:

> Dysphonia caused by UMN damage tends to be strained, harsh, and loud. Dysphonia caused by ataxia may have adequate vocal quality, but pitch and loudness control are often aberrant. Respiratory support is uneven, contributing to the loudness variability. On sustained phonation, a slow tremor is heard.

If the dysarthria has no UMN involvement, muscle tone is low and there is no strained vocal quality. If there is UMN involvement, however, a strained voice quality usually predominates, although it is inconsistent. (Cohen et al., 2009)

Trigeminal Neuralgia

Trigeminal neuralgia (TN, *tic doloreaux*) is more common in patients with MS (Jensen et al., 1982). It is defined clinically by sudden, usually unilat-eral, severe, brief, stabbing or lancinating, recur-rent episodes of pain in the distribution of one or more branches of the fifth cranial (trigeminal) nerve (Merskey et al., 1994). A recent paper described six patients with symptoms of TN and lesions in the fifth nerve entry zone and three patients with lesions involving trigeminal brain-stem nuclei. The authors conclude that central demyelination at the pontine entry zone of the sensory fibers can be responsible for TN in these patients (Gass et al., 1997).

Tinnitus and Hearing Loss

Involvement of the eighth cranial nerve can lead to symptoms of tinnitus and hearing loss. The incidence of hearing loss in persons with MS is estimated at about 5%, and rarely, hearing loss may be the initial manifestation of the dis-ease (Commins and Chen, 1997; Szymanska et al., 2004). Partial lesions of the brainstem nuclei lead to diminished acuity for high tones associated with tinnitus. Unilateral lesions in the brainstem nuclei or higher connections are not associated with loss of hearing secondary to bilat-eral connections.

Facial Nerve Palsy

A unilateral peripheral seventh cranial nerve palsy (Bell palsy) may be caused by MS. In one large series of patients with MS ($n = 483$) it was reported to occur in about 4% of patients, and occasionally may be the presenting symptom of MS (Zadro et al., 2008). It is thought to be due to the pres-ence of a plaque at the facial nerve nucleus or root exit zone the nerve, which may not always be able to be visualized on MRI (Commins and Chen, 1997).

TREATMENT OF MULTIPLE SCLEROSIS–RELATED BRAINSTEM AND CEREBELLAR DYSFUNCTION

Tremor

Pharmacologic

Treatment of tremor can involve pharmacologic, rehabilitative, or surgical intervention. A key step is to correctly diagnose the type of tremor present as treatments vary according to type. A mild tremor in MS may respond to different types of medication, including some antiepileptic drugs (AEDs) such as carbamazepine, benzodiazepines, topiramate, and primidone (Sechi et al., 2003). Other agents that have been used with mixed success include carbamazepine, propranolol, tetrahydrocannabinol, clonazepam, and isoniazid (Alusi et al., 2001; Schapiro, 2002). However, these drugs may have considerable side effects (Alusi et al., 2001).

Fourteen MS patients, aged 27 to 57 years, with cerebellar-type tremor and duration ranging from 3 to 14 years, were given levetiracetam 500 mg twice daily for 1 week followed by increments of 500 mg twice daily each week up to the target dose of 50 mg/kg/day. Although only 11 patients were analyzed, the medication administration was associated with subjective and objective improvement of the tremor, with significant lowering of all tremor measurements' sum of scores as well as of ADL mean score between the baseline and follow-up (Striano et al., 2006). Tetrahydrocannabinol (THC), a component of marijuana, showed a non-significant trend toward subjective benefit in MS tremor in one study (Wade et al., 2004). Beta blockers work primarily by eliminating any essential tremor superimposed on the rubral tremor.

Botulinum toxin is approved for use to treat limb spasticity, but it also may help dampen tremor. It inhibits the vesicular release of acetylcholine in the neuromuscular junction and thus may weaken the muscles that are contributing to the tremor in patients with MS. There have not been any randomized trials looking at the use of botulinum toxin in tremor associated with MS, but information can be extrapolated from work in other neurological disorders (Henderson et al., 1996).

Rehabilitation

In severe cases, upper-limb intention tremor can be an enormous problem, often resulting in an almost insurmountably disabling condition. Severe upper limb tremors are often the precipitating cause for institutional care of persons with MS. Weighted wrist cuffs and weighted walkers are the most practical methods for dampening ataxic tremor (Kraft, 1984; Aisen et al., 1993). The best method is the employment of a heavy weight (3 to 5 lb) on the distal limb, which may help reduce the excursion of the extremity by dampening its movement (Kraft, 1984). Fortunately, in most cases of severe MS intention tremor, strength is generally well preserved; a heavy weight can be well tolerated. Other simple techniques that can be assessed in the MS specialist's office include simply assessing the synchrony of the tremor in each hand. If they are even a bit out of synchrony, then the physician can assess whether movements with the fingers interdigitated produce a reduced tremor excursion. If so, then the patient can use one hand to stabilize the other.

Other techniques that can be tried for upper limb intention tremor include stabilization of the joint proximal to that being moved (e.g., stabilization of the elbow when using the hand), keeping the trunk well supported, training in using only one joint at a time, and not looking directly at the object being manipulated. For lower limb tremor, use of a weighted walker or wheeled walker and trying tai chi or other "control/relaxation" exercises can be helpful.

One study of in-patient rehabilitation for the treatment of MS-related ataxia and tremor involved eight half-hour sessions of occupational therapy (postural dynamics, adaptive equipment, and damping and weighting) and physical therapy for 8 working days (Jones et al., 1996). The intervention group significantly improved relative to a wait-listed control group on one ADL scale but not on two impairment scales. However, intervention subjects had significantly greater improvement in activity and fatigue.

Surgery

For severe cases of tremor, stereotactic thalamo-tomy and deep brain thalamic stimulation (DBS) can be performed. Accurate diagnosis and patient selection greatly influence outcome. Deep brain stimulation is indicated for patients with relatively stable disease and disabling upper limb tremor (Schulder et al., 2003). A review found that DBS relieved tremor in >80% and improved daily func-tioning in >70% of reported MS cases (Wishart et al., 2003). However, long-term hardware com-plications occur in about one-fourth of patients (Lyons et al., 2004). With careful patient selec-tion, unilateral thalomotomy has been used with success rates between 69% and 96% (Speelman et al., 2002). With both of these procedures, there is a 20% risk of tremor recurrence within a year. The target area for neurosurgical treatment of tremor is the nucleus ventralis posterior, which is the cerebellar input nucleus of the thalamus. More recently, the area of interest is the nucleus ventralis oralis posterior, which is the basal gan-glia output center. This suggests that MS tremors may be generated from the basal ganglia despite the cerebellar appearance of the tremor (Stein et al., 1999). Complications from thalomotomy include worsening of gait, hemiparesis, confu-sion, and lethargy (Alusi et al., 1999). Also, there should always be caution applied to operating on the brain of a patient with active disease. The authors vividly recall an MS patient with disabling intention tremor who had the development of new MS lesions along the thalomotomy route, presumably as a result of the physical breaking down of the blood–brain barrier in the region.

Other treatments for tremor

An exciting new development to treat tremor, dys-metria, and weakness is virtual reality. Such sys-tems work on the adaptive ability of neuroplasticity in the brain (Steffin, 1997a). Haptic systems are currently being developed that are cued by the patient's environment. The system then provides patients with cues and provides "force corridors" to help guide the patient's wrist and hand move-ments. There is ongoing research on developing sensory augmentation for visual and propriocep-tive loss (Steffin, 1997b).

Ataxia and Other Movement Disorders

At the present time, the most practical manage-ment of ataxia involves either broadening the base of support with a cane or crutch or, more optimally, a walker for greater stability. When this is not suf-ficient, the avoidance of bipedal ambulation is the goal and patients need to be taught to function in a scooter or wheelchair. Patients with MS with ataxia tend to prefer three-wheeled electric scoot-ers as they are typically not weak but have prob-lems with motor control. These scooters are relatively easy to disassemble for the trunk of a car and do not require the purchase of a special van.

Approximately three-quarters of individuals with MS have some degree of ambulatory impair-ment (Kraft et al., 1986; LaBan et al., 1998). Gait impairment in MS can be caused by weakness, spasticity, fatigue, proprioceptive loss, cerebellar or vestibular dysfunction, visual loss, or inability to multitask.

Compared with healthy people, patients with MS show decreased stride length, increased steps per minute (cadence), slower free-speed walking rates, less rotation at the hips, knees and ankles (stiffer gait), increased trunk flexion, and reduced vertical lift in center of gravity. Overall, they take short quick steps and lack full range of motion (Gehlsen et al., 1986). A survey conducted in 1983 indicated that 60% of people with MS needed some assistance with ambulation (Baum and Rothschild, 1983). Most relied on a wheelchair or physical assistance from another person. Falls are the most important sequelae of gait and balance disturbances. In one cross-sectional study of ambu-latory patients with MS, 54% reported at least one fall over the previous 2 months and 32% were recurrent fallers. Impaired balance was the best predictor of falls, followed by use of an assistive device (Cattaneo et al., 2002). Recommendations for mobility aids should focus on enhancing gait stability, rather than on the cosmesis and conve-nience of walking.

Studies suggest that nonspecific exercise pro-grams without some ambulation component are ineffective for enhancing gait (Gehlsen et al., 1986; Rodgers et al., 1999; DeBolt and McCubbin, 2004). Continual programs are necessary to maintain good mobility and balance in this disease. One way to make this affordable is to provide group therapy using task-oriented or kinesiology techniques. All patients who trip and fall do not need an orthosis. Evaluation for heel cord tightness, spasticity, clonus, and weakness should be carried out, and corrective measures should be taken. In cases of intermittent falling, the examiner should inquire about the conditions under which it occurs. Falls occurring when the patient is occupied with other activities (such as talking with a companion) may be related to the difficulty MS patients have with multitasking. Because loss of proprioceptive function results in the use of compensatory visual, auditory, tactile, and cognitive cues, multitasking diminishes the MS patient's ability to "focus" on walking (Kraft, 2005).

Vertigo

Vestibular symptoms like vertigo and ocular symptoms partially respond to medications that suppress the vestibular input like antihistamines, phenothiazines, and benzodiazepienes. These drugs have anticholinergic effects and benzodiazepienes modulate the GABA pathway. The phenothiazines may have extrapyramidal side effects, and all these medications have sedating side effects. If the vertigo is caused by a central lesion, vestibular rehabilitation exercises work less well than for a peripheral lesion. These exercises are aimed at promoting central adaptation. In a retrospective review, there was benefit from a specific vestibular physical therapy program for patients with central lesions (Brown et al., 2006).

Dysarthria, Dysphagia, and Dysphonia

General speech performance registers in the normal range in the majority of individuals with MS. The most common speech problem in MS is controlling the volume of speech (either too soft or too loud). Dysarthria is reported in 14%–19% and it is most often found in more neurologically impaired cases (Darley et al., 1972). It has been characterized as a mixed spastic cerebellar dysarthria, although flaccid dysarthrias are also encountered. Apraxia, anomia, and aphasia are much less common (Lacour et al., 2004). Speech problems associated with MS are severe enough to limit comprehensibility in about 4% of cases (Beukelman et al., 1985). Evaluation by speech therapy is advised in all such cases. The immediate goal is compensated intelligibility. The ultimate result is rarely if ever normal speech. When verbal communication is less than 50% intelligible, one should try one of the many augmentative communication devices. Speech pathology treatment strategies for MS dysarthria are to control speech rate, voice emphasis, and phrase shifts and to reduce phase length and increase voice power (Merson and Rolnick, 1998). Lee Silverman Voice Therapy focuses on tasks to maximize phonatory and respiratory functions, encouraging patients to "think loud," and it can be useful for patients with flaccid dysarthria (Hartelius and Nord, 1997; Sapir et al., 2001).

Dysphagia is a potentially life-threatening manifestation of MS. A quantitative water test detected dysphagia in 43% of an MS cohort, almost half of whom had no related complaints (Thomas and Wiles, 1999). Using fiberoptic nasopharyngeal endoscopy, dysphagia was found in 48% of non-ambulatory individuals and 11% of ambulatory individuals (Calcagno et al., 2002). When video fluoroscopy has been used, most asymptomatic MS individuals have been found to have abnormalities (Wiesner et al., 2002). The oral phase of swallowing is more frequently abnormal than the pharyngeal and esophageal phases. Fluids can be more problematic than solids, but for the majority of dysphasic individuals, both are abnormal (De Pauw et al., 2002). Questions about choking, aspiration, or swallowing difficulty should be asked as part of the routine review of systems. If the risk factors mentioned previously are present, clinicians should have a low threshold for a speech and swallowing referral. When dysphagia is reported and the individual has an abnormal clinical swallow study, video fluoroscopy is recommended. Postural techniques such as making the head and neck more upright during initial oral stage of swallowing as well as implementing a chin tuck maneuver during the pharyngeal phase of swallowing can be helpful. Modification of intake volume and consistency by adding thickening agents to liquids may enable mildly to moderately dysphagic individuals to improve swallowing.

Trigeminal Neuralgia

According to the AAN practice parameter, medical treatment for trigeminal neuralgia has evidence to support its use. Carbamazepine (Level A) or oxcarbazepine (Level B) should be offered for pain control while baclofen and lamotrigine (Level C) may also be considered. Starting doses of Carbamazepine are 100–200 mg oral twice a day and are titrated based upon patient response. Other pharmacologic approaches to treating trigeminal neuralgia are discussed in Chapter 20.

For patients with TN refractory to medical therapy, Gasserian ganglion percutaneous techniques, gamma knife, and microvascular decompression may be considered (Level C) (Gronseth et al., 2008).

Facial Nerve Palsy (Bell Palsy)

An acute peripheral facial nerve palsy due to MS may be treated in the same manner as any other MS exacerbation, that is, with a brief course of corticosteroids.

NOTES

1   It is time that the pejorative term "*confined* to a wheelchair" no longer be used. "Wheelchair reliant" or "wheelchair dependant" is much more fitting for mobility and independence facilitated by twenty-first century mobility aids.

REFERENCES

Aisen ML, Arnold A, Baiges I, Maxwell S, Rosen M. The effect of mechanical damping loads on disabling action tremor. *Neurology*. 1993;43(7):1346–1350.

Alusi SH, Glickman S, Aziz TZ, Bain PG. Tremor in multiple sclerosis. *J Neurol Neurosurg Psychiatry*. 1999; 66(2):131–134.

Alusi SH, Worthington J, Glickman S, Bain PG. A study of tremor in multiple sclerosis. *Brain*. 2001;124(pt 4): 720–730.

Baum HM, Rothschild BB. Multiple sclerosis and mobility restriction. *Arch Phys Med Rehabil*. 1983;64(12): 591–596.

Beukelman DR, Kraft GH, Freal J. Expressive communication disorders in persons with multiple sclerosis: a survey. *Arch Phys Med Rehabil*. 1985;66(10):675–677.

Brown KE, Whitney SL, Marchetti GF, Wrisley DM, Furman JM. Physical therapy for central vestibular dysfunction. *Arch Phys Med Rehabil*. 2006;87(1):76–81.

Calcagno P, Ruoppolo G, Grasso MG, De Vincentiis M, Paolucci S. Dysphagia in multiple sclerosis - prevalence and prognostic factors. *Acta Neurol Scand*. 2002; 105(1):40–43.

Cattaneo D, De Nuzzo C, Fascia T, et al. Risks of falls in subjects with multiple sclerosis. *Arch Phys Med Rehabil*. 2002;83(6):864-867.

Cohen SM, Elakattu A, Noordzij JP, Walsh MJ, Langmore SE. Palliative treatment of dysphonia and dysarthria. *Otolaryngol Clin N Am*. 2009;42:107–121.

Commins D, Chen J. MS: a consideration in acute cranial nerve palsies. *Am J Otol*. 1997;18:590–595.

Cunningham DJ. *Cunningham's Text-Book of Anatomy*. 9th ed. New York: Oxford University Press; 1951.

Darley FL, Brown JR, Goldstein NP. Dysarthria in multiple sclerosis. *J Speech Hearing Res*. 1972;15(2):229–245.

DeBolt LS, McCubbin JA. The effects of home-based resistance exercise on balance, power, and mobility in adults with multiple sclerosis. *Arch Phys Med Rehabil*. 2004;85(2):290–297.

De Pauw A, Dejaeger E, D'Hooghe B, Carton H. Dysphagia in multiple sclerosis. *Clin Neurol Neurosurg*. 2002; 104(4):345–351.

Frohman EM, Kramer PD, Dewey RB, Kramer L, Frohman TC. Benign paroxysmal positioning vertigo in multiple sclerosis: diagnosis, pathophysiology and therapeutic techniques. *Mult Scler*. 2003;9(3):250–255.

Gass A, Kitchen N, MacManus DG, et al. Trigeminal neuralgia in patients with multiple sclerosis: lesion localization with magnetic resonance imaging. *Neurology*. 1997;49(4):1142–1144.

Gehlsen G, Beekman K, Assmann N, et al. Gait characteristics in multiple sclerosis: progressive changes and effects of exercise on parameters. *Arch Phys Med Rehabil*. 1986;67(8):536–539.

Grant JCB. *An Atlas of Anatomy*. 4th ed. Baltimore: Williams & Wilkins Company; 1956.

Gronseth G, Cruccu G, Alksne J, et al. Practice parameter: the diagnostic evaluation and treatment of trigeminal neuralgia (an evidence-based review): report of the Quality Standards Subcommittee of the American Academy of Neurology and the European Federation of Neurological Societies. *Neurology*. 2008;71(15): 1183–1190.

Hartelius L, Nord L. Speech modification in dysarthria associated with multiple sclerosis: an intervention based on vocal efficiency, contrastive stress, and verbal repair strategies. *J Med Speech-lang Pathol*. 1997;5: 113–140.

Henderson JM, Ghika JA, Van Melle G, Haller E, Einstein R. Botulinum toxin A in non-dystonic tremors. *Euro Neurol*. 1996;36(1):29–35.

Jensen TS, Rasmussen P, Reske-Nielsen E. Association of trigeminal neuralgia with multiple sclerosis: clinical and pathological features. *Acta Neurol Scand*. 1982; 65(3):182–189.

Jones L, Lewis Y, Harrison J, Wiles CM. The effectiveness of occupational therapy and physiotherapy in multiple sclerosis patients with ataxia of the upper limb and trunk. *Clin Rehabil*. 1996;10(4):277–282.

Kraft GH. Movement disorders. In: Basmajian JV, Kirby RL, eds. *Medical Rehabilitation*. Baltimore: Williams and Wilkins; 1984: 162–165.

Kraft GH. Multiple sclerosis: a paradigm shift. In: Kraft GH, Brown T, eds. *Physical Medicine and Rehabilitation Clinics of North America: Multiple Sclerosis: A Paradigm Shift*. Philadelphia: Saunders; 2005: 513–557.

Kraft GH, Freal JE, Coryell JK. Disability, disease duration, and rehabilitation service needs in multiple sclerosis: patient perspectives. *Arch Phys Med Rehabil.* 1986; 67(3):164–168.

Kutzelnigg A, Faber-Rod JC, Bauer J, et al. Widespread demyelination in the cerebellar cortex in multiple sclerosis. *Brain Pathol.* 2007;17(1):38–44.

LaBan MM, Martin T, Pechur J, Sarnacki S. Physical and occupational therapy in the treatment of patients with multiple sclerosis. In: Kraft GH, ed. *Physical Medicine and Rehabilitation Clinics of North America.* Philadelphia: Saunders; 1998: 603–614, vii.

Lacour A, De Seze J, Revenco E, et al. Acute aphasia in multiple sclerosis: a multicenter study of 22 patients. *Neurology.* 2004;62(6):974–977.

Lyons KE, Wilkinson SB, Overman J, Pahwa R. Surgical and hardware complications of subthalamic stimulation: a series of 160 procedures. *Neurology.* 2004;63(4): 612–616.

Mayo Clinic. *Clinical Examinations in Neurology.* 2nd ed. Philadelphia: W.B. Saunders Company; 1963.

Merskey H, Bogduk N, Sload PA. *Classification of Chronic Pain: Descriptions of Chronic Pain Syndromes and Definitions of Pain Terms.* 2nd ed. Seattle, WA: IASP Press; 1994: 59.

Merson RM, Rolnick MI. Speech-language pathology and dysphagia in multiple sclerosis. *Phys Med Rehabil Clin N Am.* 1998;9(3):631–641.

Moore KL, Dalley AF, Agur AMR. *Clinically Oriented Anatomy.* 6th ed. Philadelphia: Lippincott Williams & Wilkins; 2009.

Nociti V, Bentivoglio AR, Frisullo G, et al. Movement disorders in multiple sclerosis: Causal or coincidental association? *Mult Scler.* 2008;14(9):1284–1287.

Rodgers MM, Mulcare JA, King DL, et al. Gait characteristics of individuals with multiple sclerosis before and after a 6-month aerobic training program. J Rehabil Res Dev. 1999;36(3):183–188.

Sapir S, Pawlas AA, Ramig LO, et al. Effects of intensive phonatory-respiratory treatment (LSVT) on voice in two individuals with multiple sclerosis. *J Med Speechlang Pathol.* 2001;5:141–151.

Schapiro RT. Pharmacologic options for the management of multiple sclerosis symptoms. *Neurorehabil Neural Repair.* 2002;16(3):223–231.

Schulder M, Sernas TJ, Karimi R. Thalamic stimulation in patients with multiple sclerosis: long-term follow-up. *Stereotact Funct Neurosurg.* 2003;80(1–4):48–55.

Sechi G, Agnetti V, Sulas FM, et al. Effects of topiramate in patients with cerebellar tremor. *Prog Neuropsychopharmacol Bio Psychiatry.* 2003;27(6):1023–1027.

Speelman JD, Schuurman R, de Bie RM, Esselink RA, Bosch DA. Stereotactic neurosurgery for tremor. *Mov Disord.* 2002;17(suppl 3):S84–S88.

Steffin M. Computer assisted therapy for multiple sclerosis and spinal cord injury patients application of virtual reality. *Stud Health Technol Inform.* 1997a;39:64–72.

Steffin M. Virtual reality therapy of multiple sclerosis and spinal cord injury: design consideration for a haptic-visual interface. *Stud Health Technol Inform.* 1997b;44: 185–208.

Stein JF, Aziz TZ. Does imbalance between basal ganglia and cerebellar outputs cause movement disorders? *Current Op Neurol.* 1999;12(6):667–669.

Striano P, Coppola A, Vacca G, et al. Levetiracetam for cerebellar tremor in multiple sclerosis: an open-label pilot tolerability and efficacy study. *J Neurol.* 2006; 253(6):762–766.

Szymanska M, Gerwel A, Cieszynska J. Sudden sensorineural hearing loss as the first symptom of MS. Review of the literature and case report. *Otolarngol Pol.* 2004;58(6):1143–1149.

Thomas FJ, Wiles CM. Dysphagia and nutritional status in multiple sclerosis. *J Neurol.* 1999;246(8):677–682.

Wade DT, Makela P, Robson P, House H, Bateman C. Do cannabis-based medicinal extracts have general or specific effects on symptoms in multiple sclerosis? A double-blind, randomized, placebo-controlled study on 160 patients. *Mult Scler.* 2004;10(4):434–441.

Wiesner W, Wetzel SG, Kappos L, et al. Swallowing abnormalities in multiple sclerosis: correlation between video fluoroscopy and subjective symptoms. *Euro Radiol.* 2002;12(4):789–792.

Wishart HA, Roberts DW, Roth RM, et al. Chronic deep brain stimulation for the treatment of tremor in multiple sclerosis: review and case reports. *J Neurol Neurosurg Psychiatry.* 2003;74(10):1392–1397.

Zadro I, Barun B, Habrek N, Brinar V. Isolated cranial nerve palsies in MS. *Clin Neurol Neurosurg.* 2008;110:886–888.

Disorders of Mobility in Multiple Sclerosis

Thomas E. McNalley and Jodie K. Haselkorn

What walks on four legs in the morning, two legs in afternoon, and three legs at night?

Answer: Man—who crawls on all fours as a baby, then walks on two feet as an adult, and then walks with a cane in old age.

—*Riddle of the Sphinx*

Upright ambulation is a defining characteristic of *Homo sapiens*. The riddle above occupies a central place in Western thought and suggests how mobility is archetypal to human experience. Among the most treasured milestones of the developing child are the first steps; we have even named a period of life after a kind of mobility: toddling. While the acquisition of standing and first steps delights both child and family, the loss of safe, independent ambulation is associated with fear, grief, and concern about family and community roles.

Multiple sclerosis (MS) has been called a disorder of mobility. Most directly, loss of muscle strength and control can make the coordinated movements of walking impossible. Further impairments of sensation, proprioception, balance, fatigue, and vision can singly or in concert limit the ability to walk. Development of spasticity from the upper motor neuron syndrome can further undermine motor control and at the very least restrict fluidity of movement.

Restricted mobility can be associated with increased risks of joint contracture, osteoporosis, weight gain, injuries from falls, skin breakdown, limitations in activities and participation, as well as decreased overall quality of life. Fortunately, medical and rehabilitation interventions can slow the progression of disability.

WEAKNESS

Research suggests that gait impairment can begin quite early in the course of MS (Givon et al., 2009).

Weakness may result from disuse, fatigue, denervation, or side effects of medications; lesions in either the brain or spinal cord can diminish muscle strength. Loss of strength seems primarily to derive from neurologic changes, but one study has also shown changes in muscle cross-bridging and isoform expression (Garner and Widrick, 2003).

Researchers have investigated the use of various pharmaceutical agents to specifically address weakness. Disease-modifying agents have been associated with decreased relapse rate, magnetic resonance imaging (MRI) activity, and reduction in disability. High-dose corticosteroids as well as ACTH have been used to accelerate recovery from attacks of MS (Goodin et al., 2002; Frohman et al., 2007). Long-term benefits have not been demonstrated and these agents can have side effects that include muscle weakness and osteopenia (Zorzon et al., 2005). Intravenous immunoglobulin (IVIG) has also been suggested as an intervention that might reduce the number and severity of relapses. A Cochrane review in 2003 did not find adequate evidence to strongly support use of IVIG, as the trials reviewed did not adequately correlate with the reviewers' preferred outcome measures (Gray et al., 2003). The reviews suggested more trials be conducted, using MRI and other endpoints to evaluate efficacy.

Of renewed interest is the use of 4-aminopyridine to treat weakness. This agent is a potassium-channel blocker that increases acetylcholine release at the neuromuscular junction and in the central nervous system (CNS) (Hollander et al., 1986). In individuals with MS, 4-aminopyridine benefits appear to be related to improvement of nerve conduction and the frequency response in demyelinated nerve fibers via prolongation of the repolarization phase of the action potential (van Diemen et al., 1993). Use of the short-acting

4-aminopyridine was limited by the side effects, especially seizures. Dalfampridine (AMPYRA) is a sustained release preparation of 4-aminopyridine recently approved by the Federal Drug Administration to improve walking speed in individuals with all types of MS. The effectiveness of the agent was demonstrated in two controlled clinical trials involving a total of 540 participants. Individuals with all types of MS were included in these trials if they were able to perform a Timed 25-foot Walk (T25W) in 8-45 seconds. Participants had average disease duration of 13 years and a mean Kurtzke Expanded Disability Status Score of 6. The primary measure of efficacy in both trials was walking speed (in feet per second) as measured by T25FW. Responders, participants who showed faster walking speed for a least three visits out of a possible four during the double-blind intervention period compared to the maximum value achieved in five non-double-blind non-intervention visits. A significantly greater proportion of participants taking dalfampridine were responders, compared to those taking placebo (Trial 1: 34.8% vs. 8.3%; Trial 2: 42.9% vs. 9.3%). The increased response rate in the active group was observed across all four major types of MS disease course and was not affected by the presence or absence of a disease modifying agent. Effectiveness was independent of degree of impairment, age, gender, and body mass index. (Goodman et al., 2008). Dalfampridine 10 mg should be administered orally twelve hours apart. The medication should be swallowed whole and not broken or chewed. Adverse reactions that occurred during the clinical trials more frequently in the actively treated group with an incidence >5% in the active group included: urinary tract infection, insomnia, headache, nausea, asthenia, back pain, balance and balance disorder. Other adverse events meeting above criteria with an incidence <5% in the active group included MS relapse, paresthesia, nasopharyngitis, constipation, dyspepsia, and pharygolarygeal pain. Dalfampridine is contraindicated in individuals with a prior history of seizures or renal impairment (Creatinine Clearance <50mL/min).

SPASTICITY

Spasticity can be a serious secondary impairment of MS that limits mobility. Spasticity is usually considered an abnormal resistance in muscle to a quick externally induced stretch. Clinically, spasticity is associated with increased tonus in muscles, exaggerated deep tendon and cutaneous reflexes, spread of motor activity to distant muscles, co-contraction of agonist muscle groups, clonus with sustained stretch, and spasms in major muscle groups. These findings plus other symptoms of upper motor neuron syndrome—weakness, decreased coordination, decreased rapid alternating movements, and fatiguability contribute to the decreased mobility in MS. The pathophysiology is not well characterized and findings are likely related to changes in the brain, the spinal cord, as well as the periphery (Haselkorn and Loomis, 2005).

The clinician should assess for spasticity or a change in spasticity at each visit. A home or community-based flexibility program can prevent interference in usual activities for some individuals with MS. If the spasticity interferes with function and is focal, treatment with nerve- or muscle-blocking agents, such as botulinum toxin or alcohol, improves specific functions. If the spasticity is generalized, antispasticity oral agents such as baclofen, tizanidine, diazepam, and dantrolene can be beneficial. These agents have side effects, including fatigue and weakness, that may limit use in MS. Although there have been numerous individual clinical trials that support the use of individual agents and the medications are widely used to manage symptoms, the Cochrane Collaboration calls for higher quality research before comment on the absolute and comparative efficacy as well as tolerability of antispasticity agents (Shakespeare, 2003). For persons with advanced disease and severe spasticity, intrathecal baclofen can help manage symptoms of pain and muscle tightness (Smail et al., 2006). See Table 14-1 for a summary of oral agents.

REHABILITATION

While we await neuroregenerative agents, rehabilitation strategies are successful in the restoration of function in people with MS (Patti et al. 2002; Craig et al., 2003; Patti et al., 2003; Khan et al., 2007). Individuals with complex or rapid deterioration of mobility should be seen by a specialist in MS rehabilitation. Rehabilitation strategies in MS frequently involve a team of providers, including physical therapy, occupational therapy, recreational therapy, vocational therapy, and social work.

TABLE 14-1 Common Anti-Spasticity Agents, Doses, and Side Effects

Generic (Trade)	Starting Dose	Maximum Dose	Side Effects
Baclofen (Lioresal)	5 mg PO three times a day	80 mg per day (some patients may need and tolerate more)	Somnolence; Dizziness; Headache Nausea/vomiting/constipation; Weakness
Tizanidine (Zanaflex)	4 mg daily (usually at bedtime)	36 mg per day	Hypotension; Somnolence; Dizziness Dry mouth; Weakness; Abnormal LFTs; Constipation/diarrhea
Dantrolene (Dantrium)	25 mg daily	100 mg four times a day	Liver disease (requires monitoring); Constipation/diarrhea; Lightheadedness; Asthenia, dizziness, headache; Somnolence; Fatigue, malaise; Diplopia
Diazepam (Valium)	2–10 mg orally 3–4 times per day	Not known; death from overdose is rare	Hypotension; Fatigue; Somnolence; Weakness; Rash; Diarrhea; Ataxia/dyscoordination

Adapted from Haselkorn and Loomis, 2005.

Many MS centers organize clinics that include neurologists, physiatrists, and therapists along with other relevant specialists to coordinate and centralize care.

A history and physical examination are essential to determine the sources of mobility impairments before instituting a program. The history should include questions about specific instances that limit activities. For instance, does the person have difficulty with bed mobility, transferring from bed to standing, toileting or showering, getting around the home, walking to the car, getting up or down stairs, walking on uneven ground, playing with children, getting to and from work, enjoying usual leisure activities, as well as participating in a regular exercise program? Physical examination should include a neurological examination including postural function and observation of transfers and gait. A loss of mobility may be due to impairments such as a loss of lower extremity motor or sensory function, proprioceptive deficits, ataxia, reduced balance, spasticity, and pain. Other secondary impairments seen in MS such as a reduction in vision, bladder urgency, a neurogenic bowel, fatigue, and depression may also contribute to mobility problems. Additionally, other unrelated impairments such as benign positional vertigo or degenerative joint disease may further limit ambulation. Identifying the specific causes and

customizing a treatment program can result in a restoration of function. Additional information about the home, workplace, and avocational activities is important to address safety and quality of life.

Falls are common in MS (Cattaneo et al., 2002; Finlayson et al., 2006). Persons with MS may normalize falls, even falls that result in injury (Peterson et al., 2008). Routine questions about specific situations that lead to walking difficulty, how often an individual "wobbles," has a "near miss" or falls, as well as the circumstances of the last fall, can be informative. It is not uncommon to have individuals report falls into burners, the refrigerator, the stove, the shower, down stairs, and so on. Routine assessment for falls can identify problems and interventions to prevent injury and enhance mobility (Cattaneo et al., 2006).

Therapy

Ideally, at the time of diagnosis the individual would be engaged in a regular fitness program. If not, her clinician would work with her to identify a program in the community or refer her to therapy to establish a safe exercise program.

Sometimes the person is not referred to therapy until there is a mobility problem. At this point, the person with MS should receive a functional evaluation and a guided program of flexibility, strengthening, endurance, and gait training. The goals of therapy are to address disuse and specific impairments to restore function, as well as to provide a safe home exercise program to maintain function. A program of range of motion along with resisted movement and strengthening can proceed to activity-specific training. For example, the person with MS who is an avid hiker but experiencing new weakness can stretch to maintain optimal range at lower-extremity joints, strengthen unaffected muscles, and gradually increase activity until it is possible to return to hiking. An assessment and prescription for appropriate footwear can increase stability at the ankle and prevent injury and falls. If the impairment progresses, the use of an assistive device or orthotic may be warranted for a portion of time or for regular use.

Occupational therapy also plays a vital role in rehabilitation of persons with MS who experience mobility limitations. An evaluation starts with a history and assessment of basic self-care activities such as transfers, toileting, dressing, and bathing, along with instrumental activities such as shopping, housekeeping, and meal preparation. A home safety assessment considers factors such as lighting, floor surfaces, and work areas. Treatment strategies include techniques for safe transfers, a plan to improve energy efficiency that optimizes basic and instrumental activities of daily living, and modifications to improve safety. Assessment and provision of adaptive aides such as mattress loops, reachers, grab bars, transfer poles, raised toilet seats, shower chairs, and tub benches can enhance the safety of basic activities of daily living.

Mobility impairments can limit an individual's ability to work. A vocational counselor working with the individual and others on the team can optimize the individual's function and make worksite recommendations in order to maintain employment. Some simple strategies that limit the impact of mobility impairments include locating an office near a bathroom, scheduling meetings on the same floor, using a cart to optimize energy efficiency, and using transfer poles at key transition points.

Orthotics and Functional Electrical Stimulation

Bracing may include an ankle-foot orthosis (AFO) that provides mediolateral stability and limits the impact of dorsiflexion weakness or footdrop. An AFO assists with toe clearance in the setting of reasonable hip and knee flexion as well as preventing inversion injuries at the ankle due to weakness, sensory or proprioceptive loss. This orthotic can be helpful with transfers, but is especially useful for ambulation in the home and outdoors.

Ankle-foot orthoses come in a wide variety of appearances, weights, designs, and desired outcomes. Premolded, "off-the-shelf" AFOs can be quite effective for some persons and are the least expensive. A custom fabricated AFO is desirable if the orthotic will be used regularly or to address specific functional issues. Individualized designs can adjust trim lines, balancing comfort and weight with mediolateral stability. The ankle joint can be hinged using a variety of different materials. A hinged joint simulates more normal ankle movement. This may not only improve toe pick up but may also make it rising from a chair more comfortable. Increased plantar flexion can be limited with a plantar flexion stop. This can substitute for weak dorsiflexors and improve push off. The foot plates can also be customized to potentially minimize spasticity and maximize push off. Customized orthotics come in a variety of materials and colors that optimize function and also acceptance, similar to the function and comfort seen with custom eyeglass prescriptions.

The best prescription may not be immediately apparent during a clinic visit. A detailed evaluation with physical therapist and orthotist can result in an optimal recommendation to achieve goals of fit, function, and acceptance. Driving can be affected by an AFO, and this should be considered in the prescription and training. As with eyeglasses, a person who is getting a new customized AFO should be advised to anticipate a need for adjustment after initial delivery and receive instructions on wearing schedule.

Functional electrical stimulation (FES) involves the use of surface electrodes to stimulate weak muscles. Coordinating this assistance with the normal gait cycle, stimulation over the deep fibular nerve substitutes for weak dorsiflexors and facilitates toe clearance and eccentric control of the tibia. Typically, a physician will request an evaluation by a physical therapist or orthotist who is specifically trained in the evaluation for, fitting of, and gait training with these devices. Several follow-up visits may be necessary to optimize gait. One study has shown improved speed of walking and reduced energy cost in gait when using FES (Paul et al., 2008).

Other Approaches

Using functionally based retraining while eliminating restrictions of gravity and friction in ambulation is intuitively appealing (Paul et al., 2008). A recent pilot study suggests that the use of body-weight-supported treadmill training was both tolerated and may increase efficiency of walking as measured in several domains (Giesser et al., 2007). The intervention supplied locomotor training to patients with EDSS scores of 7 to 7.5 and showed improvement in muscle strength, spasticity, endurance, balance, walking speed, and quality of life. Another pilot study compared BWSTT alone to robotic-assisted BWSTT and found improvements in both groups, although there was no difference between treatment groups (Lo and Triche, 2008).

Assistive Technology

The range of assistive technology for ambulation is broad, spanning from canes to power wheelchairs. In general, canes and crutches add to the base of support and contribute to stability. Canes come in single-point and four-point or "quad" canes. Increasing the number of points contacting the ground improves stability and support. Forearm crutches, sometimes referred to as "Lofstrand" or "Canadian" crutches, further increase support and may free up hand function to do daily activities while standing. These crutches require excellent upper-extremity strength and proper coordination of gait. The elderly man of the Sphinx riddle uses a cane, and frequently persons requiring any assistive device express concern that they may "look old." The compassionate physician will recognize the barriers to accepting assistive devices and attempt to help the person adjust. For example, many people prefer using customized walking sticks or hiking poles instead of canes, and these can be effective if the poles provide adequate stability.

Walkers also are very effective in providing stability for weak lower extremities or ataxia. Standard, front-wheeled, and seated walkers provide different levels of stability and support. The standard walker is the most stable and least mobile. Within wheeled walkers, tire size and type affect the ability to navigate irregular surfaces. Seated walkers can be particularly helpful for persons with MS who experience fatigue, as the ability to take breaks and sit on the walker may conserve energy for longer community outings. The use of a walker may be limited if the person has upper-extremity weakness, ataxia, or pain. In all cases, a physical therapist should review with the user the proper use of the walker and ensure safety in a variety of terrains.

As ability to ambulate decreases, a person with MS may require a wheeled mobility device for longer distances or all of the time. People with MS relate that knowing that there is a variety of interventions available to address mobility problems well ahead of the experience of any dysfunction reduces the fear of activity limitations and social participation, even if it does not encourage early acceptance. They also point out that even when they have experienced improved functioning associated with other adaptive aides, they may be reluctant to use a wheeled mobility device. The use of a wheeled mobility device part time to enhance interaction in the community frequently drives the decision to accept this option full time.

It can be tricky to determine the right moment to prescribe wheeled mobility. Initiating a prescription too early can result in disuse and increase mobility impairments. Reviewing and adapting a home exercise program at this time reinforces the need to maintain joint mobility, muscle strength, and endurance. Waiting too long increases risk of injury due to falls and associated injury. When the clinician and individual with MS have together found the right time to move to part -time or full-time wheeled mobility, an evaluation by a physical therapist that specializes in mobility is ideal. If the use of a wheelchair is planned for most of the time, a customized prescription is necessary. Consideration of the person's disease course, other impairments, and medical conditions, along with her personal goals, access at home, work, and the community, as well as the type of vehicle used are essential.

The person with MS, the therapist, and the physician should consider the pros and cons of a manual wheelchair, scooters, and power wheelchair. Wheelchairs offer many more seating options than scooters and are generally more comfortable for someone who needs most-of-the-day, long-term use. Most manual chairs are smaller and lighter than the power options. Manual chairs can be customized with a power assist (Karmarkar et al., 2008). Scooters may offer more portability than a power chair but offer a limited range of seating options and other customization. Powered wheelchair mobility may be the best choice in the setting of disabling fatigue, severe weakness, positioning difficulty, or when it is necessary to regularly move over rough ground. The choices for customized wheeled mobility are numerous. Tilt-in-space chairs provide for optimal pressure relief and skin protection (Arva et al., 2009; Dicianno et al., 2009). Chairs that change heights are available, permitting eye-to-eye contact with non–chair users and preventing cervical loading in the wheelchair user (Arva et al., 2009). Robotic chairs equipped with sensors are available to be used in a regular mode or, when the situation demands it, climb stairs or even drive themselves with a verbal command. Robotic chairs are increasingly able to navigate safely in the community through a variety of environmental conditions, to identify hazards, and to access information from the nearby landmarks. In addition, advanced systems are able to cue the user in a specific context to optimize performance and to do meaningful self-care (Cooper, 2009). All of the options at face value can be somewhat to very expensive, but they are also associated in savings in secondary complications and additional services required from care partners. A power chair can be difficult to transport in a vehicle. Careful consideration of numerous factors, including home, vehicle, worksite, and leisure, results in optimized function at the best value for many years.

Exercise and Activity Restriction

Heat exposure and elevated body temperature have been implicated in worsening of symptoms and MS exacerbations. Classically, changes in vision—Uhthoff sign—have accompanied heat-related pseudo-exacerbations. As a result, some persons with MS have not been as active as might be ideal due to concern that exercise may actually worsen their symptoms. Furthermore, some persons with MS experience autonomic instability with changes in heart rate and blood pressure. Nonetheless, exercise clearly benefits the cardiovascular and musculoskeletal systems; improves balance, strength, and stability; and likely contributes to overall well-being and mood (Mostert and Kesselring, 2002; White and Dressendorfer,

2004; Rampello et al., 2007). Using a precooling regimen, adapting exercise to limit overheating with a long warm-up period, and monitoring for changes in cardiovascular parameters can support a successful exercise program. Participants should monitor their fatigue levels and adjust accordingly. Water exercise in a "cool pool" (not more than 85°F) is particularly well suited for persons with MS, and weights can increase the strength-building benefits of hydrotherapy.

COMPLICATIONS OF IMMOBILITY

As limitations of mobility progress, so do the risks of adverse consequences of these limitations. For clinicians caring for persons with MS, the transition from full ambulation to reduced mobility to wheelchair use should trigger vigilance for a number of complications. Preventive measures and early intervention can help prevent the most dire sequelae of the loss of mobility.

Skin

The combination of prolonged sitting or lying along with reduced sensation creates a likely scenario for skin breakdown, a scenario complicated further by moisture exposures and changes in bony architecture wrought by contracture or joint tightness. With skin breakdown comes risk of pain, increased spasticity, and in extreme cases, infection, sepsis, and death. Prevention of skin breakdown is the most effective intervention, as healing can be prolonged and complicated in persons who have multiple comorbidities. Proper seating, alignment, padding, and frequent inspection all play roles in prevention, as do adequate nutrition and education of patients and caregivers.

Skin breakdown can arise from prolonged sitting in one position as well as from shearing forces from transfers. Persons who have reduced ability to ambulate along with reduced sensation should learn to do timed pressure-releases to allow adequate blood flow and relief of compression over bony prominences. Regular inspection should be part of the person's or caregiver's day. Transfer techniques are critical, and they should be reviewed both if mobility impairments progress and periodically over the course of illness. Moisture from bowel or bladder incontinence or perspiration can macerate skin and accelerate skin breakdown. Decreased nutritional status can also increase the risk of decubitus ulcers. Aggressive treatment of these impairments can protect skin integrity.

If skin does break down, the clinician should investigate the contributing factors and seek to alleviate them. Consultation with a wound care specialist may be helpful. There are numerous types of dressings and varieties of topical enzymatic preparations that can assist in wound healing. Sharp or mechanical debridement may be necessary as well for wounds with necrotic tissue. Caregivers and the person with MS should be provided with specific instructions or a home health nurse can assist with wound management. In extreme cases, surgery may be necessary to repair profound decubitus ulcers.

Osteoporosis

Known risk factors for osteoporosis are heredity, reduced activity, female gender, lower body-mass index, smoking, chronic use of corticosteroids and postmenopausal status. Persons with MS are at theoretically greater risk for osteoporosis because of female predominance, decreased mobility, and use of corticosteroids (Cosman et al., 1999). Cosman et al. (1999) showed that patients with MS have a higher frequency of adulthood atraumatic fractures than do age- and gender-matched control subjects. A small study showed an odds' ratio of 2.6 of having osteopenia in those with MS vs. controls (Zorzon et al., 2005).

Management of waning bone mineral density can manifest in both preventive and therapeutic paradigms. Persons with MS should receive counseling on adequate intake of calcium (1200 mg daily) and vitamin D (2000 IU for adults). The dietary reference values may change in the future as more research is done (Yetly et al., 2009). For individuals in high-risk geographic regions with limited sunlight, those who may not get enough sun exposure, or those on medications that interfere with vitamin D, measurement of serum vitamin D can guide therapy. Adequate weight-bearing and resistive exercise can also help maintain bone health. Counseling patients to quit smoking and to use alcohol in moderation has also shown benefit in the general population.

Once osteoporosis has been established diagnostically, options for treatment include estrogens, bisphosphonates, and selective estrogen receptor modulators (SERMs). No specific guidelines exist for treatment of those with MS and osteoporosis. Use of the above pharmaceutical interventions should occur with consultation of an endocrinologist.

Contracture

Prolonged sitting and/or lying frequently results in joint contracture. Once having transitioned to a wheelchair, the person with MS is at risk for both hip and knee flexion contractures. The risk is increased in those with spasticity or increased muscle tone. Plantarflexion and inversion deformity at the ankle, known as equinovarus, is the most common musculoskeletal deformity and is particularly likely in the bedbound individual.

Contractures can make positioning difficult, contribute to skin breakdown, and cause pain and reduce functional mobility. Treatment includes preventive stretching, use of antispasticity medications, neurolytic block with botulinum toxin or phenol, and bracing. In advanced cases, surgical release with tendon lengthening or z-plasty can restore range of motion. Aggressive intervention may be needed post surgery to preserve the range recaptured.

Quality of Life

As noted initially, loss of ambulation can be a symbolically powerful moment in the progress of disability from MS. Anticipatory guidance from the earliest stages of disease can in some cases prepare the individual for the transition. If the time arrives that independent ambulation is either unsafe or impossible, the clinician should anticipate the attendant grief that comes with loss of this ability. Individuals with MS may re-experience these emotions with each prescription of an assistive device. The clinician can contribute to the positive aspects of change by highlighting that a manual or power wheelchair can increase participation in some activities and reduce fatigue. Furthermore, recommendations for participation in adaptive sports and activities may open new venues for persons with MS to enjoy various activities.

REFERENCES

Arva J, Paleg G, Lange M, et al. RESNA Position on the Application of Wheelchair Standing Devices. *Assist Technol.* 2009;21(3):161–168.

Cattaneo D, Nuzzo C, Fascia T, Macalli M, Pisoni I, Cardini R. Risks of falls in subjects with multiple sclerosis. *Arch Phys Med Rehabil.* 2002;83(6):864–867.

Cattaneo D, Regola A, Meotti M. Validity of six balance disorders scales in persons with multiple sclerosis. *Disabil Rehabil.* 2006;28(12):789–795.

Cooper RA. SMARTWheel: from concept to clinical practice. *Prosthet Orthot Int.* 2009;33(3):198–209.

Cosman F, Nieves J, Komar L, et al. Fracture history and bone loss in patient with MS. *Neurology.* 1999; 51(4):1161–1165.

Craig J, Young CA, Ennis M, Baker G, Boggild M. A randomised controlled trial comparing rehabilitation against standard therapy in multiple sclerosis patients receiving intravenous steroid treatment. *J Neurol Neurosurg Psychiatry.* 2003;74(9):1225–1230.

Dicianno BE, Arva J, Lieberman JM, RESNA Position on the Application of Tilt, Recline, and Elevating Legrests for Wheelchairs. *Assist Technol.* 2009;21(1): 13–22.

Finlayson ML, Peterson EW, Cho CC. Risk factors for falling among people aged 45 to 90 years with multiple sclerosis. *Arch Phys Med Rehabil.* 2006;87(9): 1274–1279.

Frohman EM, Shah A, Eggenberger E Metz L, Zivadinov R, Stüve O. Corticosteroids for multiple sclerosis: I. Application for treating exacerbations. *Neurotherapeutics.* 2007;4(4):618–626.

Garner DJP, Widrick JJ. Cross-bridge mechanisms of muscle weakness in multiple sclerosis. *Muscle Nerve.* 2003;27(4):456–464.

Giesser B, Beres-Jones J, Budovitch A, Herlihy E, Harkema S. Locomotor training using body weight support on a treadmill improves mobility in persons with multiple sclerosis: a pilot study. *Mult Scler.* 2007;13(2):224–231.

Givon U, Zeilig G, Achiron A. Gait analysis in multiple sclerosis: characterization of temporal-spatial parameters using GAITRite functional ambulation system. *Gait Posture.* 2009;29(1):138–142.

Goodin DS, Frohman EM, Garmany GP Jr., Halper J Likosky WH, Lublin FD, et al. Disease modifying therapies in multiple sclerosis: report of the Therapeutics and Technology Assessment Subcommittee of the American Academy of Neurology and the MS Council for Clinical Practice Guidelines. *Neurology.* 2002; 58(2):169–178.

Goodman A, Brown T, Krupp LB, et al. Sustained-release oral fampridine in multiple sclerosis: a randomised, double-blind, controlled trial. *Lancet.* 2009;373(9665): 732–738.

Goodman AD, Brown TR, Cohen JA, et al. Dose comparison trial of sustained-release fampridine in multiple sclerosis. *Neurology.* 2008;71(15):1134–1141.

Gray O, McDonnell GV, Forbes RB. Intravenous immunoglobulins for multiple sclerosis. *Cochrane DB Sys Rev.* 2003;DOI: 10.1002/14651858.CD002936.

Haselkorn JK, Loomis S. Multiple sclerosis and spasticity. *Phys Med Rehab Clin N Am.* 2005; 16(2):467–482.

Hollander E, Mohs RC, Davis KL. Cholinergic approaches to the treatment of Alzheimer's disease. *Br Med Bull.* 1986;42(1):97–100.

Karmarkar A, Cooper RA, Liu H, Connor S, Puhlman J. Evaluation of Pushrim-Activated Power Assisted Wheelchairs (PAPAW) using ANSI/RESNA standards. *Arch Phys Med Rehabil.* 2008;89(6):1191–1198.

Khan F, Turner-Stokes L, Ng L, Kilpatrick T. Multidisciplinary rehabilitation for adults with multiple sclerosis. *Cochrane DB Sys Rev.* 2007;DOI: 10.1002/14651858.CD006036.pub2.

Lo AC, Triche EW. Improving gait in multiple sclerosis using robot-assisted, body weight supported treadmill training. *Neurorehabil Neural Repair.* 2008;22(6): 661–671.

Mostert S, Kesselring J. Effects of a short-term exercise training program on aerobic fitness, fatigue, health perception and activity level of subjects with multiple sclerosis. *Mult Scler.* 2002;8(2):161–168.

Patti F, Ciancio MR, Cacopardo M, et al. Effects of a short outpatient rehabilitation treatment on disability of multiple sclerosis patients. *J Neurol.* 2003;250(7): 861–866.

Patti F, Ciancio MR, Reggio E, et al. The impact of outpatient rehabilitation on quality of life in multiple sclerosis. *J Neurol.* 2002;249(8):1027–1033.

Paul L, Rafferty D, Young S, Miller L, Mattison P, McFadyen A. The effect of functional electrical stimulation on the physiological cost of gait in people with multiple sclerosis. *Mult Scler.* 2008;14(7):954–961.

Peterson EW, Cho CC, von Koch L, Finlayson ML. (2008). Injurious falls among middle aged and older adults with multiple sclerosis. *Arch Phys Med Rehabil.* 2008; 89(6):1031–1037.

Rampello A, Franceschini M, Piepoli M, et al. Effect of aerobic training on walking capacity and maximal exercise tolerance in patients with multiple sclerosis: a randomized crossover controlled study. *Phys Ther.* 2007;87(5):545–555.

Shakespeare D, Boggild M, Young C. Anti-spasticity agents for multiple sclerosis. *Cochrane DB Sys Rev.* 2003; 4(CD001332).

Smail DB, Peskine A, Roche N, Mailhan L, Thiebaut JB, Bussel B. Intrathecal baclofen for treatment of spasticity of multiple sclerosis patients. *Mult Scler.* 2006;12(1): 101–103.

van Diemen HA, Polman CH, van Dongen M, et al. 4-aminopyridine induces functional improvement in multiple sclerosis patients: a neurophysiological study. *J Neurol Sci.* 1993;116(2):220–226.

White LJ, Dressendorfer RH. Exercise and multiple sclerosis. *Sports Med.* 2004;34(15):1077–1100.

Yetly EA, Brulé D, Cheney MC, et al. Dietary reference intakes for vitamin D: justification for a review of the 1997 values. *Am J Clini Nutr.* 2009;89:719–727.

Zorzon M, Zivadinov R, Locatelli L, et al. Long-term effects of intravenous high dose methylprednisolone pulses on bone mineral density in patients with multiple sclerosis. *Eur J Neurol.* 2005;12(7):550–556.

15 Management of Urinary and Bowel Dysfunction in Multiple Sclerosis

Ja-Hong Kim

Bladder and bowel manifestations of multiple sclerosis (MS) are common and can be a source of considerable distress to the patient's quality of life, with significant social and economic consequences. It is estimated that about 50% to 90% of the MS patient population develops some form of lower urinary tract and/or bowel dysfunction during the course of the disease (Goldstein et al., 1982; Sirls et al., 1994; Bakke et al., 1996). Interestingly, voiding dysfunction may comprise the initial presenting symptom in up to 15% of MS patients, usually in the form of acute urinary retention or as a new onset of urgency and frequency, secondary to overactivity (Wyndaele et al., 2005). Since micturition and defecation require proper coordination between the afferent fibers entering the S3-5 segments of the spinal cord and the brainstem centers critical to neurologic control, any demyelination along the central nervous system (particularly in the spinal cord) can cause disconnection of these pathways, resulting in various combinations of voiding and bowel symptoms.

The severity of the dysfunction and the degree of bother are closely related to the patient's general neurologic disability, and therefore effective management options should be based on the overall functional status and updated periodically as the disease progresses.

Achieving satisfactory control of urinary and bowel symptoms can have a major impact on a patient's quality of life, as some patients consider incontinence to be one of the worst aspects of the disease (Hemmett, 2004). There is also substantial health-care cost associated with urinary and/or fecal incontinence in terms of additional nursing care, supplies, and increased office and hospital visits due to secondary complications, such as urinary retention and recurrent infections. Clearly, addressing bladder and bowel dysfunction is essential to the overall MS patient management and ideally performed by a suitably trained specialist as part of a multidisciplinary team.

The goal of this chapter is to provide a comprehensive algorithm for the diagnosis and management of urinary and bowel symptoms based on focused literature review of the various treatment modalities and expert opinion. Brief overview of the relevant anatomy and physiology will be presented to enhance the understanding of the current therapeutic guidelines.

BLADDER MANAGEMENT

Structure and Function of the Lower Urinary Tract

The key function of the urinary tract system is to filter the blood and excrete waste in the form of urine, which is then collected and eliminated by volitional effort. This is accomplished by two structurally separate yet dependent components: *(1)* the upper tract consisting of the kidneys and ureters and *(2)* the lower urinary tract (LUT), which includes the bladder and urethra (Fig. 15-1). The main task of micturition is performed by the bladder, a muscular reservoir that distends to store urine at low pressure without leakage and pumps to expel urine efficiently and voluntarily. Histologically, it is made up of three layers: the outer adventitial connective tissue layer, a middle smooth muscle layer comprising the functional detrusor, and an innermost urothelial lining that provides an elastic and impervious barrier.

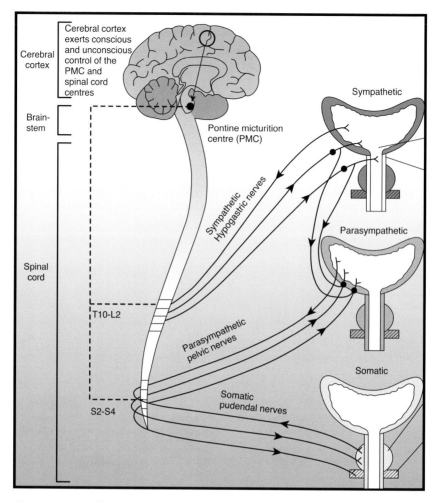

Figure 15-1 Neuroanatomy of lower urinary tract symptoms.

Continence is maintained by the proximal and the distal urethral sphincter mechanisms, which are anatomically and functionally different in men and women. In males, the proximal urethral sphincter includes the bladder neck and the prostatic urethra, which consist of powerful smooth muscle layers contiguous with the trigone and bladder base. Conversely, the female bladder neck is a weaker structure with poorly defined smooth muscle fibers and plays a less significant role in continence. The distal urethral sphincter is an integral part of the continence mechanism for both genders composed of inner smooth and outer striated muscle layers. Some refer to this circular striated muscle as the rhabdosphincter, which is primarily located at the level of postprostatic or membranous urethra in males and middle third in the female urethra. The LUT functions are also influenced by other anatomic factors such as integrity of the pelvic floor musculature and dynamic relationship of the bladder and its outlet to various points in the bony pelvis, especially in women.

Neuroanatomy of the Lower Urinary Tract

Local innervation of the LUT is chiefly by parasympathetic and sympathetic autonomic and peripheral somatic motor and sensory systems (Fig. 15-1). The parasympathetic efferents originate from the S2 to S4 spinal cord segments and emerge as preganglionic fibers in the ventral roots. After leaving the sacral foramina, they unite together to form the pelvic splanchnic nerves, which course deep in the pelvis running on each side of the rectum. These nerve bundles meet up with the hypogastric nerves near the bladder and the urethra to form the pelvic plexus, which is sometimes referred to as the inferior hypogastric plexus. This is a freely interconnected set of nerves located between the peritoneum and the endopelvic fascia which branch out to innervate the pelvic organs. The hypogastric and pelvic nerves also carry afferent autonomic nerve impulses to the dorsal column of the lumbosacral spinal cord.

The sympathetic innervation to the LUT originates in the thoracolumbar spinal cord from T10 to L2 and traverses the lumbar sympathetic ganglion to join the presacral nerve. They form a fenestrated network of nerve fibers called the superior hypogastric plexus, which lies anterolateral to the great vessels and bifurcates into paired hypogastric nerves at the sacral promontory. The superior hypogastric plexus and hypogastric nerves are mainly sympathetic, the pelvic splanchnic nerves are mainly parasympathetic, and the inferior hypogastric plexus contains both types of fibers. The afferent sensory pathways from the pelvic organs are conveyed by both the pelvic and hypogastric nerves.

The somatic innervation is important in regard to the musculature of the pelvic floor and the striated urethral sphincter. The somatic supply to the distal urethral sphincter arises from motorneurons in the anterior horn of S2–S4, in an area known as Onuf nucleus, via the efferents in the pudendal nerve. Although there is some controversy regarding the neural supply of the striated sphincter, most will agree that it is innervated only through motor end plates, implying pure somatic control. Recent neuroanatomic dissection of the male cat showed evidence of cholinergic and adrenergic autonomic innervation of the intramural striated sphincter (Elbadawi, 1985), but the clinical applicability of this finding to humans remains unclear.

Neurophysiology of Micturition

Although the bladder function of urine storage and voiding may be conceptually simple, the process of micturition involves a sophisticated integration of peripheral autonomic, somatic, and central nervous systems on the smooth and striated musculature of the LUT. Failure to coordinate these neural pathways can manifest in various degrees of LUT dysfunction, such as incontinence or elevated postvoid residual urine with high resting pressures in the bladder. These conditions are often associated with chronic urinary tract infections (UTIs), which can cause acute neurologic deterioration in the MS patients especially when coupled with pyrexia. Moreover, retrograde transmission of high intravesical pressures can be damaging to the upper tracts. Considering the serious clinical implications of neurogenic voiding dysfunction, it is therefore essential to understand the neural mechanisms controlling the lower urinary tract function for optimal investigation and treatment of patients with neuropathic voiding dysfunction.

The complex events of micturition have been studied for over a century and still not fully appreciated. Most of our contemporary knowledge on neurophysiology of the LUT is based on animal studies, which were pioneered by Barrington (1931, 1941) and others (Bradley et al., 1976; Mahoney et al., 1977) who described several micturition reflexes and feedback loops in the cat. Detailed discussion of the various theories on neural circuits, neurotransmitters, and reflex centers is beyond the scope of this chapter, but most experts would agree that neurologic control that regulates continence and voiding in humans involves two key micturition centers: the sacral micturition center (SMC) and the pontine micturition center (PMC).

During filling, distension of the bladder wall triggers afferent activity and stimulates the reflex sympathetic outflow to the bladder outlet and pudendal outflow to the distal urethral sphincter. These responses promote continence by three mechanisms that are facilitated largely in the SMC: (1) increasing accommodation in the bladder body via ß-adrenergic receptors, (2) increasing outlet resistance by stimulation of predominantly α-adrenergic receptors in the bladder base and proximal urethra and by causing an increase in activity of striated muscle of the pelvic floor ("spinal guarding reflex"), and (3) inhibiting bladder contractility by blocking effect on parasympathetic ganglionic transmission (De Groat and Lalley 1972; Blaivas et al., 1977; Castkeden and Morgan, 1980;

Ishizuka et al., 1996). During voiding, intense vesical afferent activity activates the PMC, which inhibits the spinal guarding reflexes (sympathetic and pudendal outflow to the urethra) and stimulates the sacral parasympathetic pathways outflow to the bladder and sphincter smooth muscle. The expulsion phase consists of an initial relaxation of the urethral sphincter followed in a few seconds by a contraction of the bladder, an increase in bladder pressure, and the flow of urine. These reflexes require the integrative action of the PMC, which serves as the final common pathway for all bladder motor neurons. Disruptions in any of these pathways can lead to voiding dysfunction categorized into a failure of either storage or emptying. In the MS patient population, LUT manifestations can be unpredictable and challenging to categorize since the disease involves multifocal deficits along the central and peripheral nervous system with a variable course.

Lesions Responsible for Lower Urinary Tract Symptoms in Multiple Sclerosis

The demyelinating lesions responsible for LUT dysfunction in patients with MS show a tendency to fluctuate and change over time and often progress with the disease. In 18 MS patients restudied in follow up, 55% showed a urodynamic pattern different from that seen at baseline (Wheeler et al., 1983). The demyelinating process most commonly involves the posterolateral columns of the spinal cord, with the majority of patients having cervical cord involvement (Oppenheimer, 1978). In other studies based on autopsy findings, about 40% of patients have lumbar cord involvement

and 18% have sacral cord involvement (Blaivas and Kaplan, 1988). Thus, it is not surprising that voiding dysfunction and sphincter dysfunction is so frequent in the MS patient population. Although it is difficult to predict who will develop lower urinary tract symptoms (LUTS), it is most common in the presence of pyramidal tract dysfunction (Betts et al., 1994).

Types of Bladder Dysfunction and Urodynamic Findings in Multiple Sclerosis

There are several ways to classify neuropathic voiding dysfunction, most commonly based on neuroanatomy (upper motor neuron vs. lower motor neuron), urodynamic findings, or functional deficits. Due to the complex and variable neuropathic involvement in the MS patient population, the most practical and clinically useful system is to categorize according to functional deficit: (1) failure to store, (2) failure to empty, or (3) combined dysfunction (Table 15-1). Failure to store results from small spastic bladder and reflects an inability of the detrusor to inhibit contractions until a reasonable amount of urine has accumulated. This type of dysfunction is often associated with a urodynamic finding of detrusor hyperreflexia, which involves overactivity of the detrusor muscle and results in symptoms of frequency, urgency, nocturia, and often urge incontinence. Failure to empty is often associated with a flaccid or acontractile bladder resulting from demyelination in the area of the SMC. The bladder overfills from lack of awareness due to the disruption of message transmission to the brain, and there is very little voluntary or reflex control over micturition since

TABLE 15-1 Categories of Bladder Dysfunction

Type of Dysfunction	Pathology	Symptoms	Urodynamic Findings
Failure to store	Small spastic bladder	Frequency, urgency, nocturia, and urge incontinence	Detrusor hyperreflexia
Failure to empty	Flaccid acontractile bladder	Incomplete emptying, chronic retention, hesitancy, dribbling, frequency, urgency, and overflow incontinence	Detrusor areflexia
Combined dysfunction	Spastic bladder with uncoordinated sphincter activity	Frequency, urgency, hesitancy, urge incontinence, incomplete emptying	Detrusor hyperreflexia with sphincter dyssynergia

the SMC cannot send messages to the bladder and sphincter. Patients with a contractile bladder may present with chronic retention, hesitancy, dribbling, frequency, and overflow incontinence. Combined dysfunction exhibits features of both storage and emptying disorders and results from detrusor-sphincter dyssynergia (DSD), or lack of coordination between detrusor contraction and sphincter relaxation. Patients in this group tend to have wide range of symptoms, including recurrent UTIs, prolonged voiding, extreme hesitancy, and incontinence. Distinguishing between the different types of bladder dysfunction is essential when attempting to provide effective therapy.

Algorithm for evaluation of voiding dysfunction

Urinary symptoms occur in 50% to 80% of MS patients and can be a source of significant morbidity (Goldstein et al., 1982; Gallien et al., 1998). Thus, each person with MS who complains of LUTS should be systematically assessed by a health-care professional who is knowledgeable about MS and its effects on voiding function. Investigation should be appropriate for the patient's current needs and level of disability. Although the urodynamic testing may be an important part of the evaluation for neuro-urologic patients, it may not be necessary as the initial step for MS patients with mild symptoms, since upper tract complications are much less common in patients with MS than in spinal cord injury. Thorough history and physical is an excellent starting point to categorize the degree and type of voiding dysfunction, since persons with MS can have variable clinical presentation and tend to have complex, unpredictable, and fluctuating courses. It is imperative to include a focused neurologic exam to check the viability of the sacral arc pathway by assessing the base anal sphincter tone, perineal musculature contraction, and bulbocavernosal reflex. Evaluation of the patient's coordination, cognitive function, and manual dexterity is also crucial to determine the patient's ability to self-catheterize.

Interpreting Lower Urinary Tract Symptoms

Various terms are used to describe symptoms associated with voiding dysfunction but are oftentimes interpreted differently by clinicians and patients. In order to end the confusion and have a universal language for the scientific community at large, the International Continence Society (ICS) defined these commonly used terms (Abrams et al., 2003).

Frequency refers to an increase in number of voiding occurring throughout the day, usually specified as *daytime frequency* or *nocturia* depending on time of the day. It is important to establish that there is no set number of voids which qualifies as daytime frequency or nocturia, and that the focus is on the effect that the urinary frequency has on the patient's quality of life. Usually daytime frequency of greater than every hour or getting up more than once at night is considered bothersome enough for patients to seek an evaluation. It must be emphasized that the frequency of urination depends on the rate at which urine is formed and the ability of the bladder to store it.

Urgency is the complaint of a sudden compelling desire to pass urine, which is difficult to defer. People who experience this problem have little time to reach a bathroom and often have urge-related incontinence or dribbling. *Dribbling* is the leakage of small amounts of urine from the bladder and can occur with urgency or without sensation. Complaints of frequency, urgency, and nocturia with or without dribbling are considered "irritative" symptoms indicating a storage problem. These are the most common symptoms among MS patients with voiding dysfunction and may correlate with detrusor hyperreflexia in urodynamic studies (UDS).

Hesitancy involves difficulty in initiating urinary stream and may be the result of interrupted spinal pathways which coordinate normal voluntary voiding. When hesitancy is accompanied by decreased force of stream or interrupted flow, it usually indicates an emptying problem and associated with hyporeflexic or acontracile bladder on urodynamic studies. Detrusor hyperreflexia with dyssynergic sphincter may also be demonstrated on UDS.

Urinary *incontinence* is the complaint of any involuntary leakage of urine and is considered to be a storage symptom. This is often socially embarrassing and impacts negatively on a patient's quality of life and complicates management. There are different types of incontinence that need to be distinguished for optimal treatment. *Urge urinary incontinence* is always precipitated by strong urge to urinate or involuntary bladder contraction, which may occur at low volumes in the MS patient with small contracted bladder. Sometimes urge incontinence is entirely affected by the patient's disability status; ambulatory patients with detrusor hyperreflexia are able to get to the toilet on time to avoid incontinence episodes.

Stress urinary incontinence is the complaint of involuntary leakage on effort or exertion, or on sneezing or coughing. In female MS patients, it is important to assess for this type of leakage, which can be effectively addressed with various minimally invasive anti-incontinence procedures such as midurethral sling or injectible therapy. Some patients have a very complex picture with *mixture of both urge and stress*-related incontinence. These patients would benefit from formal urodynamic evaluation to measure leak point pressures, functional capacity, and various other parameters, since they may require different treatment modalities to address their mixed incontinence.

Overflow incontinence is any involuntary loss of urine associated with overdistension of the bladder. This is an emptying problem and should not be mistaken for urge incontinence that is treated with an anticholinergic or other therapies which can impair detrusor function and exacerbate the patient's inability to efficiently void.

Urine Testing

The initial screening for any new or change in urinary symptoms in MS patients is to rule out UTI by microscopic urinalysis with culture and sensitivity testing. Although the dipstick test has excellent negative predictive value for excluding UTI (>98%), the positive predictive value for confirming UTI is only 50% (Fowlis, 1994). It should therefore be emphasized that the diagnosis of UTI is made by a urine culture, and the presence of bacteria in urine does not necessarily mean that there is infection. Many MS patients, especially those who perform intermittent catheterization or have an indwelling catheter, have chronic bacteriuria which can be carefully watched in absence of fever, pain, or generalized deterioration. Presence of blood in urine in otherwise asymptomatic patients more than 50 years of age should always be fully investigated by a urologist with upper tract imaging and cystoscopy to rule out genitourinary malignancy.

Measurement of Postvoid Residual

Postvoid residual (PVR) measurement should be part of the preliminary assessment in all MS patients. Measuring the amount of urine voided and the PVR usually enables the distinction to be made between problem of storage and emptying. This can be obtained by bladder ultrasound or by in-out catheterization after the patient has voided to his or her best ability. Elevated PVR (e.g., <150 cc) indicates emptying problem and possibly DSD and puts the patient at risk for recurrent UTI and incontinence. Minimizing the residual urine is a major component of successful management of voiding dysfunction and should be checked at every office visit. This is especially relevant in patients who are placed on antimuscarinic treatment, which impairs detrusor contraction and increases PVR.

Imaging

Baseline upper urinary tract imaging study should be performed in all MS patients with LUTS. Usually a renal ultrasound is adequate to assess for hydronephrosis, which indicates improper drainage of the kidneys. A recent metanalysis of over 2000 MS patients found only 7 patients with upper tract abnormalities (Koldewijn et al., 1995). The low incidence of hydronephrosis and reflux has led many urologists to abandon routine yearly upper urinary tract imaging unless baseline studies are abnormal or clinical status dictates repeat imaging (Sirls et al., 1994). Patients with hematuria and over age 50 should undergo more detailed upper tract imaging to evaluate the collecting system. Computed tomography with excretory phase urography (CTU) has replaced intravenous pyelogram as the imaging test of choice to workup hematuria for its superior visualization of renal parenchyma as well as the entire collecting system to effectively rule out genitourinary malignancy.

Urodynamic Studies

Urodynamic evaluation is an important process in MS patients with complex LUTS. It is particularly useful in patients who have urinary incontinence, failed initial conservative management, or experience worsening symptoms. Multichannel urodynamics consisting of cystometry and pressure/flow studies with fluoroscopic imaging (videourodynamics) provide invaluable information regarding the presence of detrusor hyperreflexia, elevated filling pressures (indicative of poor compliance), DSD, functional capacity, and urethral competence. In women whom surgical treatment is being considered for stress urinary incontinence, videourodynamics is necessary because of the complexity of the various mechanisms that may be contributing to her symptomatology.

Several studies have confirmed that the most common urodynamic finding in MS patients is detrusor hyperreflexia, occurring in 34% to 99% of case series (Blaivas and Kaplan, 1988; Sirls et al., 1994; Litwiller et al., 1999). Of the patients with hyperreflexia, concomitant DSD was noted in 30% to 65% and impaired detrusor contractility or areflexia in 12% to 38% (Wyndaele et al., 2005). Similarly, Chancellor et al. summarized the urodynamic findings in MS patients after reviewing several series and categorized them into three basic patterns: *(1)* detrusor overactivity, striated sphincter synnergia: 26% to 50% (average 38%); *(2)* detrusor overactivity, striated sphincter dyssynergia: 24% to 46% (average, 29%); and *(3)* detrusor areflexia: 19% to 40% (average, 26%) (Chancellor and Blaivas, 1993). Another urodynamic finding is sphincteric flaccidity seen in less than 15% of patients (Litwiller et al., 1999) and can result in sphincteric incontinence. One study observed weakened pelvic floor contraction in nearly all 30 MS female patients (DeRidder et al., 1998), which can have a significant impact on management of incontinence.

Management of Lower Urinary Tract Symptoms

The goals of treatment are to relieve LUTS, avoid or stabilize upper tract dysfunction, prevent UTI, and re-establish continence. Because the course of MS can be unpredictable, the treatment plan should be as flexible and conservative as possible and tailored to suit the patient's overall disability status. General lifestyle changes should be recommended in all MS patients with LUTS, which include limiting fluid intake to 1–2 liters a day, eliminating caffeine, timed voiding, and pelvic floor exercises (for those patients who have minimal disability). Although usually used to treat stress incontinence, pelvic floor exercises, if performed correctly, can enhance the inhibitory effect of pelvic floor contraction on the detrusor, thus improving urgency and urge-related incontinence. Bladder training, which involves incrementally delaying urination for longer periods, often supervised by physiotherapists with or without biofeedback, can further improve detrusor overactivity. There is good evidence suggesting both these modalities may be effective and they are certainly safe (Vahtera et al., 1997; McClurg et al., 2006).

Treatment of failure to store bladder

Antimuscarinic medication is the mainstay treatment option in managing storage dysfunction based on its theoretical efficacy and encouraging clinical experience. Several antimuscarinic medications have exploded the market, and some of them have been systematically investigated in small studies to show efficacy in reducing frequency, urgency, and incontinence in MS (Gajewski and Awad, 1986; Ethans et al., 2004). However, a recent Cochrane Database review concluded that there is lack of data to advocate the use of anticholinergics in MS patients after reviewing 33 randomized controlled studies assessing the absolute and comparative efficacy, tolerability, and safety of these agents (Nicholas et al., 2009). Nonetheless, clinicians continue to prescribe antimuscarinics as first-line treatment for patients with storage dysfunction. In most cases, antimuscarinic medications and clean intermittent catheterizations (CICs) are used together to maximize the capacity and ensure complete emptying. Patients and their caregivers should be warned of the side effects of antimuscarinics, which includes dry mouth, constipation, and cognitive deterioration, especially in those patients with baseline impairment. Other oral medications, such as imipramine, terodiline, and propantheline, have also been used with some success. Imipramine has both anticholinergic and alpha-stimulating properties, which can be useful in female patients with a combination of detrusor hyperreflexia and intrinsic sphincter deficiency.

Terodiline was shown to have dual anticholinergic and calcium antagonistic action on detrusor muscle, but it was withdrawn from use due to serious cardiac arrhythmias reported in the elderly patients (Andersson, 1984). There are older data on the use of propantheline in MS patients, but it has lost favor among clinicians after it was shown to be less efficacious than oxybutynin (Gajewski and Awad, 1986; Nicholas et al., 2009).

Intravesical therapy has been instituted with some MS patients refractory to oral agents. There is some evidence showing efficacy of intravesical oxybutynin in patients who were unrelieved with standard oral therapy (Weese et al., 1993; Gillberg and Sundquist, 1998). Other agents, such as capsaicin and resiniferatoxin, have also been shown to improve clinical and urodynamic parameters of detrusor overactivity in patients with spinal cord damage, including MS population (de Seze et al., 1998; Kim et al., 2003). This may be a good alternative for those debilitated patients with leakage despite indwelling catheters due to severe detrusor hyperreflexia.

Patients with mainly bothersome nocturia have been prescribed desmopressin (DDAVP) with caution (Bosma et al., 2005). One pilot study of eight patients assessed the efficacy of intranasal DDAVP on intractable nocturia and reported five patients with complete relief and two with considerable benefit, with 6 to 8 hours of antidiuresis (Valiquette et al., 1992). In patients with dependent edema and nocturnal polyuria, some clinicians have given a daytime dose of diuretic with reduction in nocturia (Reynard et al., 1998).

Patients who fail conservative therapy of antimuscarinics with or without CIC may require surgical management to treat severe neurogenic detrusor overactivity and poorly compliant bladder. There is now level III evidence suggesting that botulinum toxin A injection into detrusor muscle in MS patients is highly efficacious in improving symptoms, urodynamic parameters, and quality of life (Kalsi et al., 2007). However, almost all these patients needed to perform CIC, more so than the nonneurogenic population. Nevertheless, this may be a viable option for those patients with leakage despite the indwelling catheter who are poor surgical candidates for bladder augmentation.

In MS patients with refractory storage problem who have a stable benign neurologic status, surgical options such as sacral neuromodulation and augmentation cystoplasty have been tried in small studies. In 1997, the Food and Drug Administration approved Medtronic Interstim therapy for the treatment of nonobstructive urinary retention and symptoms of bladder overactivity, including urgency, frequency, and urge incontinence. Its mechanism of action is incompletely understood, but it probably interferes with or interrupts abnormal reflex arcs, which control the symptom pattern at the sacral nerve roots S3 and S4. A multicenter, international, prospective study of 581 patients found that Interstim therapy resulted in a greater than 50% decrease in intractable LUTS and incontinence episodes, but this study excluded patients with underlying neurologic disorders. Since then, several studies have looked at the efficacy of this treatment for neurogenic bladder, and a recent study observed 81% success rate in MS patients with refractory detrusor overactivity who noted greater than 50% reduction in leakage episodes, nocturia, or pad usage (Wallace et al., 2007). Few other studies have showed similar promising results (Chartier-Kastler et al., 2000; Wallace et al., 2007), but thus far there is limited long-term efficacy data in patients with progressive neurologic diseases such as MS. Moreover, the need for repeat MRI sometimes precludes this treatment option for MS patients.

Augmentation cystoplasty has become an established treatment option for neurogenic and nonneurogenic LUTS in patients with hyperactive or small-capacity bladders who have failed conservative management. This invasive surgical therapy must be approached with caution in the MS patient population with dynamic neurologic conditions that can affect the postoperative course. In one study, nine MS patients (seven with relapse-remitting and two with secondary-progressive form of disease) underwent bladder augmentation with ileum and were noted to have bladder capacity increased by mean of 600 ml, maximal detrusor pressure decreased to 30 cm H_2O, and overall improvement in continence (Zachoval et al., 2003). All patients needed to perform CIC after surgery, which must be considered prior to considering this surgical option. Although rare, complications, such as bowel obstruction, perforation of augmented bladder, metabolic disorders, UTI, and stone formation, are real concerns in this special group of patients with heavy reliance on caregivers. Nonetheless, augmentation cystoplasty can be lifesaving in patients with high-pressure small-capacity bladders with renal deterioration and refractory urge-related incontinence.

Another treatment option for those MS patients with severe detrusor instability with incontinence who cannot tolerate an invasive surgery is indwelling catheterization. This is not an optimal form of management since it can ultimately lead to urethral erosion and recurrent UTI in the long term. Suprapubic tube (SPT) is an alternative to urethral catheters, but some patients have urge-related leakage despite indwelling drainage. These patients may benefit from procedures that increase the outlet resistance, such as obstructive urethral slings for women or artificial urethral sphincters for men. In patients who have severe urethral erosion or necrosis for long-term Foley catheterization, formal bladder neck closure transvaginally for women or transperineally for men may be considered.

Treatment of failure to empty

Improving bladder drainage is a crucial part of effective management of voiding dysfunction in MS patients because incomplete emptying can exacerbate detrusor hyperreflexia and irritative LUTS. One common method to facilitate bladder emptying is Crede maneuver or suprapubic tapping of the bladder, which can stimulate sacral reflex activity and elicit a bladder contraction. This technique involves applying smooth, even downward pressure to the lower abdomen from the umbilicus to the pubis with both hands while performing simultaneous valsalva maneuvers after a natural void attempt. It is not recommended in patients with dyssynergia because the increased pressure on the bladder can be generated to the upper tracts. Some patients, especially women, have successfully utilized this approach to empty the bladder and minimize or avoid CIC altogether. Unfortunately, this is not effective in most circumstances since urethral relaxation remains a problem for MS patients. Furthermore, there is little data about the possible long-term effects using this technique in MS patients, and its use remains controversial in spinal cord patients (Abrams et al., 2008).

Pharmacologic agents to stimulate detrusor contraction such as bethanechol is essentially ineffectual when taken orally. In patients with DSD, adding an alpha blocker can improve bladder emptying, but it must be administered with caution since it can lower blood pressure. One study evaluated the role of alpha blocker in MS patients and showed a significant reduction in PVR (O'Riordan et al., 1995). This medication can be particularly effective in male patients with prostatic obstruction of the bladder neck when used in combination with 5-alpha reductase inhibitors (McConnell et al., 2003). Striated muscle relaxants such as baclofen and diazepam have been prescribed with variable success, but these medications may exacerbate muscle weakness and are not commonly utilized for bladder management.

Clean intermittent catherization performed by the patient or the caregiver is the most effective management for patients with incomplete emptying or chronic urinary retention. There is no formal evidence based on large randomized control studies because it would be considered unethical to untreat patients with elevated PVR. Based on generally accepted expert opinion, CIC is recommended for MS patients with PVR that is consistently greater than 100 cc on repeat measurements taken at separate visits. It is usually well tolerated by patients and allows them to empty the bladder at planned intervals, thus avoiding dribbling or incontinence. The frequency of catheterizations should be tailored for each patient based on the patient's ability to void naturally, but it is usually performed every 4 to 6 hours. If the patient has overflow or urge incontinence between catheterizations, simply increasing the frequency can improve the leakage. Adding anticholinergic medication can also decrease incontinence episodes.

Indwelling catheterization is offered to MS patients when CIC is not possible and is considered a last resort. It is associated with increased incidence of UTI and can cause urethral necrosis in the long term. Therefore, SPT should be placed rather than urethral catheter and changed monthly. Colonization with bacteria or yeast is inevitable, and bacteriuria can be safely watched unless there is development of fever, chills, malaise, or neurologic deterioration. If the patient has incontinence due to severe detrusor hyperreflexia despite indwelling catheterization and anticholinergic medication, intravesical injection of botulinum toxin A injection has been used with some success (Lekka and Lee, 2006).

BOWEL MANAGEMENT

Bowel dysfunction, such as constipation, evacuation urgency, and incontinence, is common in MS and reported in about 50% of patients with MS (Hinds et al., 1990). The mechanism of defecation is analogous to micturition, involving afferent fibers S3–S5. Bowel movement is initiated by a reflex process that is stimulated by rectal wall distention that leads to smooth muscle contraction and internal anal sphincter relaxation. Abdominal wall muscle contraction and voluntary relaxation of the external anal sphincter further facilitate evacuation and require intact T6–T12 spinal cord segments. Demyelination in any of these areas may cause defecatory disorders, which can have a major impact on the patient's quality of life. Fortunately, these bothersome issues can be effectively managed with a comprehensive bowel regimen incorporating dietary adjustments, behavioral modifications, and various combinations of pharmacologic agents.

Types of Bowel Dysfunction

As with urinary dysfunction, MS patients will develop some type of bowel dysfunction during the course of the disease, including constipation, diarrhea, and incontinence. *Constipation* is the most common problem in MS and can be caused or exacerbated by several factors: decreased mobility, weakened abdominal muscles, functional outlet obstruction due to pubococcygeal spasticity or impaired anal sphincter relaxation, inadequate fluid intake, insufficient dietary bulk, and medications. *Fecal incontinence* can result from several pathologic situations: sphincter dysfunction, constipation with rectal overload and overflow, and/or diminished rectal sensation. Presence of chronic *diarrhea* or loose stools is a major health concern and precipitating factor for incontinence. This debilitating condition must be effectively addressed by treating any existing viral or bacterial infection and eliminating medications or dietary irritants. Medications used to treat spasticity of

striated muscles, such as baclofen and tizanidine, can also contribute to incontinence by relaxing the external anal sphincter and should be adjusted accordingly. There are several other categories of drugs that can precipitate defecatory dysfunction, and a thorough review of the patient's medication list should be the first step in evaluating and managing bowel dysfunction (Table 15-2). This is especially relevant for MS patients with concomitant LUTS, since they are usually on anticholinergics and fluid restriction that can exacerbate constipation and make it more challenging to manage both problems. After careful review of the patient's medication list, substitution or dosage adjustments must be done one item at a time, allowing a sufficient interim period to assess the impact of each oral agent.

Nutritional and Fluid Intake Guidelines

Good dietary regimen and fluid intake are absolutely critical to achieving optimal stool consistency and bowel control. The recommended liquid intake is about 8 to 12 cups or 2000 ml per day. However, the increased fluid intake can exacerbate LUTS in patients with detrusor overactivity so this must be carefully considered in MS patients with urinary storage problems. Dietary irritants such as caffeine and alcohol can contribute to rectal urgency and incontinence, as well as LUTS, and should be eliminated.

The addition of fiber to the diet can significantly improve stool consistency and decrease the transit time. The Recommended Daily Allowance is at

TABLE 15-2 Drugs That Exacerbate Bowel Dysfunction

Antihypertensives
Analgesics/narcotics
Anticholinergics
Sedatives/tranquilizers
Diuretics
Tricyclic antidepressants
Anatacids
Iron supplements
Muscle relaxants

least 15 g daily taken in gradually increasing doses through the consumption of raw fruits, vegetables, legumes, flaxseed, and whole-grain breads and cereals rather than fiber concentrates (Subcommittee, National Research Council, 1989). If a high-fiber diet cannot be tolerated, bulking agents such as Metamucil, FiberCon, and Citrucel can be taken with one or two glasses of liquid. This combination distends the gastrointestinal tract and defecation usually occurs within 12 to 24 hours, although the desired effect may be delayed for up to 3 days. Patients may experience bloating, gas, and diarrhea from a high-fiber diet and may require few weeks for dissipation. This can be avoided by gradually incorporating foods rich in high fiber. Finally, establishing a sensible, balanced diet eaten at regular times in a relaxed atmosphere is important to everyone, including the most debilitated MS patient.

Pharmacologic

Stool softeners, such as Colace (dioctyl sodium sulfasuccinate-DSS, 100 mg), Surfak (40 mg), and chronulac syrup, are useful adjuncts to treat dessicated stools. These agents draw increased amounts of water from body tissues into the bowel, thereby decreasing hardness and facilitating elimination. They must be used consistently for maximal benefit and are not habit forming like laxatives. It is important to note that these do not stimulate motility and work only on the stool consistency.

If stool softeners are not effective, the addition of mild laxatives is the next step. Laxatives act as chemical irritants to the bowel and can be habit forming. Gentle over-the-counter laxatives such as pericolace or perdiem taken at bedtime will induce bowel movement within 8 to 12 hours. An ounce of milk of magnesia at bedtime can also be effective.

Constipation that is refractory to oral agents can be treated with rectal suppositories, which provide both chemical and mechanical stimulation combined with lubrication to promote stool elimination. The onset of action is within 15 minutes to an hour and can be used on an as-needed basis. Most commonly used agents are glycerin suppositories (act as lubrication and less habit forming), dulcolax suppositories (stimulates rectal contraction that facilitates evacuation), and therevac mini-enemas, which stimulate and lubricate to aid emptying. Fleet or tap water enemas should be reserved for severe episodes of obstipation or for debilitated patients with atonic bowel. In general, enemas should not be used routinely because they are habit forming and may deplete sodium. It is important to insert the suppository against the rectal wall and not in the stool for it to be effective.

Although diarrhea is much less common than constipation in MS patients, it has a significant impact on a person's quality of life because it is often associated with urge-related fecal incontinence. It is thought that the diarrhea results from a reflex-like activity due to demyelinating lesions similar to urinary frequency and leads to recurrent emptying even though the rectum is not full. Controlling diarrhea is best achieved with bulking agents taken at lower doses. Anticholinergic medications given for urinary symptoms can be helpful when a hyperactive bowel is the underlying cause of diarrhea and incontinence. In refractory cases, antimotility agents such as loperamide have been very effective in controlling diarrhea. Other causes for diarrhea such as infectious diarrhea or occult malignancy must be considered and appropriately managed prior to giving antimotility agents.

Physical Activity and Timed Evacuations

Establishing a regular bowel program in conjunction with dietary measures and pharmacologic agents is essential to successful bowel management. The first step is to set up a schedule for 15 to 30 minutes of uninterrupted time for elimination that is most convenient for the patient. The most effective time for bowel movement is shortly after a meal due to the gastrocolic reflex. Once a convenient time has been selected, it is important to adhere to this routine on a daily basis. Valsalva maneuvers, digital stimulation, and drinking warm liquid such as coffee can enhance the evacuation effort. Maintaining physical activity is also crucial to promote regular elimination schedule as well as improving overall fitness and quality of life.

In summary, many over-the-counter medications are available to treat bowel dysfunction associated with MS. Combination of carefully selected agents can significantly improve defecatory symptoms, but indiscriminate use should be avoided to prevent bowel dependency. Establishing consistent bowel regimen with focus on regular physical activity, balanced high-fiber diet, and adequate fluid intake can effectively manage most bowel symptoms.

KEY POINTS

Neuropathic bladder and bowel dysfunction secondary to MS is common and requires multidisciplinary approach to treatment. The severity and type of dysfunction are unpredictable and dynamic, much like the disease itself. Effective management is best formulated and executed with a specialist based on the patient's level of overall disability and symptom severity.

The goal of management of genitourinary manifestations of MS is to optimize continence, protect kidney function, minimize complications (such as infections), and improve the patient's quality of life. Initial workup should include thorough evaluation of bothersome symptoms and a physical exam to assess for surgically correctable anatomic abnormalities such as prolapse, urinalysis, and PVR. Referral to a specialist for videourodynamics should be considered for those patients who have urinary incontinence, failed initial conservative management, or have worsening symptoms. Baseline upper tract evaluation with renal ultrasound should be performed in all MS patients with LUTS, but there is no evidence to support annual radiologic follow-up in stable patients with normal baseline studies. The most common type of MS voiding dysfunction is detrusor hyperreflexia with or without sphincter dyssynergia, resulting in urinary frequency, urgency, and incomplete emptying due to ineffectual detrusor spasms. In these patients, a combination of pharmacologic agent and CIC regimen can satisfactorily address majority of bladder problems. Several other treatment modalities, including botulinum toxin, sacral neuromodulation, and augmentation cystoplasty, have shown good outcomes in select group of patients who fail initial conservative management.

Bowel issues, such as constipation, evacuation urgency, and incontinence, commonly coexist with urinary symptoms in MS patients. Most bowel difficulties can be successfully managed with consistent bowel regimen, which includes a combination of bulking agents, timed eliminations, optimal nutrition and fluid intake, physical activity, and rectal stimulants. Invasive options, such as surgical bowel diversion, are rarely indicated.

REFERENCES

Abrams P, Agarwal M, Drake M, et al. A proposed guideline for the urological management of patients with spinal cord injury. *BJU Int.* 2008;101:989–994.

Abrams P, Cardozo L, Fall M, et al. The standardization of terminology in lower urinary tract function: report from the standardization sub-committee of the International Continence Society. *Urology.* 2003; 61(1):37–49.

Andersson K-E. Terodiline in the treatment of urinary frequency and motor urge incontinence. *Scand Urol Nephrol Suppl.* 1984;87:13–16.

Bakke A, Myhr KM, Gronning M, Nland H. Bladder, bowel and sexual dysfunction in patients with multiple sclerosis – a cohort study. *Scand J Urol Nephrol Suppl.* 1996;179:61–66.

Barrington FJF. The component reflexes of micturition in the cat: I and II. *Brain.* 1931;54:177.

Barrington FJF. The component reflexes of micturition in the cat: III. *Brain.* 1941;64:239.

Betts CD, D'Mellow MT, Fowler CJ. Urinary symptoms and the neurological features of bladder dysfunction in multiple sclerosis. *Brain.* 1994;117(pt 6):1303–1310.

Blaivas JG and Kaplan SA. Urologic dysfunction in patients with multiple sclerosis. *Semin Urol.* 1988; 8:159–164.

Blaivas JG, Labib KL, Bauer SB, Retik AB. A new approach to electromyography of the external urethral sphincter. *J Urol.* 1977;117:773.

Bosma R, Wynia K, Havlikova E, et al. Efficacy of desmopressin in patients with multiple sclerosis suffering from bladder dysfunction: a meta-analysis. *Acta Neurol Scand.* 2005;112:1–5.

Bradley WE, Rockswold GL, Timm GW, Scott FB. Neurology of micturition. *J Urol.* 1976;115:481–486.

Cappellano F, Bertapelle P, Spinelli M, et al. Quality of life assessment in patients who undergo sacral neuromodulation implantation for urge incontinence: an additional tool for evaluating outcome. *J Urol.* 2001; 166:2277–2280.

Castkeden CM, Morgan B. The effect of beta-adrenoceptor agonists on urinary incontinence in the elderly. *Br J Clin Pharmacol.* 1980;10(6):619.

Chancellor MB, Blaivas JG. Multiple sclerosis. *Probl Urol.* 1993;7:15–33.

Chartier-Kastler EJ, Ruud Bosch JL, Perrigot M, et al. Long-term results of sacral nerve stimulation (S3) for the treatment of neurogenic refractory urge incontinence related to detrusor hyperreflexia. *J Urol.* 2000; 164:1476–1480.

De Groat WC and Lalley PM. Reflex firing in lumbar sympathetic outflow to activation of vesical afferent fibers. *J Physiol.* 1972;226:289.

DeRidder D, Vermeulen C, DeSmet E, et al. Clinical assessment of pelvic floor dysfunction in multiple sclerosis. *Neurourol Urodyn.* 1998;17:337–542.

de Seze M, Wiart L, Joseph PA, et al. Capsaicin and neurogenic detrusor hyperreflexia: a double-blind placebo-controlled study in 20 patients with spinal cord lesions. *Neurourol Urodyn.* 1998;17:513–523.

Elbadawi A. Ultrastructure of vesicourethral innervation. III. Anoaxonal synapses between postganglionic cholinergic axons and probably SIF cell derived processes in the feline lissosphincter. *J Urol.* 1985;133–524.

Ethans KD, Nance PW, Bard RJ, et al. Efficacy and safety of tolterodine in people with neurogenic detrusor overactivity. *J Spinal Cord Med.* 2004;27:214–218.

Fowlis GA, Waters J, Williams G. The cost effectiveness of combined rapid tests (Multistix) in screening for urinary tract infections. *J R Soc Med.* 1994;87: 681–682.

Gajewski JB, Awad SA. Oxybutynin versus propantheline in patients with multiple sclerosis and detrusor hyperreflexia. *J Urol.* 1986;135:966–968.

Gallien P, Robineu S, Nicolas B, et al. Vesicouretral dysfunction and urodynamic findings in multiple sclerosis: a study of 194 cases. *Arch Phys Med Rehabil.* 1998; 79:25–27.

Gillberg PG, Sundquist S. Comparison of the in vitro and in vivo profiles of tolterodine with those of subtype-selective muscarinic receptor antagonists. *Eur J Pharm.* 1998;349(2–3):285–292.

Goldstein I, Siroky MB, Sax DS, Krane RJ. Neurourologic abnormalities in multiple sclerosis. *J Urol.* 1982;128: 541–545.

Hemmett L, Holmes J, Barnes M, et al. What drives quality of life in multiple sclerosis? *QJM.* 2004;97: 671–676.

Hinds JP, Eidelman BH, Wald A. Prevalence of bowel dysfunction in multiple sclerosis: a population survey. *Gastroenterology.* 1990;98:1538–1542.

Ishizua O, Persson K, Mattiasson A, et al. Micturition in conscious rats with and without bladder outlet obstruction: role of spinal alpha adrenoceptors. *Br J Pharmacol.* 1996;117:962–966.

Kalsi V, Gonzales G, Popat R, et al. Botulinum injections for the treatment of bladder symptoms of multiple sclerosis. *Ann Neurol.* 2007;62:452–457.

Kim JH, Rivas DA, Shenot PJ, et al. Intravesical resiniferatoxin for refractory detrusor hyperreflexia: a multicenter, blinded, randomized, placebo-controlled trial. *J Spinal Cord Med.* 2003;26:358–363.

Koldewijn EL, Hommes OR, Lemmens WAJG, et al. Relationship between lower urinary tract abnormalities and disease-related parameters in multiple sclerosis. *J Urol.* 1995;154:169–173.

Lekka E, Lee LK. Successful treatment with intradetrusor botulinum-A toxin for urethral urinary leakage (catheter bypassing) in patients with end-staged multiple sclerosis and indwelling suprapubic catheters. *Eur Urol.* 2006;50:806–809.

Litwiller SE, Frohman EM, Zimmern PE. Multiple sclerosis and the urologist. *J Urol.* 1999;61:743–757.

Mahoney DT, Laberte RO, Blais DJ. Integral storage and voiding reflexes: neurophysiological concept of continence and micturition. *Urology.* 1977;10:95–106.

McClurg D, Ashe RG, Marshall K, et al. Comparison of pelvic floor muscle training, electromyography biofeedback, and neuromuscular electrical stimulation for bladder dysfunction in people with multiple sclerosis: a randomized pilot study. *Neurourol Urodyn.* 2006; 25:337–348.

McConnell JD, Roehrborn CG, Bautista OM, et al. The long-term effect of doxazosin, finasteride, and combination therapy on the clinical progression of benign prostatic hyperplasia. *N Engl J Med.* 2003;349:2387–2398.

Nicholas RD, Friede T, Hollis S, Young CA. Anticholinergics for urinary symptoms in multiple sclerosis. *The Cochrane Library* 2009; Issue 4.

Oppenheimer DR. The cervical cord in multiple sclerosis. *Neuropathol Appl Neurobiol.* 1978;4:151–162.

O'Riordan JI, Doherty C, Javed M, et al. Do alpha-blockers have a role in lower urinary tract dysfunction in multiple sclerosis? *J Urol.* 1995;153:1114–1116.

Reynard JM, Cannon A, Yang Q, et al. A novel therapy for nocturnal polyuria: a double-blind randomized trial of furosemide against placebo. *Br J Urol.* 1998;81:215–218.

Sirls LT, Zimmern PE, Leach GE. Role of limited evaluation and aggressive medical management in multiple sclerosis: a review of 113 patients. *J Urol.* 1994;151: 946–950.

Subcommittee on the 10th Ed of the RDAs, Food and Nutrition Board, Commission on Life Sciences, National Research Council. Recommended dietary Allowances, Washington, DC: National Academy Press; 1989.

Vahtera T, Haaranen M, Viramo-Koskela AL, et al. Pelvic floor rehabilitation is effective in patients with multiple sclerosis. *Clin Rehabil.* 1997;11:211–219.

Valiquette G, Abrams G, Herbert J. DDAVP in the management of nocturia in multiple sclerosis. *Ann Neurol.* 1992;31:577.

Wallace PA, Lane FL, Noblett KL. Sacral nerve neuromodulation in patients with underlying neurologic disease. *Am J Obstet Gynecol.* 2007;197:96, e91–e95.

Weese DL, Roskamp DA, Leach GE, et al. Intravesical oxybutynin chloride: experience with 42 patients. *Urology.* 1993;41:527–530.

Wheeler JS, Siroky MB, Pavlakis AJ, et al. The changing neurourologic pattern of multiple sclerosis. *J Urol.* 1983;130:1123–1126.

Wyndaele JJ, Castro D, Madersbacher H, et al. *Neurogenic and faecal incontinence.* In: Abrams P, et al ed. *Incontinence.* Paris: Health Publications;2005:1059–1162.

Zachoval R, Pitha J, Medova E, et al. Augmentation cystoplasty in patients with multiple sclerosis. *Urol Int.* 2003;70:21–26.

16 Assessment and Treatment of Sexual Dysfunction in Multiple Sclerosis

Frederick W. Foley

There have been few large-scale epidemiological studies on sexual dysfunction in persons with multiple sclerosis (MS). In the general population, studies have indicated that women experience higher rates of sexual dysfunction than men, with 43% of women and 31% of men aged 18 to 59 years experiencing at least occasional sexual dysfunction (Laumann et al., 1999). Age and any physical or mental illness increases risk. The most common sexual problems reported for men include erectile dysfunction and premature ejaculation. A 5% occurrence rate of erectile dysfunction in healthy 40-year-old men has been reported, with a 15%–25% occurrence rate after age 65. For women in the general U.S. population, low or absent libido and lubrication difficulties were the most frequent problems (Laumann et al., 1999, 2005, 2009).

Among persons with MS, fewer large-scale studies have been conducted. Several smaller studies have indicated that a wide variety of sexual concerns are present, ranging in frequency between 40% and 80% (Lilius et al., 1976; Minderhoud et al., 1984; Valleroy and Kraft, 1984; Zorzon et al., 1999; McCabe, 2002; Norvedt et al., 2007). The most common complaints were decreases in genital sensation, fatigue, decrease in libido and vaginal lubrication, and difficulties with orgasm. In several studies, a correlation was found between sexual difficulties and overall level of disability. However, in one study, the rates of sexual dysfunction in MS were higher than a non-MS comparison group only on genital numbness interfering with sexuality (McCabe, 2002). Sexual dysfunction in MS has been strongly linked to how patients perceive their overall quality of life (Norvedt et al., 2007).

An interim analysis of a subset of MS patients (*n* = 5868) in a recent large epidemiology study in the United States found that 67.2% endorsed a sexual problem that was present *always* or *almost always* during the preceding 6-month period (Foley et al., 2007). The most common persistent problems reported for men included erectile dysfunction (52.1%), loss of sexual confidence (37.6%), orgasmic dysfunction (36.5%), and genital numbness (31.4%). Among women, the most common persistent problems reported during the previous 6-month period included orgasmic dysfunction (39.9%), loss of libido (35.9%), inadequate vaginal lubrication (34.2%), and genital numbness (27.8%). Numerous other persistent sexual problems were reported in both men and women with MS, albeit with lower frequencies.

PRIMARY, SECONDARY, AND TERTIARY SEXUAL DYSFUNCTION

The traditional way of evaluating sexual dysfunction is to classify disorders according to aspects of the sexual response cycle, such as disorders of libido, arousal, and orgasm. However, because of the complex ways in which MS can affect sexuality and expressions of intimacy, the MS literature in part has described sexual dysfunctions from primary, secondary, and/or tertiary perspectives (Sanders et al., 2000; Christopherson et al., 2006; Foley, 2006; Foley et al., 2007; Foley and Werner, 2007). Primary sexual dysfunction results from central nervous system lesions that directly affect the sexual response. Spinal cord lesions in the S-2 to S-4 region are highly correlated with sexual dysfunction. In both men and women, primary problems may include loss of libido, decreased, absent, or unpleasant genital sensations, and diminished capacity for orgasm. Men may experience difficulty achieving or maintaining an erection, and a decrease in, or loss of, ejaculatory force or frequency. Women may experience decreased or absent vaginal lubrication.

Secondary sexual dysfunction stems from nonsexual MS symptoms that can also affect the sexual response, such as bladder and bowel problems, fatigue, depression, spasticity, muscle weakness, body or hand tremors, impairments in attention and concentration, sexual side effects from symptomatic treatments, and nongenital sensory paresthesias.

Tertiary sexual dysfunction is the result of disability-related psychosocial and cultural issues that can interfere with one's sexual feelings and experiences. Examples include body-image concerns, performance anxiety, changes in self-esteem secondary to disability-related role changes, and inhibitions about sexual communication and problem solving with one's partner or health-care providers.

OBSTACLES TO SCREENING AND ASSESSMENT FOR SEXUAL DYSFUNCTION IN MULTIPLE SCLEROSIS

A survey of MS specialty health-care professionals (primarily neurologists and nurses) investigated reasons for not inquiring about sexual function during patient visits (Griswald et al., 2003). The survey found the following reasons listed: limited time with patients (44%), "outside my role" (15.3%), patient discomfort (12.5%), lack of professional training or comfort (6.9%), other priorities (5.6%), limited medical coverage so they cannot afford treatment (2.8%), too intrusive for patients (2.8%), and 8.3% of the sample did not answer the question. Discussion of how MS health-care providers can address some of these obstacles occurs in the remainder of the chapter.

SCREENING AND ASSESSMENT FOR SEXUAL DYSFUNCTION

There are many ways MS practitioners can screen for sexual dysfunction in the office or clinic setting. If a review of physical symptoms is conducted via patient report or interview as part of the

evaluation, a question about sexual functioning can be asked when inquiring about bladder and bowel function. A 19-item self-report sexual dysfunction screen developed specifically for persons with MS can be filled out by the patient in about 2 minutes (Foley et al., 2007). Following a positive screen for sexual dysfunction, the patient can be asked if he or she would like help with these symptoms. In one randomized study, simply providing educational materials on MS and sexual dysfunction was associated with improvements in reported symptoms on follow-up (Foley, 2006).

Increased comfort level with asking about sexual questions comes with practice. Many patients rely on the physician or nurse to bring up questions about sexuality, yet they are grateful the topic was addressed (Foley, 2006). Putting sexual questions into a clear context for the patient eases potential discomfort in the discussion. For example, when taking a medical history with a new patient, asking about gynecological history, history of sexually transmitted diseases, or general difficulties with sexual function or satisfaction are important aspects of history. Likewise, when bladder or bowel problems are reported by the patient, sexual dysfunction or discomfort is present most of the time. Inquiry into bladder or bowel function should be accompanied by sexual function inquiry. When prescribing symptomatic medicines that may potentially affect sexual functioning, it represents an opportunity to educate the patient while having a more general conversation about any sexual concerns.

If patients respond positively that they experience sexual problems, there are many ways of addressing the concerns, depending on available time, resources, and scope of practice. At a minimum, having physician and counseling referral resources that specialize in sexual dysfunction is important. Since time with patients and reimbursement for services are critical practice issues (Kaufman et al., 2005/2006), giving patients a more detailed questionnaire to fill out at home and setting a follow-up appointment to specifically address sexual concerns may be necessary. Providing educational materials has demonstrated benefit in a randomized study of women with MS with sexual dysfunction (Christopherson et al., 2006).

PRIMARY SEXUAL DYSFUNCTION IN MULTIPLE SCLEROSIS

Assessment and Treatment

The evaluation process may include a physical history and examination, a review of current medications for their potential effects on sexual functioning, a detailed sexual history, and perhaps some specialized tests of bladder and/or sexual function. The sexual history thoroughly examines the current problem and investigates both present and prior sexual relationships and behaviors. It is also advantageous to conduct a joint interview of the person who has MS and his or her sex partner in order to gain a better understanding of the problem as it is experienced by both persons. Asking questions regarding the couple's communication, problem solving, and overall relationship satisfaction helps obtain a balanced view of the strengths and weaknesses of their relationship. Once the information from the history, physical, and sexual history interview has been completed, treatment typically begins with feedback from the assessment process, education about the effects of MS on sexual function, and suggestions for managing these symptoms.

Orgasmic Dysfunction

As mentioned previously, epidemiology data indicate that almost 40% of women with MS and 36% of men experience chronic orgasmic dysfunction. Multiple sclerosis can interfere directly or indirectly with orgasm. In women and men, orgasm depends on nervous system pathways in the brain (the center of emotion and fantasy during masturbation or intercourse), and pathways in the sacral, lumbar, thoracic, and cervical areas of the spinal cord. Spinal cord lesions are highly associated with disturbances in genital sensation, sexual arousal, and orgasm. In addition, orgasm can be inhibited by secondary (indirect physical) symptoms, such as nongenital sensory changes, cognitive problems, fatigue, and other MS symptoms. Tertiary (psychosocial or cultural) orgasmic dysfunction stems from anxiety, depression, and loss of sexual self-confidence or sexual self-esteem.

Treatment of orgasmic loss in MS depends on understanding the factors that are contributing to the loss, as well as appropriate symptom management of the interfering problems.

Decreased Vaginal Lubrication

Similar to the erectile response in men, vaginal lubrication is controlled by multiple pathways in the brain and spinal cord. Decreased vaginal lubrication that interferes in sexual function is very common in MS (34% of women) (Foley et al., 2007). Using generous amounts of water-soluble lubricants, such as K-Y Jelly, Replens, or Astroglide, frequently ameliorates this condition. Some trial and error is necessary, as the reported satisfaction with the sensation associated with different lubricants is variable. Lubricants that contain menthol or other vasoactive agents can sometimes improve sensation. The use of petroleum-based jellies (e.g., Vaseline) for vaginal lubrication is not advised because of increased risk of bacterial infection with their use.

Decreased Libido

Persistently decreased libido is much more common in women with MS than in men (Foley et al., 2007). To date, there are no published clinical trials of medications that restore libido in MS. However, there are a number of medicines in various stages of development that specifically target hypoactive sexual desire disorder in women. Phase III studies of more than 2000 premenopausal women with low libido have been conducted with flibanserin (Boehringer Ingelheim). Although the preliminary findings are encouraging, the results have not yet been published, and the medicine has not yet been approved in the United States or Europe. Flibanserin is a 5-HT1a serotonin receptor agonist, a 5-HT2a serotonin receptor antagonist, and a dopamine D4 receptor partial agonist. It works in the central nervous system (CNS) by blocking serotonin release, which increases dopaminergic activity after several weeks (Borsini et al., 2002; Jolly et al., 2008). Bremelanotide (Palatin Technologies) is a compound that is undergoing Phase II trials. It functions as a melanocortin receptor agonist in the CNS, is delivered by subcutaneous injection, and may increase libido in both women and men. However, Phase III studies have not yet been conducted. Neither of these compounds has been tested with persons with MS. For postmenopausal women, hormone replacement therapies that contain a small amount of testosterone have helped, although there are no studies to date of women with MS. Testosterone replacement in postmenopausal women or persons with abnormally low physiological levels has been tried in non-MS populations. Similarly, there is research evaluating an FDA-approved clitoral vacuum device (Eros) and vibrators to see whether blood flow, libido, and sensation can be enhanced in women with MS.

There are some medicines prescribed off-label for which there is some anecdotal data that suggest they may improve libido and orgasm in women, although there is an absence of clinical trial data in MS. The general strategy with using these medicines is to increase dopaminergic neurotransmission in the CNS, since dopamine pathways are critical in the sexual response cycle for both men and women. Some of these medicines include buspirone, buproprion, deprenyl, mirapax, and trazodone.

Pelvic floor exercises (Kegel exercises) are sometimes prescribed to enhance female sexual responsiveness, although they have not been tested in a clinical trial in MS. In women with significantly reduced sensation, electromyogram (EMG) biofeedback is required to help them identify and contract the appropriate pelvic floor muscles in the prescribed manner. The rationale for pelvic floor exercises is that they improve muscle tone and genital blood flow, which can enhance arousal and orgasm.

When loss of desire is due to secondary sexual dysfunction (for example, as a result of fatigue) or tertiary sexual dysfunction (for example, as a result of depression), treatment of the interfering secondary or tertiary symptoms frequently restores libido. When a person's libido is diminished by MS, he or she may begin to avoid situations that were formerly associated with sex and intimacy. Sexual avoidance serves as a source of misunderstanding and emotional distress within a relationship. The partner may feel rejected, and the person with MS may experience anxiety, guilt, and reduced self-esteem. Misunderstandings surrounding sexual avoidance frequently compound the loss of desire and diminish emotional intimacy in relationships.

Some men and women who have sustained loss of libido report that they continue to experience sexual enjoyment and orgasm even in the absence of sexual desire. They may initiate or be receptive to sexual activities without feeling sexually aroused, knowing that they will begin to experience sexual pleasure with sufficient emotional and physical stimulation. This adaptation requires developing new internal and external "signals" associated with wanting to participate in sexual activity. In other words, instead of experiencing libido as an internal "signal" to initiate sexual behaviors, one can experience the anticipation of closeness or pleasure as an internal cue that may lead to initiating sexual behaviors and the subsequent enjoyment of sexual activity.

Changing one's sexual signals or cues to initiate sexual activity can be assisted by conducting a body mapping exercise, which constitutes modified sensate focus exercises that take into account MS symptoms (Sanders et al., 2000). Body mapping is typically used to help compensate for primary (genital) or secondary (nongenital) sensory changes, but it can be a useful first step in the enhancement of physical pleasure and emotional closeness, as well as sexual communication and intimacy.

Diminished libido is frequently associated with a decrease in sexual fantasies, which can sometimes be stimulated by increasing sexual imagery and fantasy. Historically, most sexual literature, videos, and magazines have been developed to appeal to a male rather than female audience. Recently, however, sexual videos are being marketed to appeal to couples and women, such as those made by Candida Royalle and other producers of feminist erotica. They include fewer closeups of genitals during orgasm and have more emotional and romantic content and imagery. When libido is partially intact but difficulty sustaining arousal and/or having orgasms occurs, sharing sexual fantasies or watching sexually oriented videos together may help sustain arousal. Similarly, introducing new kinds of sexual play into sexual behavior can help maintain arousal and trigger orgasms.

Decreased Genital Sensation and Sensory Paresthesias

Decreased sensation interferes significantly with sexual arousal and orgasm. In part, it can generally be addressed with more vigorous genital stimulation.

The use of vibrators can be helpful, as the stimulation frequently needs to be more prolonged. Oral sex (for women) is generally more stimulating than intercourse. Some report anecdotally that applying nonprescription topical gels or creams that contain menthol, L-Arginine, niacin, or ergotamine improves sensation and arousal. In women without MS, topical applications of prescription alprostadil cream improved sensation and arousal (Liao et al., 2008), but this has not been tried in MS to date. Exploring alternative sexual touches, positions, and behaviors, while searching for those that are the most pleasurable, is often very helpful. Masturbation with a partner observing or participating can provide important information about ways to enhance sexual interactions.

For complete lack of genital sensation, there is no treatment currently available. Counseling can help a person maintain a sexual relationship with complete genital numbness, as emotional and nongenital physical pleasure can still be derived from a sexual relationship.

Uncomfortable genital sensory disturbances, including burning, pain, or tingling, can sometimes be relieved with gabapentin (Neurontin), carbamazepine (Tegretol), phenytoin (Dilantin), or divalproex (Depakote) or by a tricyclic antidepressant such as amitriptyline (Elavil). Alternatively, the application of a cold gel pack to the genital area prior to sexual activity has been reported sometimes to reduce genital sensory paresthesias.

Erectile Problems

There are a number of oral FDA-approved PDE-5 (phosphodiesterase-type-5) inhibitors to treat erectile dysfunction. The mechanism of action involves active inhibition of the PDE-5 enzyme with subsequent increases in cyclic guanosine monophosphate (cGMP), which maintains smooth muscle relaxation and venous compression in the penis. These medicines include sildenafil (Viagra), vardenafil (Levitra), and tadalafil (Cialis). To date, only sildenafil has been evaluated in clinical trials with men who have MS, although the other medicines are very similar and may be prescribed (Fowler et al., 2005). PDE-5 inhibitors do not improve libido, but they are associated with increased frequency and satisfaction of erections and intercourse. These medicines are contraindicated for use with nitrate-based cardiac medicines, since they interact and can lower blood pressure excessively.

In addition to the PDE-5 inhibitors, there are other oral medicines in development for erectile dysfunction. For example, apomorphine SL (Uprima) is a dopaminergic agonist with affinity for D1 and D2 dopamine receptor sites in the brain, and it has been found in clinical trials to improve erectile function in non-MS populations. Apomorphine induces activation in the nucleus paraventricularis leading to erection. It has not been tried to date in MS.

Injectable medications for erectile dysfunction in MS include prostaglandin E1 (alprostadil; Prostin VR), which has been approved by the FDA for the management of erectile problems. Autoinjectors are available that work with a simple push-button mechanism. Dose titration is done in the urologist's office, to establish the lowest effective dose and minimize the probability of priapism (an overly prolonged erection), a potentially serious side effect. A second potential side effect is scarring at the injection site. Injectable prostaglandin E1 has been widely used in neurologic populations, including MS (Hirsch et al., 1994).

Alprostadil can also be delivered via a urethral suppository (Muse). The drug is then absorbed into the penile tissues, stimulating an erection. However, approximately one-third of the men who tried the drug reported penile discomfort. As with the injectable alprostadil, priapism can occur.

Phentolamine (Regitine in the United States; Rogitine in Canada) is sometimes used in combination with either prostaglandin E1 and/or papaverine to heighten medication efficacy. Phentolamine is an alpha-adrenergic blocking agent and will not induce erections without the presence of another medication (most frequently prostaglandin E1 and/or papaverine). Depending on the type of symptoms the man is experiencing, a urologist may prescribe different combinations of these medications.

One noninvasive way to achieve an erection is to use a vacuum assistive device. With this method, a plastic tube is fitted over the flaccid penis, and a pump creates a vacuum that subsequently produces an erection. Then, a latex constriction band is slipped from the base of the tube onto the base of the penis. The band maintains engorgement of the penis for sexual activities, although it cannot be used for more than 30 minutes.

A more invasive form of treatment for erectile problems is the penile prosthesis. There are two types of penile prostheses: semirigid and inflatable. With the semirigid type, flexible rods are surgically implanted in the corpus cavernosa of the penis. These rods can be bent upward when an erection is desired and bent downward at other times. Following insertion of the rods, the penis remains somewhat enlarged, with a permanent semierection. With the inflatable type, a fluid reservoir and pump are surgically implanted in the abdomen and scrotum, with inflatable reservoirs inserted into the penis that inflate when an erection is desired. This type of prosthesis is barely noticeable, but the potential risks are significant. Surgical complications, infection, scarring, and difficulty operating the pump can create long-term problems. Approximately 80% of the men who use these types of prostheses find them satisfactory. In general, a penile prosthesis is only recommended when other efforts to manage erectile dysfunction have not been successful.

The efficacy of any treatment depends on the ability of both partners to communicate openly about sexual issues and decide on methods that are comfortable and enjoyable for both. Education about treatment options provides persons who have MS and their partners with the language and knowledge that enables discussion and informed decision making.

SECONDARY SEXUAL DYSFUNCTION IN MULTIPLE SCLEROSIS

In multiple sclerosis, the incidence of fatigue, muscle tightness or spasms, bladder and bowel dysfunction, and pain, burning, or other discomfort can have adverse effects on the experience of sexual activity. The interference of these symptoms with sexual function can often be alleviated by taking an aggressive approach to symptom management.

Fatigue

One of the most common secondary sexual symptoms in MS is fatigue. Fatigue greatly interferes with sexual desire and the physical ability to initiate and sustain sexual activity. Fatigue can be managed in a number of ways. Pharmacologic management generally involves prescribing stimulants such as modafinil (Provigil), methylphenidate (Ritalin), or antidepressants with an energizing effect, such as bupropion (Welbutrin), when they are not contraindicated (e.g., history of cardiac problems or seizures).

Nonpharmcologic management may include setting aside some time in the morning for sexual activity because this is often when MS fatigue is at its lowest ebb. Energy conservation techniques, such as taking naps and using ambulation aids, can preserve the energy needed for sexual activities. Choosing sexual activities and positions that are less physically demanding or weight-bearing for the partner with MS may minimize fatigue during sex.

Bladder and Bowel Symptoms

Pharmacologic interventions have also been used to manage bladder and bowel symptoms in MS. Some common symptoms of bladder dysfunction include incontinence and urinary urgency and frequency. Anticholinergic medications help manage incontinence by reducing spasms of the bladder and the urethra. One side effect of anticholinergics is dryness of the vagina. However, as previously mentioned, vaginal dryness can be alleviated by using generous amounts of a water-soluble lubricant, such as K-Y Jelly. A physician may be able to help modify daily medication schedules to allow for maximum effectiveness at the time of planned sexual activity.

Restricting fluid intake for an hour or two before sex and conducting self-catheterization just before sexual activity will also minimize incontinence. For men who are concerned about small amounts of urinary leakage, wearing a condom during sex is advised. If an indwelling catheter is used, health-care providers may be able to offer tips for handling or temporarily removing catheters. If a woman needs to keep the catheter in place, she can move it out of the way by folding it over and taping it to her stomach with paper tape. It is a good idea to experiment with different sexual positions and activities to find those that feel the most comfortable with the catheter in place.

Spasticity

Spasticity can make changing leg positions for sexual activity, or straightening the legs, uncomfortable or painful. Active symptomatic management of spasticity will minimize its impact on sexuality. Range of motion and other physical therapy exercises are commonly employed, as well as antispasticity medications, such as baclofen (Lioresal) and tizanidine (Zanaflex). Taking an antispasticity medication 30 minutes before anticipated sexual activity can be helpful. Exploring alternative sexual positions for intercourse is frequently necessary when spasticity is a problem. Women who have spasticity of the adductor muscles may find it difficult or painful to separate their legs. Changing positions (e.g., lying on one side with the partner approaching from behind, in a "nestled spoons" position) to accommodate this symptom can help minimize the impact.

Weakness

Weakness is a common MS symptom, and it frequently necessitates finding new positions for satisfactory sexual activities. Sustained myotonia (increased muscle tension) is part of the sexual response cycle that helps lead toward orgasm, and muscle weakness can interfere with it. Reclining (non-weight-bearing) positions do not place as much strain on muscles and are therefore less tiring. Pillows can be used to improve positioning and reduce muscle strain. Inflatable wedge-shaped pillows are specifically designed to provide back support during sexual activity and can be purchased by mail order. Oral sex requires less movement than intercourse, and using a hand-held or strap-on vibrator can help compensate for hand weakness while providing sexual stimulation.

Distractibility and Cognitive Changes

Epidemiology studies on the frequency of cognitive changes have indicated that approximately 43%–65% of persons with MS sustain changes in cognition (Rogers and Panegyres, 2007). Sustained attention helps sexual feelings to build progressively toward orgasm. Multiple sclerosis can cause impairments in attention and concentration that may interfere with maintaining sexual desire during sexual activities. Cognitive changes may also lead to partners misinterpreting each other or having difficulty in communication, underscoring the importance in determining whether such changes are present (Foley et al., 1994). Providing pharmacological intervention (prescribing stimulants) may help this symptom and reduce its impact in relationships, although there is little empirical evidence as of yet. From a rehabilitation counseling perspective, one of the main strategies to deal with distractibility is to minimize nonsexual stimuli and maximize sensual and sexual stimuli. Creating a romantic mood and setting, using sensual music and lighting, talking in sexy ways, and engaging in erotic touching provide multisensory stimuli that minimize "cognitive drift" during sex. Introducing humor at those moments when the person "loses attention" allows mutual acceptance of this frustrating symptom and helps minimize its impact.

TERTIARY SEXUAL DYSFUNCTION IN MULTIPLE SCLEROSIS

The physical changes experienced by people who have MS can alter their view of themselves as sexual beings, as well as their perception of the way others view them. The psychological and cultural context in which physical changes occur can adversely affect self-image, mood, sexual and intimate desire, and the ease or difficulty with which persons with MS communicate with their partners.

Self-Image and Body Image

Women with MS have greater body image–related sexual dysfunction (28%) than men (14%) (Foley et al., 2007). In Western societies, women are particularly susceptible to having a negative body image. The media's depiction of women as unrealistically thin and oozing with sensuality is at odds with the reality of most women's personal experience. The extremely high prevalence of diagnosed eating disorders, the variety of commercially packaged diet programs and cosmetic surgery centers, and the multibillion-dollar cosmetics industry targeting women all reflect the efforts of women to reconcile their sensual and sexual self-image with the unrealistic cultural feminine mystique. Women with MS may have difficulty enjoying their sensual and sexual nature because of the gap between their internalized cultural images of the "sensual woman" and their MS-related physical changes.

Similar cultural pressures affect men. Internalized cultural images of men as potent, aggressive, and powerful are at odds with the illness experience. Changes associated with MS in erectile capacity or employment can be associated with an internal sense of failure or defectiveness as the discrepancy between culturally induced self-expectations and one's personal experience grows wider. Sex therapy or counseling with couples that targets tertiary causes of sexual dysfunction has demonstrated efficacy in MS (Foley et al., 2001).

Changing Roles

Changes in family and societal roles secondary to disability can affect one's capacity for intimacy and sexuality. The person with MS who has difficulty fulfilling his or her designated work and household roles may no longer feel like an equal partner. The partner of a severely disabled individual may feel overburdened by additional caregiving, household, and employment responsibilities. The couple's intimate relationship can be threatened by the growing tension that results from these feelings.

In addition, the caregiving partner (either male or female) may have trouble switching from the nurturing role of caretaker to the more sensual role of lover. As a sexual partner of a woman (or man) with a disability, a man may begin to think of his partner as too fragile or easily injured, or as a "patient" who is ill and therefore unable to be sexually expressive. If it is practical or culturally acceptable, having non-family members perform caretaking activities helps minimize this "role conflict." When caretaking must be performed by the sexual partner, separating caretaking activities from times that are dedicated to romantic and sexual activities can minimize this conflict.

Accompanying these role changes may be an increasing sense of isolation in the relationship and less understanding of the partner's struggles and perspectives. The diminishing capacity to understand and work through these issues creates greater isolation and misunderstanding, leading to increasing resentments.

Cultural Expectations Regarding Sexual Behavior

The religious, cultural, and societal influences in our lives help shape our thoughts, views, and expectations about sexuality. One of the notions about sexuality that prevails in Western culture is a "goal-oriented" approach to sex. In this approach, the sexual activity is done with the goal of having penile-vaginal intercourse, ultimately leading to orgasm. Here, the sexual behaviors labeled as foreplay, such as erotic conversations, touching, kissing, and genital stimulation, are seen as steps that inevitably lead to intercourse rather than as physically and emotionally satisfying sexual activities in their own right. Hence, couples are not thought to be having "real" sex until they are engaging in coitus, and sex is typically not considered "successfully completed" until orgasm occurs.

This Western view of sexuality leads to spending a great deal of time and energy worrying about the MS-related barriers to intercourse and orgasm ("the goal") rather than seizing the opportunity to explore physically and emotionally satisfying alternatives to intercourse. The capacity to discover new and fulfilling ways to compensate for sexual limitations requires that couples be able to let go of preconceived notions of what sex should be and focus instead on openly communicating their sexual needs and pleasures without fear of ridicule or embarrassment.

Clinical Depression and Other Multiple Sclerosis–Related Emotional Challenges

Major depressive disorder is common in MS, with lifetime risk estimates as high as 50% (Mohr et al., 2001). Depression is highly associated with sexual dysfunction. Although depression treatment has proven effective in MS with antidepressant therapy and cognitive-behavioral psychotherapy (Mohr et al., 2001), sexual side effects from antidepressant treatments, especially the selective serotonin reuptake inhibitors (SSRIs) and serotonin norepinephrine reuptake inhibitors (SNRIs) compromise depression treatment efficacy for sexual dysfunction. The SNRIs (e.g., venlafaxine, desvenlafaxine, duloxetine, etc.) have reportedly slightly lower sexual side effects than the SSRIs (e.g., fluoxetine, paroxetine, sertraline, citalapram, etc). Antidepressants that serve primarily as dopamine agonists (e.g., buproprion) reportedly have few or no sexual side effects. When it comes to prescribing an antidepressant, selecting one of the latter agents (if there is not a history of seizures or significant anxiety present) would decrease the probability of sexual side effects. In addition, since in one major clinical trial of MS patients with major depression, cognitive-behavioral psychotherapy was as equally effective as sertraline, referring to a psychologist or psychiatrist expert in this approach may be a viable alternative (Mohr et al., 2001). If prescribing an SSRI is necessary to adequately treat depression, anecdotal clinical experience suggests that adding a small amount of buproprion or prescribing PDE-5 inhibitors concomitantly may help ameliorate SSRI-induced orgasmic dysfunction.

The MS experience is frequently associated with emotional challenges besides depression, including grief, demoralization, and coping with an uncertain future (Lode et al., 2009). These emotional struggles may temporarily dampen interest in sex or the ability to give and receive sexual pleasure. Education and counseling are approaches that typically address these issues.

REFERENCES

Borsini F, Evans K, Jason K, Rohde F, Alexander B, Pollentier S. Pharmacology of flibanserin. *CNS Drug Rev.* 2002;8(2):117–142.

Christopherson JM, Moore K, Foley FW, Warren KG. A comparison of written materials vs. materials and counseling for women with sexual dysfunction and multiple sclerosis. *J Clin Nurs.* 2006;15:742–750.

Foley FW. Sexuality. In: Kalb RC, ed. *Multiple Sclerosis: A Guide for Families.* 3rd ed. New York: Demos Medical Publishing; 2006:53–80.

Foley FW, Dince W, Bedell JR, et al. Psychoremediation of communication skills for cognitively impaired persons with multiple sclerosis. *J Neurol Rehabil.* 1994;7(6):165–176.

Foley FW, LaRocca NG, Sorgen A, Zemon V. Rehabilitation of intimacy and sexual dysfunction in couples with multiple sclerosis. *Mult Scler Clin Lab Res.* 2001;7(6):417–421.

Foley FW, Werner M. How MS affects sexuality and intimacy. In: Kalb RC, ed. *Multiple Sclerosis: The Questions You Ask, The Answers You Need.* 4th ed. New York: Demos Medical Publishing; 2007:172–198.

Foley FW, Zemon V, Campagnolo D, et al. *The epidemiology of sexual dysfunction in multiple sclerosis in the United States.* Platform presentation at: The 21st Annual Meeting of the Consortium of Multiple Sclerosis Centers, May 31 2007; Washington DC.

Fowler CJ, Miller JR, Sharief MK, Hussain IF, Stecher VJ, Sweeney M. A double blind, randomized study of sildenafil citrate for erectile dysfunction in men with multiple sclerosis. *J Neurol Neurosurg Psychiatry.* 2005;76(5):700–705.

Griswald G, Foley FW, Zemon V, LaRocca NG, Halper J. MS health professionals' comfort, training, and practice patterns regarding sexual dysfunction. *Int J Mult Scler Care.* 2003;5(2):3–10.

Hirsch IH, Smith RL, Chancellor MB, Bagley DH, Carsello J, Staas WE, Jr. Use of intracavernous injection of prostaglandin E1 for neuropathic erectile dysfunction. *Paraplegia.* 1994;32(10):661–664.

Jolly E, Clayton A, Thorp J, Lewis-D'Agostino D, Wunderlich G, Lesko L. Design of phase II pivotal trials of flibanserin in female hypoactive sexual desire disorder. *Sexologies.* 2008;17(suppl 1):S133–S134.

Kaufman M, Cutter G, Schwid S, et al. (2005/2006). Longitudinal assessment of multiple sclerosis patients and reimbursement issues. *Int J Mult Scler Care.* 2005/2006;7(4):29–31.

Laumann EO, Glasser DB, Neves RC, Moreira ED, GSSAB Investigators' Group. A population-based survey of sexual activity, sexual problems and associated help-seeking behavior patterns in mature adults in the United States of America. *Int J Impotence Res.* 2009; 21(3):171–178.

Laumann EO, Nicolosi A, Glasser DB, et al. Sexual problems among women and men aged 40-80: prevalence and correlates identified in the Global Study of Sexual Attitudes and Behaviors. *Int J Impotence Res.* 2005; 17(1):39–57.

Laumann EO, Paik A, Rosen RC. Sexual dysfunction in the United States: prevalence and predictors. *JAMA.* 1999;281(6):537–544.

Liao Q, Zhang M, Geng L, et al. Efficacy and safety of alprostadil cream for the treatment of female sexual arousal disorder: a double-blind, placebo-controlled study in Chinese population. *J Sex Med.* 2008;5(8): 1923–1931.

Lilius HG, Valtonen EJ, Wikstrom J. Sexual problems in patients suffering from multiple sclerosis. *J Chron Dis.* 1976; 29:643–647.

Lode K, Bru E, Klevan G, Myhr KM, Nyland NH, Larsen JP. Depressive symptoms and coping in newly diagnosed patients with multiple sclerosis. *Mult Scler Clin Lab Res.* 2009;15(5):638–643.

McCabe MP. Relationship functioning and sexuality among people with MS. *J Sex Res.* 2002;39:302–309.

Minderhoud JM, Leemhuis JG, Kremer J, Laban E, Smits PM. Sexual disturbances arising from multiple sclerosis. *Acta Neurolog Scandinav.* 1984;70(4): 299–306.

Mohr DC, Boudewyn AC, Goodkin DE, Bostrom A, Epstein L. Comparative outcomes for individual cognitive-behavior therapy, supportive-expressive group psychotherapy, and sertraline for the treatment of depression in multiple sclerosis. *J Consult Clin Psychol.* 2001;69(6):942–949.

Norvedt M, Rilse T, Frugard J, et al. Prevalence of bladder, bowel, and sexual problems among multiple sclerosis patients two to five years after diagnosis. *Mult Scler.* 2007;13(1):106–112.

Rogers JM, Panegyres PK. Cognitive impairment in multiple sclerosis: evidence-based analysis and recommendations. *J Clin Neurosci.* 2007;14(10):919–927.

Sanders A, Foley FW, LaRocca NG, Zemon V. The multiple sclerosis intimacy and sexuality questionnaire–19. *Sexual Disabil.* 2000;18(1):3–26.

Valleroy ML, Kraft GH. Sexual dysfunction in multiple sclerosis. *Arch Phys Med Rehabil.* 1984;65(3):125–128.

Zorzon M, Zivadinov R, Boxco A, et al. Sexual dysfunction in multiple sclerosis: a case-control study. I. Frequency and comparison of groups. *Mult Scler Clin Lab Res.* 1999;5(6):428–431.

Gender and Reproductive Issues in Multiple Sclerosis

Rhonda Voskuhl and Barbara S. Giesser

For decades it has been known that women are more susceptible than men to multiple sclerosis (MS). Sex hormones and/or sex-linked gene inheritance may be responsible for this enhanced susceptibility of women. In general, it has been documented that women have more robust immune responses than men (Whitacre et al., 1999). However, an effect of sex on the immune response does not preclude additional effects of sex on the target organ in MS, the central nervous system (CNS) (Cerghet et al., 2006; Spring et al., 2007).

In this chapter, we will consider the gender bias in MS with respect to effects of sex hormones and sex chromosomes on both the immune system and the CNS. Clinical issues pertaining to reproductive function will also be discussed.

SEX DIFFERENCES IN MULTIPLE SCLEROSIS

During reproductive ages, there is a distinct female preponderance of autoimmune diseases, including MS (Whitacre et al., 1999). Sex hormones and/or sex chromosomes may be responsible for this enhanced susceptibility. In men, the onset of MS tends to be relatively later in life (30s–40s), coinciding with the beginning of the decline in bioavailable testosterone (T) (Weinshenker, 1994). Thus, the female to male ratio is greater in patients presenting with MS before age 20 (3.2:1) as compared to the ratio in the MS population as a whole (2:1) (Duquette et al., 1992). Interestingly, a recent Canadian study found a disproportionate increase in the incidence of MS in women (Orton et al., 2006). This increase in the sex ratio, approaching 4:1, was theorized to possibly be of environmental origins. Notably, relatively higher sex ratios in MS

as recently reported remain consistent with the sex ratios that were previously known in other autoimmune diseases such as rheumatoid arthritis (RA) and systemic lupus erythematosus (SLE).

While it is clear that there is an increase in the incidence of MS in women as compared to men, a different question is whether established disease progresses at a different rate in women versus men. Clinical neurologists have had the impression that men progress more rapidly than women. However, this may be confounded by the fact that their assessments have included primary progressive multiple sclerosis (PPMS). Primary progressive MS is genetically distinct from relapsing-remitting multiple sclerosis (RRMS) and secondary progressive multiple sclerosis (SPMS) in that there is no sex bias in its incidence. It also differs with respect to genetic association loci, site of the MS lesions, rate of progression and response to anti-inflammatory treatments. Primary progressive MS primarily affects the spinal cord, is associated with relatively rapid progression of motor deficits, and is less responsive to anti-inflammatory treatments. Since the ratio of women to men is 1:1 in PPMS, there are relatively more men with PPMS when comparing it with the male:female ratio in RRMS and SPMS. This would make it appear as though men have a more severe course of MS. However, many propose that PPMS is a different disease pathologically than RRMS and SPMS, and that it should be considered as such. Then the question becomes, Do men and women with RRMS or SPMS progress at different rates? Unfortunately most studies did not assess their data according to sex, and the answer to this question is currently unknown. A National Multiple Sclerosis Society Task Force on Gender and MS has suggested that placebo-treated

MS patients in clinical trials should be assessed for effects of gender on their disease course (Whitacre et al., 1999).

Existing data suggest that early predictors of future disability in MS include sex, age of onset, and degree of recovery from first episode (Runmarker et al., 1994; Confavreux et al., 2003). These are not mutually exclusive. Men tend to have later age of onset. Further, while women develop MS more frequently, there are some magnetic resonance imaging (MRI) and clinical data that suggest that when men develop MS, their disease is more severe, as evidenced by more destructive lesions (T1 holes on MRI) and a clinical course that is more progressive (less relapses and more permanent disability) (Confavreux et al., 2003; Pozzilli et al., 2003). Thus, women spend more years in an early relapsing-remitting phase before transitioning to the secondary progressive phase, while men have a shorter time in the relapsing-remitting phase before transitioning to the secondary progressive phase. Interestingly, once the transition to a progressive course or given stage of disability has been reached, there is no sex difference in the rate of further progression (Confavreux et al., 2003). A possible hypothesis for what may be occurring is that there is an interaction between the aging CNS and the transition to SPMS. Women with an onset of MS at age 20–30 will spend approximately 15 years in the RRMS phase before approaching the transition at ages 40–45, while men with age of onset at ages 35–40 will spend much less time in the RRMS phase before beginning the transition to SPMS at ages 40–45. Thus, the transition tends to occur at approximate ages 40–45 regardless of sex. Future neuropathologic studies should consider the role of the aging CNS on the development of SPMS. Future studies should also address why many relatively young men, ages 20–30, remain asymptomatic during their early years as compared to women who are already experiencing clinical relapses and remissions. Our group has postulated that relatively high levels of testosterone in young men may be playing a temporarily protective role in men who are otherwise genetically predisposed to ultimately developing MS (Sicotte et al., 2007).

Given that the clinical picture of disease progression in women versus men is complex, neuroimaging studies were conducted in 413 MS subjects, comparing women and men with MS, in an effort to reveal some insights based on subclinical biomarkers of disease. Men had fewer contrast enhancing lesions than women, but a higher likelihood for them to evolve into T1 "black holes" (Pozzilli et al., 2003). Since enhancing lesions are considered a biomarker for relapses, these data were consistent with the observation that men are less likely to develop early RRMS. Further, since T1 black holes are thought to be destructive and potentially associated with permanent neurological damage, these data were also consistent with the suggestion that when men develop MS, it tends to be more severe clinically (Weinshenker, 1994; Hawkins and McDonnell, 1999; Confavreux et al., 2003). However, in a follow-up study of 35 women and 25 men with RRMS, the finding of fewer enhancing lesions in men was confirmed, but the increased likelihood for lesions to evolve into T1 black holes in men was not, perhaps due to the smaller sample size (Tomassini et al., 2005). Together, the data appear to confirm that men are less likely to develop clinical relapses and enhancing lesions on MRI at an early age, but it remains unclear as to whether the course of MS in men is more severe as compared to age-matched women with MS.

Sex Differences in the Murine Model of Multiple Sclerosis

While there is no perfect animal model of MS, experimental autoimmune encephalomyelitis (EAE) is the most widely used animal model for studying the pathogenesis of MS. EAE models vary depending upon the species and strain of the animal used as well as upon the method of EAE induction. Some models are monophasic, some are relapsing, and others are chronic progressive. Monophasic models (B10.PL strain) are best suited for studying mechanisms involved in downregulation of autoimmune responses, while relapsing models (SJL strain) are amenable to studying mechanisms involved in relapses. Chronic disability models (C57BL/6 strain) are suitable for studying mechanisms of inflammation-mediated neuronal degeneration (Voskuhl, 1996). It is of importance that genetic background appears to dictate in large measure what type of disease course will be induced.

Decades of work have described the immunology and the neuropathology of EAE. Immunologic studies have focused on myelin protein–specific immune responses, including those directed against myelin basic protein (MBP), proteolipid protein (PLP), and myelin oligodendrocyte protein (MOG). Much of what has been theorized in MS with respect to immune responses was based on initial findings in EAE, including the role for pro-inflammatory cytokines, chemokines, adhesion molecules, and costimulatory molecules. Regarding the neuropathology of EAE, past studies have focused on detailed characterization of lesions with respect to the inflammatory infiltrate composition, the level of demyelination, the level of oligodendrocyte loss, microglial activation, and astrocytic scar formation (Brown et al., 1982; Mokhtarian et al., 1984; Raine et al., 1980, 1999). Less attention has focused on neurons, with only recent descriptions of a relationship between axonal loss and disability (Wujek et al., 2002). Central nervous system pathology "beyond the lesion" has been described in normal-appearing white matter (NAWM) characterized by decreases in axon densities in white matter tracts of the dorsal spinal cord (Morales et al., 2006; Deboy et al., 2007; Tiwari-Woodruff et al., 2007). Another study has described motor neuron dendritic abnormalities in gray matter of spinal cords of mice with EAE (Bannerman et al., 2005), and neuronal staining in spinal cord gray matter has been shown to be abnormal even early during the course of EAE (Morales et al., 2006). Regarding neuroimaging "beyond the lesion" in EAE, diffusion tensor imaging (DTI) changes have been described in dorsal cord and optic nerve (Kim et al., 2006; Deboy et al., 2007), and cerebellar gray matter atrophy has also been described (Mackenzie-Graham et al., 2006). Thus, while EAE has been the prototypic inflammation mediated disease tool used by immunologists for decades, more recently EAE has also been characterized with respect to its neurodegenerative component.

As is the case for MS, since EAE has both an inflammatory and a neurodegenerative component, sex differences must be considered with respect to effects on both the immune system and the CNS in EAE. In the relapsing murine model, EAE has been characterized to have a sex bias that parallels that of MS, with males being less susceptible to disease than females (Bebo et al., 1996,

1998a, 1999; Voskuhl et al., 1996; Kim and Voskuhl, 1999). In part, this difference may result from the protective effects of testosterone in male mice. This has been suggested by studies demonstrating that the removal of physiologic levels of testosterone from male mice via castration increases disease susceptibility (Bebo et al., 1998b; Smith et al., 1999). Also, in animal models of other autoimmune diseases where a similar gender dimorphism exists (nonobese diabetic mice, thyroiditis, and adjuvant arthritis), castration was shown to increase the disease prevalence and/or the disease severity (Ahmed and Penhale, 1982; Fitzpatrick et al., 1991; Fox, 1992; Harbuz et al., 1995). Furthermore, testosterone levels have been shown to be decreased in male mice during EAE relapse (Foster et al., 2003). Together these data support the hypotheses that endogenous androgens may be protective at physiologic levels.

Notably, however, while some strains of mice have increased susceptibility to EAE in females as compared to males, other strains have either more susceptibility to disease in males as compared to females (Papenfuss et al., 2004), or there is no sex bias (Okuda et al., 2002; Palaszynski et al., 2004b). Effects of removal of androgens in EAE have previously been shown to be dependent upon genetic background (Palaszynski et al., 2004b), and some autosomal gene linkages to susceptibility to MS have been identified in one gender but not the other (Kantarci et al., 2005). Thus, in the outbred human population, the genetic background of some, but not all, individuals may be permissive to effects of sex. Importantly, since overall there is a gender difference in many autoimmune diseases in humans, we hypothesize that the incidence of relatively permissive genetic backgrounds is likely to be prevalent, not rare, in occurrence.

Ovarian Hormones: Estrogen Treatment Ameliorates Experimental Autoimmune Encephalomyelitis

Sex differences in MS and the EAE model may be related to sex hormones, sex chromosomes, or both. With respect to sex hormones, female sex hormones or male sex hormones may play a role. Since pregnancy changes include alterations in female sex hormones, the changes in disease during pregnancy are consistent with a potential role of female sex hormones in disease.

It was shown over a decade ago that EAE in guinea pigs, rats, and rabbits improved during pregnancy (Abramsky, 1994). Further, it was shown that relapsing-remitting EAE improved during late pregnancy (Voskuhl and Palaszynski, 2001; Langer-Gould et al., 2002). The EAE model was then used to determine whether an increase in levels of a certain hormone during pregnancy might be responsible for disease improvement. Since estrogens and progesterone increase progressively during pregnancy to the highest levels in the third trimester, these hormones were candidates for possibly mediating a protective effect. Two estrogens, estradiol and estriol, increase progressively during pregnancy. Estradiol is otherwise present at much lower fluctuating levels during the menstrual cycle in nonpregnant women and female mice. Estriol, in contrast, is made by the fetal placental unit and is not otherwise present in nonpregnant states. Over the last 10 years it has been shown in numerous studies that estrogen treatment (both estriol and estradiol) can ameliorate both active and adoptive EAE in several strains of mice (Jansson et al., 1994; Kim et al., 1999; Bebo et al., 2001; Ito et al., 2001; Matejuk et al., 2001; Liu et al., 2002, 2003; Polanczyk et al., 2003; Subramanian et al., 2003). Estriol treatment has also been shown to be effective in reducing clinical signs in EAE when administered after disease onset (Kim et al., 1999). Finally, both estradiol and estriol have been shown to be efficacious in both female and male mice with EAE (Palaszynski et al., 2004a).

Estrogen type and dose in ameliorating experimental autoimmune encephalomyelitis

A clinical amelioration of EAE occurred when estriol was used at doses to induce serum levels that were physiologic with pregnancy. On the other hand, estradiol had to be used at doses severalfold higher than pregnancy levels in order to induce the same degree of disease protection (Jansson et al., 1994). Thus, while it is clear that high doses of estradiol are protective in EAE, it has not yet been clearly established whether low doses of estradiol are protective. Some reports have found that ovariectomy of female mice makes EAE worse

(Matejuk et al., 2001), while others have found that ovariectomy does not have a significant effect on disease (Voskuhl and Palaszynski, 2001). Thus, it is controversial whether low levels of endogenous estradiol, which fluctuate during the menstrual cycle, have a significant influence on EAE.

Estrogen treatment in experimental autoimmune encephalomyelitis: effects on the immune system

Protective mechanisms of estrogen treatment (both estriol and estadiol) in EAE clearly involve anti-inflammatory processes, with estrogen-treated mice having fewer inflammatory lesions in the CNS (Kim et al., 1999). Estrogen treatment has also been shown to downregulate chemokines in the CNS of mice with EAE and may affect expression of matrix matalloprotease-9 (MMP-9), each leading to impaired recruitment of cells to the CNS (Matejuk et al., 2001; Subramanian et al., 2003). In addition, estrogen treatment has been shown to impair the ability of dendritic cells to present antigen (Liu et al., 2002; Zhang et al., 2004). Finally, estrogen treatment has recently been shown to induce certain regulatory T cells in EAE (Matejuk et al., 2004; Polanczyk et al., 2004). Thus, estrogen treatment has been shown to be anti-inflammatory through a variety of mechanisms.

Estrogen treatment in experimental autoimmune encephalomyelitis: effects on the central nervous system

An anti-inflammatory effect of estrogen treatment in EAE does not preclude an additional more direct neuroprotective effect. Estrogens are lipophilic, readily traversing the blood–brain barrier, with the potential to be directly neuroprotective (Brinton, 2001; Garcia-Segura et al., 2001; Wise et al., 2001). Numerous reviews have described estrogen's neuroprotective effects, both in vitro and in vivo (Garcia-Segura et al., 2001; Wise et al., 2001; Sribnick et al., 2003) in other model systems. Given the neuroprotective effect of estrogen treatment in other disease models, it was determined whether estrogen treatment might be neuroprotective in EAE. Estradiol treatment not only reduced clinical disease severity and was anti-inflammatory with respect to cytokine production in peripheral immune cells, it also decreased CNS white matter inflammation and demyelination. In addition, decreased neuronal staining, accompanied by increased immunolabeling of microglial/monocyte cells surrounding these abnormal neurons, was observed in gray matter of spinal cords of placebo-treated EAE mice at the earliest stage of clinical disease, and treatment with estradiol significantly reduced this gray matter pathology. Thus, estradiol treatment was not only anti-inflammatory but also neuroprotective in the prevention of both white and gray matter pathology in spinal cords of mice with EAE (Morales et al., 2006).

Estrogen receptors that mediate protection from experimental autoimmune encephalomyelitis

Determining which estrogen receptor mediates the protective effect of an estrogen treatment in disease is of central importance for future development of selective estrogen receptor modifiers that aim to maximize efficacy and minimize toxicity. The actions of estrogen are mediated primarily by nuclear estrogen receptors, ERα and ERβ, although nongenomic membrane effects have also been described (Weiss and Gurpide, 1988). Both ERα and ERβ are expressed in both the immune system and the CNS (Kuiper et al., 1998; Enmark and Gustafsson, 1999; Erlandsson et al., 2001; Igarashi et al., 2001). Estrogen receptor knockout mice have been used to show that the protective effect of estrogen treatment (estradiol and estriol) in EAE was dependent upon the presence of ERα, not ERβ (Liu et al., 2003; Polanczyk et al., 2003). A highly selective ERα ligand (Harrington et al., 2003) was then shown to alleviate clinical disease in this MS model while being both anti-inflammatory and neuroprotective (Morales et al., 2006). It was also shown that estrogens may act in vivo during EAE via direct actions on cells within the CNS (Garidou et al., 2004). Interestingly, differential neuroprotective and anti-inflammatory effects were found using ERα versus ERβ ligand treatment in EAE (Tiwari-Woodruff et al., 2007). Clinically, ERα ligand treatment abrogated disease at the onset and throughout the disease course. In contrast, ERβ ligand treatment had no effect at disease onset but promoted recovery during the chronic phase of the disease. ERα ligand treatment was

anti-inflammatory in the systemic immune system, while ERβ ligand treatment was not. Also, ERα ligand treatment reduced CNS inflammation, while ERβ ligand treatment did not. Interestingly, treatment with either the ERα or the ERβ ligand was neuroprotective as evidenced by reduced demyelination and preservation of axon numbers in white matter. Thus, by using the ERβ selective ligand, it was shown that neuroprotective effects of estrogen treatment were not necessarily dependent upon anti-inflammatory properties.

A pilot trial of estriol treatment in multiple sclerosis

Since estriol is the major estrogen of pregnancy and since an estriol dose that yielded a pregnancy level in mice was protective in EAE (Kim et al., 1999), estriol was administered in a prospective pilot clinical trial to women with MS, in an attempt to recapitulate the protective effect of pregnancy on disease (Sicotte et al., 2002). A crossover study was used whereby patients were followed for 6 months pretreatment to establish baseline disease activity, which included cerebral MRI every month and neurologic exam every 3 months. The patients were then treated with oral estriol (8 mg/day) for 6 months, then observed for 6 more months in the posttreatment period. Six RR patients and four SP patients finished the 18-month study period. The RRMS subjects were then retreated with oral estriol and progesterone in a 4-month extension phase. Estriol treatment resulted in serum estriol levels that approximated levels observed in untreated healthy control women who were 6 months pregnant. When PBMCs were stimulated ex vivo, a favorable shift in cytokine profile (decreased pro-inflammatory cytokines and increased anti-inflammatory cytokines) was observed during treatment as compared to baseline (Soldan et al., 2003). On serial MRIs, the RR patients demonstrated an 80% reduction in gadolinium-enhancing lesions within 3 months of treatment, as compared to pretreatment (Sicotte et al., 2002), and this improvement in enhancing lesions correlated with the favorable shift in cytokine profiles (Soldan et al., 2003). Importantly, gadolinium-enhancing disease activity gradually returned to baseline in the posttreatment period, and the favorable cytokine shift also returned to baseline. Further, in the 4-month extension phase of the study, both the decrease in brain-enhancing lesions and the favorable immune shift returned upon retreatment with estriol in combination with progesterone in the RRMS group. These latter data have important translational implications, since progesterone treatment is needed in combination with estrogen treatment to prevent uterine endometrial hyperplasia when estrogens are administered for a year or more in duration. These results indicate that treatment with progesterone in combination with estriol did not neutralize the beneficial effect of estriol treatment on these biomarkers of disease. A multicenter, double-blind, placebo-controlled trial of estriol treatment in RRMS is now ongoing.

The effect of estrogens in multiple sclerosis: summary

A protective effect of relatively high doses of estrogens (estradiol and estriol) within the late pregnancy range has been shown in the MS model, while a role for lower endogenous fluctuating levels of estrogens during the menstrual cycle is controversial. Mechanisms underlying the protective effects of high-dose estrogens include both anti-inflammatory and neuroprotective properties. Anti-inflammatory properties of estrogen treatment in EAE are mediated primarily by ERα, not ERβ. However there is a role for ERβ in the neuroprotective properties. Whether treatment with supplemental estrogens may be protective in women with MS is currently being investigated through clinical trials.

Testicular Hormones: The Effect of Endogenous Androgens in the Mouse Model of Multiple Sclerosis

Sex differences in MS and the EAE model may be related to sex hormones, sex chromosomes, or both. With respect to sex hormones, female sex hormones or male sex hormones may play a role. This section will discuss a possible role for male sex hormones. To begin to test the role of endogenous androgens in MS, the EAE model was used. Since EAE in the relapsing-remitting murine model had previously been characterized to have a sex difference that paralleled that of MS, with males being less susceptible to disease than females (Voskuhl et al., 1996; Kim and Voskuhl,

1999), the SJL strain was used. Protective effects of testosterone in male mice were shown by studies demonstrating that the removal of physiologic levels of testosterone from male mice via castration increased disease susceptibility (Bebo et al., 1998b; Palaszynski et al., 2004b). Also, testosterone levels were shown to be decreased in male mice during EAE relapse (Foster et al., 2003). Together these data support the hypotheses that endogenous androgens are protective at physiologic levels in this MS model.

Androgen treatment in the mouse model of multiple sclerosis

Treatment of EAE was done using either testosterone or 5α-dihydrotestosterone (DHT). The latter form of testosterone was used since it cannot be converted to estrogen. Indeed, not only were both androgen treatments shown to be protective in gonadally intact males of a strain in which endogenous androgens are protective, but they were also protective in a strain in which endogenous androgens are not protective (Palaszynski et al., 2004b). These data indicated that, even in genetic backgrounds that are not permissive to a protective effect of endogenous androgens, protection can still be provided by supplemental exogenous androgen treatment. This suggested that the mechanisms of disease protection may differ between endogenous physiologic androgens and supplemental supraphysiologic androgen treatment. These preclinical data laid the groundwork for clinical trials designed to treat men in the heterogeneous MS population with testosterone.

Testosterone levels in men with multiple sclerosis

Onset of MS in women typically occurs soon after puberty. In men, disease onset usually occurs later in life (age 30–40), coinciding with the age at which serum testosterone levels begin to decline in normal healthy men (Nankin and Calkins, 1986; Tenover et al., 1987; Gray et al., 1991; Vermeulen, 1991; Morley et al., 1997). Interestingly, this phenomenon may be true of other autoimmune diseases as well. The onset of rheumatoid arthritis in men also takes place later in life with a reported four-fold increase in incidence rates in older men (ages 35–74) as compared to younger men (ages 18–34). Furthermore, the sex difference of RA in women versus men is 4:1 between ages 35–44, which decreases to 1.1:1, by age 75 (Doran, 2002 et al). Together these observations suggest that relatively high levels of testosterone in young men after puberty may provide temporary protection from autoimmune disease onset in those men who were genetically predisposed to ultimately develop disease.

Additionally, it has been reported that 24% of male MS patients tested had significantly lower levels of testosterone as compared to age-matched healthy men (Wei and Lightman, 1997). The reason for the decreased testosterone levels remains unclear. It may be due to gonadal failure or due to effects on the hypothalamic-pituitary axis (HPA) such as stress or hypothalamic lesions (Foster et al., 2003). In men with MS and sexual dysfunction, low testosterone levels have been previously shown to be associated with low luteinizing hormone levels, thereby ruling out gonadal failure (Foster et al., 2003). Interestingly, a decrease in free testosterone levels has been reported in untreated men with new onset RA (Kanik et al., 2000), making the possibility of hypothalamic lesions in the brain as an explanation for low serum testosterone levels in men with MS less likely. An effect of the stress of chronic illness on the HPA may be the most likely explanation for the relatively lower levels of testosterone in men with chronic autoimmune diseases.

Testosterone treatment in multiple sclerosis

Data in EAE has suggested that supplemental, exogenous testosterone treatment may provide protection across genetic backgrounds in men of the heterogeneous MS population (Palaszynski et al., 2004b). To investigate possible effects of testosterone treatment in MS, testosterone was administered via transdermal application (AndroGel) to men with RRMS in a small pilot trial (Sicotte et al., 2007). Ten grams of the gel containing 100 mg of testosterone was used topically daily. A crossover design, using a within-arm comparison of 6 months pretreatment to 12 months treatment, was employed to reduce the effect of disease heterogeneity given the small sample size (Stone et al., 1997).

Ten subjects with RRMS completed the study. The subjects were relatively mildly affected with MS having a median EDSS score was 2.0 (range: 1.5 to 2.5). At baseline, all subjects had testosterone levels in the lower range of normal with a mean of 493 ng/dl (range: 321–732). During daily treatment with testosterone, serum testosterone levels rose 50% on average to the higher range of normal. Lean body mass (muscle mass) increased significantly during treatment.

Scores from the Paced Auditory Serial Addition Task (PASAT) component of the Multiple Sclerosis Functional Composite (MSFC), a commonly used cognitive test in MS, remained stable during the first 6 months of treatment (months 3 and 6), trended upward after 9 months, and were significantly improved by the twelfth month of treatment. There was also a trend for improvement in spatial memory. These findings were consistent with previous reports of testosterone-mediated improvements in working and spatial memory in healthy nonhypogonadal elderly men (Janowsky et al., 2000; Cherrier et al., 2001). No significant changes were observed in classic MS disability measures (i.e., the EDSS, 9-hole peg test, or the 25" timed walk), which was not surprising given the short treatment duration.

The 10 subjects had low levels of enhancing lesion activity on brain MRI at baseline, and this low level was not significantly increased or decreased with treatment. The lack of a decrease in measures of inflammatory activity on MRI during treatment with testosterone may be due to the relatively low levels of inflammatory activity present at baseline. The exclusion of subjects on disease-modifying treatments likely created a selection bias toward subjects with relatively milder clinical disease and less inflammatory activity on MRI. Thus, in this subject group, it could only be concluded that testosterone treatment did not significantly increase inflammatory activity on otherwise relatively quiescent MRIs.

The most interesting finding of the study was the effect on brain atrophy. During the first 9 months of the study, brain volumes decreased at an annualized rate of −0.81% ($p = 0.0001$). This mean annualized brain atrophy rate of −0.81% observed during the first 9 months of this study was consistent with previous rates observed in MS patients (Miller et al., 2002). During the subsequent

9 months of testosterone treatment, brain atrophy slowed to an annualized rate of –0.26%. This represented a 67% reduction in the rate of brain volume loss compared to the pretreatment period. Interestingly, the timing of the cognitive improvements coincided with the slowing of brain atrophy on MRI. The protective effect of testosterone treatment on brain atrophy was observed in the absence of an appreciable anti-inflammatory effect, possibly suggesting direct neuroprotective effects. Larger placebo-controlled trials of testosterone treatment in men with MS are warranted.

The effect of testicular hormones in multiple sclerosis: summary

In the MS model EAE, endogenous androgens are protective in some strains but not others. However, exogenous supplemental treatment with testosterone is protective across genetic backgrounds. An immunomodulatory role has been shown, while direct effects on the CNS have not been studied in the model. In humans with MS, we hypothesize that some, but not all, men may be of a genetic background that is permissive to a protective effect of relatively high physiologic levels of testosterone that exist in young men. This may mask the early presentation of the relapsing-remitting phase of the disease. As these men age, testosterone levels gradually decline and clinical MS onset is observed. Later during the course of disease, it is possible that the stress of chronic disease may affect the hypothalamic pituitary axis to suppress testosterone levels further, to within the low normal range. Whether treatment with supplemental testosterone may offer some protection in men with MS is currently being investigated through clinical trials.

SEX CHROMOSOME EFFECTS IN MULTIPLE SCLEROSIS

A non-mutually exclusive alternative to sex hormone–induced differences in EAE and MS is a direct genetic effect. That is, specific gene products, which are not induced by gonadal hormones, yet are expressed in a sexually dimorphic manner in either the immune system or the CNS, could induce sex-specific patterns of immune system or CNS development or function. Data using the informative transgenic mice model indicated that the XX sex chromosome complement was disease promoting as compared to the XY$^-$ complement with respect to both immune responses (Palaszynski et al., 2005) and disease severity in the animal model of MS (Smith-Bouvier et al., 2008). It remains to be determined whether this effect is due to (1) gene(s) unique to the Y chromosome, (2) a higher dose of X genes that escape X-inactivation in XX mice, or (3) paternal imprinting of X genes that are present in XX, but not XY$^-$, mice (Arnold and Burgoyne, 2004). Candidate autoimmune regulatory genes on the X chromosome include IL-13Rα, CD40 ligand, FoxP3, and Toll Like Receptor 7 (TLR 7), to name a few. Further studies mapping the gene on either X or Y are needed to discern mechanisms underlying direct sex chromosome effects in the MS model.

The Effect of Pregnancy on Clinical Multiple Sclerosis

Sex hormones and/or sex-linked gene inheritance may be responsible for the enhanced susceptibility of women to MS. Evidence consistent with a role for sex hormones as a disease modifier comes from well-documented effects of pregnancy on MS. Effects of pregnancy have been better characterized in the RRMS phase than in the SPMS phase, likely due to the age of the patients in each group and their respective childbearing capacities. Subsequent effects of prior pregnancies can be assessed in both RRMS and SPMS groups. It has been appreciated for decades that symptoms of patients with autoimmune diseases are affected by pregnancy and the postpartum period. The most well-characterized observations include those in MS, RA, and psoriasis. These patients experience clinical improvement during pregnancy with a temporary "rebound" exacerbation postpartum (Birk et al., 1990; Da Silva and Spector, 1992; Nelson et al., 1992; Abramsky, 1994; Runmarker and Andersen, 1995; Damek and Shuster, 1997; Confavreux et al., 1998; Whitacre et al., 1999). Interestingly, and in contrast, women with SLE may experience an exacerbation of symptoms with gestation (Jungers et al., 1982). This differential effect of pregnancy on these diseases is thought to reflect the difference in immunopathogenesis of SLE as compared to MS, RA, and psoriasis.

Multiple sclerosis, RA, and psoriasis are principally cell-mediated diseases, whereby autoimmune cell infiltrates into target organs cause the damage. In contrast, in SLE significant damage is mediated by auto-antibodies deposited in the target organs.

The Effect of Pregnancy on Relapses

What is the precise effect of pregnancy on MS? During decades of observations that MS improved during late pregnancy, the early studies did not separate the MS patients into RR and SP groups (Birk et al., 1988, 1990; Abramsky, 1994). However, what was generally described was that there was a period of relative "safety" with regard to relapses during pregnancy followed by a period of increased relapses postpartum. These clinical observations were supported by a small study of two patients who underwent serial cerebral MRIs during pregnancy and postpartum. In both women there was a decrease in MR disease activity (T2 lesion number) during the second half of pregnancy and a return of MR disease activity to prepregnancy levels in the first months postpartum (van Walderveen et al., 1994). Other studies found that in addition to having a decrease in disease activity in patients with established MS, the risk of developing the first episode of MS was decreased during pregnancy as compared to nonpregnant states (Runmarker and Andersen, 1995). The most definitive study of the effect of pregnancy on MS came in 1998 by the Pregnancy in Multiple Sclerosis (PRIMS) Group (Confavreux et al., 1998). Relapse rates were determined in 254 women with MS during 269 pregnancies and for up to 1 year after delivery. Relapse rates were significantly reduced from 0.7 per woman year in the year before pregnancy to 0.2 during the third trimester. Rates then increased to 1.2 during the first 3 months postpartum before returning to prepregnancy rates. No significant changes were observed between relapse rates in the first and second trimester as compared to the year prior to pregnancy. Together these data clearly demonstrated that the latter part of pregnancy is associated with a significant reduction in relapses, while there is a rebound increase in relapses postpartum.

In a 2-year follow-up report by the PRIMS group, clinical factors that predicted postpartum flares were examined. Neither breastfeeding nor epidural anesthesia affected likelihood to relapse postpartum. The best predictor of which subjects would relapse postpartum was their prepregnancy relapse rates. Those with the most active disease before pregnancy were the most likely to relapse postpartum (Vukusic et al., 2004).

The Effect of Pregnancy on Disability

Since latter pregnancy is associated with a reduction in relapses and the postpartum period with a transient increase in relapses, what is the net effect of pregnancy on the accumulation of disability? Using a short-term 2-year follow-up, no net effect of a single pregnancy on disability accumulation was observed (Vukusic et al., 2004). However, long-term follow-up studies suggested that disability accumulation may be reduced significantly in those with pregnancies after the onset of MS (Verdru et al., 1994). A study by Damek and Shuster indicated that a full-term pregnancy increased the time interval to reach a common disability endpoint (walking with the aid of a cane or crutch). In essence, pregnancy increased the time interval to having a secondary progressive course (Damek and Shuster, 1997). Runmarker compared the risk of transition from a relapsing-remitting to a secondary progressive course in women who were pregnant after MS onset, with that in women who were not pregnant after MS onset. Importantly, the two groups were matched for neurological deficit, disease duration, and age. There was a significantly decreased risk of a progressive course in women who became pregnant after MS onset as compared to those who were not pregnant (Runmarker and Andersen, 1995). The fact that the patients were matched for neurologic deficit, disease duration, and age is extremely important in this latter study, for one might predict that there might be a selection bias such that women with less disability would be more likely to become pregnant and a difference in baseline disability could explain the longer time interval to reach a secondary progressive course. Careful matching of the groups made this explanation unlikely and therefore the study indeed provided support for a net beneficial effect of pregnancy on the accumulation of disability in MS.

While there is clearly a short-term effect of pregnancy on decreasing relapse rates and possibly a long-term effect of pregnancy on increasing the time interval to reach a given level of disability, there appear to be no conclusive data supporting a long-term effect of pregnancy in healthy individuals and their subsequent risk to develop MS. One study reported that women of parity 0–2 developed MS twice as often as women of parity 3 or more, thereby implying a protective effect of multiple pregnancies, but the difference did not reach statistical significance (Villard-Mackintosh and Vessey, 1993). Another found no association between parity and the subsequent risk of developing MS (Hernan et al., 2000). Together these data indicate that pregnancy in healthy women has no long-lasting effects with regard to reducing their risk of developing MS in the future. However, if women with MS become pregnant, it will indeed be associated with a temporary reduction in relapses during the pregnancy, with a transient increase in relapse rate for several months postpartum.

Given that late pregnancy is a state of temporary immunomodulation lasting 4–5 months, one then returns to the question of whether multiple pregnancies would be expected to have permanent effects on disability. Since it is known that up to 8 years of continuous treatment with immunomodulatory treatments have only a modest impact disability in MS (Johnson et al., 1995; Kappos et al., 2006), a temporary anti-inflammatory effect of the third trimester of pregnancy would not be expected to impact long-term disability. However, an as yet unidentified pregnancy-associated neuroprotective effect, combined with the temporary anti-inflammatory effect, could reconcile the finding of a beneficial effect of pregnancy on long-term disability.

The Effect of Pregnancy on the Immune System

Since mechanisms of action of the approved disease-modifying therapies for MS involve anti-inflammatory effects and since these treatments result primarily in a reduction in relapse rates, it is logical to hypothesize that mechanisms underlying the protective effect of pregnancy on MS relapses involve anti-inflammatory effects. Indeed, pregnancy has been shown to have significant effects on the immune system.

Pregnancy is a challenge for the immune system. From the mother's standpoint, the fetus is an allograft since it harbors antigens inherited by the father. It is evolutionarily advantageous for the mother to transiently suppress cytotoxic, cell-mediated, Th1 type immune responses involved in fetal rejection during pregnancy. However, not all immune responses should be suppressed since humoral, Th2 type immunity is needed for passive transfer of antibodies to the fetus. Thus, a shift in immune responses with a downregulation of Th1 and an upregulation of Th2 is thought to be necessary for fetal survival (Wegmann et al., 1993; Formby, 1995; Hill et al., 1995; Raghupathy, 1997). Two recent studies have been completed whereby MS subjects were followed longitudinally for immune responses during pregnancy and postpartum. Gilmore et al. demonstrated that peripheral immune cells had increased Th1 cytokines postpartum as compared to the third trimester, while cells derived from subjects in the third trimester produced more Th2 cytokine (Gilmore et al., 2004). Al-Shammri et al. also found that six of the eight MS patients' immune cells showed a distinct shift from a Th2 cytokine bias during pregnancy, toward a Th1 cytokine bias after delivery (Al-Shammri et al., 2004). In light of these data demonstrating a relative shift to Th2 systemically during pregnancy, with a rebound back to Th1 postpartum, it becomes highly plausible that these alterations in the immune response could underlie the improvement in putative Th1-mediated autoimmune diseases during pregnancy, as well as the exacerbation postpartum.

The Effect of Pregnancy on the Central Nervous System

Pregnancy is a complex event characterized by changes in numerous factors that may impact the CNS. These include increases in estriol, estadiol, progesterone, and prolactin, to name a few (Voskuhl, 2003). Potential neuroprotective effects of estrogens have already been discussed. Recently, it was shown that pregnant mice have an enhanced ability to remyelinate white matter lesions, and that prolactin regulates oligodendrocyte precursor proliferation and mimics this regenerative effect of pregnancy (Gregg et al., 2007). This finding may be potentially exploited in pursuit of a therapeutic repair strategy to increase remyelination. However, when considering the effect of prolactin treatment in neuroimmunologic diseases such as MS, one must consider that prolactin has pro-inflammatory properties that could potentially exacerbate disease, as has been shown in the MS model, EAE (Riskind et al., 1991). Thus, when considering any pregnancy factor, its effects on both the CNS and the immune system must be considered. Notably, breastfeeding, which would be associated with a prolonged state of increased levels of prolactin, was not associated with an increased relapse rate as compared to no breastfeeding (Vukusic et al., 2004). This lack of a difference in relapse rate may suggest that the proinflammatory properties of increased prolactin during breastfeeding may not be clinically significant. On the other hand, relapse rate is a relatively insensitive, albeit important, outcome measure. Future studies should compare immune responses, enhancing lesions on MRI, and prolactin levels in MS women who are or are not breastfeeding postpartum.

The Effect of Pregnancy on Multiple Sclerosis: Conclusions from Research

In summary, what is striking about pregnancy is that it represents a state that is characterized by two important changes. First, there is a downregulation of cellular immune responses. This relative immunosuppression likely occurs to prevent fetal rejection. Second, pregnancy is characterized by the presence of potentially neuroprotective hormones such as estrogens, progesterone, and prolactin. It would seem evolutionarily advantageous to have such neuroprotective factors present as neuronal and oligodendrocyte lineage cells in the fetus progress through critical developmental windows (Craig et al., 2003). Together, the combined anti-inflammatory and neuroprotective state of pregnancy, which is perhaps aimed at protecting the fetus, is precisely what is needed to protect the CNS during inflammatory attack in MS. The relapse rate is significantly reduced during pregnancy, with an increase in the first 3–6 months postpartum, but parity is not associated with increased long-term disability and may in fact increase time to reach disability.

CLINICAL REPRODUCTIVE ISSUES

Medical Management of Multiple Sclerosis during Pregnancy

Basic research and clinical observations as outlined previously suggest that late pregnancy is beneficial in MS and that the postpartum period is characterized by vulnerability to increased relapses. Given these insights, what is the current best medical management of women with MS who are pregnant?

The first consideration regarding pregnancy is that women and men with MS do not suffer from infertility problems as part of the natural history of the disease process (Giesser, 2002). Despite theoretical possibilities of effects of MS on fertility due to abnormalities in the hypothalamic-pituitary-adrenal axis or the hypothalamic-pituitary-gonadal axis (Grinsted et al., 1989), observations thus far indicate that women and men with MS are normal with respect to their ability to bear children (Giesser, 2002; Cavalla et al., 2006). The fact that the natural history of untreated MS disease is not associated with infertility does not, however, preclude the fact that some disease-modifying drugs used in MS can be associated with infertility. Mitoxantrone and cyclosphosphamide, for example, are known to impact fertility (Cavalla et al., 2006).Young men and women with MS who need to have immunosuppressive therapy may need to be counseled about sperm and egg banking before starting this therapy. Beta-interferon has been associated with menstrual irregularities, but whether this has any effect on fertility remains unknown. There are no reports of negative effects of Copaxone use on fertility. Further, one must keep in mind that women with MS have infertility issues at a rate consistent with the normal age-matched population. In those MS women who pursue in vitro fertilization (IVF) treatments, the question is often posed as to whether infertility treatments may alter hormonal balance and thereby affect MS disease activity. To date there are too few cases of MS women undergoing IVF to warrant firm conclusions. Anecdotal reports exist, however, which suggest that IVF may be associated with an exacerbation of relapse in MS (Laplaud et al., 2007; Hellwig et al., 2008). The increased relapse rate mainly occurred in patients treated with gonadotrophin-releasing hormone (GnRH) agonists, but not the patients treated by GnRH antagonists. A mechanism whereby these treatments might lead to relapse remains unknown and further study is needed on larger numbers of MS patients to determine whether certain forms of IVF indeed exacerbate MS. Currently there are no large studies establishing that this is necessarily the case.

There are no data that suggest that offspring of persons with MS have a higher rate of congenital malformations, but a few studies have indicated that babies born to women with MS may be subject to lower birth weight (Dahl et al., 2008; Hellwig et al., 2008a; Chen et al., 2009). Children born to parents with MS have 20–50 times the risk of the general population of developing the disease, but the absolute rate itself is low (1%–5%) (Sadovnick and Ebers, 1995). Women with MS have not been reported to have higher rates of miscarriage, eclampsia, premature delivery, or stillbirth compared to the general population (Argyriou and Makris, 2008).

Another consideration entails the management of MS disease-modifying drugs in women who wish to become pregnant (see Table 17-1). Copaxone is pregnancy Category B, while the interferons (Rebif, Avonex, and Betaseron) are Category C (see Table 17-2). An increased potential for spontaneous abortion has been reported for the interferons (Boskovic et al., 2005; Sandberg-Wollheim et al., 2005). Lower birth weight of babies with in utero exposure to beta interferon was observed in some studies (Boskovic et al., 2005; Patti et al., 2008; Weber-Schoendorfer and Schaefer, 2009), but not in others (Sandberg-Wollheim et al., 2005; Hellwig et al., 2009). Women with MS who plan to become pregnant should be informed of the potential hazards of interferon use with respect to their fetus. Copaxone

treatment appears to be safer since to date there is no documentation of Copaxone treatment–related negative outcomes on pregnancy. Nevertheless, there are still insufficient data to assume that Copaxone treatment is safe during pregnancy. Thus, the current recommendation is that women with MS who plan to become pregnant should discontinue use of disease-modifying drugs for one to two menstrual cycles prior to attempting conception, particularly if they are on an interferon (Ferrero et al., 2004). The greatest risk for relapses is during the time when women have discontinued use of disease-modifying treatments and have not yet become pregnant or are in the early stages of pregnancy, since the latter half of pregnancy appears to provide some natural protection from MS relapses. Based on clinical trial designs, there is approximately a 3-month washout period from when disease-modifying drugs are discontinued to when the majority of their disease protection potential is lost. Thus, those women with MS who discontinue disease-modifying treatments, and then cannot become pregnant within a few months, are at risk for relapse during this time.

During the postpartum period, there is an increased susceptibility for relapses that occurs principally within 3–6 months postpartum (Confavreux et al., 1998). To prevent relapses during this postpartum period, many women with MS will choose to resume disease-modifying drugs within 2 weeks after delivery of their child. This is based on the idea that it will generally take up to 3 months for disease-modifying drugs to provide protection from relapses, depending on the particular disease-modifying therapy. For example, based on the temporal window of effects of various treatments on inflammation as assessed by enhancing lesions on MRI, high-dose interferons may act more rapidly (1–3 months) upon

TABLE 17-1 FDA Pregnancy Risk Categories

A: No evidence of fetal harm in human studies

B: No evidence of fetal harm in animal studies

C: Evidence of fetal harm in animal studies or no data available

D: Evidence of fetal harm in humans; use may be justified in some circumstances

X: Evidence of fetal harm in humans; not indicated for use in pregnancy

TABLE 17-2 Pregnancy Categories of Disease-Modifying Therapies

Agent	Pregnancy Risk Category
Beta-interferon 1-b	C
Beta-interferon 1-a	C
Glatiramer acetate	B
Natalizumab	C
Mitoxantrone	D
Cyclophosphamide	D
Azathioprine	D
IVIG	C

initiation of treatment as compared to Copaxone (6–9 months). How aggressive one chooses to be in preventing postpartum relapses should principally be driven by insights into how frequent relapses occurred prior to pregnancy. Indeed, it is the prepregnancy relapse rate, not breastfeeding, method of delivery, or anesthesia that has been shown to be the best predictor of postpartum relapse (Vukusic et al., 2004). In general, if relapses were relatively well controlled with a given disease-modifying treatment prior to pregnancy, then one generally resumes the given treatment based on this prior responsiveness. If relapses were poorly controlled with a given treatment prior to pregnancy, then one might consider switching to a different disease-modifying treatment postpartum. Small studies that were not placebo controlled have suggested that treatment with intravenous immunoglobulin (IVIG) might prevent postpartum relapses (Achiron et al., 2004), but larger studies that are well controlled are needed before establishing this as an efficacious treatment option.

The desire to breastfeed confounds decisions concerning the resumption of disease-modifying therapies postpartum. It is not currently known whether disease-modifying treatments may pass through the mother's milk to the baby, so none of these treatments are generally recommended for use in women who are nursing. In addition, consideration of the type of breastfeeding warrants attention since one small study has reported that exclusive breastfeeding, as opposed to breastfeeding supplemented with formula, may offer some protection against relapses in the immediate postpartum period (Langer-Gould et al., 2009).

Symptom Management during Pregnancy

Several of the symptoms that women with MS experience when they are not pregnant may be aggravated in the gravid condition. These include fatigue, urinary frequency and urgency, and gait problems. Most of the medications used to treat these symptoms are Category C, that is, not indicated for use during pregnancy (see Table 17-3). Nonpharmacologic strategies such as energy conservation techniques, assistive devices, and frequent timed voiding may safely ameliorate these symptoms until the patient delivers.

Management of Acute Relapse during Pregnancy

As mentioned previously, relapse during pregnancy is uncommon. If an exacerbation during pregnancy does occur and affects function severely enough to warrant treatment, in general, a brief course of corticosteroids may safely be given, in collaboration with the obstetrician, but it should be avoided during the first trimester. Methylprednisolone is metabolized before crossing the placenta (in contrast to dexamethasone, and may therefore be preferable (Ferrero et al., 2004). Intravenous immunoglobulin (IVIG) has not been reported to have adverse effects on the developing fetus and may also be considered for treatment of an acute relapse during pregnancy (Ferrero et al., 2004). Glucocorticoids are excreted in breast milk, and so treatment of postpartum relapses may obviate nursing during, and briefly after, steroid administration. A highly supportive environment, put in

TABLE 17-3 Pregnancy Categories of Symptom Management Agents

Agent	Symptom	Pregnancy Risk Category
Corticosteroid	Acute exacerbation*	C
Baclofen	Spasticity	C
Diazepam	Spasticity*, anxiety	D
Tizanidine	Spasticity	C
Gabapentin	Seizure, pain*, spasticity*	C
Amantadine	Fatigue*	C
Modafinil	Fatigue*	C
Oxybutinin	Overactive bladder	B
Tolterodine	Overactive bladder	C

*No FDA indication for this use, or no indication for use in multiple sclerosis. (From Giesser, B., 'Gender Issues in Multiple Sclerosis', *The Neurologist*, 8(6), 351–356, 2002, with permission.)

place ahead of time, is advisable to not only reduce fatigue of the mother but also to have assistance readily available in case the mother experiences a relapse.

Management of Labor and Delivery

Generally, women with MS may be managed through labor and delivery similarly to women without MS. Women who have chronically been on long-term steroids may require additional steroid administration during labor. Women with a profound sensory deficit may not be able to feel contractions or push effectively and so may require mechanical assistance. General and epidural anesthesia are both considered safe for women with MS. Older literature has suggested that spinal anesthesia may be more neurotoxic, but there are insufficient data to support this (Argyriou and Makris, 2008). The PRIMS study found no correlation between administration of epidural anesthesia and postpartum relapse rate (Vukusic et al., 2004).

Interaction of Multiple Sclerosis and the Menstrual Cycle

Self-report studies suggest that premenopausal women with MS commonly experience transient worsening of neurologic symptoms premenstrually and may be more likely to have exacerbations during this time frame (Smith and Studd, 1992;

Zorgdrager and De Keyser, 1997; Giesser, 2002; Zorgdrager and De Keyser, 2002). One case report cited three women with premenstrual pseudo-exacerbations who responded to prophylactic treatment with aspirin (Wingerchuk and Rodriguez, 2006). Interestingly, the effect appeared to be independent of body temperature. The mechanisms for these observations are unclear. Two small studies have attempted to correlate hormone levels during different phases of the menstrual cycle with gadolinium-enhancing lesion activity on MRI with inconsistent results (Bansil et al., 1999; Pozzilli et al., 1999).

Only one small study to date has been reported about the effects of menopause on MS (Smith and Studd, 1992), with 54% of 19 post menopausal women reporting worsening of neurologic symptoms coincident with menopause. There are currently no guidelines for use of hormone replacement therapy in women with MS, but as there are no data to suggest that this is either beneficial or contraindicated; until further information appears, this decision is best made on gynecologic grounds.

Estrogen Treatment in Multiple Sclerosis: Oral Contraceptive Use

Levels of estrogens that are lower than those which occur during pregnancy, such as levels induced by doses in oral contraceptives or hormone replacement therapy, may or may not be high enough to be protective in MS. While some studies have attempted to simulate a situation of treatment with oral contraceptives in EAE mice and have shown an effect on disease (Bebo et al., 2001; Subramanian et al., 2003), doses used in mice are not readily translatable to humans. In fact the data in humans thus far have suggested that treatment with oral contraceptives is not likely to suppress MS. The incidence rate of MS onset in both former and current oral contraceptive users is not different from that in never-users (Thorogood and Hannaford, 1998). It is not surprising that former use of oral contraceptives in healthy women would have no effect on subsequent risk to develop MS, since one would not anticipate that the effect of treatment on the immune system would be permanent. However, the fact that incidence rates for MS in current oral contraceptive pill users were not decreased, as compared to never-users, suggests that the estrogens in oral contraceptives are not of sufficient type or dose to ameliorate the immunopathogenesis of MS even temporarily during current use. This remains an unresolved issue as controversial results emerge with respect to the use of oral contraceptives and MS risk during current use (Hernan et al., 2000; Alonso et al., 2005). Studies of hormone replacement therapy and effects on disease activity in rheumatoid arthritis can provide further clues with respect to which doses of estrogens could potentially be protective in MS (Da Silva and Hall, 1992). In a randomized placebo-controlled trial of transdermal estradiol in 200 postmenopausal RA patients, who continued other antirheumatic medications, it was found that those who achieved a serum estradiol level >100 pmol/ liter had significant improvements in articular index, pain scores, morning stiffness, and sedimentation rates, while those with lower estradiol levels did not demonstrate improvement (Hall et al., 1994). There has been no consistent correlation between disease markers in MS or RA and hormone levels during the menstrual cycle in females. Together these reports suggest that it is likely that a sustained level of a sufficient dose of an estrogen will be necessary to ameliorate disease activity in MS and RA.

These data indicate that choice of hormonal contraception for women with MS should be made on gynecologic rather than neurologic criteria.

CONCLUSIONS

Sex differences in autoimmune diseases are prevalent across numerous human diseases, including MS, as well as in numerous animal models of these diseases, including EAE. Effects of sex hormones (estrogens and androgens) and sex chromosomes (XX and XY) have been shown in the immunopathogenesis of EAE. Further study is needed to determine the extent of these effects in the CNS.

Sex hormones and sex chromosomes can have synergistic or antagonistic effects with respect to each other depending on the processes and the tissues being studied. Furthermore, some hormone effects and sex chromosome complement effects are more readily observed on some autosomal genetic backgrounds as compared to others. While this is a complex system, it is not surprising given prior precedent of numerous genetic contributions to complex polygenetic diseases with some genes serving to enhance disease and others serving to suppress disease.

Autoimmune diseases have classically been thought to be due to an interaction between environmental and genetic factors, with the latter generally referring to autosomal genetic background. Newer data indicate that autoimmune diseases should now be considered to be due to an interaction between the environment, autosomal genetic background, and sex-specific factors such as sex hormones and sex chromosomes.

Multiple sclerosis does not appear to affect fertility or increase risk of congenital abnormalities or pregnancy complications, with the possible exception of a risk for low birth weight. Pregnancy is a relatively protected time for risk of relapse, with a increase in relapses occurring 3–6 months postpartum.

The best predictor of postpartum relapse in a given patient is their prepregnancy relapse rate. Decisions regarding resuming use of disease-modifying therapies after pregnancy need to be made on an individual basis.

REFERENCES

Abramsky O. Pregnancy and multiple sclerosis. *Ann Neurol.* 1994;36(suppl):S38–S41.

Achiron A, Kishner I, Dolev M, et al. Effect of intravenous immunoglobulin treatment on pregnancy and postpartum-related relapses in multiple sclerosis. *J Neurol*. 2004;251:1133–1137.

Ahmed SA, Penhale WJ. The influence of testosterone on the development of autoimmune thyroiditis in thymectomized and irradiated rats. *Clin Exp Immunol*. 1982;48:367–374.

Alonso A, Jick SS, Olek MJ, Ascherio A, Jick H, Hernan MA. Recent use of oral contraceptives and the risk of multiple sclerosis. *Arch Neurol*. 2005;62: 1362–1365.

Al-Shammri S, Rawoot P, Azizieh F, et al. Th1/Th2 cytokine patterns and clinical profiles during and after pregnancy in women with multiple sclerosis. *J Neurol Sci*. 2004;222:21–27.

Argyriou AA, Makris N. Multiple sclerosis and reproductive risks in women. *Reprod Sci*. 2008;15:755–764.

Arnold AP, Burgoyne PS. Are XX and XY brain cells intrinsically different? *Trends Endocrinol Metab*. 2004; 15:6–11.

Bannerman PG, Hahn A, Ramirez S, et al. Motor neuron pathology in experimental autoimmune encephalomyelitis: studies in THY1-YFP transgenic mice. *Brain*. 2005;128:1877–1886.

Bansil S, Lee HJ, Jindal S, Holtz CR, Cook SD. Correlation between sex hormones and magnetic resonance imaging lesions in multiple sclerosis. *Acta Neurol Scand*. 1999;99:91–94.

Bebo BF, Jr., Adlard K, Schuster JC, Unsicker L, Vandenbark AA, Offner H. Gender differences in protection from EAE induced by oral tolerance with a peptide analogue of MBP-Ac1-11. *J Neurosci Res*. 1999; 55:432–440.

Bebo BF, Jr., Fyfe-Johnson A, Adlard K, Beam AG, Vandenbark AA, Offner H. Low-dose estrogen therapy ameliorates experimental autoimmune encephalomyelitis in two different inbred mouse strains. *J Immunol*. 2001;166:2080–2089.

Bebo BF, Jr., Schuster JC, Vandenbark AA, Offner H. Gender differences in experimental autoimmune encephalomyelitis develop during the induction of the immune response to encephalitogenic peptides. *J Neurosci Res*. 1998a;52:420–426.

Bebo BF, Jr., Vandenbark AA, Offner H. Male SJL mice do not relapse after induction of EAE with PLP 139–151. *J Neurosci Res*. 1996;45:680–689.

Bebo BF, Jr., Zelinka-Vincent E, Adamus G, Amundson D, Vandenbark AA, Offner H. Gonadal hormones influence the immune response to PLP 139–151 and the clinical course of relapsing experimental autoimmune encephalomyelitis. *J Neuroimmunol*. 1998b; 84:122–30.

Birk K, Ford C, Smeltzer S, Ryan D, Miller R, Rudick RA. The clinical course of multiple sclerosis during pregnancy and the puerperium. *Arch Neurol*. 1990;47:738–42.

Birk K, Smeltzer SC, Rudick R. Pregnancy and multiple sclerosis. *Semin Neurol*. 1988;8:205–213.

Boskovic R, Wide R, Wolpin J, Bauer DJ, Koren G. The reproductive effects of beta interferon therapy in pregnancy: a longitudinal cohort. *Neurology*. 2005;65: 807–811.

Brinton RD. Cellular and molecular mechanisms of estrogen regulation of memory function and neuroprotection against Alzheimer's disease: recent insights and remaining challenges. *Learn Mem*. 2001;8: 121–133.

Brown A, McFarlin DE, Raine CS. Chronologic neuropathology of relapsing experimental allergic encephalomyelitis in the mouse. *Lab Invest*. 1982;46:171–185.

Cavalla P, Rovei V, Masera S, et al. Fertility in patients with multiple sclerosis: current knowledge and future perspectives. *Neurol Sci*. 2006;27:231–239.

Cerghet M, Skoff RP, Bessert D, Zhang Z, Mullins C, Ghandour MS. Proliferation and death of oligodendrocytes and myelin proteins are differentially regulated in male and female rodents. *J Neurosci*. 2006;26: 1439–1447.

Chen YH, Lin HL, Lin HC. Does multiple sclerosis increase risk of adverse pregnancy outcomes? A population-based study. *Mult Scler*. 2009;15:606–612.

Cherrier MM, Asthana S, Plymate S, et al. Testosterone supplementation improves spatial and verbal memory in healthy older men. *Neurology*. 2001;57:80–88.

Confavreux C, Hutchinson M, Hours MM, Cortinovis-Tourniaire P, Moreau T. Rate of pregnancy-related relapse in multiple sclerosis. Pregnancy in Multiple Sclerosis Group. *N Engl J Med*. 1998;339:285–291.

Confavreux C, Vukusic S, Adeleine P. Early clinical predictors and progression of irreversible disability in multiple sclerosis: an amnesic process. *Brain*. 2003; 126:770–782.

Craig A, Ling Luo N, Beardsley DJ, et al. Quantitative analysis of perinatal rodent oligodendrocyte lineage progression and its correlation with human. *Exp Neurol*. 2003;181:231–240.

Dahl J, Myhr KM, Daltveit AK, Gilhus NE. Pregnancy, delivery and birth outcome in different stages of maternal multiple sclerosis. *J Neurol*. 2008;255: 623–627.

Damek DM, Shuster EA. Pregnancy and multiple sclerosis. *Mayo Clinic Proceed*. 1997;72:977–989.

Da Silva JA, Hall GM. The effects of gender and sex hormones on outcome in rheumatoid arthritis. *Baillieres Clin Rheumatol*. 1992;6:196–219.

Da Silva JA, Spector TD. The role of pregnancy in the course and aetiology of rheumatoid arthritis. *Clin Rheumatol*. 1992;11:189–194.

Deboy CA, Zhang J, Dike S, et al. High resolution diffusion tensor imaging of axonal damage in focal inflammatory and demyelinating lesions in rat spinal cord. *Brain*. 2007;130(pt 8):2199–2210.

Doran MF, Pond GR, Crowson CS, O'Fallon M, Gabriel SE. Trends in incidence and mortality in rheumatoid arthritis in Rochester, Minnesota, over a forty-year period. *Arthritis Rheum*. 2002;46:625–631.

Duquette P, Pleines J, Girard M, Charest L, Senecal-Quevillon M, Masse C. The increased susceptibility of women to multiple sclerosis. *Can J Neurol Sci*. 1992; 19:466–471.

Enmark E, Gustafsson JA. Oestrogen receptors - an overview. *J Intern Med*. 1999;246:133–138.

Erlandsson MC, Ohlsson C, Gustafsson JA, Carlsten H. Role of oestrogen receptors alpha and beta in immune organ development and in oestrogen-mediated effects on thymus. *Immunology.* 2001;103:17–25.

Ferrero S, Pretta S, Ragni N. Multiple sclerosis: management issues during pregnancy. *Eur J Obstet Gynecol Reprod Biol.* 2004;115:3–9.

Fitzpatrick F, Lepault F, Homo-Delarche F, Bach JF, Dardenne M. Influence of castration, alone or combined with thymectomy, on the development of diabetes in the nonobese diabetic mouse. *Endocrinology.* 1991; 129:1382–1390.

Formby B. Immunologic response in pregnancy. Its role in endocrine disorders of pregnancy and influence on the course of maternal autoimmune diseases. *Endocrinol Metab Clin N Am.* 1995;24:187–205.

Foster SC, Daniels C, Bourdette DN, Bebo BF, Jr. Dysregulation of the hypothalamic-pituitary-gonadal axis in experimental autoimmune encephalomyelitis and multiple sclerosis. *J Neuroimmunol.* 2003;140:78–87.

Fox HS. Androgen treatment prevents diabetes in non-obese diabetic mice. *J Exp Med.* 1992;175:1409–1412.

Garcia-Segura LM, Azcoitia I, DonCarlos LL. Neuroprotection by estradiol. *Prog Neurobiol.* 2001;63:29–60.

Garidou L, Laffont S, Douin-Echinard V, et al. Estrogen receptor alpha signaling in inflammatory leukocytes is dispensable for 17beta-estradiol-mediated inhibition of experimental autoimmune encephalomyelitis. *J Immunol.* 2004;173:2435–2442.

Giesser BS. Gender issues in multiple sclerosis. *Neurologist.* 2002;8:351–356.

Gilmore W, Arias M, Stroud N, Stek A, McCarthy KA, Correale J. Preliminary studies of cytokine secretion patterns associated with pregnancy in MS patients. *J Neurol Sci.* 2004;224:69–76.

Gray A, Berlin JA, McKinlay JB, Longcope C. An examination of research design effects on the association of testosterone and male aging: results of a meta-analysis. *J Clin Epidemiol.* 1991;44:671–684.

Gregg C, Shikar V, Larsen P, et al. White matter plasticity and enhanced remyelination in the maternal CNS. *J Neurosci.* 2007;27:1812–1823.

Grinsted L, Heltberg A, Hagen C, Djursing H. Serum sex hormone and gonadotropin concentrations in premenopausal women with multiple sclerosis. *J Intern Med.* 1989;226:241–244.

Hall GM, Daniels M, Huskisson EC, Spector TD. A randomised controlled trial of the effect of hormone replacement therapy on disease activity in postmenopausal rheumatoid arthritis. *Ann Rheum Dis.* 1994; 53:112–116.

Harbuz MS, Perveen-Gill Z, Lightman SL, Jessop DS. A protective role for testosterone in adjuvant-induced arthritis. *Br J Rheumatol.* 1995;34:1117–1122.

Harrington WR, Sheng S, Barnett DH, Petz LN, Katzenellenbogen JA, Katzenellenbogen BS. Activities of estrogen receptor alpha- and beta-selective ligands at diverse estrogen responsive gene sites mediating transactivation or transrepression. *Mol Cell Endocrinol.* 2003;206:13–22.

Hawkins SA, McDonnell GV. Benign multiple sclerosis? Clinical course, long term follow up, and assessment of prognostic factors. *J Neurol Neurosurg Psychiatry.* 1999;67:148–152.

Hellwig K, Agne H, Gold R. Interferon beta, birth weight and pregnancy in MS. *J Neurol.* 2009;256: 830–831.

Hellwig, K, Beste C, Brune N, Haghikia A, Muller T, Schimrigk S, Gold R. Increased MS relapse rate during assisted reproduction technique. *J Neurol.* 2008; 255:592–593.

Hellwig K, Brune N, Haghikia A, et al. Reproductive counselling, treatment and course of pregnancy in 73 German MS patients. *Acta Neurol Scand.* 2008a; 118:24–28.

Hernan MA, Hohol MJ, Olek MJ, Spiegelman D, Ascherio A. Oral contraceptives and the incidence of multiple sclerosis. *Neurology.* 2000;55:848–854.

Hill JA, Polgar K, Anderson DJ. T-helper 1-type immunity to trophoblast in women with recurrent spontaneous abortion. *JAMA.* 1995;273:1933–1936.

Igarashi H, Kouro T, Yokota T, Comp PC, Kincade PW. Age and stage dependency of estrogen receptor expression by lymphocyte precursors. *Proc Natl Acad Sci USA.* 2001;98:15131–15136.

Ito A, Bebo BF, Jr., Matejuk A, et al. Estrogen treatment down-regulates TNF-alpha production and reduces the severity of experimental autoimmune encephalomyelitis in cytokine knockout mice. *J Immunol.* 2001;167: 542–552.

Janowsky JS, Chavez B, Orwoll E. Sex steroids modify working memory. *J Cogn Neurosci.* 2000;12: 407–414.

Jansson L, Olsson T, Holmdahl R. Estrogen induces a potent suppression of experimental autoimmune encephalomyelitis and collagen-induced arthritis in mice. *J Neuroimmunol.* 1994;53:203–27.

Johnson KP, Brooks BR, Cohen JA, et al. Copolymer 1 reduces relapse rate and improves disability in relapsing-remitting multiple sclerosis: results of a phase III multicenter, double-blind placebo-controlled trial. The Copolymer 1 Multiple Sclerosis Study Group. *Neurology.* 1995;45:1268–1276.

Jungers P, Dougados M, Pélissier C, et al. Lupus nephropathy and pregnancy. Report of 104 cases in 36 patients. *Arch Intern Med.* 1982;142:771–776.

Kanik KS, Chrousos GP, Schumacher HR, Crane ML, Yarboro CH, Wilder RL. Adrenocorticotropin, glucocorticoid, and androgen secretion in patients with new onset synovitis/rheumatoid arthritis: relations with indices of inflammation. *J Clin Endocrinol Metab.* 2000; 85:1461–1466.

Kantarci OH, Goris A, Hebrink DD, et al. IFNG polymorphisms are associated with gender differences in susceptibility to multiple sclerosis. *Genes Immun.* 2005; 6(2):153–161.

Kappos L, Traboulsee A, Constantinescu C, et al. Long-term subcutaneous interferon beta-1a therapy in patients with relapsing-remitting MS. *Neurology.* 2006; 67:944–953.

Kim JH, Budde MD, Liang HF, et al. Detecting axon damage in spinal cord from a mouse model of multiple sclerosis. *Neurobiol Dis.* 2006;21:626–632.

Kim S, Liva SM, Dalal MA, Verity MA, Voskuhl RR. Estriol ameliorates autoimmune demyelinating disease: implications for multiple sclerosis. *Neurology.* 1999;52: 1230–1238.

Kim S, Voskuhl RR. Decreased IL-12 production underlies the decreased ability of male lymph node cells to induce experimental autoimmune encephalomyelitis. *J Immunol.* 1999;162:5561–5568.

Kuiper GG, Shughrue PJ, Merchenthaler I, Gustafsson JA. The estrogen receptor beta subtype: a novel mediator of estrogen action in neuroendocrine systems. *Front Neuroendocrinol.* 1998;19:253–286.

Langer-Gould A, Garren H, Slansky A, Ruiz PJ, Steinman L. Late pregnancy suppresses relapses in experimental autoimmune encephalomyelitis: evidence for a suppressive pregnancy-related serum factor. *J Immunol.* 2002;169:1084–1091.

Langer-Gould A, Huang SM, Gupta R, et al. Exclusive breastfeeding and the risk of postpartum relapses in women with multiple sclerosis. *Arch Neurol.* 2009; 66(8):958–963.

Laplaud DA, Lefrere F, Leray E, Barriere P, Wiertlewski S. Increased risk of relapse in multiple sclerosis patients after ovarian stimulation for in vitro fertilization. *Gynecol Obstet Fertil.* 2007;35:1047–1050.

Liu HB, Loo KK, Palaszynski K, Ashouri J, Lubahn DB, Voskuhl RR. Estrogen receptor alpha mediates estrogen's immune protection in autoimmune disease. *J Immunol.* 2003;171:6936–6940.

Liu HY, Buenafe AC, Matejuk A, et al. Estrogen inhibition of EAE involves effects on dendritic cell function. *J Neurosci Res.* 2002;70:238–248.

Mackenzie-Graham A, Tinsley MR, Shah KP, et al. Cerebellar cortical atrophy in experimental autoimmune encephalomyelitis. *Neuroimage.* 2006;32(3):1016–1023.

Matejuk A, Adlard K, Zamora A, Silverman M, Vandenbark AA, Offner H. 17beta-estradiol inhibits cytokine, chemokine, and chemokine receptor mRNA expression in the central nervous system of female mice with experimental autoimmune encephalomyelitis. *J Neurosci Res.* 2001;65:529–542.

Matejuk A, Bakke AC, Hopke C, Dwyer J, Vandenbark AA, Offner H. Estrogen treatment induces a novel population of regulatory cells, which suppresses experimental autoimmune encephalomyelitis. *J Neurosci Res.* 2004; 77:119–126.

Miller DH, Barkhof F, Frank JA, Parker GJ, Thompson AJ. Measurement of atrophy in multiple sclerosis: pathological basis, methodological aspects and clinical relevance. *Brain.* 2002;125:1676–1695.

Mokhtarian F, McFarlin DE, Raine CS. Adoptive transfer of myelin basic protein-sensitized T cells produces chronic relapsing demyelinating disease in mice. *Nature.* 1984;309:356–358.

Morales LB, Loo KK, Liu HB, Peterson C, Tiwari-Woodruff S, Voskuhl RR. Treatment with an estrogen receptor alpha ligand is neuroprotective in experimental autoimmune encephalomyelitis. *J Neurosci.* 2006;26:6823–6833.

Morley JE, Kaiser FE, Perry HM, III, et al. Longitudinal changes in testosterone, luteinizing hormone, and follicle-stimulating hormone in healthy older men. *Metab Clin Exper.* 1997;46:410–413.

Nankin HR, Calkins JH. Decreased bioavailable testosterone in aging normal and impotent men. *J Clin Endocrinol Metab.* 1986;63:1418–1420.

Nelson JL, Hughes KA, Smith AG, Nisperos BB, Branchaud AM, Hansen JA. Remission of rheumatoid arthritis during pregnancy and maternal-fetal class II alloantigen disparity. *Am J Reprod Immunol.* 1992;28: 226–227.

Okuda Y, Okuda M, Bernard CC. Gender does not influence the susceptibility of C57BL/6 mice to develop chronic experimental autoimmune encephalomyelitis induced by myelin oligodendrocyte glycoprotein. *Immunol Lett.* 2002;81:25–29.

Orton SM, Herrera BM, Yee IM, et al. Sex ratio of multiple sclerosis in Canada: a longitudinal study. *Lancet Neurol.* 2006;5:932–936.

Palaszynski KM, Liu H, Loo KK, Voskuhl RR. Estriol treatment ameliorates disease in males with experimental autoimmune encephalomyelitis: implications for multiple sclerosis. *J Neuroimmunol.* 2004a;149:84–89.

Palaszynski KM, Loo KK, Ashouri JF, Liu H, Voskuhl RR. Androgens are protective in experimental autoimmune encephalomyelitis: implications for multiple sclerosis. *J Neuroimmunol.* 2004b;146:144–152.

Palaszynski KM, Smith DL, Kamrava S, Burgoyne PS, Arnold AP, Voskuhl RR. A yin-yang effect between sex chromosome complement and sex hormones on the immune response. *Endocrinology.* 2005;146(8): 3280–3285.

Papenfuss TL, Rogers CJ, Gienapp I, et al. Sex differences in experimental autoimmune encephalomyelitis in multiple murine strains. *J Neuroimmunol.* 2004;150:59–69.

Patti F, Cavallaro T, Lo Fermo S, et al. Is in utero early exposure to interferon beta a risk factor for pregnancy outcomes in MS? *J Neurol.* 2008;255:1250–1253.

Polanczyk MJ, Carson BD, Subramanian S, et al. Cutting edge: estrogen drives expansion of the CD4+CD25+ regulatory T cell compartment. *J Immunol.* 2004;173: 2227–2230.

Polanczyk M, Zamora A, Subramanian S, et al. The protective effect of 17beta-estradiol on experimental autoimmune encephalomyelitis is mediated through estrogen receptor-alpha. *Am J Pathol.* 2003;163: 1599–1605.

Pozzilli C, Falaschi P, Mainero C, et al. MRI in multiple sclerosis during the menstrual cycle: relationship with sex hormone patterns. *Neurology.* 1999;53:622–624.

Pozzilli C, Tomassini V, Marinelli F, Paolillo A, Gasperini C, Bastianello S. 'Gender gap' in multiple sclerosis: magnetic resonance imaging evidence. *Eur J Neurol.* 2003;10:95–97.

Raghupathy R. Th1-type immunity is incompatible with successful pregnancy. *Immunol Today.* 1997;18:478–482.

Raine CS, Barnett LB, Brown A, Behar T, McFarlin DE. Neuropathology of experimental allergic encephalomyelitis in inbred strains of mice. *Lab Invest.* 1980; 43:150–157.

Raine CS, Cannella B, Hauser SL, Genain CP. Demyelination in primate autoimmune encephalomyelitis and acute multiple sclerosis lesions:a case for antigen-specific antibody mediation. *Ann Neurol.* 1999;46:144–160.

Riskind PN, Massacesi L, Doolittle TH, Hauser SL. The role of prolactin in autoimmune demyelination: suppression of experimental allergic encephalomyelitis by bromocriptine. *Ann Neurol.* 1991;29:542–547.

Runmarker B, Andersen O. Pregnancy is associated with a lower risk of onset and a better prognosis in multiple sclerosis. *Brain.* 1995;118:253–261.

Runmarker B, Andersson C, Odén A, Andersen O. Prediction of outcome in multiple sclerosis based on multivariate models. *J Neurol.* 1994;241:597–604.

Sadovnick AD, Ebers GC. Genetics of multiple sclerosis. *Neurol Clin.* 1995;13:99–118.

Sandberg-Wollheim M, Frank D, Goodwin TM, et al. Pregnancy outcomes during treatment with interferon beta-1a in patients with multiple sclerosis. *Neurology.* 2005;65:802–806.

Sicotte NL, Giesser BS, Tandon V, et al. Testosterone treatment in multiple sclerosis: a pilot study. *Arch Neurol.* 2007;64:683–688.

Sicotte NL, Liva SM, Klutch R, et al. Treatment of multiple sclerosis with the pregnancy hormone estriol. *Ann Neurol.* 2002;52:421–428.

Smith ME, Eller NL, McFarland HF, Racke MK, Raine CS. Age dependence of clinical and pathological manifestations of autoimmune demyelination. Implications for multiple sclerosis. *Am J Pathol.* 1999;155:1147–1161.

Smith R, Studd JW. A pilot study of the effect upon multiple sclerosis of the menopause, hormone replacement therapy and the menstrual cycle. *J R Soc Med.* 1992; 85:612–613.

Smith-Bouvier DL, Divekar AA, Sasidhar M, et al. A role for sex chromosome complement in the female bias in autoimmune disease. *J Exp Med.* 2008;205: 1099–1108.

Soldan SS, Retuerto AI, Sicotte NL, Voskuhl RR. Immune modulation in multiple sclerosis patients treated with the pregnancy hormone estriol. *J Immunol.* 2003;171: 6267–6274.

Spring S, Lerch JP, Henkelman RM. Sexual dimorphism revealed in the structure of the mouse brain using three-dimensional magnetic resonance imaging. *Neuroimage.* 2007;35:1424–1433.

Sribnick EA, Wingrave JM, Matzelle DD, Ray SK, Banik NL. Estrogen as a neuroprotective agent in the treatment of spinal cord injury. *Ann N Y Acad Sci.* 2003;993:125–133, 159–160.

Stone LA, Frank JA, Albert PS, et al. Characterization of MRI response to treatment with interferon beta-1b: contrast-enhancing MRI lesion frequency as a primary outcome measure. *Neurology.* 1997;49:862–869.

Subramanian S, Matejuk A, Zamora A, Vandenbark AA, Offner H. Oral feeding with ethinyl estradiol suppresses and treats experimental autoimmune encephalomyelitis in SJL mice and inhibits the recruitment of inflammatory cells into the central nervous system. *J Immunol.* 2003;170:1548–1555.

Tenover JS, Matsumoto AM, Plymate SR, Bremner WJ. The effects of aging in normal men on bioavailable testosterone and luteinizing hormone secretion: response to clomiphene citrate. *J Clin Endocrinol Metab.* 1987; 65:1118–1126.

Thorogood M, Hannaford PC. The influence of oral contraceptives on the risk of multiple sclerosis. *Br J Obstet Gynaecol.* 1998;105:1296–1299.

Tiwari-Woodruff S, Morales LB, Lee R, Voskuhl RR. Differential neuroprotective and antiinflammatory effects of estrogen receptor (ER){alpha} and ERbeta ligand treatment. *Proc Natl Acad Sci USA.* 2007; 104:14813–14818.

Tomassini V, Onesti E, Mainero C, et al. Sex hormones modulate brain damage in multiple sclerosis: MRI evidence. *J Neurol Neurosurg Psychiatry.* 2005;76: 272–275.

van Walderveen MA, Tas MW, Barkhof F, et al. Magnetic resonance evaluation of disease activity during pregnancy in multiple sclerosis. *Neurology.* 1994;44:327–329.

Verdru P, Theys P, D'Hooghe MB, Carton H. Pregnancy and multiple sclerosis: the influence on long term disability. *Clin Neurol Neurosurg.* 1994;96:38–41.

Vermeulen A. Clinical review 24: Androgens in the aging male. *J Clin Endocrinol Metab.* 1991;73:221–224.

Villard-Mackintosh L, Vessey MP. Oral contraceptives and reproductive factors in multiple sclerosis incidence. *Contraception.* 1993;47:161–168.

Voskuhl R. Sex hormomes and other pregnancy-related factors with therapeutic potential in multiple sclerosis. In: Cohen D, Rudick R, eds. *Multiple Sclerosis Therapeutics.* Vol 32. London: Martin Dunitz Ltd., 2003:535–549.

Voskuhl RR. Chronic relapsing experimental allergic encephalomyelitis in the SJL mouse: relevant techniques. *Methods.* 1996;10:435–439.

Voskuhl RR, Palaszynski K. Sex hormones and experimental autoimmune encephalomyelitis: implications for multiple sclerosis. *Neuroscientist.* 2001;7:258–270.

Voskuhl RR, Pitchekian-Halabi H, MacKenzie-Graham A, McFarland HF, Raine CS. Gender differences in autoimmune demyelination in the mouse: implications for multiple sclerosis. *Ann Neurol.* 1996;39:724–733.

Vukusic S, Hutchinson M, Hours M, et al. Pregnancy and multiple sclerosis (the PRIMS study): clinical predictors of post-partum relapse. *Brain.* 2004;127:1353–1360.

Weber-Schoenderfer C, Schaefer C. MS, immunomodulators and pregnancy outcome: a prospective observational study. *Mult Scler.* 2009;15(9):1037–1042.

Wegmann TG, Lin H, Guilbert L, Mosmann TR. Bidirectional cytokine interactions in the maternal-fetal relationship: is successful pregnancy a TH2 phenomenon?. *Immunol Today.* 1993;14:353–356.

Wei T, Lightman SL. The neuroendocrine axis in patients with multiple sclerosis. *Brain.* 1997;120:1067–1076.

Weinshenker BG. Natural history of multiple sclerosis. *Ann Neurol.* 1994;36:S6–S11.

Weiss DJ, Gurpide E. Non-genomic effects of estrogens and antiestrogens. *J Steroid Biochem.* 1988;31:671–676.

Whitacre CC, Reingold SC, O'Looney PA. A gender gap in autoimmunity. *Science.* 1999;283:1277–1278.

Wingerchuk DM, Rodriguez M. Premenstrual multiple sclerosis pseudoexacerbations: role of body temperature and prevention with aspirin. *Arch Neurol.* 2006;63:1005–1008.

Wise PM, Dubal DB, Wilson ME, Rau SW, Bottner M. Minireview: neuroprotective effects of estrogen-new insights into mechanisms of action. *Endocrinology.* 2001;142:969–973.

Wujek JR, Bjartmar C, Richer E, et al. Axon loss in the spinal cord determines permanent neurological disability in an animal model of multiple sclerosis. *J Neuropathol Exp Neurol.* 2002;61:23–32.

Zhang QH, Hu YZ, Cao J, Zhong YQ, Zhao YF, Mei QB. Estrogen influences the differentiation, maturation and function of dendritic cells in rats with experimental autoimmune encephalomyelitis. *Acta Pharmacol Sin.* 2004;25:508–513.

Zorgdrager A, De Keyser J. Menstrually related worsening of symptoms in multiple sclerosis. *J Neurol Sci.* 1997;149:95–97.

Zorgdrager A, De Keyser J. The premenstrual period and exacerbations in multiple sclerosis. *Eur Neurol.* 2002;48:204–206.

Cognitive Impairment and Mood Disturbances

Nicholas G. LaRocca

There is marked enfeeblement of the memory; conceptions are formed slowly; the intellectual and emotional faculties are blunted in their totality.

—*Charcot, Lectures on the Diseases of the Nervous System Delivered at La Salpetriere (1877)*

Charcot wisely recognized the existence of cognitive changes in his multiple sclerosis (MS) patients. However, subsequent generations did not generally heed his wise counsel. In the early 1980s, patients were still being told that MS does not cause memory problems. This surprising stance toward a common MS symptom was driven in part by a small number of studies that grossly underestimated the prevalence of the problem (Cottrell and Wilson, 1926; Kurtzke, 1970) and by a desire to shield patients from the grim reality of cognitive decline. The result was that MS cognitive impairment was a taboo topic and patients experiencing these problems received short shrift if they brought up the subject.

Cracks began to appear in this wall of silence in the early 1990s when the National MS Society's Cognitive Function Study Group published a paper estimating the prevalence of MS cognitive impairment to be 54%–65% (Peyser et al., 1990). Since that time research and clinical care focused on cognitive impairment has grown exponentially. Most importantly, MS patients experiencing cognitive changes are now taken seriously as family members, employers, and health-care professionals adopt strategies to help compensate for MS-related cognitive changes. This chapter will discuss many of the strategies that can be used in day-to-day work with people with MS to help ensure successful communication and implementation of treatment plans.

FREQUENCY AND SEVERITY

When Peyser et al. (1990) published their estimate that 54%–65% of persons with MS were cognitively impaired, most of the cited prevalence studies had used clinic rather than community-based samples. The concern was that clinic samples might be more disabled and therefore have a higher frequency of cognitive changes. Two subsequent studies that used community-based samples did indeed find slightly lower figures for prevalence, 43% (Rao et al., 1991) and 46% (McIntosh-Michaelis et al., 1991). In the intervening years, as more and more studies of cognitive impairment have been completed, the pendulum seems to have swung back to some extent and 50% or more is the figure most commonly cited today.

Although MS can produce a severe dementia, this is rare. By far the most common presentation of cognitive impairment is in the mild to moderate range. In terms of everyday activities, this means that the patient experiences some difficulty performing daily activities such as remembering names, processing information, and so on but is able to live independently and, in some cases, even continue to work. Part of the reason for this relatively positive picture arises from the fact that MS tends to selectively affect some cognitive functions while sparing others. As a result, patients are often able to compensate for weakness in one area by capitalizing on strengths in another.

ETIOLOGY

There are many forces at work to compromise the cognitive function of persons with MS. These include structural and chemical changes in the brain, untoward effects of medications used to treat MS symptoms, disabling fatigue, and emotional states.

Demyelination, Axonal Transection, and Cerebral Atrophy

Modern neuroimaging methodologies, especially magnetic resonance imaging (MRI) and its variants, have provided powerful tools to study the relationships between brain structures and processes and cognitive impairments as observed in MS. A full discussion of the substantial body of research on this subject is beyond the scope of this chapter. However, Table 18-1 summarizes some of the more important findings. This is not intended to be an exhaustive listing but rather to be a sampling of the considerable research in this area.

Biochemical Changes

With the major focus on demyelinative lesions, the myelinated areas of the brain that appear to be lesion free on MRI have long been known as normal–appearing white matter (NAWM). However, magnetic resonance spectroscopy (MRS) has been used to examine these areas and has shown abnormalities that are correlated with impairment in attention and memory tasks (Christodoulou et al., 2003).

Medication Side Effects

The list of medications commonly used in MS is a long one and some may compromise cognitive function. Intravenously administered steroids have been shown to compromise both verbal and visual memory in MS patients, although these effects are transient and the long-term impact on cognition may be positive (Uttner et al., 2006).

Although many other medications commonly used in MS may compromise cognitive function, research on these effects is lacking. However, the clinician should be alert to the possibility of such side effects, especially with regard to selective serotonin reuptake inhibitors, muscle relaxants, antispasticity agents, antiseizure medications, benzodiazepines, opiates, and anticholinergics. The list could go on and the clinician needs to be vigilant concerning the possible side effects of any medication used with persons with MS. It is particularly important to use care in treating patients who already have cognitive changes. Their cognitive "reserve" is diminished and a medication that causes drowsiness or other cognition-challenging effects may be enough to precipitate more severe dysfunction.

Genetics

Several studies have linked the presence of the gene for apolipoprotein E (APOE) to a more negative outcome in MS. However the evidence of a role for APOE in cognitive changes in MS has been equivocal (Feinstein, 2007; Parmenter et al., 2007; Shi et al., 2008) and there is some suggestion that the effect is mostly in men (Savettieri et al., 2004). Although research continues to expand our understanding of the genetic underpinnings of MS, no susceptibility genes for MS-related cognitive function have been positively identified.

Fatigue

Although patients report that fatigue interferes with the performance of cognitive tasks, the truth appears to be more complex. DeLuca (2006) provides a lucid explanation of these complexities. He points out that when patients are tested following *prolonged* (but not necessarily sustained or constant) mental effort, for example, over the course of a work day, they do *not* show a decrement in cognitive performance despite reporting that they feel fatigued. In contrast, cognitive performance does decline in the face of *sustained* mental effort on a challenging task, even though such a task is not performed over an extended period of time such as a work day. The take-away message seems to be to punctuate challenging cognitive tasks with periodic breaks, especially if it is noticed that performance is deteriorating.

Anxiety, Stress, and Depression

It is common for patients to be told that their cognitive impairment is just due to depression. Although cognition can certainly be adversely affected by a major depressive episode, depression is not generally the underlying cause of these deficits. Studies have indicated that those cognitive functions requiring the most effort such as speed of information processing are the most likely to be affected by depression (Arnett et al., 1999).

TABLE 18-1 Relationship between Lesion Areas and Impaired Cognitive Functions in Multiple Sclerosis

Area	Impairment	Citation
Total lesion area	Overall impairment	(Rao et al., 1989)
	Verbal memory	
	Abstract reasoning	
	Visuospatial problem solving	
	Overall impairment	(Comi et al., 1995)
	Visual memory*	(Feinstein et al., 1992)
	Verbal memory	(Ryan et al., 1996)
	Visual memory	
	Verbal fluency	
Atrophy	Attention	(Benedict et al., 2002a)
	Conceptual reasoning	
	Visual memory	
	Verbal memory	
	Verbal memory	(Amato et al., 2008b)
	Sustained attention and concentration	
	Processing speed	(Lazeron et al., 2006)
	Attention	(Piras et al., 2003)
	Memory	
	Visual memory	
Frontal	Executive functions	(Arnett et al., 1994)
	Attention	(Nebel et al., 2007)
	Attention	(Benedict et al., 2002a)
	Conceptual reasoning	
	Visual memory	
	Verbal memory	
	Processing speed	(Lazeron et al., 2006)
	Processing speed	(Genova et al., 2009)
	Attention	(Piras et al., 2003)
	Memory	
	Visual memory	
	Sustained attention and concentration	(Amato et al., 2008b)
Occipital	Attention	(Nebel et al., 2007)
	Processing speed	(Lazeron et al., 2006)
	Attention	(Piras et al., 2003)
	Memory	
	Sustained attention and concentration	(Amato et al., 2008b)
Parietal	Attention	(Nebel et al., 2007)
	Verbal memory	(Ryan et al., 1996)
	Processing speed	(Genova et al., 2009)
Temporal	Attention	(Piras et al., 2003)
	Memory	
	Verbal memory	(Amato et al., 2008b)
Corpus callosum	Information processing	(Rao et al., 1989)
	Dichotic listening	
	Verbal fluency	(Pozzilli et al., 1991)
	Visual memory	(Ryan et al., 1996)
Hippocampus	Visual memory	(Roosendaal et al., 2009)
	Verbal memory	(Sicotte et al., 2008)

*Included patients with both multiple sclerosis and clinically isolated syndrome.

FUNCTIONS MOST COMMONLY AFFECTED

When considering the potential impact of MS on cognition, there are three important points. First, there are some functions that are more likely to be affected than others. Second, even among the functions most commonly affected, some functions will be impaired while others are partially or completely intact. Third, the pattern of impaired and intact functions tends to vary from patient to patient.

Learning and Memory

Memory is the function most frequently cited as impaired in MS and was even mentioned by Charcot over 100 years ago. From the standpoint of the patient and family, memory impairment is probably the most sentinel of deficits since the use of memory pervades virtually every daily activity.

Memory is a complex process and considerable research has been devoted to understanding the types of memory most likely to be affected by MS and under what conditions. *Procedural memory* refers to the mental storehouse for skills such as riding a bike or tying shoelaces. Because procedural memory is not generally conscious, people find it hard to communicate procedural memory skills in words, for example, it is difficult to explain to someone how to tie a shoelace. Procedural memory tends not to be affected in MS. *Semantic memory*, in which is stored general knowledge and understanding of words, concepts, and the world in general, is similarly rarely affected in MS. On the other hand, *working memory* and *long-term memory* are frequently impaired in persons with MS. Working memory refers to the short-term storage of information for just a few seconds, while that information is being processed, either for immediate use or eventual long-term storage. Impairment of working memory interferes with the ability to adequately process information and encode information for later retrieval. Long-term memory refers to the storage and retrieval of information over a more protracted period of time, that is, a few minutes to indefinitely. Although long-term memory tends to be impaired in MS, information learned prior to the onset of the disease tends not to be affected.

For some time it was the prevailing theory that the long-term memory deficits seen in MS were primarily due to defective *retrieval* of information that had been adequately learned and retained. However, some researchers have challenged this hypothesis by showing that if the original learning of information is enhanced, retrieval will be normal or near normal in MS patients. For example, DeLuca et al. (1998) trained both MS patients and healthy controls to memorize a list of words. The MS patients took more trials to learn the list. However, when tested later, there was no difference in the number of words recalled between the patients and controls, even after a week's delay. The implications of this research for the healthcare professional are obvious: to ensure that MS patients remember information about the disease or medication regimens, the information should be repeated more than once at the very least.

Complex Attention

We live in an age of multitasking; it is considered routine to divide our attention between two or more activities, for example, watching TV and surfing the Web. Everyday life presents myriad situations that call for divided, that is, complex attention such as preparing a meal while keeping an eye on youngsters. The term *multitasking* is somewhat of a misnomer because the process mainly involves *switching* between two or more tasks and screening out the irrelevant information from one task while focusing on the other. Although people with MS do not seem to have much of a problem with attention and concentration when one stream of information is involved, for example, reading a book, complex attention does tend to suffer (Paul et al., 1998; Nebel et al., 2007; Prakash et al., 2008). The underlying problem seems to be slowed information processing (Balsimelli et al., 2007), and partial solutions include avoiding multitasking whenever possible and reducing unnecessary distractions.

Information Processing Speed

Persons with MS will vividly describe the fact that they are just not able to process information as rapidly as they did before MS. Myriad studies have documented the fact that processing of information is likely to be slowed in MS (De Luca et al., 2004; Balsimelli et al., 2007; Macniven et al., 2008). This deficit has wide-ranging implications, particularly for memory. If processing of information is slowed, people with MS are likely to have difficulty learning and remembering information because they cannot process the incoming information quickly enough to "get" it all and store it for later retrieval. Slowed information processing also contributes to difficulties with complex attention. In addition, slowed information processing can have an adverse impact on a variety of daily tasks that demand rapid processing of information such as driving and conversation. For the clinician doing patient education or providing instructions or information, the implications are to keep the flow of information at a modest pace and check periodically to make sure that the patient has really absorbed what has been said.

Visual-Perceptual Skills

Visual-perceptual skills refer to a complex set of functions involving both the perception of objects and the ability to represent them and manipulate them in consciousness. When someone drives toward a specific destination, she is following a mental representation of the route that she has seen on a previous occasion. Obviously other factors weigh in to this process as well, such as primary sensation (vision), proprioception, memory, and speed of information processing. Rao et al. (1991) have estimated that visual-perceptual deficits affect approximately 20% of MS patients. These deficits may affect everyday activities such as recognition of faces, driving, putting things together (e.g, those pieces of furniture that are sold with "some assembly required"), recognizing the difference between similar objects, and navigating in unfamiliar surroundings. For the clinician who is trying to explain some complex information to an MS patient that involves diagrams or similar materials, extra time and written explanations may be crucial.

Executive Functions

Executive functions include planning, prioritizing, organizing, problem solving, reasoning, decision making, and judgment. Executive functions are typically manifest in the ability to plan and initiate a complex, multistep task or project, organize the steps involved, implement the steps according to a set of priorities and time frame, and bring the task to completion. Executive functions are often affected in MS but due to the complexity of these abilities and the many factors that contribute to them, it is difficult to estimate the frequency of these problems in MS (Amato et al., 2008a; Kalmer et al., 2008; Simioni et al., 2009). It is impairment of executive functions that is most likely to get persons with MS into trouble. Bad financial decisions, disorganization, the inability to cope with a complex set of tasks in the workplace are possible implications. The individual so affected may need assistance with the organization and implementation of tasks, particularly with planning. Since decision making can be affected, a collaborative model should be adopted, if it is not already in place, in which the spouse or other responsible family member shares responsibility for important decisions.

Word Finding

Most people find that from time to time they are unable to come up with a word that they would like to use during the course of a conversation. However, for many people with MS this "tip of the tongue" phenomenon is a true scourge that makes normal conversation a frustrating obstacle course. Like memory and speed of information processing, patients are likely to report this problem along with the related problem of verbal fluency deficits, both of which have long been known to exist in MS (Rao et al., 1991). Patients tend to become anxious when, in the course of a conversation, word-finding difficulty occurs. This anxiety probably exacerbates the problem. Helping patients to slow down and try to avoid getting overly anxious may help them to carry on with the conversation and perhaps substitute another word for the one they cannot retrieve.

Functions Generally Intact

- As was noted previously, *basic attention* tends not to be affected in MS, while complex or divided attention is. In other words, the basic ability to focus on a task and not become distracted is generally intact.

- *Basic verbal skills* likewise tend to be intact (Wishart and Sharp, 1997). These skills include the ability to understand words and sentences and to express oneself verbally. Of course, word-finding problems—the "tip of the tongue" phenomenon—may interfere with self-expression in many MS patients.

- Given the number of cognitive functions that can be affected in MS, it may seem contradictory to say that *general intelligence* is usually preserved in MS (Bobholz and Rao, 2003). Multiple sclerosis tends to affect some cognitive abilities while leaving others intact, particularly basic verbal skills and, in some cases, reasoning ability. Thus, an MS patient may have trouble remembering things but is just as "smart" as ever. Actual scores on standard IQ tests may decline anyway because these tests have several sections that place demands on speed of information processing and visual-perceptual skills. In addition, those patients with very severe cognitive impairment are likely to show declines in virtually all areas of intellectual functioning.

Impact on Quality of Life

- *Self-esteem* is likely to be affected by any of the myriad symptoms of MS such as difficulty walking, bladder dysfunction, fatigue, and so on. However, the most devastating turn of events for an MS patient is probably the feeling of "losing one's marbles." In defining who they are, different people emphasize different things. However, for most people, "smarts" in some form play a critical role in defining who they are, be it street smarts, social intelligence, or just basic cognitive functions. When cognitive functions decline, self-esteem suffers.

- Rao et al. (1991) provided convincing evidence that cognitive impairment accounts for much of the high rate of unemployment among people with MS. The damaging effect of cognitive impairment is not confined to MS patients in highly sophisticated jobs. Difficulties with memory, speed of information processing, and visual-perceptual skills can adversely affect ability to remain employed even for workers in much less sophisticated positions. These effects are particularly problematic for younger patients who are still in school and who really need to be able to process quickly, learn, and remember vast amounts of information.

- While it may be no surprise that many people with MS have difficulty driving, it is only in recent years that research has demonstrated that MS-related cognitive impairments can adversely affect driving performance (Schultheis et al., 2001, 2002; Shawaryn et al., 2002). Speed of information processing, working memory, and visual-perceptual skills all play important roles in driving and, as we have seen, are often impaired in MS. Because driving is an important component of independence and may be necessary in certain jobs, it is often difficult for patients to either give up driving or cut back on where and under what conditions they drive. The health-care professional may need to broach this topic and referral to a professional driving evaluation program in a rehabilitation center may be in order.

- Cognitive impairment does not just affect the patient. *Family and social life* are also affected. Many families of MS patients are not aware that MS can cause cognitive impairments. When a patient begins to forget things, family members may become angry, thinking that the person with MS is lazy or does not care. Family members need to be educated concerning the nature of the cognitive changes that occur in MS and how the family can help. Family life may change as the person with MS requires some help with remembering things, organizing, and avoiding situations that place too many demands on complex attention. Most families will need to set up a family calendar in order to record the appointments and activities of all members of the household. More than ever, important decisions will need to be shared, particularly if executive functions have been impaired. Social life may become more awkward if the person with MS experiences severe problems with word finding, memory, and/or speed of information processing. The key will be to assist the patient to remain active and involved in both family and social life because isolation will only add to the burden already created by the disease.

Relationship to Other Aspects of the Disease

- The *duration* of the disease is not predictive of whether a patient will have cognitive impairment. Although cognitive impairment tends to progress over time in MS (Amato et al., 2001), it can and does appear at any time during the course of the illness, even as the first symptoms (Rao et al., 1991). Conversely, patients who have had MS for many years may be completely free of cognitive deficits. Similar to other MS symptoms, cognitive impairment can worsen during an exacerbation and then improve as a remission takes place. However, it is rare for cognitive changes to disappear completely once they have appeared.
- *Physical disability* is likewise not predictive of cognitive impairment and cognitive changes can occur even when physical symptoms are absent or very mild. Moreover, patients with substantial physical disability may be free of cognitive changes. It does appear, however, that if a patient has had MS for a long time *and* is severely disabled physically, the probability of cognitive impairment is increased to some extent (Amato et al., 2001). In the past it was thought that the *course* of the disease was highly predictive of cognitive impairment with chronic progressive patients at greater risk (Rao, 1987). However, later studies have found that cognitive impairment may occur with any course, even in otherwise mildly affected relapsing-remitting patients (Amato et al., 2006) and that the extent of lesion load is a better predictor (Feinstein, 2007). Because secondary progressive patients *on average* are likely to have a greater lesion load, they are at somewhat greater risk to be cognitively impaired. However, the important idea to keep in mind is that cognitive impairment can and does occur with any course, even in so-called benign patients (Amato et al., 2008b; Rovaris et al., 2008).

ASSESSMENT

Subjective Observation

Diagnosis and treatment of cognitive dysfunction is likely to begin with subjective observation either on the part of the patient, family or friends, an employer, or a health-care professional. These observations may be triggered by memory lapses, poor judgment, a health-care provider's history taking, or other similar event. However, in many cases, these observations are less than accurate.

Subjective observation tends to be severely limited even as a preliminary screening tool. Benedict et al. (2003a, 2004) developed and administered two versions of a brief questionnaire to screen for cognitive changes, a patient version and an informant version, the MS Neuropsychological Screening Questionnaire. The patients were also given a battery of cognitive tests. They found that patients' scores tended to correlate with depression scores and that the informant scores were more predictive of the patients' actual performance on the cognitive tests. In other words, some patients who were cognitively impaired did not report any problems while others who were not cognitively impaired did. Therefore, screening for cognitive impairment is likely to be more effective if patient self-report is supplemented by a family member or other informant and objective testing.

Mental Status Examination

The mental status examination or its more formal versions such as the mini mental state examination (MMSE) (Folstein et al., 1975) are often used to screen for cognitive impairment in MS. Unfortunately, because MS-related cognitive changes can be subtle and vary from patient to patient, these techniques are likely to miss as many as half of patients with cognitive impairment (Peyser et al., 1980; Rao et al., 1989). Many studies have attempted to "rescue" the MMSE for use in MS by experimenting with different cut-off scores and other manipulations, but in the end, the MMSE has been found to lack the sensitivity and specificity to serve as a useful screen. The lack of utility of these generic bedside mental status techniques has led to attempts to develop short screening batteries that specifically address the unique characteristics of MS.

Brief Cognitive Batteries

The term *brief* seems to mean different things to different people and what might be a brief screening battery to one would represent an unacceptable interval of poorly reimbursed or unreimbursed time for another. In addition, what may be feasible in a research setting could be impossible in the clinic.

Although there have been many attempts to develop brief screening batteries for use in MS, two stand out: the Screening Examination for Cognitive Impairment (SEFCI) and the Brief Repeatable Neuropsychological Battery (BRNB).

The SEFCI was developed by Beatty et al. (1995), takes about a half-hour to administer, tests functions frequently affected in MS, and has good sensitivity and specificity. Since the SEFCI has only one version, it is not well suited to longitudinal administration.

The BRNB was developed by Rao (Rao, S.M. A Manual for the Brief, Repeatable Battery of Neuropsychological Tests in Multiple Sclerosis. Unpublished paper, 1991) takes about three-quarters of an hour to administer, tests functions frequently affected in MS, and has good sensitivity and specificity (Strober et al., 2009). However, unlike the SEFCI, the BRNB has 15 equivalent versions, making longitudinal administration feasible. In addition, normative data from healthy controls exist (Boringa et al., 2001). Although longer to administer, the existence of alternate forms gives the BRNB somewhat of an edge over the SEFCI and as a result it has seen wider use, especially in clinical trials.

A relatively recent development in short batteries for MS has been the fielding of computerized neuropsychological assessment methods. Wilken et al. (2003) evaluated the Automated Neuropsychological Assessment Metrics (ANAM), a computerized battery developed by the U.S. Department of Defense. The ANAM consists of eight subtests that assess some of the functions most frequently affected in MS (e.g., processing speed, memory, etc.). The investigators examined the extent to which the ANAM could correctly classify relapsing-remitting MS patients as cognitively impaired, using a traditional battery of tests as the reference standard. The ANAM was able to correctly classify 95.8% of the patients in the study, and the individual subtests making up the ANAM demonstrated moderate to high correlations with the tests in the traditional battery.

Full Neuropsychological Batteries

Multiple sclerosis can produce a variety of different cognitive impairments that can vary from patient to patient, and range from mild to severe. Such a configuration of impairments requires a comprehensive and sensitive approach to assessment. This is especially the case when a goal of the assessment is to obtain a picture of the patient's strengths and weaknesses. While efforts to develop abbreviated test batteries continue, an adequate cognitive test battery for use in MS still entails two or more hours of testing and, in many cases, much more time than that.

LaRocca and Caruso (2006) have summarized the most important functions that should be included in a cognitive battery for use in MS:

- Depression and other personality issues
- General intellectual ability
- Conceptual reasoning
- Processing speed
- Attention and concentration, especially complex attention
- Verbal and visual memory
- Expressive language
- Receptive language
- Visuospatial ability
- Dexterity

One test battery developed for MS that captures the above functions and is relatively brief compared to more traditional assessments is the Minimal Assessment of Cognitive Function in MS (MACFIMS; Benedict et al., 2002b). The MACFIMS was the result of a consensus conference of leading experts in MS, is evidence-based, and takes about 2 hours to administer. The clinician can add additional tests to the MACFIMS as needed to address particular issues.

The MACFIMS is provided as an example of a comprehensive, sensitive, and scientifically sound assessment battery. However, it is not the only sound approach to assessment in MS. Assessment of cognitive function in MS may be performed by neuropsychologists, clinical psychologists, speech-language pathologists, and occupational therapists.

Each of these professions tends to use slightly different tests and to emphasize evaluation of different functions. The key to a good assessment is the evaluation of the key functions most likely to be affected in MS by a professional who is experienced with the disease. Although a cognitive assessment can be expensive and time consuming, in many instances, it is the only way to adequately evaluate cognitive impairment.

Other Assessment Issues

Some other issues to keep in mind regarding the assessment of cognitive impairment in MS:

- Feedback to the patient and family is a very important part of the assessment and should be done by the professional who interpreted the tests.
- Some follow-up is likely to be needed if impairments are found. These may include counseling, cognitive rehabilitation, vocational rehabilitation, or other measures.
- Although cognitive impairment correlates well with lesion load, serial MRI is not an effective way to judge whether cognitive impairment is getting worse. Only cognitive assessment can determine this.
- Emotional, familial, and social issues are almost always involved when there is cognitive impairment. The clinician needs to be prepared to address these issues along with the cognitive changes.

ADDRESSING COGNITIVE IMPAIRMENT

Practical Strategies for the Health-Care Provider

If cognitive impairments are present, the health-care professional can do a number of things to ensure that the interaction with patients will be more productive. See Table 18-2 for a summary of some strategies that the clinician, patient, and family members can use to address impairments in cognitive functions.

- When *memory* problems are present, information conveyed to the patient should be repeated and wherever possible presented

both verbally and in writing. It is also helpful to determine through questions whether the patient really "got it." Having a family member present for these communications is also helpful. Dates and times of follow-up appointments should always be written down and the patient should receive a reminder call the day before the appointment. The patient should receive written information and instructions concerning any diagnostic procedures to be performed and a written report of the results afterwards.
- If *processing speed* has slowed, it is a good idea to keep the flow of information to the patient at a modest pace and to check periodically to make sure there are no gaps in understanding.
- For patients with *attention* problems, communication with the health-care professional should take place in a quiet environment that is free of unnecessary distractions. The focus should be on the conversation without the simultaneous distraction of a physical examination or other procedure.
- Perhaps most crucial, the health-care professional needs to be on the lookout for cognitive changes and should always broach the subject along with queries about other symptoms. Although self-report of cognitive impairment leaves much to be desired, if the subject is seen by the patient and family as worthy of discussion, it is at least a starting point.

Multiple Sclerosis Disease-Modifying Drugs

The hypothetical rationale for a beneficial effect of MS disease-modifying agents (DMAs) on cognition is compelling: since cognitive impairment is associated with lesion load and atrophy, treatments that slow the development of these changes should slow the progression of cognitive impairment. In practice, however, there is only limited evidence to support this hypothesis. Studies have shown a modest positive effect for interferon beta-1b (Pliskin et al., 1996; Barak and Achiron, 2002), interferon beta-1a (Fischer et al., 2000), and natalizumab (Stephenson et al., 2009) but not for glatiramer acetate (Weinstein et al., 1999). However, there were methodological issues with

TABLE 18-2 Strategies to Address Impaired Cognitive Functions in Multiple Sclerosis

Function Impaired	Strategies for Clinicians, Patients, and Families
Learning and memory	Repeat information
	Provide information in writing
	Check to see if the individual "got it"
	Convey information to both patient and family member
	Use organizer book or electronic organizer
	Use a family calendar to keep track of everyone's activities
	Use a well-organized filing system at home
	Try to keep house organized and things in their place
	Use lists for shopping, packing for trips, tasks, etc.
	Take notes concerning people, places, things, etc.
Complex attention	Seek out quiet environments
	Avoid distractions
	Avoid multitasking
	Try to get the "main idea" when reading, listening, or watching things
Speed of information processing	Covey information at a modest pace
	Check to see if the individual "got it"
	Ask family, friends, co-workers to "slow down" if necessary
	See strategies for complex attention impairments
Visual-perceptual skills	Take extra time to explain things involving visual material
	Take extra time to do things involving V-P skills
	Plan routes ahead when driving
	Avoid distractions when driving or whenever using V-P skills
Executive functions	Use planning tools that break projects up into a step-by-step process
	Make major decisions collaboratively with family members
	Learn to organize and manage time wisely
	Use to-do lists with item prioritized

all of these studies: none were really designed to evaluate impact on cognitive impairment and the patients in the studies generally had little or no cognitive impairment at the outset. However, despite the lack of direct evidence, because these treatments slow the development of factors thought to cause cognitive changes, for example, MS lesions and cerebral atrophy, use of DMAs may in the long-term help to slow the progression of cognitive impairment (Bagert et al., 2002).

Symptomatic Treatments

Given the sheer variety of agents that have been tested, it is surprising that so few have shown any value at all. The most consistently successful drug in treating cognitive impairment in MS has been donepezil hydrochloride, an acetylcholinesterase inhibitor. Krupp et al. (2004) have shown that donepezil can produce a modest improvement in verbal memory in MS patients with memory deficits and that this effect appears to have some practical significance for everyday life. In a recently published study, investigators showed that a single does of methylphenidate could temporarily improve performance on a task involving attention, working memory, and processing speed (Harel et al., 2009). However, since this study did not involve ongoing treatment, it is not yet known how these effects carry over to daily life. Studies examining the effect of corticosteroids on cognitive impairment have shown both positive and negative effects (Oliveri et al., 1998; Patzold et al., 2002). Another recent study examined the potential benefits of ginkgo biloba on a variety of cognitive impairments in MS patients but did not produce a statistically significant change in cognitive function (Lovera et al., 2007). Positive results have been found with methylphenidate (Harel et al., 2009) and L-amphetamine sulfate (Morrow et al., 2009), and anecdotal reports suggest that many physicians are prescribing attention-enhancing drugs to their MS patients with cognitive impairment.

A number of other agents have shown some preliminary promise in small studies, including testosterone gel (Sicotte et al., 2007), monthly treatments with a combination of cyclophosphamide and corticosteroids (Zéphir et al., 2005), modafinil in combination with interferon beta-1a (Wilken et al., 2004), and erythropoietin (Ehrenreich et al., 2007). However, these agents require much more research before definite conclusions about their efficacy in treating cognitive impairment can be reached.

The list of treatments that have not been successful in treatment cognitive impairment in MS is a long one. Space does not permit a discussion of these, but they are listed below for reference:

- 3,4-diaminopyridine
- 4-aminopyridine
- Amantadine
- Cooling
- Magnetic fields
- Memantine: a dose of 30 mg per day can produce revisible *worsening* in neurological symptoms in MS patients (Villoslada et al., 2009)
- Pemoline
- Prokarin

Cognitive Rehabilitation and Strategies

Cognitive rehabilitation in MS has seen significant growth in recent years both clinically and in terms of its evidence base. Sometimes referred to as cognitive "remediation," cognitive rehabilitation can be roughly divided into *restorative* vs. *compensatory* approaches. Most comprehensive cognitive rehabilitation programs combine elements of both approaches.

The *restorative* approach attempts to improve cognitive function through various exercises that challenge affected skills. For example, verbal memory might be targeted through the use of computer delivered exercises that require the patient to memorize lists of words that gradually increase in terms of the difficulty of the words and the length of the list. Video games focused on cognitive skills generally fall into this category. The underlying assumption of this approach is that the human brain is characterized by a certain amount of "plasticity" or adaptability and, if challenged in the right ways, can improve functionally, perhaps by rerouting cognitive tasks through different parts of the brain.

Unfortunately, evidence for the value of restorative approaches in MS has been limited. While some studies have found computer-mediated exercises and related approaches effective in improving attention, memory, and other functions (Plohman et al., 1998; Tesar et al., 2005; Brenk et al., 2008), others have had disappointing results (Mendozzi et al., 1998; Solari et al., 2004). Despite these mixed results, research continues to try to identify restorative approaches that may be more effective than those that have been tried thus far. In addition, newer approaches, including video games and exercise, are beginning to be explored and may hold promise for the future.

In contrast to the restorative approach, the *compensatory* approach does not attempt to restore impaired abilities but rather to work around those impairments using substitution to achieve functional success. For example, if memory impairment is present, rather than using memory exercise (a restorative approach) the compensatory approach would train the patient to utilize memory aids such as a notebook, a smartphone, a family calendar, a filing system, better organization, and so on.

Despite the self-evident nature of compensatory approaches, evidence for their utility in MS has been mixed at best. Some comprehensive cognitive rehabilitative programs have proven beneficial for a variety of functions, including executive functions, spatial abilities, and memory (Tesar et al., 2005), visual memory (Jonsson et al., 1993), verbal memory and reasoning (Rodgers et al., 1996), and cognitive function in general (Khan et al., 2008). However, other studies have failed to show any effect at all on cognitive functions (Shepko and Hollenbeck, 1997; Allen et al., 1998; Benedict et al., 2000; Lincoln et al., 2002).

Fortunately, the research on both restorative and compensatory approaches is mixed rather than uniformly negative, suggesting that as studies become more refined, it may be possible to identify the most effective approaches in both areas. In the meantime MS patients need assistance in coping with the cognitive changes that for many are a life-changing experience. At the very least, patients need to learn basic, compensatory strategies that will allow them to function as independently as possible in daily life. In addition, when cognitive impairment occurs, intervention generally needs to include not only measures addressing the cognitive changes but also attention to the emotional, familial, and social ramifications. Indeed, there is some hint in the research that the most successful approaches to cognitive rehabilitation in MS are those that address more than just cognition. In working with MS patients on memory remediation, it is often observed that sessions may be interrupted periodically because patients need to talk about family issues, depression, or similar topics.

MOOD DISTURBANCES

Although MS is not a psychiatric disorder per se, it is often accompanied by a variety of mood disturbances, many of which appear to be the direct result of the disease. In addition, MS does not confer immunity to the psychiatric conditions that appear in the population at large. Therefore, the management of MS entails comprehensive attention to a wide assortment of mood disturbances beginning when symptoms first appear.

Depression and Dysphoria

Frequency and severity

Charcot (1877) is generally regarded as the first to document depression as integral to MS. The term *depression* is used to refer to a spectrum of conditions ranging from major depressive disorder to dysphoric symptoms. The diagnosis of depression among MS patients is important because depression can have a serious impact on quality of life, may lead to suicide, and is treatable using medication and/or psychotherapy.

The lifetime prevalence of major depressive disorder in persons with MS has been estimated to be approximately 50% (Minden and Schiffer, 1990) with 12-month prevalence estimated at approximately 25% (Patten et al., 2003) and current prevalence at 14% (Minden and Schiffer, 1990), all of which exceed that observed in the general population (Patten et al., 2003).

Suicidal ideation and suicide are important complications of depression in MS. In a study of Veterans Health Administration patients with MS, investigators found that 29.4% reported suicidal ideation during the past 2 weeks and that in 7.9% this ideation was persistent (Turner et al., 2006). Among MS clinic attendees the rate of suicides was 7.5 times greater than in the general population (Sadovnick et al., 1991). Patients early in the course of the disease seem to be at particular risk (Fredrickson et al., 2003). Patients with an anxiety disorder have also been found to be at greater risk of suicidal ideation (Korostil and Feinstein, 2007).

Etiology and course

Structural MRI studies have indicated that depression in MS patients is not associated with overall lesion load or cerebral atrophy but rather with lesions in specific frontal areas and with gray matter atrophy and increased cerebrospinal fluid (CSF) volume in the temporal region (Zorzon et al., 2001; Feinstein et al., 2004). However, it is important to note that these structural changes only partially account for the variance in depression, suggesting that other factors are also at work (Foley et al., 1992).

Genetic susceptibility is likely to be an additional etiological factor. Patten et al. (2000) found a familial pattern to major depression among MS patients, suggesting that there is some genetic susceptibility at work.

Given the many stresses that MS can introduce into a person's life, it would not be surprising to find a number of psychosocial factors associated with depression. This has indeed been the case with research supporting an association with uncertainty, disability, emotion-focused coping, and hope (Feinstein, 2007). However, whether these are causes, reactions, or a combination of the two is unclear at this time. There can be little doubt, however, that MS can be a devastating disease to which patients may have strong emotional reactions.

Controversy has existed for many years concerning the possibility that interferon beta could trigger depression or even suicide in MS patients. In the pivotal clinical trial of interferon beta-1b, there were four suicide attempts among the patients in the treated group and none in the placebo group. While this difference did not reach statistical significance, it did raise concerns about interferons, especially given the already high risk of depression among MS patients. However, most subsequent research did not find an increased risk of depression in patients treated with interferon beta-1b (Feinstein et al., 2002) or interferon beta-1a (Patten and Metz, 2002; Zephir et al., 2003) and that depression during the course of treatment tends to be associated with pretreatment mood rather than interferon treatment itself (Mohr et al., 1997). Patten's (2006) review of the literature supported this conclusion and also found that when psychiatric side effects do arise with the interferons, they can be adequately managed while treatment continues.

Relationship to other aspects of the disease

Depressive symptoms can affect patients with any type of MS, at any time during the course of the illness, and regardless of degree of physical disability. As a result, the clinician needs to be vigilant at all times to screen for possible depression. That being said, certain types of patients appear to be at greater risk for experiencing depressive symptoms, including those with recent-onset MS and more severe physical disability (Chwastiak et al., 2002; Patten et al., 2005; Hyphantis et al., 2008).

Symptoms and assessment

In MS, the term *depression* can refer to a number of conditions ranging from a major depressive episode (Table 18-3) to mild symptoms of dysphoria. Throughout this spectrum of conditions, a long-standing concern has been whether depressive symptoms that overlap with MS symptoms render the assessment and diagnosis of depression problematic. Sleep disruption, fatigue, and difficulty

concentrating are common in both depression and MS. Possible ways to handle this issue have included simply ignoring the symptoms in question and developing scales specifically geared to medically ill populations, for example, the Chicago Multiscale Depression Inventory (Nyenhuis et al., 1998). However, research has indicated that concern about the confounding effect of these vegetative symptoms is largely exaggerated and that attempts to ignore or exclude them are generally not warranted (Randolph et al., 2000).

Other issues in the assessment of depression in MS patients include the question of whether depression presents in the same way as it does in the general population. For example, there is some evidence that among MS patients depression presents less with guilt, disinterest, and withdrawal and more with anger and irritability (Minden et al., 1987). Feinstein (2007) has also pointed out the importance of so-called subthreshold depression, that is, that which does not quite meet diagnostic criteria for a major depressive episode. While such subthreshold depression may be less severe than the full-blown variety, its psychosocial ramifications may be no less daunting.

The reference standard for diagnosing depression is a diagnostic interview with a psychiatrist or other equally qualified mental health professional. However, performing such an assessment on more than a tiny proportion of patients would be impractical. As a result, there has been considerable discussion of various screening methods using brief, self-report instruments (Goldman Consensus Group, 2005). The ultimate in brief depression screen is the Yale Single Question Screen (Lachs et al., 1990). Unfortunately the Yale Single Question Screen lacks sensitivity in MS (Avasarala et al., 2003). A more appropriate choice is the Beck Fast Screen for Medically Ill Patients (Beck et al., 2000), which has been validated for use in MS (Benedict et al., 2003b).

In screening for depression in MS it is important to keep in mind that many MS patients experience a grieving process in which they mourn the losses that MS has visited upon them. The characteristics of grief can at times mimic the symptoms of depression, but the implications from a therapeutic standpoint may be quite different. For a complete discussion of the phenomenon of grief as it plays out in MS, see Chapter 26.

TABLE 18-3 Criteria for a "major depressive episode" in the *Diagnostic and Statistical Manual*, 4th edition

Criterion	Features
A	Five (or more) of the following symptoms have been present during the same two-week period and represent a change from previous functioning; at least one of the symptoms is either (1) depressed mood or (2) loss of interest or pleasure
	(i) Depressed mood most of the day, as indicated by either subjective report (e.g. feels sad or empty) or observation made by others (e.g. appears tearful). **Note**: in children or adolescents, can be irritable mood
	(ii) Markedly diminished interest or pleasure in all, or almost all, activities of the day, nearly everyday (as indicated by either subjective account or observation made by others)
	(iii) Significant weight loss when not dieting or weight gain (e.g. change of more than 5% of body weight in a month), or decrease or increase in appetite nearly everyday. **Note**: in children, consider failure to make expected weight gains
	(iv) Insomnia or hypersomnia nearly every day
	(v) Psychomotor agitation or retardation nearly every day (observable by others, not merely subjective feelings of restlessness or being slowed down)
	(vi) Fatigue or loss of energy nearly every day
	(vii) Feelings of worthlessness or excessive or inappropriate guilt (which may be delusional) nearly every day (not merely self-reproach or guilt about being sick)
	(viii) Diminished ability to think or concentrate, or indecisiveness, nearly every day (either by subjective account or observed by others)
	(ix) Recurrent thoughts of death (not just fear of dying), recurrent suicidal ideation without specific plan, or a suicide attempt or a specific plan for committing suicide
B	The symptoms do not meet the criteria for a mixed episode
C	The symptoms cause clinically significant distress or impairment in social occupational, or other important areas of functioning
D	The symptoms are not due to the direct physiological effects of a substance (e.g., a drug of abuse, a medication) or a general medical condition (e.g., hypothyroidism)
E	The symptoms are not better accounted for by bereavement, i.e. after the loss of a loved one; the symptoms persist for longer than 2 months or are characterized by marked functional impairment, morbid preoccupation with worthlessness, suicidal ideation, psychotic symptoms or psychomotor retardation

Source: with permission from American Psychiatric Association,1994.

Whatever approach is used in screening for depression, the important point is that depression and suicide are both more common in MS than in the general population and that it is essential for the clinician to address these issues.

Treatment

Given the high prevalence of depression and suicide among MS patients, there has been surprisingly little research concerning treatment. What little research has been completed suggests that the treatments that are effective in the general population are also viable for MS patients.

There is evidence that standard antidepressants are effective in MS, but side effects are an important consideration, especially if they aggravate MS symptoms such as sexual dysfunction (Schiffer and Wineman, 1990; Mohr et al., 2001). The best course is probably to choose psychopharmacologic agents based on individual patient needs and side effect profile.

Psychotherapy, both individual and group, has been shown to be effective in MS. Mohr et al. (2001) showed that cognitive behavior therapy (CBT) was just as effective as sertraline and could even be effective when conducted by phone (Mohr et al., 2000). Foley et al. (1987) also showed that CBT delivered in a "stress inoculation" format was effective against depression in MS patients.

Following a review of the literature and consensus conference of experienced MS mental health clinicians and researchers, the Goldman Consensus Group (2005) recommended that the standard of treatment for moderate to severe depression in MS should include both medication and psychotherapy.

Electroconvulsive therapy (ECT) has been used to treat depression and other disorders in MS but has never been subject to adequate study as to its safety and efficacy. The literature on the subject is based on uncontrolled case reports with small numbers of patients; for example, Mattingly et al. (1992) and Rasmussen and Keegan (2007) were both based on only three cases. The presence of contrast enhancing lesions are thought to put patients at risk for neurological deterioration following ECT, although this is based on very limited evidence (Mattingly et al., 1992). The advice offered by Feinstein (2007) seems wise: to exhaust other treatment options before resorting to ECT. And as Rasmussen and Keegen (2007) advise, a thorough neurological examination and full informed consent should precede treatment.

Bipolar Disorder

Bipolar disorder may be manifest as one or more manic (Table 18-4) or hypomanic (Table 18-5) episodes, or of a mixed type in which such episodes alternate with depressive episodes. Although bipolar disorder is not very common in MS, there is evidence that lifetime prevalence for the disorder among MS patients (13%) is higher than that for the general population (1%) (Schiffer et al., 1986; Joffe et al., 1987).

It is unclear why the comorbidity between MS and bipolar disorders should be so great, and relatively few studies have addressed this question. Some sort of shared brain pathology has been

TABLE 18-4 Criteria for a manic episode in DSM-IV

Criterion	Features
A	A distinct period of abnormally and persistently elevated, expansive or irritable mood lasting at least one week (or any duration if hospitalization is necessary)
B	During the period of mood disturbance, three or more of the following symptoms have persisted (four if the mood is only irritable) and have been present to a significant degree:
	(i) inflated self-esteem or grandiosity
	(ii) decreased need for sleep(e.g. feels rested after only 3 hours of sleep)
	(iii) more talkative than usual or pressure to keep talking
	(iv) flight of ideas or subjective experience that thoughts are racing
	(v) distractibility (i.e. attention too easily drawn to unimportant or irrelevant external stimuli)
	(vi) increase in goal-directed activity (either socially, at work or school, or sexually) or psychomotor agitation
	(vii) excessive involvement in pleasurable activities that have a high potential for painful consequences (e.g. engaging in unstrained buying sprees, sexual indiscretions, or foolish business investments)
C	The mood disturbance is sufficiently severe to cause marked impairment in occupational functioning or in usual social activities or relationships with others, or to necessitate hospitalization to prevent harm to self or others, or there are psychotic features.

Source: With permission from the American Psychiatric Association, 1994.

TABLE 18-5 Criteria for a hypomanic episode in DSM-IV

Criterion	Features
A	A distinct period of persistently elevated, expansive or irritable mood lasting throughout at least four days, that is clearly different from the usual non-depressed mood.
B	As in the criteria for manic episode
C	The episode is associated with an unequivocal change in functioning that is uncharacteristic of the person when not symptomatic
D	The disturbance in mood and the change in functioning are observable by others
E	The episode is not severe enough to cause marked impairment in social or occupational functioning, or to necessitate hospitalization, and there are no psychotic features

Source: With permission from the American Psychiatric Association, 1994.

raised as a possibility (Feinstein, 2007) but evidence for this is very limited and unconvincing. Steroids can induce a manic or hypomanic state in many MS patients (Minden et al., 1988), but this could not explain more than a small part of the high prevalence of bipolar disorder among MS patients. There is some limited evidence for a genetic susceptibility to bipolar disorder in certain families of MS patients (Schiffer et al., 1988), but additional studies are needed using the more precise tools available today.

Symptoms and assessment

The caveats mentioned previously in regard to the diagnosis of depression are also applicable to bipolar disorder when it is of the mixed type. The diagnosis of mania or hypomania is the critical element and this follows the *DSM-IV* criteria. However, in some cases, the clinician may need to differentiate between a manic or hypomanic episode and the classic MS symptom of euphoria (discussed later).

Treatment

Treatment of bipolar disorder in MS is at present based on anecdotal experience as there are no controlled studies on which to lean. Persons with MS generally respond to outpatient therapy with appropriate psychopharmacologic agents, although in extreme cases hospitalization may be needed. In addition, psychotherapy and family counseling may be helpful in assisting the patient and family to deal with the ramifications of this troubling condition.

Euphoria

Although euphoria may in some instances be confused with mania, it is a distinct clinical entity quite characteristic of MS. Although at one time it was thought to be common in MS, modern estimates place its prevalence at around 10% (Fishman et al., 2004). Euphoric patients are unrealistically optimistic and unconcerned, often in the face of devastating circumstances (Minden, 1999) and may appear excessively cheerful. Euphoria is generally seen in patients with moderate to severe physical disability, extensive brain lesions, and, particularly, cognitive impairment.

Euphoria and its associated conditions, for example, cognitive impairment, can place great stress on the family and euphoric patients may be, in certain circumstances, a danger to themselves because of their poor grasp of their situation and cognitive impairment. Unfortunately there is no recognized treatment for euphoria, although family counseling may be helpful in coping with the situation. When neuropsychiatric symptoms that accompany euphoria such as disinhibition, lack of insight, cognitive impairment, and disagreeableness (Fishman et al., 2004) become serious, these symptoms can be treated, although the literature is at present silent on the efficacy of such treatment.

Emotional Lability

The issue of "mood swings" is a frequent and often troubling one for people with MS and their families. The term *emotional lability* is used rather loosely and can refer to a wide variety of behaviors ranging from mild bouts of irritability and/or sadness to extreme fluctuations in mood. When these mood swings are extreme and beyond the individual's control, they may be referred to as emotional lability.

Emotional lability involves rapid, sudden, and extreme changes in mood that seem to be out of proportion to the situation. They may pass as quickly as they appear and be followed by long periods of relative calm. The emotions expressed could include anger, irritability, sadness, despair, happiness, or other emotions. There is almost always a specific precipitating event or set of events and the emotions expressed are appropriate to the event but exaggerated in terms of intensity and expression.

It is not known how common this phenomenon is among people with MS and it can be difficult to distinguish it from more normal reactions to life stress. It has been hypothesized that emotional lability is caused by lesions in those parts of the brain responsible for the control and expression of emotion, but data testing this idea are lacking at present (LaRocca, 2000).

In addressing emotional lability, it is generally useful to help the family understand that these outbursts are likely to be manifestations of the disease and not readily controlled by the individual. In some cases it may be possible to work with the person who has MS to develop strategies to minimize the impact of emotional lability. These strategies may include building greater awareness of the warning signs that an emotional flare-up is in the offing, learning stress management techniques to help interrupt the flare-up, avoiding situations that tend to trigger these episodes, and removing oneself from the scene when an episode begins in order to avoid untoward social repercussions. In some cases, mood-stabilizing drugs may be useful (Iannaccone and Ferini-Strambi, 1996).

Pseudobulbar Affect

Although sometimes confused with emotional lability, pseudobulbar affect is a more serious and extreme condition in which uncontrollable bouts of laughing and/or crying arise suddenly and without warning and seem to have no connection to the actual feelings of the individual or the current situation. It is as though the experience of emotions and the expression of emotions have become disconnected. Pseudobulbar affect can be extremely upsetting and embarrassing to both patient and family and can disrupt social situations in a way that is uniquely awkward.

At one time it was thought that pseudobulbar affect was a very common symptom in MS, but recent work has estimated the prevalence to be around 10% (Feinstein et al., 1997). Disease characteristics associated with pseudobulbar affect include longer duration of MS, greater physical disability, a progressive course, and cognitive impairment (Feinstein et al., 1997).

Pseudobulbar affect is not unique to MS and has been reported in amyotrophic lateral sclerosis, stroke, Alzheimer's disease, and other disorders. It is now widely accepted that pseudobulbar affect is the result of insult to the structural integrity of the brain in which voluntary control of the expression of emotion becomes partially or completely disconnected from the experience of emotion. MRI studies with MS patients have identified a number of associations with pseudobulbar affect, including lesions in the prefrontal cortex (Feinstein et al., 1999), bilateral medial inferior frontal, left medial superior frontal, bilateral inferior parietal, and brain stem (Ghaffer et al., 2008).

Studies with MS patients have shown benefits from treatment with amitriptyline (Schiffer et al., 1985) and fluoxetine (Seliger et al., 1992). Mood stabilizing drugs have also been suggested as a possible treatment (Udaka et al, 1984). With the right treatment it is possible to achieve complete elimination of symptoms. (Feinstein, 2007). A potential new treatment combines dextromethorphan with quinidine (Zenvia). In a double-blind study this combination was shown to reduce episodes of laughing and crying and improve quality of life (Panitch et al., 2006). As of this writing, the sponsor was completing phase III studies of the drug with FDA filing expected in the next few months.

Anxiety

Compared to depression, anxiety has received relatively little attention from MS researchers. However, clinical experience indicates that anxiety in various forms tends to be a major feature of the experience of living with MS and that it begins with the very first symptoms, long before a diagnosis is established. There are many obvious drivers for MS-related anxiety, including uncertainty, unpredictability, physical and psychological limitations, social and financial strain, exacerbations, and the complexities of treatment.

Feinstein et al. (1999) found that one in four MS patients who attended an outpatient neurology clinic reported significant symptoms of anxiety. Korostil and Feinstein (2007) determined the lifetime prevalence of several anxiety disorders, including generalized anxiety disorder (18.6%), panic disorder (10.0%), obsessive-compulsive disorder (8.6%), and social phobia (7.8%). With the exception of social phobia, these figures were significantly higher than those for the general population. Hyphantis et al. (2008) found that patients with recent onset MS were more likely that those with long-standing MS to be assessed with a wide variety of psychiatric diagnoses.

An extremely important issue in MS is the relationship between anxiety, depression, and suicidal ideation and action. Quesnel and Feinstein (2004) found that the combination of depression with anxiety was associated with increased suicidal ideation. Other vulnerable times tend to be when disease activity flares up during exacerbation.

The reasons for the high frequency of anxiety disorders in MS are unclear. There are a number of obvious factors at work such as the unpredictability of MS, uncertainty about the future, financial insecurity, social and family strain, changes in self image, and so on. However, some researchers have suggested that at least some of the personality change observed in MS may be due to direct effects of MS such as cerebral atrophy (Benedict et al., 2008). Research concerning this aspect of MS is at a relatively early stage of development and for the time being, there are truly more questions than answers.

Appropriate treatment of anxiety and anxiety disorders in MS requires adequate screening and diagnosis. The first step as always is to open a dialogue concerning what has been happening in a patient's life and how he or she has been handling things. Referral to a mental health professional is a logical next step in order to do a more in-depth assessment. From there, treatment may be recommended and may include medication, psychotherapy,

and/or supportive counseling. There is a massive literature on the pharmacologic treatment of anxiety disorders in the general population but unfortunately no studies specific to MS. However, there is every reason to believe that standard treatments should work as well in MS.

Short-term psychotherapy can be useful, particularly when oriented toward problem-solving strategies. Support groups or other supportive models may also be helpful, particularly those that offer dialogue with peers. Because MS is relapsing-remitting for most people, at least at onset, psychotherapy and supportive counseling can be conceptualized as a cyclical process in which feelings and issues related to the disease are successfully worked through until a flare-up occurs, at which point the process repeats itself.

Since MS is a disease that affects the family as well as the patient, family counseling or, in some cases, individual psychotherapy or counseling for family members may be useful. There is also a wide range of other treatment options to address specific issues in MS such as rehabilitation, vocational counseling, financial planning, and so on. These other interventions may yield additional benefits in terms of relieving some of the underlying causes of anxiety.

REFERENCES

Allen DN, Goldstein G, Heyman RA, Rondinelli T. Teaching memory strategies to persons with multiple sclerosis. *J Rehabil Res Dev.* 1998;35(4):405–410.

Amato MP, Ponziani G, Siracusa G, Sorbi S. Cognitive dysfunction in early-onset multiple sclerosis: a reappraisal after 10 years. *Arch Neurol.* 2001;58(10):1602–1606.

Amato MP, Zipoli V, Goretti B, et al. Benign multiple sclerosis: cognitive, psychological and social aspects in a clinical cohort. *J Neurol.* 2006;253:1054–1059.

Amato MP, Zipoli V, Portaccio E. Cognitive changes in multiple sclerosis. *Exp Rev Neurother.* 2008a;8:1585–1596.

Amato MP, Portaccio E, Stromillo ML, et al. Cognitive assessment and quantiative magnetic resonance metrics can help to identify benign multiple sclerosis. *Neurology.* 2008b;71:632–638.

Arnett PA, Rao SM, Bernardin L, Grafman J, Yetkin FZ, Lobeck L. Relationship between frontal lobe lesions and Wisconsin Card Sorting Test performance in patients with multiple sclerosis. *Neurology.* 1994;44: 420–425.

Arnett PA, Higginson CI, Voss WD, Bender WI, Wurst JM, Tippin JM. Depression in multiple sclerosis: relationship to working memory capacity. *Neuropsychology.* 1999;13(4):548–556.

Avasarala JR, Cross AH, Trinkaus, K. Comparative assessment of the Yale Single Question and Beck Depression Inventory Scale in screening for depression in multiple sclerosis. *Mult Scler.* 2003;9:307–310.

Bagert B, Camplair P, Bourdette D. Cognitive dysfunction in multiple sclerosis : natural history, pathophysiology and management. *CNS Drugs.* 2002;16(7): 445–455.

Balsimelli S, Mendes MF, Bertolucci PH, Tilbery CP. Attention impairment associated with relapsing-remitting multiple sclerosis patients with mild incapacity. *Arq Neuro-Psiquiatr.* 2007;65(2A):262–267.

Barak Y, Achiron A. Effect of interferon-beta-1b on cognitive functions in multiple sclerosis. *Eur Neurol.* 2002; 47(1):11–14.

Beatty WW, Paul RH, Wilbanks SL, Hames KA, Blanco CR, Goodkin DE. Identifying multiple sclerosis patients with mild or global cognitive impairment using the Screening Examination for Cognitive Impairment (SEFCI). *Neurology.* 1995;45(4):718–723.

Beck AT, Steer RA, Brown GK. *BDI-Fast Screen for Medical Patients Manual.* San Antonio, TX: The Psychological Corporation; 2000.

Benedict RH, Bakshi R, Simon JH, Priore R, Miller C, Munschauer F. Frontal cortex atrophy predicts cognitive impairment in multiple sclerosis. *J Neuropsychiatry Clin Neurosci.* 2002a;14(1):44–51.

Benedict RH, Cox D, Thompson LL, Foley R, Weinstock-Guttman B, Munschauer F. Reliable screening for neuropsychological impairment in multiple sclerosis. *Mult Scler.* 2004;10(6):675–678.

Benedict RH, Fischer JS, Archibald CJ, et al. Minimal neuropsychological assessment of MS patients; a consensus approach. *Clin Neuropsychol.* 2002b;16: 381–397.

Benedict RH, Fishman I, McClellan MM, Bakshi R, Weinstock-Guttman B. Validity of the Beck Depression Inventory-Fast Screen in multiple sclerosis. *Mult Scler.* 2003b;9:393–396.

Benedict RH, Hussein S, Englert J, et al. (2008). Cortical atrophy and personality in multiple sclerosis. *Neuropsychology.* 2008;22(4):432–441.

Benedict RH, Munschauer F, Linn R, Miller C, Murphy E, Foley F, Jacobs L. Screening for multiple sclerosis cognitive impairment using a self-administered 15-item questionnaire. *Mult Scler.* 2003a;9:95–101.

Benedict RH, Shapiro A, Priore R, Miller C, Munschauer F, Jacobs L. Neuropsychological counseling improves social behavior in cognitively-iimpaired multiple sclerosis patients. *Mult Scler.* 2000;6(6):391–396.

Bobholz JA, Rao SM. Cognitive dysfunction in multiple sclerosis: a review of recent developments. *Curr Opin Neurol.* 2003;16:283–288.

Boringa JB, Lazeron RHC, Reuling IEW, et al. The Brief Repeatable Battery of Neuropsychological Tests: normative values allow application in multiple sclerosis practice. *Mult Scler.* 2001;7:263–267.

Brenk A, Laun K, Haase CG. Short-term cognitive training improves mental efficiency and mood in patients with multiple sclerosis. *Eur Neurol.* 2008;60(6):304–309.

Charcot J-M. *Lectures on the Diseases of the Nervous System Delivered at La Salpetriere.* London: New Sydenham Society; 1877.

Christodoulou, C, Krupp, LB, Liang, Z, et al. Cognitive performance and MR markers of cerebral injury in cognitively impaired MS patients. *Neurology.* 2003; 60(11):1793–1798.

Chwastiak L, Ehde DM, Gibbon LE, Sullivan M, Bowen JD, Kraft GH. Depressive symptoms and severity of illness in multiple sclerosis: epidemiologic study of a large community sample. *Am J Psychiatry.* 2002; 159(11):1862–1868.

Comi, G, Filippi, M, Martinelli, V, et al. Brain MRI correlates of cognitive impairment in primary and secondary progressive multiple sclerosis. *J Neurol Sci.* 1995; 132:222–227.

Cottrell SS, Wilson SAK. The affective symptomatology of disseminated sclerosis. *J Neurol Psychopathol.* 1926; 7:1–30.

DeLuca J. What do we know about cognitive changes? In: LaRocca N, Kalb R, eds. *Multiple sclerosis: Understanding the Cognitive Challenges.* New York: Demos Medical Publishing; 2006: pp. 17–40.

DeLuca J, Chelune GJ, Tulsky D, Lengenfelder J, Chiaravalloti ND. Is processing speed or working memory the primary information processing deficit in multiple sclerosis? *J Clin Exp Neuropsychol.* 2004; 26(4):550–562.

DeLuca J, Gaudino E, Diamond BJ, Christodoulou C, Engel RA. Acquisition and storage deficits in multiple sclerosis. *J Clin Exp Neuropsychol.* 1998;20:376–390.

Ehrenreich H, Fischer B, Norra C, et al. Exploring recombinant erythropoietin in chronic progressive multiple sclerosis. *Brain.* 2007;130:2577–2588.

Fassbender K, Schmidt R, Mössner R. Mood disorders and dysfunction of the hypothalamic-pituitary-adrenal axis in multiple sclerosis: association with cerebral inflammation. *Arch Neurol.* 1998;55(1):66–72.

Feinstein A. *The Clinical Neuropsychiatry of Multiple Sclerosis.* 2nd ed. New York: Cambridge University Press; 2007.

Feinstein A, Kartsounis LD, Miller DH, Youl BD, Ron MA. Clinically isolated lesions of the type seen in multiple sclerosis: a cognitive, psychiatric, and MRI follow up study. *J Neurol, Neurosurg Psychiatry.* 1992;55: 869–876.

Feinstein A, Feinstein KJ, Gray T, O'Connor P. The prevalence and neurobehavioral correlates of pathological laughter and crying in multiple sclerosis. *Arch Neurol.* 1997;54:1116–1121.

Feinstein A, O'Connor P, Gray T, Feinstein K. The effects of anxiety on psychiatric morbidity in patients with multiple sclerosis. *Mult Scler.* 1999;5:323–326.

Feinstein A, Roy P, Lobaugh N, Feinstein KJ, O'Connor P. Structural brain abnormalities in multiple sclerosis patients with major depression. *Neurology.* 2004;62: 586–590.

Feinstein A, O'Connor P, Feinstein KJ. Multiple sclerosis, interferon beta-1b and depression: a prospective investigation. *J Neurol.* 2002;249:815–820.

Fischer JS, Priore RL, Jacobs LD, et al. Neuropsychological effects of interferon beta-1a in relapsing multiple sclerosis. Multiple Sclerosis Collaborative Research Group. Ann Neurol. 2000;48(6):885–892.

Fishman I, Benedict RHB, Bakshi R, Priore R, Weinstock-Guttman B. Construct validity and frequency of euphoria sclerotica in multiple sclerosis. J Neuropsychiatry Clin Neurosci. 2004;16:350–356.

Foley FW, Bedell JR, LaRocca NG, Scheinberg LC, Reznikoff M. Efficacy of stress-inoculation training in coping with multiple sclerosis. J Consul Clin Psychol. 1987;55:919–922.

Foley FW, Traugott U, LaRocca NG. et al. A prospective study of depression and immune dysregulation in multiple sclerosis. Arch Neurol. 1992;49:238–244.

Folstein MF, Folstein SE, McHugh PR. Mini-mental state: a practical method for grading the cognitive state of patients for the clinician. J Psychiatric Res. 1975;12:189–198.

Fredrikson S, Cheng Q, Jiang GX, Wasserman D. Elevated suicide risk among patients with multiple sclerosis in Sweden. Neuroepidemiology. 2003;22(2):146–152.

Genova HM, Hillary FG, Wylie G, Rypma B, DeLuca J. Examination of processing speed deficits in multiple sclerosis using functional magnetic resonance imaging. Int J Neuropsychol Soc. 2009;15:383–393.

Ghaffar O, Chamelian L, Feinstein A. The neuroanatomy of pseudobulbar affect: a quantitative MRI study in multiple sclerosis. J Neurol. 2008;255(3):406–412.

Goldman Consensus Group. The Goldman consensus statement on depression in multiple sclerosis. Mult Scler. 2005;11:328–337.

Harel Y, Appleboim N, Lavie M, Achiron A. Single dose of methylphenidate improves cognitive performance in multiple sclerosis patients with impaired attention process. J Neurol Sci. 2009;276(1–2):38–40.

Hyphantis TN, Christou K, Kontoudaki S, et al. Disability status, disease parameters, defense styles, and ego strength associated with psychiatric complications of multiple sclerosis. Int J Psychiatry Med. 2008;38(3):307–327.

Iannaccone S, Ferini-Strambi L. Pharmacologic treatment of emotional lability. Clin Neuropharmacol. 1996;19(6):532–535.

Joffe RT, Lippert GP, Gray TA, Sawa G, Horvath Z. Mood disorder and multiple sclerosis. Arch Neurol. 1987;44(4):376–378.

Jønsson A, Korfitzen EM, Heltberg A, Ravnborg MH, Byskov-Ottosen E. Effects of neuropsychological treatment in patients with multiple sclerosis. Acta Neurol Scand. 1993;88(6):394–400.

Kalmar JH, Gaudino EA, Moore NB, Halper J, DeLuca J. The relationship between cognitie deficits and everyday functional activities in multiple sclerosis. Neuropsychology. 2008;22(4):442–449.

Khan F, Pallant JF, Brand C, Kilpatrick TJ. Effectiveness of rehabilitation intervention in persons with multiple sclerosis. J Neurol Neurosurg Psychiatry. 2008;79(11):1230–1235.

Korostil M, Feinstein A. Anxiety disorders and their clinical correlates in multiple sclerosis patients. Mult Scler. 2007;13:67–72.

Krupp LB, Christodoulou C, Melville P, Scherl WF, MacAllister WS, Elkins LE. Donepezil improved memory in multiple sclerosis in a randomized clinical trial. Neurology. 2004;63(9):1552–1553.

Kurtzke JF. Neurologic impairment in multiple sclerosis and the disability status scale. Acta Neurol Scand. 1970;46:493–512.

Lachs MS, Feinstein AR, Cooney LM, Jr., et al. A simple procedure for general screening for functional disability in elderly patients. Ann Intern Med. 1990;112(9):699–706.

LaRocca N. Cognitive and emotional disorders. In: Burks JS, Johnson KP, eds. Multiple Sclerosis: Diagnosis, Medical Management, and Rehabilitation. New York: Demos Medical Publishing; 2000: 405–424.

LaRocca N, Caruso L. Assessment of cognitive changes. In: LaRocca N, Kalb R, eds. Multiple Sclerosis: Understanding the Cognitive Challenges. New York: Demos Medical Publishing; 2006: 42–45.

Lazeron RH, de Sonneville LM, Scheltens P, Polman CH, Barkhof F. Mult Scler. 2006;12:760–768.

Lincoln NB, Dent A, Harding J, et al. Evaluation of cognitive assessment and cognitive intervention for people with multiple sclerosis. J Neurol Neurosurg Psychiatry. 2002;72(1):93–98.

Lovera J, Bagert B, Smoot K, et al. Ginkgo biloba for the improvement of cognitive performance in multiple sclerosis: a randomized, placebo-controlled trial. Mult Scler. 2007;13(3):376–385.

Macniven JA, Davis C, Ho MY, Bradshaw CM, Szabadi E, Constantinescu CS. Stroop performance in multiple sclerosis; information processing, selective attention, or executive functioning? J Int Neuropsychol Soc. 2008;14(5):805–814.

Mattingly G, Baker K, Zorumski CF, Figiel GS. Multiple sclerosis and ECT: Possible value of gadolinium-enhanced magnetic resonance scans for identifying high-risk patients. J Neuropsychiatry Clin Neurosci. 1992;4(2):145–151.

McIntosh-Michaelis SA, Roberts MH, Wilkinson SM, et al. The prevalence of cognitive impairment in a communitiy survey of multiple sclerosis. Br J Clin Psychol. 1991;30(pt 4):333–348.

Mendozzi L, Pugnetti L. Computer assisted memory retraining of patients with multiple sclerosis. Ital J Neurol Sci. 1998;19:S431–S438.

Minden S. Treatment of mood and affective disorders. In: Rudick R, Goodkind D, eds. Multiple Sclerosis Therapeutics. New York: Martin Dunitz; 1999: 517–541.

Minden SL, Orav J, Reich P. Depression in multiple sclerosis. Gen Hosp Psychiatry. 1987;9(6):426–434.

Minden SL, Orav J, Schildkraut JJ. Hypomanic reactions to ACTH and prednisone treatment for multiple sclerosis. Neurology. 1988;38:1631–1634.

Minden SL, Schiffer RB. Affective disorders in multiple sclerosis: review and recommendations for clinical research. Arch Neurol. 1990;47:98–104.

Mohr DC, Goodkin DE, Likosky W, Gatto N, Baumann KA, Rudick RA. Treatment of depression improves adherence to interferon beta-1b therapy for multiple sclerosis. *Arch Neurol.* 1997;54:531–533.

Mohr DC, Boudewyn AC, Goodkin D, Bostrom A, Epstein L. Comparative outcomes for individual cognitive-behavior therapy, supportive-expressive therapy, and sertraline for the treatment of depression in multiple sclerosis. *J Consult Clin Psychol.* 2001;69:942–949.

Mohr DC, Likosky W, Bertagnolli A, et al. Telephone-administered cognitive-behavioral therapy for the treatment of depressive symptoms in multiple sclerosis. *J Consult Clin Psychol.* 2000;68(2):356–361.

Morrow SA, Kaushik T, Zarevics P, Erlanger D, Bear MF, Munschauer FE. The effects of L-amphetamine on cognition in MS patients: results of a randomized controlled trial. *J Neurol.* 2009;256:1432–1459.

Nebel K, Wiese H, Seyfarth J, et al. Activity of attention related structures in multiple sclerosis patients. *Brain Res.* 2007;1151:150–160.

Nyenhuis DL, Luchetta T, Yamamoto C, et al. The development, standardization, and initial validation of the Chicago Multiscale Depression Inventory. *J Personality Assess.* 1998;70(2):386–401.

Oliveri RL, Sibilia G, Valentino P, Russo C, Romeo N, Quattrone A. Pulsed methylprednisolone induces a reversible impairment of memory in patients with relapsing-remitting multiple sclerosis. *Acta Neurol Scand.* 1998;97(6):366–369.

Panitch, H.S., Thisted, R.A., Smith, R.A., Wynn, D.R., Wymer, J.P., Achiron, A, Vollmer, T.L., Mandler, R.N., Dietrich, D.W., Fletcher, M., Pope, L.E., Berg, J.E., Miller, A. Psuedobulbar Affect in Multiple Sclerosis Study Group. Randomized, controlled trial of dextromethorphan/quinidine for pseudobulbar affect in multiple sclerosis. *Ann Neurol.* 2006;59(5):780–787.

Parmenter BA, Denney DR, Lynch SG, Middleton LS, Harlan LM. Cognitive impairment in patients with multiple sclerosis: association with the APOE gene and promoter polymorphisms. *Mult Scler.* 2007;13:25–32.

Patten SB. Psychiatric side effects of interferon treatment. *CDS.* 2006;1(2):143–150.

Patten SB, Beck CA, Williams JVA, et al. Major depression in multiple sclerosis: a population-based perspective. *Neurology.* 2003;61:1524–1527.

Patten SB, Lavorato DH, Metz LM. Clinical correlates of CES-D depressive symptom ratings in an MS population. *Gen Hosp Psychiatry.* 2005;27:439–445.

Patten SB, Metz LM, SPECTRIMS Study Group. Interferon beta-1a and depression in secondary progressive MS: data from the SPECTRIMS trial. *Neurology.* 2002;59(5):744–746.

Patten SB, Metz LM, Reimer MA. Biopsychosocial correlates of lifetime major depression in a multiple sclerosis population. *Mult Scler.* 2000;6:115–120.

Patzold T, Schwengelbeck M, Ossege LM, Malin JP, Sindern E. Changes of the MS functional composite and EDSS during and after treatment of relapses with methylprednisolone in patients with multiple sclerosis. *Acta Neurol Scand.* 2002;105(3):164–168.

Paul RH, Beatty WW, Schneider R, Blanco C, Hames K. Impairments of attention in individuals with multiple sclerosis. *Mult Scler.* 1998;4(5):433–439.

Peyser JM, Edwards KR, Poser CM, Filskov SB. Cognitive function in patients with multiple sclerosis. *Arch Neurol.* 1980;377:577–579.

Peyser JM, Rao SM, LaRocca NG, Kaplan E. Guidelines for neuropsychological research in multiple sclerosis. *Arch Neurol.* 1990;47:94–97.

Piras MR, Magnano I, Canu ED, et al. *J Neurol Neurosurg Psychiatry.* 2003;74:878–885.

Pliskin NH, Hamer DP, Goldstein DS, et al. Improved delayed visual reproduction test performance in multiple sclerosis patients receiving interferon beta-1b. *Neurology.* 1996;47(6):1463–1468.

Plohmann AM, Kappos L, Ammann W, et al. Computer assisted retraining of attentional impairments in patients with multiple sclerosis. *J Neurol Neurosur Psychiatry.* 1998;64(4):455–462.

Pozzilli C, Bastianello S, Padovani A, et al. Anterior corpus callosum atrophy and verbal fluency in multiple sclerosis. *Cortex.* 1991;27:441–445.

Prakash RS, Erickson KI, Snook EM, Colcombe SJ, Motl, RW, Kramer AF. Cortical recruitment during selective attention in multiple sclerosis: an fMRI investigation of individual differences. *Neuropsychologia.* 2008;46(12):2888–2895.

Quesnel S, Feinstein A. Multiple sclerosis and alcohol: a study of problem drinking. *Mult Scler.* 2004;10:197–201.

Randolph JJ, Arnett PA, Higginson CI, Voss WD. Neurovegetative symptoms in multiple sclerosis: relationship to depressed mood, fatigue and physical disability. *Arch Clin Neuropsychol.* 2000;15:387–398.

Rao SM, Hammeke TA, Speech TJ. Wisconsin Card Sorting Test performance in relapsing-remitting and chronic-progressive multiple sclerosis. *J Consult Clin Psychol.* 1987;55(2):263–265.

Rao SM, Leo GJ, Bernardin L, Unverzagt F. Cognitive dysfunction in multiple sclerosis: frequency, patterns and prediction. *Neurology.* 1991;41:685–691.

Rao SM, Leo GJ, Haughton VM, St. Aubin-Faubert P, Bernardin L. Correlation of magnetic resonance imaging with neuropsychological testing in multiple sclerosis. *Neurology.* 1989;39:161–166.

Rasmussen KG, Keegan BM. Electroconvulsive therapy in patients with multiple sclerosis. *J ECT.* 2007;23(3):179–180.

Rodgers D, Khoo K, MacEachen M, Oven M, Beatty WW. Cognitive therapy for multiple sclerosis: a preliminary study. *Altern Ther Health Med.* 1996;2(5):70–74.

Roosendaal SD, Moraal B, Pouwels PJ, et al. Accumulation of cortical lesions in MS: relation with cognitive impairment. *Mult Scler.* 2009;15:708–714.

Rovaris M, Riccitelli G, Judica, E, et al. Cognitive impairment and strutural brain damage in benign multiple sclerosis. *Neurology.* 2008;71:1521–1526.

Ryan L, Clark CM, Klonoff H, Li D, Paty D. Patterns of cognitive impairment in relapsing-remitting multiple sclerosis and their relationship to neuropathology on magnetic resonance images. *Neuropsychology.* 1996;10: 176–193.

Sadovnick AD, Eisen K, Ebers GC, Paty DW. Cause of death in patients attending multiple sclerosis clinics. *Neurology.* 1991;41(8):1193–1196.

Savettieri, G, Messina, D, Andreoli, V, et al. Gender-related effect of clinical and genetic variables on the cognitive impairment in multiple sclerosis. *Neurology.* 2004;251: 1208–1214.

Schiffer RB, Herndon RM, Rudick RA. Treatment of pathologic laughing and weeping with amitriptyline. *N Engl J Med.* 1985;312:1480–1482.

Schiffer RB, Weitkamp LR, Wineman M, Guttormsen S. Multiple sclerosis and affective disorder: family history, sex and HLA-DR antigens. *Arch Neurol.* 1988; 45:1345–1348.

Schiffer RB, Wineman NM. Antidepressant pharmacotherapy of depression associated with multiple sclerosis. *Am J Psychiatry.* 1990;147(11):1493–1497.

Schiffer RB, Wineman M, Weitkamp LR. Association between bipolar affective disorder and multiple sclerosis. *Am J Psychiatry.* 1986;143:94–95.

Schultheis MT, DeLuca J, Garay E. The influence of cognitive impairment on driving performance in multiple sclerosis. *Neurology.* 2001;56:1089–1094.

Schultheis MT, Garay E, Millis SR, DeLuca J. Motor vehicle crashes and violations among drivers with multiple sclerosis. *Arch Phys Med Rehabil.* 2002;83:1175–1178.

Seliger GM, Hornstein A, Flax J, Herbert J, Schroder K. Fluoxetine improves emotional incontinence. *Brain Injury.* 1992;6:267–270.

Shawaryn MA, Schultheis MT, Garay E, DeLuca J. Assessing functional status: The relationship between the Multiple Sclerosis Functional Composite and driving. *Arch Phys Med Rehabil.* 2002;83(8):1123–1129.

Shepko AG, Hollenbeck MA. Comparison of treatment duration for remediation of memory impairment in individuals with multiple sclerosis. *Mult Scler.* 1997; 3:208.

Shi J, Zhao CB, Vollmer TL, Tyry TM, Kuniyoshi SM. APOE epsilon 4 allele is associated with cognitive impairment in patients with multiple sclerosis. *Neurology.* 2008;70:185–190.

Sicotte NL, Giesser BS, Tandon V, et al. Testosterone treatment in multiple sclerosis: a pilot study. *Arch Neurol.* 2007;64:683–688.

Sicotte NL, Ker, KC, Giesser BS, et al. Regional hippocampal atrophy in multiple sclerosis. *Brain.* 2008;131: 1134–1141.

Simioni S, Ruffieux C, Kleeberg J, et al. Progressive decline of decision-making performances during multiple sclerosis. *J Int Neuropsychol Soc.* 2009;15(2): 291–295.

Solari A, Motta A, Mendozzi L, et al. Computer-aided retraining of memory and attention in people with multiple sclerosis: a randomized, double-blind controlled trial. *J Neurol Sci.* 2004;222(1–2):99–104.

Stephenson, J., Kamat, S., Rajagopalan, K. Agarwal, S. Singer, J. Early Effects of Natalizumab on Patient Reported Fatigue and Cognitive Function. Poster presented at the annual meeting of the American Academy of Neurology, 2009:(P02.142), Seattle, WA.

Strober L, Englert J, Munschauer F, weinstock-Guttman B, Rao S, Benedict R. Sensitivity of conventional memory tests in multiple sclerosis: comparing the Rao Brief Repeatable Neuropsychological Battery and the Minimal Assessment of Cognitive Function in MS. *Mult Scler.* 2009;15(9):1077–1084.

Tesar N, Bandion K, Baumhackl U. Efficacy of a neuropsychological training programme for patients with multiple sclerosis—a randomized trial. *Wiener Klinische Wochenschrift.* 2005;117(21–22):747–754.

Turner AP, Williams RM, Bowen JD, Kiviahan DR, Haselkorn JK. Suicidal ideation in multiple sclerosis. *Arch Phys Med Rehabil.* 2006;87(8):1073–1078.

Udaka F, Yamao S, Nagata H, Nakamura S, Kameyama M. Pathologic laughing and crying treated with levadopa. *Arch Neurol.* 1984;41:1095–1096.

Uttner I, Tumani H. Effects of high-dose cortisone therapy on cognition. *Nervenarzt.* 2006;77(6):647–648, 650–651.

Villoslada P, Arrondo G, Sepulcre J, Alegre M, Artieda J. Memantine induces reversible neurologic impairment in patients with MS. *Neurology.* 2009;72(19):1630–1633.

Weinstein A, Schwid SR, Schiffer RB, McDermott MP, Giang DW, Goodman AD. Neuropsychologic status in multiple sclerosis after treatment with glatiramer. *Arch Neurol.* 1999;56(3):319–324.

Wilken JA, Kane R, Sullivan CL, et al. The utility of computerized neuropsychological assessment of cognitive dysfunction in patients with relapsing-remitting multiple sclerosis. *Mult Scler.* 2003;9:119–127.

Wilken JA, Wallin MT, Sullivan CL, et al. An interim analysis of combination therapy (modafinil [PROVIGIL®] + interferon β-1a [AVONEX®] in the treatment of cognitive problems in patients with relapsing-remitting MS. Poster presented at: Annual Meeting of the Consortium of Multiple Sclerosis Centers; June, 2004; Ontario, Canada.

Wishart H, Sharpe D. Neuropsychological aspects of multiple sclerosis: a quantitative review. *J Clin Exp Neuropsychol.* 1997;19:810–824.

Zéphir H, De Seze J, Stojkovic T, et al. Multiple sclerosis and depression: influence of interferon beta therapy. *Mult Scler.* 2003;9:284–288.

Zéphir H, de Seze J, Dujardin K, et al. One-year cyclophosphamide treatment combined with methylprednisolone improves cognitive dysfunction in progressive forms of multiple sclerosis. *Mult Scler.* 2005;11: 360–363.

Zorzon M, de Masi R, Nasuelli D, et al. Depression and anxiety in multiple sclerosis: a clinical and MRI study in 95 subjects. *J Neurol.* 2001;248(5):416–421.

Lauren B. Krupp, Yashma Patel, and Christopher Christodoulou

Fatigue is an overwhelming problem for most patients with multiple sclerosis (MS). Fatigue was reported by 83% of a U.S. population-based MS cohort, and it was the most common symptom of the disease (Minden et al., 2006). Seventy-four percent reported severe fatigue in another large survey (North American Research Committee on Multiple Sclerosis, NARCOMS) (Hadjimichael et al., 2008). Patients often rate fatigue as the single most troubling aspect of the disorder, and it can be the presenting symptom at time of diagnosis (Krupp et al., 1988). The consequences of MS fatigue include unemployment (Smith and Arnett, 2005; Hadjimichael et al., 2008; Julian et al., 2008), and fatigue is closely tied to a reduced quality of life (Amato et al., 2001). The pathophysiology of MS fatigue remains poorly understood. While primary MS fatigue is thought to result from the central nervous system (CNS) and immune dysfunction associated with the disorder, additional disease features may contribute to fatigue, including sleep disturbance and depression (Scwhartz et al., 1996; Strober and Arnett, 2005). However, fatigue is also reported among some patients without depressive symptomatology (Chwastiak et al., 2005). Treatment remains difficult, but exercise programs, physical activity, and cognitive behavior therapy can be effective (Motl et al., 2005; McCullagh et al., 2008; Sauter et al., 2008; van Kessel et al., 2008). Some medications can also attenuate fatigue. Overall, our understanding and treatment of MS fatigue remains incomplete. Further elucidation of the pathophysiology of fatigue should hopefully lead to more effective interventions.

DEFINITION

Fatigue can be defined as either a subjective feeling experienced by an individual or as a performance decrement observed during behavior (e.g., a decrease in performance over time) (Wessely et al., 1998). In 1998, the Multiple Sclerosis Council for Clinical Practice Guidelines established a consensus definition of fatigue as a "subjective lack of physical and/or mental energy that is perceived by the individual or caregiver to interfere with usual and desired activities" (Mutltiple Sclerosis Council for Clinical Practice, 1998). The Council distinguished chronic from acute fatigue that may follow from temporary circumstances such as physical exertion or hot weather. Chronic persistent fatigue was defined as fatigue present for any amount of time on 50% of days for more than 6 weeks, which limits functional activities or quality of life. Acute fatigue was defined as a new or significant increase in feelings of fatigue in the previous 6 weeks, which limits functional activities or quality of life. The Council also conceptualized fatigue as either primary (intrinsic to the MS disease process) or secondary to chronic illness factors such as depression or poor sleep.

CONSEQUENCES OF FATIGUE

Fatigue has a number of severe complications all of which adversely affect quality of life and have socioeconomic implications. As a result of fatigue, patients will retire early (Edgley et al., 1991) or will decrease their work hours from full time to part time (Smith and Arnett, 2005). Over a 6-month period, individuals who are working have an increased risk of becoming unemployed if among other symptoms they experience fatigue (Julian et al., 2008). Of patients with moderate to severe MS, those with fatigue are less likely to be working than individuals with similar neurological severity levels who are not fatigued (Edgley et al., 1991). Use of health-care services is also influenced by fatigue. Outpatient visits, including rehabilitation services, were increased among fatigued compared to nonfatigued patients with mild levels of MS (Johansson et al., 2009).

The multiple associations with fatigue, such as with sleep disorders and limitations in social relationships (Krupp, 2004), all contribute to a lowered quality of life in patients with fatigue (Aronson, 1997; Amato et al., 2001; Janardhan and Baksi, 2002).

DEMOGRAPHIC ASSOCIATIONS WITH FATIGUE

The relationship of fatigue to demographic factors has been somewhat inconsistent in the literature, with some factors being identified in large studies that have been less evident in smaller surveys. For example, among participants in the NARCOMS survey, those with severe fatigue were more likely to be male and to be older in age (Hadjimichael et al., 2008), though such associations have not necessarily been seen in other studies (Colosimo et al., 1995; Flachenecker et al., 2002; Lerdal et al., 2003; Chwastiak et al., 2005). There is somewhat more consistency in the observation that fatigue is more severe in those with less education (Lerdal et al., 2003; Chwastiak et al., 2005; Hadjimichael et al., 2008).

CLINICAL ASSOCIATIONS WITH FATIGUE

General Disease Features

The nature of MS-related fatigue is distinct from other types of fatigue seen in either healthy individuals or in patients with other diseases. Compared to healthy adults, individuals with MS report that fatigue interferes with meeting responsibilities, comes on easily, and prevents sustained physical functioning (Krupp et al., 1988). Fatigue related to MS can also be distinguished from that of other disorders, such as the systemic lupus erythematosus, by its marked sensitivity to heat (Krupp et al., 1989).

Fatigue occurs among patients of all MS subtypes, but it is somewhat greater in patients with secondary progressive MS than those with relapsing disease (Patrick et al. 2009), and more pronounced in individuals with greater mobility impairment

(Hadjimichael et al., 2008). People with relapsing disease and accumulating impairment tend to be more fatigued than those with a relapsing, but stable disease course (Hadjimichael et al., 2008). Some work suggests that fatigue does not correlate with disability after one controls for depression (Bakshi et al., 2000). Fatigue is also not explained by disease duration (Freal et al., 1984).

One concern for individuals with MS is whether their MS therapies contribute to fatigue. In an analysis of disease-modifying therapies and fatigue among 320 consecutive patients, no relation was noted between severe fatigue and use of immunosuppressive or immunomodulating medications compared to no treatment (Putzki et al., 2008). Of 9205 MS respondents in the NARCOMS survey, no differences in fatigue severity were identified between individuals on different disease-modifying therapies. However, respondents noting medication changes in the past 6 months reported lower fatigue levels after changing from interferon beta to glatiramer acetate (Hadjimichael et al., 2008).

Unfortunately, fatigue in MS tends to persist (Patrick et al., 2009). In a 1-year longitudinal study of 2768 patients, persistence of fatigue correlated with baseline pain, severe fatigue, depressed mood, and neurological impairment (Patrick et al., 2009).

Depression

Given that fatigue is a common symptom of depression and depression is common in MS (Sadovnick et al., 1996; Patten et al, 2003; Feinstein, 2004), it is not surprising that many (though not all) MS studies have found an association between measures of depression and fatigue (Fisk et al., 1994; Möller et al., 1994; Scwhartz et al., 1996; Ford et al., 1998; Kroencke et al., 2000). The association has also been found in studies that have excluded fatigue-related items from their depression measures (Vercoulen et al., 1996; Chwastiak et al., 2005). Many of the symptoms of depression may mimic those of fatigue, such as lack of motivation, inability to complete tasks, and sleep disturbances. In turn, fatigue may contribute to patients' feelings of loss of control over their lives, often resulting in depressed mood (Scwhartz et al., 1996).

Fatigue associated with MS can be predicted from a low sense of control over one's symptoms or environment (Scwhartz et al., 1996; Vercoulen et al., 1998; Jopson and Moss-Morris, 2003; van der Werf et al., 2003; Trojan et al., 2007). Fatigue and depression can be intricately intertwined in which depression predicts later fatigue and anxiety, while anxiety and fatigue predict later depression (Brown et al., 2009). The predictive value of baseline depression for subsequent fatigue is supported by multiple studies (Johansson et al., 2008; Brown et al., 2009; Patrick et al., 2009). Despite a strong association between depression and fatigue, there are MS patients who experience severe fatigue but lack depressive symptomatology (Chwastiak et al., 2005). As such, it is helpful to consider fatigue in part as intrinsic to the disease itself.

Anxiety

Anxiety is another common affective symptom in MS (Feinstein et al., 1999). However, its relation to fatigue has not received as much attention as depression has. Even so, the data support a relatively consistent relation between anxiety and fatigue (Ford et al., 1998; Iriarte et al., 2000; Chwastiak et al., 2005; Skerrett and Moss-Morris, 2006; Trojan et al., 2007). Anxiety may be more strongly related to mental fatigue as opposed to physical fatigue (Ford et al., 1998; Trojan et al., 2007).

Sleep Disturbances

Patients with MS often have concurrent sleep disorders. Conditions such as sleep apnea, narcolepsy, rapid eye movement (REM) sleep behavior disorder (Fleming and Pollak, 2005), periodic limb movements of sleep, and restless leg syndrome are often associated with excessive daytime sleepiness and fatigue. These conditions are more frequent in MS when compared to the general population (Tachibana et al., 1994; Fleming and Pollak, 2005). For example, nocturnal movement disorders such as periodic leg movement disorders can occur in MS patients and may be associated with cerebellar lesions (Ferini-Strambi et al., 1994). Objective measures of poor sleep, including lower sleep efficiency, wake time after sleep onset, and arousal index, have also been demonstrated more abnormalities in MS patients with fatigue compared to those without (Attarian et al., 2004;

Kaynak et al., 2006). Restless leg syndrome has also been documented in MS and has been associated with poor sleep and increased fatigue (Moreira et al., 2008).

Even in the absence of an identifiable sleep disorder, MS patients may experience disrupted sleep from symptoms associated with MS. Many individuals with MS experience nocturia, which disrupts their sleep and results in daytime somnolence (Amarenco et al., 1995; Fleming and Pollak, 2005). Other symptoms that similarly may disrupt sleep include nocturnal pain, insomnia, and muscle spasms. Such symptoms could be expected to disrupt sleep during the middle of the night. In fact, in a study of 60 patients evaluated with the FSS, sleep diary, and the Epworth Sleepiness Scale, middle insomnia occurred in over half and was significantly correlated with fatigue (Stanton et al., 2006).

Pain

Patients with MS may experience many sensory disturbances, including neuralgias, dysesthesias, and painful muscle spasms. These symptoms often inhibit restful sleep, contribute to physical deconditioning, and worsen depression. All of these factors contribute to daytime somnolence and overall fatigue. Physical pain compounded by fatigue may result in a downward spiral of functional loss for many MS patients (Stanton et al., 2006; Trojan et al., 2007).

Cognition

Despite the intuitive link between the experience of fatigue and the presence of cognitive difficulties, such a link has been difficult to establish. Numerous studies have failed to find a relation between self-reported fatigue and cognitive impairment (Johnson et al., 1997; Paul et al., 1998; Krupp and Elkins, 2000; Parmenter et al., 2003; Bailer et al., 2007). It is possible that self-report measures reflect in part the greater effort required by individuals with MS to maintain their level of performance, as compared to healthy persons (Christodoulou, 2005).

Fatigability and Motor Function

Patients with MS clearly suffer from physiological motor fatigue. Deficits in the ability to sustain muscle contraction, recruit motor pathways efficiently, and maintain normal levels of muscle metabolites during exertion are present in patients with MS (Kent-Braun et al., 1994; Sharma et al., 1995; Latash et al., 1996; Sheean et al., 1997). Unfortunately, most of these motor measures have not been shown to accurately predict self-reported fatigue. This is perhaps because the subjective measure does not adequately capture the motor aspects versus the mental aspects of fatigue.

A study involving electroencephalogram (EEG) recordings indicated that the sensorimotor areas of MS patients with fatigue were hyperactive during the execution of movement and failed to become inhibited after movement was terminated (Leocani et al., 2001). The electrophysiological correlates of self-reported fatigue in MS were further explored in a study through the use of transcranial magnetic stimulation testing (Liepert et al., 2005). The study found that with performance of a fatiguing hand-grip exercise, the MS patients with fatigue displayed reduced motor cortex inhibition compared to the MS patients without fatigue and normal controls. The degree of time to normalization of the motor threshold was also correlated with the severity of fatigue. These patients appeared to have an abnormality of the primary motor cortex, indicating an association with fatigue severity and exercise-induced reduction of membrane excitability. Impairments of inhibitory cortical circuits have also been reported in various other neurological diseases such as amyotrophic lateral sclerosis, Parkinson disease, dystonia, and stroke (Liepert et al., 2005).

FATIGUE MEASUREMENT

Fatigue is generally assessed in two ways: *(1)* questionnaires asking people about their experience of fatigue, and *(2)* measures of performance change on motor or cognitive tasks, where a decline in performance over time is presumed to be due to fatigue. In the MS community, the patient's experience of fatigue tends to be more emphasized (Multiple Sclerosis Council for Clinical Practice, 1998).

Self-Report Measures

Self-report questionnaires are by far the most common method of measuring fatigue across a variety of medical disorders. These questionnaires come in a variety of forms, from single-item visual analog scales (Krupp et al., 1989) to longer multidimensional scales (Schwartz et al., 1993; Whitehead, 2009). An extensive review of fatigue measurement is available elsewhere (Christodoulou, 2005; Whitehead, 2009). Among the more common self-report scales used in MS include the Fatigue Severity Scale (FSS) (Krupp et al., 1989) and the Modified Fatigue Impact Scale (MFIS) (Multiple Sclerosis Council for Clinical Practice, 1998). Both are relatively short, have good psychometric properties, and are sensitive to changes in fatigue due to disease progression or treatment (Whitehead, 2009). The FSS was designed as a unidimensional scale, though a recent Rasch analysis indicates that the removal of four of the nine items improves the unidimensionality of the scale (Mills et al., 2009). The Modified Fatigue Impact Scale (MFIS) uses a *multidimensional* approach to differentiate dimensions of fatigue, including cognitive, physical, and psychosocial components. The physical dimension is most associated with measures of neurologic impairment such as the EDSS. However, neuropsychological measures do not correlate well with the cognitive dimension. Other multidimensional scales include the Fatigue Descriptive Scale (FDS), which identifies three modalities of fatigue by distinguishing asthenia (fatigue at rest), from fatigability (fatigue during or after exercise), and worsening symptoms with exercise (Iriarte et al., 1999). There is also the Fatigue Scale (Chalder et al., 1993; Christodoulou, 2005), which focuses on two dimensions, a physical and mental component. A cognitive behavioral therapy intervention using the FS as an outcome showed a clear treatment effect (van Kessel et al., 2008). Fatigue can also be measured within larger or more general inventories, such as the vitality items of the SF-36 (Ware, Jr. and Sherbourne, 1992; Ware, Jr., 2000), the Fatigue-Inertia scale of the Profile of Mood States ([POMS], McHair et al., 1971), or portions of the Sickness Impact Profile ([SIP], Gilson et al., 1975).

Despite the acknowledged limitations of subjective self-report measures of fatigue, these assessments are readily available to the health-care provider and their patients and can be quickly administered. However, all self-report measures are flawed in their inability to provide information about temporal factors, as well as in their susceptibility to recall bias

(Krupp and Christodoulou, 2001; Stone and Shiffman, 2002).

Performance-Based Measures

To find more objective assessment of fatigue, investigators have developed various *performance-based measures* (Schwid et al., 1999). This assessment method uses the definition of fatigue as a quantitative decline in performance over a select period of time. This approach can be applied to both tests of motor strength and of cognitive function.

Motor fatigue can be measured with an isometric strain gauge that determines the degree of force produced by muscle contraction, creating a fatigue index (the ratio between integral of muscle strength decay over time and maximal voluntary contraction). This index was consistently elevated in patients with MS, especially those with pyramidal tract dysfunction (Djaldetti et al., 1996; Krupp and Pollina, 1996). Motor fatigue during sustained contractions can be demonstrated more readily in MS patients than in normal controls (Schwid et al., 1999). Motor fatigue can also be demonstrated in terms of motor unit firing rates or muscle metabolism (Kent-Braun et al., 1994; Sharma et al., 1995; Djaldetti et al., 1996; Latash et al., 1996; Sheean et al., 1997; Schubert et al., 1998; Schwid et al., 1999).

Objective fatigue assessment techniques have also been developed that test cognitive fatigue. Performance on psychological tests was assessed before and after a continuously effortful cognitive task (Krupp and Elkins, 2000). Performance significantly declined on neuropsychological testing among MS patients in comparison to the performance decrement observed in healthy controls. The objective changes in cognitive performance did not correlate with self-reported fatigue scales, nor was there a significant difference among those with high FSS and low FSS scores (Krupp and Elkins, 2000).

NEUROIMAGING

Structural Neuroimaging

Fatigue is a multifaceted experience that does not appear to be localizable to a single area of the CNS. With conventional magnetic resonance imaging (MRI), no one region consistently is associated with fatigue and originally studies found no relation with lesion burden (van der Werf et al., 1998; Bakshi et al., 1999). However, more sophisticated methods in larger sample sizes have revealed that MS patients with fatigue compared to those without fatigue have more atrophy of the gray and white matter and higher lesion load (Marrie et al., 2005; Tedeschi et al., 2007). In a longitudinal study, brain atrophy was noted to have a positive association between global measures of fatigue (Marrie et al., 2005). Increases in fatigue over the first 2 years was associated with greater atrophy 6 years later. Unfortunately, the study was limited in that it used items from the Sickness Impact Profile as a measure of fatigue that were related more closely to "sleepiness" rather than fatigue. More experimental imaging methods—for instance, positron emission tomography (PET) (Roelcke et al., 1997), magnetic resonance spectroscopy (MRS) (Tartaglia et al., 2004), and functional MRI (Filippi et al., 2002)—have shown that several regions of the brain have been implicated in its pathophysiology. These include the brain stem, the basal ganglia, thalamus, the limbic system, and the prefrontal cortex. Hypofunction in these areas may play a role in fatigue generation (Roelcke et al., 1997). Fluoro-deoxyglucose PET has demonstrated reduced glucose metabolism in several areas in the brains of MS patients with fatigue as compared to those without (Roelcke et al., 1997). The areas affected included the basal ganglia, the internal capsule, the posterior parietal lobe, the temporo-occipital lobe, and the prefrontal area (Roelcke et al., 1997). The reduced energy metabolism in the frontal cortex and basal ganglia may indicate that fatigue is associated with an impaired interaction between these functionally related areas as a result of the neuronal damage of MS (Roelcke et al., 1997; Sepulcre et al., 2009).

It is reasonable to consider that pathways related to complex attention would be associated with fatigue. This idea was suggested by the observation that 60 nondepressed patients with MS showed an association between self-reported fatigue and lesion burden in the right parietal-temporal region white matter (specifically parietal, juxta-ventricular white matter in the parietal lobe and callosal forceps) and left frontal white matter (specifically middle-anterior corpus callosum, anterior cingulum, and the centrum semiovale of the superior and middle frontal gyri) (Sepulcre et al., 2009). Fatigue was also associated with gray matter atrophy in the left superior frontal gyrus and bilateral frontal gyri. These are regions that include networks involved in cognitive and attentional processes.

Diffuse axonal injury has been linked to MS fatigue (Tartaglia et al., 2004; Sepulcre et al., 2009). Proton magnetic resonance spectroscopy was used to measure axonal damage in the brains of MS patients based on the resonance intensity of N-acetylaspartate (NAA), a marker of neuronal integrity. A statistically significant association between the FSS and the NAA/creatine ratio was found, implicating widespread axonal injury in the pathophysiology of fatigue in MS (Tartaglia et al., 2004). It is also possible that reductions in NAA were seen secondary to impairment of mitochondrial function in the absence of neuronal loss, and that decreased mitochondrial function is the underlying mechanism for fatigue (Tartaglia et al., 2004).

Functional Neuroimaging

Magnetic resonance imaging studies also suggest a cortical functional reorganization in MS (Rocca et al., 2007). When MS patients compared to controls performed a repetitive motor task, there was increased cortical activation in both ipsi and contralateral regions compared to healthy controls (Filippi et al., 2002). In another investigation of brain activation with functional MRI, MS patients compared to controls showed limits in the degree to which brain activation could occur during a fatiguing hand-grip exercise (White et al., 2009).

PATHOGENESIS

The pathogenesis of MS fatigue has yet to be defined. Proposed mechanisms involve both motor and nonmotor systems. Alterations in endocrine, immune, metabolic, and neurochemical regulatory processes have also been implicated in the pathogenesis of fatigue.

Neuroimmune Mechanisms

Fatigue is a common feature in a variety of immune-mediated conditions such as systemic lupus erythematosus, rheumatoid arthritis, and MS. It is reasonable to consider that the immune dysregulation common to these conditions contributes to fatigue. The observation that administration of medications with predominant effects on immune function can produce fatigue (e.g., interferon betas) further supports the link between immune regulation, cytokines, and fatigue. Another line of evidence suggesting a link between the immune system and fatigue is the observation that elevations in circulating pro-inflammatory cytokines are found in fatiguing disorders such as chronic fatigue syndrome, cancer, and viral infections (Kerr et al., 2001; Kurzrock, 2001; Patarca, 2001; Bower et al., 2002) as well as MS (Flachenecker et al., 2004).

Higher expression of TNF-α mRNA in peripheral blood cells of patients with MS related fatigue has been observed, suggesting that TNF-α may be a mediator of fatigue in MS (Flachenecker et al., 2004). Nonetheless, the association between MS-related fatigue and elevated levels of circulating cytokines has been inconsistent (Giovannoni et al., 2001; Flachenecker et al., 2004; Heesen et al., 2006). This variability is not surprising, due to the sensitivity of inflammatory cytokines to many variables.

Neuroendocrine Mechanisms

The hypothalamo-pituitary-adrenal (HPA) axis may also play a role in the pathophysiology of fatigue. Some clinical evidence exists for hyperactivity of the HPA axis in MS patients (Gottschalk et al., 2005). Significantly elevated ACTH levels indicating dysregulation of the HPA axis was demonstrated in a study involving 31 MS patients with fatigue (Gottschalk et al., 2005). This was postulated to be due to elevation of pro-inflammatory cytokines producing impairment of corticoid receptor signaling. The authors proposed that correction of corticoid receptor functioning by appropriate medications, such as antidepressants, would produce improvement patients' fatigue (Gottschalk et al., 2005). Other studies fail to recognize a correlation between fatigue and HPA axis activity (Heesen et al., 2002). On the other hand, among 73 progressive MS patients evaluated low circulating levels of dehyroepiandroterone (DHEA) and its sulphated conjugate (DHEAS) were identified in fatigue compared to nonfatigued patients (Tellez et al., 2006). Such low levels could also reflect a dysregulation of the HPA axis and low levels of DHEA are associated with increased pro-inflammatory cytokines. The low levels could also participate in further activating the HPA axis through a positive feedback mechanism.

Autonomic Nervous System Dysregulation

It has been theorized that symptoms of cardiovascular autonomic dysregulation, such as dizziness, generalized weakness, and neurocognitive complaints, bear similarities to the symptoms described in MS-related fatigue. One study of fatigued MS patients found that 20% of the patients had coexisting signs of autonomic failure (Merkelbach et al., 2001). Another study of autonomic tests and measures of heart rate variability in 60 MS patients with fatigue found impairment in the hypoadrenergic orthostatic response. This was interpreted as due to impaired sympathetic vasomotor activity (Flachenecker et al., 2003). Other studies, however, have not found a positive correlation between MS fatigue severity and autonomic dysfunction (Egg et al., 2002).

Physical Deconditioning

Without adequate exercise MS patients may become physically deconditioned and subsequently more fatigued. This can lead to a pattern of further avoidance of exercise, resulting in increased weakness. In patients who are severely disabled, respiratory function may become compromised. Physical reconditioning should always be a priority in addressing the fatigue of MS patients who fall into this category (Foglio et al., 1994).

EVALUATION

The symptom of fatigue should be investigated with a comprehensive history and examination. Self-report measures may also be helpful in distinguishing between depressive symptoms, excessive sleepiness, and fatigue. The patient should be questioned as to possible triggers such as heat or stress, the onset of the fatigue, the situations that seem to alleviate fatigue, and their current medications. Particular attention needs to be given to the possibility of depression because of its clear overlap with fatigue. Depression is often under-recognized and undertreated. In patients who exhibit signs of fatigue and depression, the first line of therapy should involve treatment of the depression. Fatigue may resolve with improvement in mood (Mohr et al., 2003; Krupp, 2004). At least at some time during their care, routine labs should be performed to rule out other causes of fatigue, such as infection or metabolic derangement (Krupp, 2004). Ruling out anemia and thyroid disease is particularly important.

TREATMENT

A variety of nonpharmacologic and medication interventions have been tried for fatigue. A meta-analysis of physical exercise and its effects on quality of life showed that exercise is mildly beneficial (Motl et al., 2005). Those measures that included fatigue and were most MS specific showed the greatest change (¼ SD improvement in quality-of-life measures). Programs that involved more than 90 minutes per week and that were aerobic rather than resistance training or yoga were most effective (Motl et al., 2005). The benefits of exercise on fatigue and quality of life appear to be sustained. On the other hand, continued participation in exercise may be difficult when patients lose motivation (McCullagh et al., 2008).

In addition to exercise, energy conservation strategies have been used to address fatigue. When treated patients were compared to a wait-listed control group, fatigue measured by the MFIS improved (Sauter et al., 2008).

Cognitive behavioral therapy (CBT) for MS fatigue has shown a striking benefit on fatigue (van Kessel et al., 2008). This study was undertaken in part based on the positive effects of CBT on patients with chronic fatigue syndrome (Deale et al., 1997; Sharpe et al., 1996; Prins et al., 2001). Both CBT and relaxation training helped fatigue in MS patients and healthy controls, but CBT was a more effective treatment for MS fatigue to the point that lowered the fatigue levels of patients to that seen in the healthy control group (van Kessel et al., 2008). The positive effects were sustained up to 6 months post intervention. Additional benefits from CBT included decreasing depression, anxiety, and stress (van Kessel et al., 2008).

Not uncommonly, nonpharmacologic interventions are coupled with medication. Medications that can be used to supplement nonpharmacologic intervention include amantadine, modafinil, and possibly aspirin. None of the research on these pharmacotherapies provides unequivocally positive results. The treatment approach should be to consider the occasional treatment success as a victory but to monitor the response and to consider drug holidays since with time the beneficial response becomes attenuated. It also remains unclear whether in many patients response to therapy is related to a placebo effect since data for the efficacy of these therapies are lacking.

A number of clinical trials on fatigue have been done with amantadine. The drug was initially used for the flu (Hayden, 1996) but also has dopaminergic effects as well as effects on glutamate receptors. Four randomized clinical trials showed positive results with different outcome assessments for fatigue (Canadian MS Research Group, 1987; Rosenberg and Appenzeller, 1988; Cohen and Fisher, 1989; Geisler et al., 1996). However, as covered in a recent Cochrane review, the studies all had limitations in design or analysis complicating the interpretation of the effect of amantadine (Pucci et al., 2007).

Modafinil is the most frequently prescribed fatigue treatment as reported by patients participating in the NARCOM registry (Hadjimichael et al., 2008). Modafinil has dual neuradrenergic/dopaminergic properties, but is not a classic sympathomimetic. A small randomized controlled trial of modafinil showed that on treatment patients had dramatic improvements in fatigue, focused attention, and dexterity (Lange et al., 2009). However, results of other controlled trials have been mixed. In one with a crossover design, the modafinil relative to the placebo group improved on the FSS. However, based on the crossover design, a placebo effect could have been responsible for the responses. Also, it was somewhat surprising that only the 200 mg dose but not the 400 mg dose was effective (Rammohan et al., 2002). In contrast, a placebo-controlled clinical trial of modafinil using a parallel group design showed no difference in improved fatigue between the placebo and actively treated group and there was more insomnia and gastrointestinal side effects in the modafinil group (Stankoff et al., 2005).

However, this study used a dose titration schedule, which may have led to fewer patients optimally dosed at 200 mg/day. Overall, it remains unclear whether modafinil is more effective than placebo, but on an individual basis a positive treatment effect may occur.

Aspirin is another medication that was studied with a randomized controlled trial for fatigue and had a treatment effect (Wingerchuk et al., 2005). While the result was positive, some have suggested that changes in other symptoms, such as pain reduction, could have contributed to the results (Schwid and Murray, 2005; Wingerchuck et al., 2005). If aspirin has a direct effect, one potential mechanism could be to alter hypothalamic output through the changes caused in neuroendocrine and autonomic responses. It is also possible that MS fatigue is cytokine induced. Aspirin and other nonsteroidal medications are effective in fatigue induced by beta interferon, which is likely mediated by cytokines (Wingerchuck et al., 2005).

Overall, no striking treatment emerges as the best intervention for fatigue. Cognitive behavioral therapy and exercise have the most documentation of a benefit but some patients also appear to respond to medication, albeit a placebo effect cannot be ruled out. Effective therapy usually requires a multidisciplinary approach.

CONCLUSION

Our understanding of MS fatigue has grown from a primarily descriptive analysis to an investigation of techniques of measurement, tests of diverse pathogenic mechanisms, and treatments. A variety of clinical trials for MS fatigue have shown some benefit with several different types of therapies. Development of more rationally based therapies should help lessen fatigue's deleterious effects on quality of life. Any step forward in improving the management of fatigue in MS will inform the treatment of fatigue associated with a wide range of medical conditions.

REFERENCES

Amato MP, Ponziani G, Rossi F, Liedl CL, Stefanile C, Rossi L. Quality of life in multiple sclerosis: the impact of depression, fatigue and disability. *Mult Scler.* 2001;7(5):340–344.

Amarenco G, Kerdraon J, Denys P. Bladder and sphincter disorders in multiple sclerosis. Clinical, urodynamic and neurophysiological study of 225 cases [in French]. *Rev Neurol (Paris)*. 1995;151(12):722–730.

Aronson KJ. Quality of life among persons with multiple sclerosis and their caregivers. *Neurology*. 1997;48(1): 74–80.

Attarian HP, Brown KM, Duntley SP, Carter JD, Cross AH. The relationship of sleep disturbances and fatigue in multiple sclerosis. *Arch Neurol*. 2004;61(4): 525–528.

Bailey A, Channon S, Beaumont JG. The relationship between subjective fatigue and cognitive fatigue in advanced multiple sclerosis. *Mult Scler*. 2007;13(1): 73–80.

Bakshi R, Miletich RS, Henschel K, et al. Fatigue in multiple sclerosis: cross-sectional correlation with brain MRI findings in 71 patients. *Neurology*. 1999;53(5):1151–1153.

Bakshi R, Shaikh ZA, Miletich RS, et al. Fatigue in multiple sclerosis and its relationship to depression and neurologic disability. *Mult Scler*. 2000;6(3):181–185.

Bower JE, Ganz PA, Aziz N, Fahey JL. Fatigue and proinflammatory cytokine activity in breast cancer survivors. *Psychosom Med*. 2002;64(4):604–611.

Brown RF, Valpiani EM, Tennant CC, et al. Longitudinal assessment of anxiety, depression, and fatigue in people with multiple sclerosis. *Psychol Psychother*. 2009; 82(pt 1):41–56.

Canadian MS Research Group. A randomized controlled trial of amantadine in fatigue associated with multiple sclerosis. *Can J Neurol Sci*. 1987;14(3):273–278.

Chalder T, Berelowitz G, Pawlikowska T, et al. Development of a fatigue scale. *J Psychosom Res*. 1993;37(2):147–153.

Christodoulou C. The assessment and measurement of fatigue. In: DeLuca J, ed. *Fatigue as a Window to the Brain*. New York: MIT Press;2005:19–35.

Chwastiak LA, Gibbons LE, Ehde DM, et al. Fatigue and psychiatric illness in a large community sample of persons with multiple sclerosis. *J Psychosom Res*. 2005; 59(5):291–298.

Cohen RA, Fisher M. Amantadine treatment of fatigue associated with multiple sclerosis. *Arch Neurol*. 1989; 46(6):676–680.

Colosimo C, Millefiorini E, Grasso MG, et al. Fatigue in MS is associated with specific clinical features. *Acta Neurol Scand*. 1995;92(5):353–355.

Deale A, Chalder T, Marks I, Wessely S. Cognitive behavior therapy for chronic fatigue syndrome: a randomized controlled trial. *Am J Psychiatry*. 1997;154(3):408–414.

Djaldetti R, Ziv I, Achiron A, Melamed E. Fatigue in multiple sclerosis compared with chronic fatigue syndrome: A quantitative assessment. *Neurology*. 1996;46(3): 632–635.

Edgley K, Sullivan M, Dehoux E. A survey of multiple sclerosis: II Determinants of employment status. *Can J Rehabil*. 1991;(4):127–132.

Egg R, Högl B, Glatzl S, Beer R, Berger T. Autonomic instability, as measured by pupillary unrest, is not associated with multiple sclerosis fatigue severity. *Mult Scler*. 2002;8(3):256–260.

Feinstein A. The neuropsychiatry of multiple sclerosis. *Can J Psychiatry*. 2004;49(3):157–163.

Feinstein A, O'Connor P, Gray T, Feinstein K. The effects of anxiety on psychiatric morbidity in patients with multiple sclerosis. *Mult Scler*. 1999;5(5):323–326.

Ferini-Strambi L, Filippi M, Martinelli V, et al. Nocturnal sleep study in multiple sclerosis: correlations with clinical and brain magnetic resonance imaging findings. *J Neurol Sci*. 1994;125(2):194–197.

Filippi M, Rocca MA, Colombo B, et al. Functional magnetic resonance imaging correlates of fatigue in multiple sclerosis. *Neuroimage*. 2002;15(3):559–567.

Fisk JD, Pontefract A, Ritvo PG, Archibald CJ, Murray TJ. The impact of fatigue on patients with multiple sclerosis. *Can J Neurol Sci*. 1994;21(1):9–14.

Flachenecker P, Bihler I, Weber F, Gottschalk M, Toyka KV, Rieckmann P. Cytokine mRNA expression in patients with multiple sclerosis and fatigue. *Mult Scler*. 2004;10(2):165–169.

Flachenecker P, Kümpfel T, Kallmann B, et al. Fatigue in multiple sclerosis: a comparison of different rating scales and correlation to clinical parameters. *Mult Scler*. 2002;8(6):523–526.

Flachenecker P, Rufer A, Bihler I, et al. Fatigue in MS is related to sympathetic vasomotor dysfunction. *Neurology*. 2003;61(6):851–853.

Fleming WE, Pollak CP. Sleep disorders in multiple sclerosis. *Semin Neurol*. 2005;25(1):64–68.

Foglio K, Clini E, Facchetti D, et al. Respiratory muscle function and exercise capacity in multiple sclerosis. *Eur Respir J*. 1994;7(1):23–28.

Ford H, Trigwell P, Johnson M. The nature of fatigue in multiple sclerosis. *J Psychosom Res*. 1998;45(1): 33–38.

Freal JE, Kraft GH, Coryell JK. Symptomatic fatigue in multiple sclerosis. *Arch Phys Med Rehabil*. 1984; 65(3):135–138.

Geisler MW, Sliwinski M, Coyle PK, Masur DM, Doscher C, Krupp LB. The effects of amantadine and pemoline on cognitive functioning in multiple sclerosis. *Arch Neurol*. 1996;53(2):185–188.

Gilson BS, Gilson JS, Bergner M, et al. The sickness impact profile. Development of an outcome measure of health care. *Am J Public Health*. 1975;65(12): 1304–1310.

Giovannoni G, Thompson AJ, Miller DH, Thompson EJ. Fatigue is not associated with raised inflammatory markers in multiple sclerosis. *Neurology*. 2001;57(4): 676–681.

Gottschalk M, Kümpfel T, Flachenecker P, et al. Fatigue and regulation of the hypothalamo-pituitary-adrenal axis in multiple sclerosis. *Arch Neurol*. 2005;62(2): 277–280.

Hadjimichael O, Vollmer T, Oleen-Burkey M. Fatigue characteristics in multiple sclerosis: the North American Research Committee on Multiple Sclerosis (NARCOMS) survey. *Health Qual Life Outcomes*. 2008; 6:100.

Hayden FG. Combination antiviral therapy for respiratory virus infections. *Antiviral Res*. 1996;29(1):45–48.

Heesen C, Gold SM, Raji A, Wiedemann K, Schulz KH. Cognitive impairment correlates with hypothalamo-pituitary-adrenal axis dysregulation in multiple sclerosis. *Psychoneuroendocrinology.* 2002;27(4):505–517.

Heesen C, Nawrath L, Reich C, Bauer N, Shultz K-H, Gold SM. Fatigue in multiple sclerosis: an example of cytokine mediated sickness behaviour? *J Neurol Neurosurg Psychiatry.* 2006;77(1):34–39.

Iriarte J, Katsamakis G, de Castro P. The Fatigue Descriptive Scale (FDS): a useful tool to evaluate fatigue in multiple sclerosis. *Mult Scler.* 1999;5(1):10–16.

Iriarte J, Subira ML, de Castro P. Modalities of fatigue in multiple sclerosis: correlation with clinical and biological factors. *Mult Scler.* 2000;6(2):124–130.

Janardhan V, Bakshi R. Quality of life in patients with multiple sclerosis: the impact of fatigue and depression. *J Neurol Sci.* 2002;205(1):51–58.

Johansson S, Ytterberg C, Gottberg K, Widen Holmqvist L, von Koch L. Use of health services in people with multiple sclerosis with and without fatigue. *Mult Scler.* 2009;15(1):88–95.

Johansson S, Ytterberg C, Hillert J, Widen Holmqvist L, von Koch L. A longitudinal study of variations in and predictors of fatigue in multiple sclerosis. *J Neurol Neurosurg Psychiatry.* 2008;79(4):454–457.

Johnson SK, Lange G, DeLuca J, Korn LR, Natelson B. The effects of fatigue on neuropsychological performance in patients with chronic fatigue syndrome, multiple sclerosis, and depression. *Appl Neuropsychol.* 1997;4(3):145–153.

Jopson NM, Moss-Morris R. The role of illness severity and illness representations in adjusting to multiple sclerosis. *J Psychosom Res.* 2003;54(6):503–511, 513–514.

Julian LJ, Vella L, Vollmer T, Hadjimichael O, Mohr DC. Employment in multiple sclerosis. Exiting and re-entering the work force. *J Neurol.* 2008;255(9):1354–1360.

Kaynak H, Altintas A, Kaynak D, et al. Fatigue and sleep disturbance in multiple sclerosis. *Eur J Neurol.* 2006;13(12):1333–1339.

Kent-Braun JA, Sharma KR, Miller RG, Weiner MW. Postexercise phosphocreatine resynthesis is slowed in multiple sclerosis. *Muscle Nerve.* 1994;17(8):835–841.

Kerr JR, Barah F, Mattey DL, et al. Circulating tumour necrosis factor-alpha and interferon-gamma are detectable during acute and convalescent parvovirus B19 infection and are associated with prolonged and chronic fatigue. *J Gen Virol.* 2001;82(pt 12):3011–3019.

Kroencke DC, Lynch SG, Denney DR. Fatigue in multiple sclerosis: relationship to depression, disability, and disease pattern. *Mult Scler.* 2000;6(2):131–136.

Krupp LB. Fatigue in Multiple Sclerosis: A Guide to Diagnosis and Management. New York: Demos Medical Publishing; 2004.

Krupp LB, Alvarez LA, LaRocca NG, Scheinberg LC. Fatigue in multiple sclerosis. *Arch Neurol.* 1988;45(4):435–437.

Krupp LB, Christodoulou C. Fatigue in multiple sclerosis. *Curr Neurol Neurosci Rep.* 2001;1(3):294–298.

Krupp LB, Elkins LE. Fatigue and declines in cognitive functioning in multiple sclerosis. *Neurology.* 2000;55(7):934–939.

Krupp LB, LaRocca NG, Muir-Nash J, Steinberg AD. The fatigue severity scale. Application to patients with multiple sclerosis and systemic lupus erythematosus. *Arch Neurol.* 1989;46(10):1121–1123.

Krupp LB, Pollina DA. Mechanisms and management of fatigue in progressive neurological disorders. *Curr Opin Neurol.* 1996;9(6):456–460.

Kurzrock R. The role of cytokines in cancer-related fatigue. *Cancer.* 2001;92(6 suppl):1684–1688.

Lange R, Volkmer M, Heesen C, Liepert J. Modafinil effects in multiple sclerosis patients with fatigue. *J Neurol.* 2009;256(4):645–650.

Latash M, Kalugina E, Nicholas J, Orpett C, Stefoski D, Davis F. Myogenic and central neurogenic factors in fatigue in multiple sclerosis. *Mult Scler.* 1996;1(4):236–241.

Leocani L, Colombo B, Magnani G, et al. Fatigue in multiple sclerosis is associated with abnormal cortical activation to voluntary movement–EEG evidence. *Neuroimage.* 2001;13(6 pt 1):1186–1192.

Lerdal A, Celius EG, Moum T. Fatigue and its association with sociodemographic variables among multiple sclerosis patients. *Mult Scler.* 2003;9(5):509–514.

Liepert J, Mingers D, Heesen C, Bäumer T, Weiller C. Motor cortex excitability and fatigue in multiple sclerosis: a transcranial magnetic stimulation study. *Mult Scler.* 2005;11(3):316–321.

Marrie RA, Fisher E, Miller DM, Lee JC, Rudick RA. Association of fatigue and brain atrophy in multiple sclerosis. *J Neurol Sci.* 2005;228(2):161–166.

McCullagh R, Fitzgerald AP, Murphy RP, Cooke G. Long-term benefits of exercising on quality of life and fatigue in multiple sclerosis patients with mild disability: a pilot study. *Clin Rehabil.* 2008;22(3):206–214.

McNair DM, Lorr M, Droppleman LF. *Profile of Mood States Manual.* San Diego, CA: Educational and Industrial Testing Service; 1971.

Merkelbach S, Dillmann U, Kölmel C, Holz I, Muller M. Cardiovascular autonomic dysregulation and fatigue in multiple sclerosis. *Mult Scler.* 2001;7(5):320–326.

Mills R, Young C, Nicholas R, Pallant J, Tennant A. Rasch analysis of the Fatigue Severity Scale in multiple sclerosis. *Mult Scler.* 2009;15(1):81–87.

Minden SL, Frankel D, Perloff J, Srinath KP, Hoaglin DC. The Sonya Slifka Longitudinal Multiple Sclerosis Study: methods and sample characteristics. *Mult Scler.* 2006;12(1):24–38.

Mohr DC, Hart SL, Goldberg A. Effects of treatment for depression on fatigue in multiple sclerosis. *Psychosom Med.* 2003;65(4):542–547.

Möller A, Wiedemann G, Rohde U, Backmund H, Sonntag A. Correlates of cognitive impairment and depressive mood disorder in multiple sclerosis. *Acta Psychiatr Scand.* 1994;89(2):117–121.

Moreira NC, Damasceno RS, Medeiros CA, et al. Restless leg syndrome, sleep quality and fatigue in multiple sclerosis patients. *Braz J Med Biol Res.* 2008;41(10): 932–937.

Motl RW, McAuley E, Snook EM. Physical activity and multiple sclerosis: a meta-analysis. *Mult Scler.* 2005; 11(4):459–463.

Multiple Sclerosis Council for Clinical Practice, Guidelines. ed. *Fatigue and Multiple Sclerosis: Evidence-Based Management Strategies for Fatigue in Multiple Sclerosis.* Washington, DC: Paralyzed Veterans Association of America; 1998.

Patten SB, Beck CA, Williams JV, Barbui C, Metz LM. Major depression in multiple sclerosis: a population-based perspective. *Neurology.* 2003;61(11):1524–1527.

Parmenter BA, Denney DR, Lynch SG. The cognitive performance of patients with multiple sclerosis during periods of high and low fatigue. *Mult Scler.* 2003; 9(2):111–118.

Patarca R. Cytokines and chronic fatigue syndrome. *Ann N Y Acad Sci.* 2001;933:185–200.

Patrick E, Christodoulou C, Krupp LB. Longitudinal correlates of fatigue in multiple sclerosis. *Mult Scler.* 2009;15(2):258–261.

Paul RH, Beatty WW, Schneider R, Blanco CR, Hames KA. Cognitive and physical fatigue in multiple sclerosis: relations between self-report and objective performance. *Appl Neuropsychol.* 1998;5(3):143–148.

Prins JB, Bleijenberg G, Bazelmans E, et al. Cognitive behaviour therapy for chronic fatigue syndrome: a multicentre randomised controlled trial. *Lancet.* 2001; 357(9259):841–847.

Pucci E, Branãs P, D'Amico R, Giuliani G, Solari A, Taus C. Amantadine for fatigue in multiple sclerosis. *Cochrane DB Sys Rev.* 2007;(1):CD002818.

Putzki N, Katsarava Z, Vago S, Diener HC, Limmroth V. Prevalence and severity of multiple-sclerosis-associated fatigue in treated and untreated patients. *Eur Neurol.* 2008;59(3–4):136–142.

Rammohan KW, Rosenberg JH, Lynn DJ, Blumenfeld AM, Pollak CP, Nagaraja HN. Efficacy and safety of modafinil (Provigil) for the treatment of fatigue in multiple sclerosis: a two centre phase 2 study. *J Neurol Neurosurg Psychiatry.* 2002;72(2):179–183.

Rocca MA, Agosta F, Colombo B, et al. fMRI changes in relapsing-remitting multiple sclerosis patients complaining of fatigue after IFNbeta-1a injection. *Hum Brain Mapp.* 2007;28(5):373–382.

Roelcke U, Kappos L, Lechner-Scott J, et al. Reduced glucose metabolism in the frontal cortex and basal ganglia of multiple sclerosis patients with fatigue: a 18F-fluorodeoxyglucose positron emission tomography study. *Neurology.* 1997;48(6):1566–1571.

Rosenberg GA, Appenzeller O. Amantadine, fatigue, and multiple sclerosis. *Arch Neurol.* 1988;45(10):1104–1106.

Sadovnick AD, Remick RA, Allen J, et al. Depression and multiple sclerosis. *Neurology.* 1996;46(3):628–632.

Sauter C, Zebenholzer K, Hisakawa J, Zeitlhofer J, Vass K. A longitudinal study on effects of a six-week course for energy conservation for multiple sclerosis patients. *Mult Scler.* 2008;14(4):500–505.

Schubert M, Wohlfarth K, Rollnik JD, Dengler R. Walking and fatigue in multiple sclerosis: the role of the corticospinal system. *Muscle Nerve.* 1998;21(8):1068–1070.

Schwartz CE, Coulthard-Morris L, Zeng Q. Psychosocial correlates of fatigue in multiple sclerosis. *Arch Phys Med Rehabil.* 1996;77(2):165–170.

Schwartz JE, Jandorf L, Krupp LB. The measurement of fatigue: a new instrument. *J Psychosom Res.* 1993; 37(7):753–762.

Schwid SR, Murray TJ. Treating fatigue in patients with MS: one step forward, one step back. *Neurology.* 2005; 64(7):1111–1112.

Schwid SR, Thornton CA, Pandya S, et al. Quantitative assessment of motor fatigue and strength in MS. *Neurology.* 1999;53(4):743–750.

Sepulcre J, Masdeu JC, Goñi J, et al. Fatigue in multiple sclerosis is associated with the disruption of frontal and parietal pathways. *Mult Scler.* 2009;15(3):337–344.

Sharma KR, Kent-Braun J, Mynhier MA, Weiner MW, Miller RG. Evidence of an abnormal intramuscular component of fatigue in multiple sclerosis. *Muscle Nerve.* 1995;18(12):1403–1411.

Sharpe M, Hawton K, Simkin S, et al. Cognitive behaviour therapy for the chronic fatigue syndrome: a randomized controlled trial. *BMJ.* 1996;312(7022):22–26.

Sheean GL, Murray NM, Rothwell JC, Miller DH, Thompson AJ. An electrophysiological study of the mechanism of fatigue in multiple sclerosis. *Brain.* 1997;120(pt 2):299–315.

Skerrett TN, Moss-Morris R. Fatigue and social impairment in multiple sclerosis: the role of patients' cognitive and behavioral responses to their symptoms. *J Psychosom Res.* 2006;61(5):587–593.

Smith MM, Arnett PA. Factors related to employment status changes in individuals with multiple sclerosis. *Mult Scler.* 2005;11(5):602–609.

Stankoff B, Waubant E, Confavreux C, et al. Modafinil for fatigue in MS: a randomized placebo-controlled double-blind study. *Neurology.* 2005;64(7):1139–1143.

Stanton BR, Barnes F, Silber E. Sleep and fatigue in multiple sclerosis. *Mult Scler.* 2006;12(4):481–486.

Stone AA, Shiffman S. Capturing momentary, self-report data: a proposal for reporting guidelines. *Ann Behav Med.* 2002;24(3):236–243.

Strober LB, Arnett PA. An examination of four models predicting fatigue in multiple sclerosis. *Arch Clin Neuropsychol.* 2005;20(5):631–646.

Tachibana N, Howard RS, Hirsch NP, et al. Sleep problems in multiple sclerosis. *Eur Neurol.* 1994;34(6): 320–323.

Tartaglia MC, Narayanan S, Francis SJ, et al. The relationship between diffuse axonal damage and fatigue in multiple sclerosis. *Arch Neurol.* 2004;61(2):201–207.

Tedeschi G, Dinacci D, Lavorgna L, et al. Correlation between fatigue and brain atrophy and lesion load in multiple sclerosis patients independent of disability. *J Neurol Sci.* 2007;263(1–2):15–19.

Tellez N, Comabella M, Juliã E, et al. Fatigue in progressive multiple sclerosis is associated with low levels of dehydroepiandrosterone. *Mult Scler.* 2006;12(4): 487–494.

Trojan DA, Arnold D, Collet JP, et al. Fatigue in multiple sclerosis: association with disease-related, behavioural and psychosocial factors. *Mult Scler.* 2007;13(8): 985–995.

van der Werf SP, Evers A, Jongen PJ, Bleijenberg G. The role of helplessness as mediator between neurological disability, emotional instability, experienced fatigue and depression in patients with multiple sclerosis. *Mult Scler.* 2003;9(1):89–94.

van der Werf SP, Jongen PJ, Lycklama à Nijeholt GJ, Barkhof F, Hommes OR, Bleijenberg G. Fatigue in multiple sclerosis: interrelations between fatigue complaints, cerebral MRI abnormalities and neurological disability. *J Neurol Sci.* 1998;160(2):164–170.

van Kessel K, Moss-Morris R, Willoughby E, Chalder T, Johnson MH, Robinson E. A randomized controlled trial of cognitive behavior therapy for multiple sclerosis fatigue. *Psychosom Med.* 2008;70(2):205–213.

Vercoulen JH, Hommes OR, Swanink CM, et al. The measurement of fatigue in patients with multiple sclerosis. A multidimensional comparison with patients with chronic fatigue syndrome and healthy subjects. *Arch Neurol.* 1996;53(7):642–649.

Vercoulen JH, Swanink CM, Galama JM, et al. The persistence of fatigue in chronic fatigue syndrome and multiple sclerosis: development of a model. *J Psychosom Res.* 1998;45(6):507–517.

Ware JE, Jr. SF-36 health survey update. *Spine (Phila Pa 1976).* 2000;25(24):3130–3139.

Ware JE, Jr., Sherbourne CD. The MOS 36-item short-form health survey (SF-36). I. Conceptual framework and item selection. *Med Care.* 1992;30(6): 473–483.

Wessely S, Hotopf M, Sharpe D. *Chronic Fatigue and Its Syndromes.* New York: Oxford University Press; 1998.

White AT, Lee JN, Light AR, Light KC. Brain activation in multiple sclerosis: a BOLD fMRI study of the effects of fatiguing hand exercise. *Mult Scler.* 2009;15(5): 580–586.

Whitehead L. The measurement of fatigue in chronic illness: a systematic review of unidimensional and multidimensional fatigue measures. *J Pain Symptom Manage.* 2009;37(1):107–128.

Wingerchuk DM, Benarroch EE, O'Brien PC, et al. A randomized controlled crossover trial of aspirin for fatigue in multiple sclerosis. *Neurology.* 2005;64(7): 1267–1269.

20   Multiple Sclerosis and Pain

Norman S. Namerow

Fifty years ago it was axiomatic that if a patient had neurological deficits with pain, then a presumptive diagnosis of multiple sclerosis (MS) could be challenged. The only exceptions to this were the retroocular pain associated with optic neuritis and trigeminal neuralgia in a patient 40 years of age or younger. In essence, pain was not considered an important part of the syndrome of MS.

As an example, in an autopsy study in 1950 Carter et al. reported pain in only 11% of their cases. By 1984, Clifford and Trotter, in a retrospective review, found pain of more than 2 weeks duration in only 29% of 315 MS patients.

Our views have changed considerably since then. In a retrospective study, Moulin et al (1988) reported acute or chronic pain in 55% of 159 patients. Forty-eight percent had a chronic pain syndrome for a mean duration of 4.9 years. Seven patients (4.2%) had paroxysmal tic-like pain diagnosed as trigeminal neuralgia. They concluded that chronic pain in MS was usually associated with a myelopathy and was more common in women, older patients, and those with disease duration greater than 5 years. The subject of neuropathic pain in central and peripheral demyelinating disorders was further reviewed by Moulin (1989), and in a subsequent article (Moulin, 1998), he reported acute pain to occur in 10% of MS patients at some point in the course of their disease, and chronic pain to occur in 50%–80% of patients. In 1996, Thompson cited an occurrence of pain in over 65% of MS patients, during all phases of the disease, and another more recent study by Osterberg and colleagues of 364 patients, showed that 57.5% reported pain during the course of their disease, including 4.9% with trigeminal neuralgia (Osterberg et al., 2005). Ehde and colleagues, in a community sample of 442 MS patients, reported 44% with persistent, bothersome pain in the 3 months prior to their survey. Twenty-seven percent reported their pain as severe and 20% reported pain of severity sufficient to interfere with their daily activities (Ehde et al., 2003).

Earlier MS studies also did not attempt to fully characterize the reported pain. Newer studies, however, have given further insight into the nature of the pain syndromes in MS (Moulin et al., 1988; Moulin, 1989; Moulin, 1998; Kerns et al., 2002; Hadjimichael et al., 2007; Kenner et al., 2007; Khan and Pallant, 2007; Piwko et al., 2007; Douglas et al., 2008; Grasso et al., 2008; O'Connor et al., 2008). These reviews have attempted to describe the pain type, duration, severity, psychosocial impact, quality-of-life effect, and pathogenesis, and they have identified those pains strictly related to MS. Boneschi et al. (2008) assessed the actual and lifetime frequency of neuropathic and "somatic" pain and headache in 428 MS patients over a 3-month period. They found a lifetime prevalence at the time of examination of at least one type of pain in 39.8% of MS patients, and 58.5% if one includes headache, and an actual prevalence of 23.8% and 39%, respectively. In contrast, Taylor (2006) estimated a 1.5% prevalence of chronic neuropathic pain in the general population. These latter two studies clearly identify the burden of pain that the MS population must carry. One study has also suggested that MS patients have a higher risk of developing a complex regional pain syndrome (CRPS) than the general population (Schwartzman et al., 2008).

Ethnicity does not appear to be a factor regarding pain. Shibasaki et al. (1981) in a limited report on the differences between British and Japanese

MS patients noted a similar prevalence of pain in 37% of British and 35% of Japanese cases.

In summary, pain is now acknowledged as a common problem in MS patients. This dramatic change in the recognition of pain as a significant factor in MS appears to be due to better data collection, a heightened awareness as to what we consider to be a painful sensation, and also the fact that newer research protocols frequently incorporate quality-of-life issues that include the occurrence of pain. With the passage of time there has also been increased attention on the issue of pain as a symptom to be monitored and documented in all patients. It has also become increasingly important with MS patients to determine the origin of the various pain generators as there has evolved a number of treatments for neuropathic pain that may have specific value in their management. These considerations become important as we focus on palliative care in MS in contrast to direct immuno-modulation therapy aimed at altering the underlying disease process. The importance of identifying and treating pain in MS goes beyond just the relief of suffering. Chronic pain in MS has a clear negative impact on the afflicted patient's quality of life and physical condition.

PAIN SYNDROMES IN MULTIPLE SCLEROSIS

It is convenient to organize pain in MS into four categories (Pollmann et al., 2005; Pollmann and Fineberg, 2008). The first category is pain caused by the demyelinating process itself and therefore specific to MS. This would include acute or paroxysmal pain such as trigeminal neuralgia, tonic spasms, optic neuritis, the L'hermitte phenomenon,

and more chronic painful dysesthesias. These would all be neuropathic pain related. The second category is pain that can be associated with chronic neurological diseases, including MS typified by spasticity, muscle spasms, joint pain, pressure-related skin pain, nerve injuries related to the use of crutches and wheelchairs, and bladder spasms and infections. Except for traumatic nerve injuries, these pains would typically be nociceptive in nature. The third category is MS therapy–related pain, specifically due to injections of an interferon or glatiramer acetate. Finally, the fourth category is pain from causes independent of neurological disease, that is, pain from causes that plague our human condition, including infections, visceral disease, headache, and inflammatory conditions such as arthritis and tendonitis.

Special reference must be made to the occurrence of headache, and migraine in particular, that appears to have a comorbidity with MS. For purposes of this review, however, we will focus on pain that is specifically related to MS, be it neuropathic or nociceptive, acknowledging the difficulty at times in differentiating the two. With this in mind, a listing of the various pain syndromes commonly associated with MS follows. This classification scheme is shown in Table 20-1.

Multiple Sclerosis–Specific Pain

Trigeminal neuralgia and other paroxysmal events

Trigeminal neuralgia is the most common and troublesome of the cranial neuralgias that occur in MS and was first identified as a paroxysmal symptom of this disease by Oppenheim in 1911.

TABLE 20-1 Classification of Multiple Sclerosis–Related Pain

Pain specific to the MS disease process

   Paroxysmal/acute: neuralgias, radicular, tonic spasms, L'hermitte sign, tic-like limb pains, dysesthesias, optic neuritis

   Chronic: dysesthesias, girdle sense, back pain, leg spasms, bladder spasms

Pain seen in chronic neurological disease, including MS: spasticity, back pain, bowel distension, infections/decubiti, limb nerve palsies

Pain that is MS treatment related: injected interferon and glateramir acetate therapy

Pain unrelated to neurological disease: cardiac, other visceral, musculoskeletal

Source: Modified from Paty and Ebers, 1998; Pollmann et al., 2005; Pollmann and Fineberg, 2008.

The presentation is similar to the tic-like facial pain of idiopathic trigeminal neuralgia that can be seen in patients without MS. The major clinical difference is the age of onset. In MS 59% of the cases occurred before the age of 50 while with idiopathic trigeminal neuralgia only 32% had symptom onset before this age (Jensen et al., 1982). This age of onset differential was further confirmed by DeSimone et al. (2005). A clinical axiom is that trigeminal neuralgia that occurs before the age of 40 is due to MS until proven otherwise (Paty and Ebers, 1998). Bilateral trigeminal neuralgia is also another presentation that suggests an MS relationship (Hooge and Redekop, 1995; Brisman, 1987). The incidence of trigeminal neuralgia in MS patients has been estimated between 4% and 7% (Paty and Ebers, 1998).

There is good evidence that MS-related trigeminal neuralgia can be attributed to a plaque of demyelination in the fifth nerve root entry zone (Gass et al., 1997). Figure 20-1 shows a postmortem pontine section from a well-documented female patient who was personally followed for many years. She had severe MS symptoms and signs including chronic tic-like facial pain diagnosed and treated as trigeminal neuralgia. A plaque in the fifth nerve root entry zone is clearly identified. In another report, magnetic resonance imaging (MRI) has shown the appearance, with gadolinium enhancement, of bilateral trigeminal nerve enlargement at the root entry zone in a patient with the sudden onset of right trigeminal neuralgia. This would appear to confirm the pathological effect of demyelination in this area (Pichiecchio et al., 2007). However, other factors may be important as demonstrated by da Silva et al. (2005). They found a high and clinically silent incidence of trigeminal involvement in MS patients and suggest a simultaneous role of both the central and peripheral myelin in trigeminal demyelination related pain.

Other cranial neuralgias have been reported, especially involving the glossopharyngeal nerve, but these are rarely seen (Minagar and Sheremata, 2000) Paroxysmal neuralgia involving retroauricular and occipital nerves has also been described. While not painful, the yearly incidence of another paroxysmal event, epileptic seizures, has been estimated to be seven times higher in MS than in the general population (Eriksson et al., 2002).

The L'hermitte phenomenon (L'hermitte et al., 1924) is typically produced by neck flexion, although it can occasionally occur spontaneously. This electric shock–like pain is spinal cord generated and may be related to mechanical stretching of the cervical cord on flexion. This mechanosensitivity is a well-identified precipitant of peripheral nerve pain associated with neuropathies and neuromas. Other structural factors such as tumors or cervical canal stenosis from degenerative spine disease must of course be ruled out.

Radiculitis

Radicular pain may be acute or chronic and may affect any limb or trunk area in a nerve root distribution. Acute radicular pain has also been reported as a presenting symptom of MS (Ramirez-Lassepas et al., 1992). An example of this is illustrated by the case of a 49-year-old woman who had a slip-and-fall accident, which reportedly caused chronic right lower extremity radicular pain despite only minimal lumbar degenerative spine disease. She was several years post a lumbar laminectomy for a prior episode of back and right leg pain. One year after her fall she developed chronic left posterior thoracic pain radiating to the axilla and anterior chest wall, and a slowly progressive left foot drop. A brain MRI showed multiple small lesions typical for MS and a thoracic scan showed a T1-2 cord level area of demyelination that confirmed the true nature of her complex underlying condition.

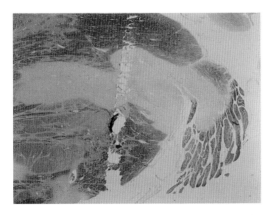

Figure 20-1 Section through pons at autopsy of a multiple sclerosis patient with trigeminal neuralgia.

Painful dysesthesias

Dysesthetic sensations are frequently described as numbness, prickling, tingling, burning, or a disagreeable perception that can be paroxysmal but also can be chronic and constant in nature. When these sensations escalate in intensity, they may be described as painful. Paroxysmal dysesthesias, including pain and itching, have also been reported as the first clinical manifestations of MS (Twomey and Espir, 1980). The incidence of acute paroxysmal pain has been variously reported to be from 4% to 24% of patients under study (Espir and Millac, 1970; Osterman and Westerberg, 1975; Twomey and Espir, 1980). Moulin et al. (1988) in their evaluation of pain syndromes in MS patients found a correlation between the prevalence of pain and the patient's age and duration of disease. The older the patient and the longer the duration of the illness, the more likely there were complaints of pain.

A "girdle sense" or the perception of a band-like constricting sensation around the trunk is typically associated with spinal demyelination and frequently involves the cord posterior columns. This sensation can be mild or very intense at which point it may be described as being very distressful if not painful.

Optic neuropathy

The pain of optic neuritis may occur with the eye immobile, but it is typically aggravated by ocular movement. In this situation, the mechanism may be related to optic nerve demyelination and edema and surround tissue reaction, including meningeal irritation, as part of the nerve inflammatory response in the process of demyelination. Study has suggested that eye motion pain is related to traction of the origins of the superior and medial ocular recti muscles on the optic nerve sheath at the orbital apex (Lepore, 1991). Up to 90% of patients with optic neuritis will have associated pain, especially on eye movement (Optic Neuropathy Study Group, 1991).

Tonic spasms

Finally, it should be stressed that the phenomenon of paroxysmal symptoms in MS is not limited to sensory or painful symptoms. Painful tonic "seizures" are well known to occur (Shibvasaki and Kuroiwa, 1974). These typically will affect a limb, but any somatic area can be affected. Pain can be associated with these events, but not all tonic spasms are described as painful. The origin of the pain may be from marked muscle spasm and occasional associated dysesthesias, but the pain may have a more central origin. Demyelination at the appropriate cord level and pontine/midbrain areas has been described. Frequent transient episodes of dysarthria have also been described which may be associated with facial paresthesias or trunkal ataxia. While the causative phenomena for all of these paroxysmal events may be neuropathic, the painful consequence of muscle spasm must also be considered.

Paroxysmal dyskinesias can also be seen. These may involve a focal area such as a hand or foot, or they may be a hemimovement disorder. More rarely a paroxysmal dyskinesia may affect both legs and the trunk. Pain frequently accompanies these movement disorders.

Headache

Headache is a unique clinical problem that must be discussed in any review of MS-related pain as there appears to be a comorbidity between MS and headache, and migraine in particular. There is limited evidence that the process of demyelination may be a factor in headache production, yet a comorbidity issue seems to be present. Rolak and Brown (1990) found that in 102 studied MS patients, 52% reported headaches compared to only 14% of a cohort of 35 patients suspected to have MS but who were subsequently found to have other disorders. In a more recent study of 238 MS patients, 51% were affected by headache while 23% of controls were so affected (Vacca et al., 2007). A significant correlation between headache and relapsing-remitting MS has also been described (D'Amico et al., 2004). Gee et al. (2005) found that overall, 154 of 277 MS patients (55.6%) also had a complaint of headache. Of this number, 61% (95 of 154) met criteria for migraine-type headache, 25.3% (39 of 154) met criteria for tension-type headache, and 13% (20 of 154) had features of both types. Of interest, MS patients with a plaque within the midbrain/periaqueductal gray area had a four-fold increase in migraine-like headaches compared to patients without such a lesion. The study suggested that that the presence of a midbrain plaque in MS patients is associated with an increased likelihood of headache with migraine characteristics. The MS and headache comorbidity issue is not totally settled however, as a recent study by Putzki et al. (2009) involving 491 patients with MS found headache prevalence rates that did not differ from controls using a German population-based, case-control study. They did find trigeminal neuralgia in 6.3% of their MS cases.

Visceral pain

There is a high incidence of bladder symptoms in MS. Between 70% and 90% of patients will experience bladder dysfunction over the course of their disease with an associated risk of urinary tract infection (Miller et al., 1965; Vickrey et al., 1999). Urinary retention, bladder spasms, and cystitis are all causes of urinary system related pain that can be chronic or acute. Urinary tract infections and in particular cystitis can present with chronic or acute pain as can the development of chronic bowel distress from constipation. Constipation is also a common problem in MS and appears to be related to debility, dehydration, and weak abdominal and pelvic muscles, but a central neuropathic cause is also highly likely as well (Corazziari et al., 2001). The diagnosis and treatment of these visceral causes of pain are beyond the scope of this review and will not be further discussed.

Other somatic pains

Nonneuropathic (nociceptive) pain syndromes are all considered to be epiphenomena related to chronic musculoligamentous weakness, stiffness, disuse, and trauma. Muscle weakness, spasticity, and spine immobility may account for chronic low back pain and the adoption of compensatory techniques that puts undue strain on joints and tendons. Arm immobility may produce a painful frozen shoulder. The use of assistive devices, such as canes, Lofstrand crutches, and wheelchairs, can bring about these secondary symptoms because of new mechanical stressors during use. Painful ulnar and median nerve injuries from wheelchair or crutch use are also well known. Pain secondary

to inflammation be it from skin, joints, connective tissue or viscera may also be seen.

It is also useful to keep in mind the potential painful effects of the currently available disease-modifying drugs for MS. This is especially important if the patient already suffers from musculoskeletal pain. The interferons can cause flu-like myalgic pains, headache, and painful injection site reactions. Careful management (ice/acetaminophen/nonsteroidal anti-inflammatory drugs/injection site rotation) can reduce these effects, however. Also the interferons can cause an increase in spasticity and possible associated muscle pain. Glatiramer acetate only occasionally produces systemic effects, but it can cause transient chest pain. It does not typically produce serious injection site reactions (Langer-Gould et al., 2004), but these also can occur.

PATHOPHYSIOLOGY

Neuropathic Pain

Neuropathic pain is pain derived from diseased or injured nerve anywhere along the neuraxis from peripheral to central locations and in MS extending from the spinal cord to subcortical areas. There can be motor as well as sensory consequences of nerve injury, but for the purposes of this review the sensory consequences are emphasized. The resultant clinical presentation can be complex with negative symptoms such as a loss of sensation, intermixed with various other symptoms of neuronal injury including paroxysmal pain, chronic pain, dysesthesias, hyperalgesia and allodynia.

The pathobiology of peripheral and central neuropathic pain is a complex and evolving science that is beyond the intent of this review. Reference is made to a review by Campbell and Meyer (2006). Basic concepts are worth discussing, however, in the context that understanding the mechanisms involved can form the basis for rational and efficacious current therapy and future pharmacotherapy strategies.

In MS the cranial neuralgias are typically associated with a plaque of demyelination at the nerve root entry zone (Fig. 20-1). Painful radicular and tic-like symptoms are also probably related to root entry zone plaques of inflammatory demyelination. The exact mechanism for these paroxysmal painful discharges is unknown, but likely it is caused by the demyelinated nerve fibers becoming hyperexcitable and characterized by spontaneous and repetitive high-frequency discharges. Such discharges have been identified in mammalian demyelinated fiber electrophysiological studies. This would be analogous to the peripheral nerve injury mechanism for inducing neuropathic pain. In this model, the inflammatory demyelinating process would produce excitatory amino acids and other neuroexcitatory proteins that stimulate an accumulation of sodium channels, which can have the effect of reducing the threshold for depolarization of the demyelinated nerves within the plaque. This circumstance would cause an increased excitability of the affected nerve fibers that is manifested by ectopic discharges and induced ephaptic discharges from nearby fibers (Campbell and Meyer, 2006). High-frequency and uncontrolled ectopic and possibly ephaptic activity would then be the putative mechanism of action for paroxysmal symptoms, including pain, in MS. While most electrophysiological studies on the mechanisms of neuropathic pain have focused on peripheral nerve, the basic principals would also seem reasonable to hold for the intramedullary fibers of dorsal root ganglion cells and their more central synaptic connections and spinocortical pathways.

This spontaneous and uncontrolled sensory input to second-order neurons has the effect of opening neuronal cell voltage-gated calcium channels and activating N-methyl-D-aspartate (NMDA) receptor sites. This occurs via the neurotransmitter glutamate acting on NMDA receptors, which are Ca^{2+} ionophores, allowing the further influx of Ca^{2+} ions. Central cellular sensitization follows, further enhancing aberrant sensory input along spino-thalmo-cortical pathways. Central sensitization may be further enhanced through activation of other neurotransmitters acting on additional receptors such as the AMPA (alpha-amino-3-hydroxy-5-methyl-4-isoxazolepropionic acid) receptors among others.

The pathophysiology of dysesthetic sensations and chronic pain is also unknown, but it has been suggested that the symptoms are related to a deafferentation syndrome further characterized by ectopic and ephaptic discharges in areas of injury.

This implies a different mechanism of symptom production in comparison to paroxysmal neuralgic symptoms. Impaired afferent nerve transmission across areas of demyelination would also account for these sensations, and slowed and blocked axonal conduction has been well identified in areas of axon demyelination (Felts, 1997). Clinically, slowed conduction has also been demonstrated by delays of somatosensory and visual evoked potential responses. The result would be a distortion of an original coherent signal as it passes through a demyelinated plaque consisting of multiple, variably affected fibers. In addition, a central plaque of demyelination may also interrupt downward projecting inhibitory activity allowing continued excitability in lower sensory neuron pools. This would then facilitate or enhance the potential for paroxysmal discharges and distorted sensory perceptions.

Just as ion channelopathies are critical for the generation of neuropathic symptoms, this downward projecting inhibitory system has its own unique contribution to the clinical presentation of pain. This inhibitory system is principally mediated by serotonin and norepinephrine neurotransmitters, although the norepinephrine-based system appears to be the more effective in this regard. This recognition has lead to the development and use of dual serotonin and norepinephrine reuptake inhibitors (SNRIs) as a means of clinically enhancing this pain inhibitory mechanism. The use of dual serotonin and norepinephrine reuptake inhibitors such as venlafaxine and duloxetine are clearly more efficacious than the purely serotonin reuptake inhibitors (SSRIs), in this regard. The pain-relieving effects of reboxitine, a selective norepinephrine reuptake inhibitor, has not yet been proven for routine use in neuropathic or nociceptive pain (Schreiber, 2009).

Paroxysmal discharges from an appropriately placed root entry zone plaque of demyelination, producing, for example, trigeminal neuralgia, is teleologically reasonable. But the exact mechanisms of central mediated pain syndromes in MS are unknown. From that discussed earlier, it would appear that paroxysmal pains and more chronic dysesthetic central pain syndromes have separate mechanisms. The first by a lesion at the brainstem and spinal cord root entry zone level and other more central areas of axon hypersensitization, and the latter by demyelinated lesions of the ascending spino-thalmo-cortical pathways as well as the descending inhibitory system. The central areas of demyelination can block or distort normal physiological axonal and neuronal communication loops producing abnormal perceived sensations.

Nociceptive Pain

Viscera, skin, joint, fascia, and tendon structures upon injury or disease produce painful sensory input over classically described sensory pathways. This discussion is beyond the needs of this review, which mainly focuses on neuropathic mechanisms intrinsic to MS. Obviously, mechanisms of pain generation, diagnosis, and treatment will vary for each tissue and organ affected. It must be stressed, however, that the borderland between nociceptive, inflammatory and neuropathic pain can be blurred and traditional nociceptive and inflammation pain treatment can have adjunctive use. Some central inhibitory pain influences are opioid related and resort to traditional pain therapies using nonsteroidal anti-inflammatory drugs (NSAIDs), and opioids can have a role in controlling pain not managed by the neuropathic pain treatments discussed.

TREATMENT

Most of the recommendations for treating neuropathic pain have been based on studies in the treatment of peripheral diabetic neuropathy, postherpetic neuralgia, and trigeminal neuralgia. Use in MS has been extrapolated from this database. Studies with MS patients have been performed, however, and the rational use of the various drugs to be discussed appears to have been verified. Central pain has also been studied in patients with complete or partial spinal cord injury and stroke, and these data have also been reviewed in the context of selecting appropriate medication for use in MS.

As more agents have been added to the armamentarium of potential therapy, a number of comprehensive reviews for a rational approach to neuropathic pain therapy have been published and reference is made to these for a more complete review (Dworkin et al., 2003, 2007; Beniczky et al., 2005; Finnerup et al., 2005, 2007; Lynch and Watson, 2006; Moulin et al., 2007). Using evidenced-based analysis of randomized clinical trials and systematic literature reviews, Dworkin et al. (2007) have listed first-line drugs for neuropathic pain to be tricyclic antidepressants (TCAs), gabapentin and pregabalin as antiepilepsy drugs (AEDs), and SNRIs. Beniczky et al. have provided a similar evidence based review for treatment options (Beniczky et al., 2005). Useful algorithms for neuropathic pain management have also been published (Finnerup et al., 2005, 2007; Dworkin et al., 2007), which allow for transition to the issue of pain in MS. Based on these studies a recommended treatment algorithm is shown in Figure 20-2.

Available evidence indicates that antiepilepsy drugs (AEDs) that modulate axon voltage-gated sodium and neuronal calcium channels and NMDA receptor sites have a role to play in the treatment of the acute, paroxysmal, and chronic causes of symptoms, including pain, following neuropathic injury and disease. This class of drugs has a long history of use for paroxysmal pain in MS. Antidepressant medications that are dual serotonin (5HT) and norepinephrine (NE) reuptake inhibitors are also readily available and have been shown to modify neuropathic pain by enhancing central inhibitory influences. The tricyclic drugs have multiple sites of action and have proved effective despite being potentially more toxic than the SNRIs. Each of these classes of medication has been shown to have a beneficial effect on pain and, in fact, they may be used in combination to produce a synergistic pain relieving response. Opioids may also play a role if pain is chronic and severe, but they should not be a first choice because of known adverse consequences.

Other medications also can be used for MS-related pain, but they are usually reserved for non-neuropathic problems such as musculoskeletal and injection site pain. NSAIDs, acetaminophen, lesser opioids such as tramadol, and muscle relaxants have had longstanding use in this regard, although tramadol has been shown to be effective in neuropathic pain as well, probably through enhancement of inhibitory influences. Caution must be exercised in using tramadol because of its propensity to cause seizures. It would be prudent to only use this in small doses or reduce or discontinue any TCA or SNRI if one or the other is also being used. Painful bladder spasms have their own specific therapy as do headaches.

ALGORITHM for PAIN MANAGEMENT

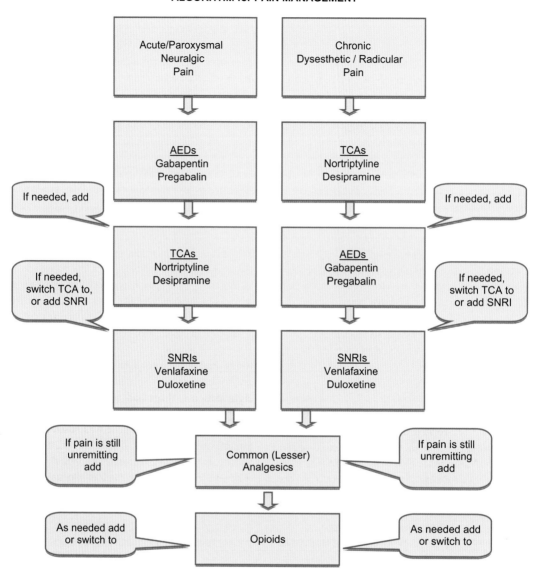

Figure 20-2 Algorithm for central pain management. The decision as to which drug to initiate therapy is somewhat arbitrary. The above represents this author's view. Others might choose to begin therapy for any central neuropathic pain syndrome with a TCA, considered a first-line drug, and subsequently layer in, as needed, gabapentin or pregabalin (first-line drugs). A second-line drug (SNRI) may be substituted for a TCA (see text for further discussion). Dworkin et al. (2003) consider SNRIs to also be first-line therapy. Third-line tramadol has serotonin and norepinephrine reuptake inhibition effects, which is of concern in view of the other agents suggested. Tramadol can precipitate seizures and should not be used if the patient has a history of seizures. If tramadol is used it would be prudent to use small doses and to reduce or eliminate any TCA or SNRI that is also being used. Acetaminophen intake must be carefully monitored. If all else fails, conventional opioids (hydrocodone, oxycodone) with or without acetaminophen can be considered. (Figure modified from Dworkin et al., 2003, Moulin et al. 2007, and Finnerup et al. (2005, 2007)

Antiepileptic Agents

Carbamazepine

The antiepilepsy drugs work by modulating neuronal membrane ion channels and thereby reducing axonal and cell excitability and sensitization. For many years it has been known that the paroxysmal symptoms of MS could be treated with anticonvulsant medications. Early on, carbamazepine evolved into the drug of choice for trigeminal neuralgia (Blom, 1962; Spillane, 1964; Espir and Millac, 1970), with limited success noted using other agents, such as phenytoin. Carbamazepine is still used for trigeminal neuralgia but does have worrisome potential side effects. Also, carbamazepine has not been shown to consistently be of value in other forms of neuropathic pain and is not recommended for this use (Gilron et al., 2006). Carbamazepine and other AEDs, excluding the calcium channel alpha 2-delta ligands gabapentin and pregabalin, have been relegated to third-line medication in the review by Dworkin et al. (2007).

Gabapentin/pregabalin

Gabapentin was first reported to successfully ameliorate MS-related dysesthetic extremity pain in 1997 (Samkoff et al., 1997) and also to relieve trigeminal neuralgia in MS (Khan, 1998). Serpell and the Neuropathic Pain Study Group (2002) also reported on the effectiveness of gabapentin in trigeminal neuralgia, and in an open-label study, Solaro et al. (1998) reported on gabapentin efficacy in treating a variety of acute painful conditions in MS, including trigeminal neuralgia.

Pregabalin has also found a role in the treatment of neuropathic pain, including diabetic peripheral neuropathy (Ricther et al., 2005), postherpetic neuralgia (Sabatowski et al., 2004), central pain (Finnerup and Jensen, 2007), and spinal injury pain (Siddall et al., 2006; Gray, 2007; Baastrup and Finnerup, 2008; Moore et al., 2009). A well-controlled study in just MS patients is wanting, however.

Other antiepilepsy medication

Lamotrigine has been shown to provide pain relief in MS patients with trigeminal neuralgia

(Lunardi et al., 1997); however, a recent Cochrane review (Wiffen and Rees, 2007) and a randomized, double-blind and placebo-controlled study by Breuer et al. (2007) concluded that there was no support for the use of this drug to treat neuropathic-related pain in MS. In studies that did not specifically include MS patients, oxcarbazepine has also been shown to be efficacious in reducing pain in refractory and newly diagnosed trigeminal neuralgia (Cruccu et al., 2008). Solaro et al. also reported on the positive effects of oxcarbazepine in treating paroxysmal symptoms in MS (Solaro et al., 2007), but this was an open-label study with only 12 patients. They could only conclude this was a possible new treatment for painful symptoms in MS but that efficacy must be confirmed with a larger study. Rossi et al. in a pilot study on the effects of levetiracetam on chronic pain in MS found sufficient cause to suggest further study to confirm its efficacy in MS-related central neuropathic pain (Rossi et al., 2009). Topiramate has also been studied with preliminary evidence to suggest a future role in treating MS-related trigeminal neuralgic pain (Zvartau-Hind et al., 2000). In a more recent but very small study with eight patients, three had complete remission of symptoms with topiramate and two had moderate relief (Domingues, 2007). It was suggested that topiramate could be an alternative treatment for trigeminal neuralgia. Gilron et al. (2001) also performed a pilot study with topiramate, using three patients with trigeminal neuralgia. All responded and the authors concluded that a larger study was necessary to more accurately assess the effectiveness of topiramate in trigeminal neuralgia therapy.

In selective cases these agents may be tried if recommended drugs have provided poor results or if the recommended drugs cannot be used because of side effects or allergic reactions. Efficacy remains an issue and the more likely use of these AEDs would be in trigeminal neuralgia. Treatment doses for these agents are variable and initial doses should be modest. However, one frequently has to increase the dosages substantially beyond initial levels to gain a therapeutic response.

Significant side effects can limit the use of these agents. Bone marrow agranulocytosis (carbamazepine), renal stones (topiramate, zonisamide), rash (lamotrigine), hyponatremia (oxcarbazepine, carbamazepine), weight gain (pregabalin) and weight loss (topiramate) are of concern, although steps can be taken to minimize these risks. Fatigue, somnolence, dizziness, and mental slowness symptoms are ubiquitous among these drugs and may prevent adequate pain-relieving doses.

Antidepressants

The central pain inhibitory system is mediated over subcorticospinal centers (periaqueductal grey, dorsolateral pontine reticular formation, nucleus raphe magnus) and pathways that utilize serotonin and norepinephrine neurotransmitters. Clinical experience has shown that the best pain treatment effect is seen with drugs that have a combined serotonin and norepinephrine reuptake inhibition action such as venlafaxine and duloxetine, in contrast to the SSRIs. Tricyclics (TCAs), which have multiple action sites, also have efficacy with neuropathic pain and have the advantage of being less expensive. Toxicity and side effects remain concerns, however, especially in the elderly patient, and there must be careful patient monitoring. The cardiac and anticholinergic effects of amitriptyline can be a limiting factor in reaching an effective drug level in some patients, an issue of particular concern in MS.

Virtually all neuropathic pain analyses, including Cochrane reviews, have endorsed the use of TCAs and SNRIs in the treatment of neuropathic pain. Clinical studies have consistently demonstrated their efficacy. More specifically, recommendations have been for nortriptyline and desipramine (avoiding amitriptyline because of toxicity issues), and the SNRIs duloxetine and venlafaxine over the SSRIs (O'Malley et al., 1999; Raskin et al., 2005; Finnerup et al., 2005, 2007; Cayley, 2006; Dworkin et al., 2007; Moulin et al., 2007; Pollmann and Fineberg, 2008; Kroenke et al., 2009).

Tricyclic therapy should begin at a low dose per day and should be slowly increased to a therapeutic effect. Rarely is treatment beyond 100 mg per day required. Other limiting side effects of the antidepressants are somnolence, fatigue, dizziness, and mental slowing. As with the anticonvulsants, treatment should start at a subtherapeutic level and be advanced slowly. Seizure-inducing concerns are nominal but should be acknowledged, especially for amitriptyline where high doses should be avoided. Patients with MS do have an increased

predilection for seizures. A list of various medication options with doses and side effects is shown in Table 20-2. Note that first-line drugs are identified by an asterisk.

Additional agents

On a theoretical basis, other modulators of central sensitization would include NMDA antagonists dextromethorphan, ketamine, and methadone; however, results do not warrant first-line treatment recommendations. Cannabinoids for central neuropathic pain have also been considered, but results do not warrant first-line use in MS (Svendsen et al., 2004; Rog et al., 2005; Russo, 2008). All of these agents have been relegated to supplemental therapy if first-line treatment fails.

For nonneuropathic pain the focus should be on using agents known to impact on the underlying painful process. For painful spasticity or tonic muscle spasms, muscle relaxants, such as baclofen and tizanidine, can be helpful (Hedley et al., 1975; Satkunam, 2003; Kamen et al., 2008). Unfortunately the necessary amount to bring about significant muscle relaxation often requires a dosage level that induces somnolence (tizanidine) and other untoward side effects such as weakness (baclofen). Intraspinal infusion pumps using baclofen can be used with good success to alleviate severe spasticity and associated pain, while avoiding unwanted side effects (Penn, 1991; Coffey et al., 1993). This technique, however, does carry its own risk profile.

NSAIDs can alleviate musculoskeletal pain, as can mild analgesics, such as acetaminophen and aspirin. Lesser opioid medication such as tramadol, and opioids such as hydrocodone or oxycodone, may also be needed on occasion. Caution should be used when considering tramadol because of its risk of inducing seizures.

RECOMMENDED THERAPY FOR NEUROPATHIC PAIN

A recommended treatment algorithm for treating MS-related neuropathic pain is shown in Figure 20-2, modified from Dworkin et al. (2003), Moulin et al. (2007) and Finnerup et al. (2007). Clinical conditions could alter the decision regarding the initial drug to use, but with the evidence for

TABLE 20-2 Medication Options for Multiple Sclerosis–Related Pain

Generic Name	Trade Name	Starting Dose	Usual Therapeutic Dose	Side Effects of Note
Oxcarbazepine	Trileptal	75 mg bid	150–375 mg bid	Hyponatremia, dizziness, fatigue, nausea, headache, somnolence, diplopia
Carbamazepine	Tegretol	100 mg bid	100–300 mg qid	Bone marrow suppression, rash, lethargy, nausea, leukopenia
Topiramate	Topamax	15 mg qd	25–150 mg bid	Renal stones, fatigue, dizziness
Lamotrigine	Lamictal	25 mg qd	100–150 mg bid	Rash, headache, dizziness, somnolence, weakness
Zonisamide	Zonegran	100 mg qd	100–400 mg qd	Renal stones, somnolence, dizziness, anorexia, nausea
Gabapentin*	Neurontin	100 mg tid	300–600 mg qid	Fatigue, somnolence, dizziness edema
Pregabalin*	Lyrica	50 mg bid	5–100 mg tid	Edema, somnolence, dizziness dry mouth, weight gain
Levetiracetam	Keppra	500 mg bid	500–1000 mg bid	Asthenia, dizziness, somnolence
Amitriptyline	Elavil	10–25 mg qhs	50–100 mg qhs	Somnolence, dry mouth, cardiac toxicity, constipation, urinary retention
Nortriptyline*	Pamelor	10–25 mg qhs	50–100 mg qhs	Somnolence, dry mouth
Desipramine*	Norpramin	10–25 mg qd	50–100 mg qd	Nausea, dry mouth, confusion
Venlafaxine*	Effexor	37.5–75 mg qd	150 mg qd	Nausea, somnolence, insomnia
Duloxetine*	Cymbalta	20–30 mg qhs	60–90 mg qd	Nausea, dry mouth, constipation
Baclofen	Lioresal	5 mg bid	5–15 mg tid	Fatigue, nausea, drowsiness leukopenia, bradycardia
Tizanidine	Zanaflex	2 mg qhs	2–6 mg tid	Dizziness, dry mouth, drowsiness, nausea, constipation
Methocarbamol	Robaxin	500 mg tid	1000 mg qid	Seizures, syncope, dizziness
Cyclobenzaprine	Flexeril	10 mg bid	10 mg qid	Constipation, fatigue, drowsiness, dry mouth,
Tramadol	Ultram	50 mg qd	50–100 mg q8h	Seizures, nausea, vertigo, constipation
Hydrocodone	Vicodin	5/325 mg bid	5–7.5/325 mg q6h	Constipation, somnolence
Hydrocodone	Norco	5/325 mg bid	5–7.5/325 mg q6h	Constipation, somnolence
Oxycodone	Percocet	5/325 mg bid	5–7.5/325 mg q6h	Constipation, somnolence Dependency

Note. The above are conservative guidelines. This is not intended to be a complete list of side effects, complications, or contraindications. Possible drug interactions must also be recognized by the treating physician. A serotonin syndrome must always be a consideration when treating with TCAs, SNRIs, and tramadol. Seizures with tramadol is a risk especially in combination with TCAs, SNRIs or SSRIs. With all of these drugs it is best to start at a low initial dose and increase slowly. In similar fashion, all of these drugs must be discontinued in slow tapering fashion to avoid withdrawal symptoms. Adjustments must be made in regard to the patient's age and the presence of renal or hepatic impairment.

*First–line drugs.

antiepilepsy drug (gabapentin and pregabalin) effectiveness with paroxysmal neuralgic pain, this warrants its own treatment track. Given the differing mechanisms of action for the recommended drugs gabapentin, pregabalin, TCAs, SNRIs, and tramadol, combined therapy can be utilized, within clinical reason, if seeking an improved response. This must be done with a degree of caution, however, especially if one combines an SNRI and a TCA. There is the risk of a serotonin syndrome with these drugs, especially if they are used together. This risk is further enhanced if tramadol, also a serotonin reuptake inhibitor, is added. For combined therapy it would be prudent to markedly reduce the dosage of the utilized TCA to a much lower level if it is planned to use this drug class in addition to an SNRI. Maximum recommended dosage levels per the manufacturers for any utilized medication are to be avoided if polypharmacy is used. It must be stressed that other potential drug interactions be kept in mind and the dosages outlined in Table 20-2 be adjusted if combined therapy is used. Medication doses must be reduced or certain drugs not used at all in patients with impaired renal or hepatic function. Reduced dosages for the elderly patient should also be acknowledged.

It must be remembered that pain may be a heralding event or may be part of an exacerbation of chronic relapsing-remitting MS. In this situation the patient would be a candidate for intravenous steroid therapy, which could ameliorate pain as well as motor and other sensory symptoms.

REFERENCES

Baastrup C, Finnerup NB. Pharmacological management of neuropathic pain following spinal cord injury. *CNS Drugs.* 2008;22(6):455–475.

Beniczky S, Tajti J, Timea Varga E, Vecsei L. Evidence based pharmacological treatment of neuropathic pain syndromes. *J Neural Transm.* 2005;112(6):735–749.

Blom S. Trigeminal neuralgia: its treatment with a new anticonvulsant drug. *Lancet.* 1962;1:839.

Boneschi FM, Colombo B, Annovazzi P, et al. Lifetime and actual prevalence of pain and headache in multiple sclerosis. *Mult Scler.* 2008;14(4):514–521.

Breuer B, Pappagallo M, Knotkova H, Guleyupoglu N, Wallenstein S, Portenoy RK. A randomized, double-blind, placebo-controlled two-period, crossover, pilot trial of lamotrigine in patients with central pain due to multiple sclerosis. *Clin Ther.* 2007;29(9):2022–2030.

Brisman R. Bilateral trigeminal neuralgia. *J Neurosurg.* 1987;67:44–48.

Campbell JN, Meyer RA. Mechanisms of neuropathic pain. *Neuron.* 2006; 52(1):77–92.

Carter S, Sciarra D, Merritt HH. The course of multiple sclerosis as determined by autopsy proven cases. *Res Publ Ass Res Nerv Ment Dis.* 1950;28:471–511.

Cayley WE. Antidepressants for the treatment of neuropathic pain. *Am Fam Phys.* 2006;73(11):1933–1934.

Clifford DB, Trotter JL. Pain in multiple sclerosis. *Arch Neurol.* 1984;41:1270–1272.

Coffey JR, Cahill D, Steers W, et al. Intrathecal Baclofen for intractable spasticity of spinal origin: results of a long term multicenter study. *J Neurosurg.* 1993; 78:226–232.

Corazziari E, Badiali D, Inghilleri M. Neurologic disorders affecting the anorectum. *Gastroenterol Clin.* 2001; 30(1):253–268.

Cruccu G, Gronseth G, Alksne J, et al. AAN-EFNS guidelines on trigeminal neuralgia management. *Eur J Neur.* 2008;15(10):1013–1028.

D'Amico D, La Mantia L, Rigamonti A, et al. Prevalence of primary headaches in people with multiple sclerosis. *Cephalalgia.* 2004;24(11):980–984.

da Silva Cj, da Rocha AJ, Mendes MF, Maia AC, Jr., Braga FT, Tilbery CP. Trigeminal involvement in multiple sclerosis: magnetic resonance imaging findings with clinical correlation in a series of patients. *Mult Scler.* 2005;11(3):282–285.

DeSimone R, Marano E, Brescia Morra V, et al. A clinical comparison of trigeminal neuralgic pain in patients with and without underlying multiple sclerosis. *Neurol Sci.* 2005;26(suppl 2):s150–s151.

Domingues RB. Treatment of trigeminal neuralgia with low doses of topiramate. *Neuropsiquiatr.* 2007;65(3B): 792–794.

Douglas C, Wollin JA, Windsor CD. Illness and demographic correlates of chronic pain among a community-based sample of people with multiple sclerosis. *Arch Phys Med Rehabil.* 2008;89(10):1923–1932.

Dworkin RH, Backonja M, Rowbotham MC, et al. Advances in neuropathic pain: diagnosis, mechanisms, and treatment recommendations. *Arch Neurol.* 2003;60:1524–1534.

Dworkin RH, O'Connor AB, Backonja M et al. Pharmacologic management of neuropathic pain: evidence-based recommendations. *Pain.* 2007;132:237–251.

Ehde DM, Gibbons LE, Chwastiak L, Bombardier CH, Sullivan MD, Kraft GH. Chronic pain in a large community sample of persons with multiple sclerosis. *Mult Scler.* 2003;9(6):605–611.

Eriksson M, Ben-Menachem E, Andersen O. Epileptic seizures, cranial neuralgias and paroxysmal symptoms in remitting and progressive multiple sclerosis. *Mult Scler.* 2002;8(6):495–499.

Espir MLE, Millac P. Treatment of paroxysmal disorders in multiple sclerosis with carbamazepine (Tegretol). *J Neurol Neurosurg Psychiatry.* 1970;33:528–531.

Felts PA. Conduction in segmentally demyelinated mammalian central axons. *J Neurosci.* 1997;17(19):7267–7277.

Finnerup NB, Jensen TS. Clinical use of pregabalin in the management of central neuropathic pain. *Neuropsychiatr Dis Treat*. 2007;3(6):885–891.

Finnerup NB, Otto M, Jensen TS, Sindrup SH. Algorithm for neuropathic pain treatment: an evidence based proposal. *Pain*. 2005;118:289–305.

Finnerup NB, Otto M, Jensen TS, Sindrup SH. An evidence based algorithm for the treatment of neuropathic pain. *Med Gen Med*. 2007;9(2):36.

Gass A, Kitchen N, MacManus DG, Moseley IF, Hennerici MG, Miller DH. Trigeminal neuralgia in patients with multiple sclerosis: lesion localization with magnetic resonance imaging. *Neurology*. 1997; 49(4):1142.

Gee JR, Chang J, Dublin AB, Vijayan N. The association of brainstem lesions with migraine-like headache: an imaging study of multiple sclerosis. *Headache*. 2005;45(6):670–677.

Gilron I, Boother SL, Rowan JS, Max MB. Topiramate in trigeminal neuralgia: a randomized, placebo-controlled multiple crossover pilot study. *Clin Neuropharmacol*. 2001;24(2):109–112.

Gilron I, Watson CP, Cahill CM, Moulin DE. Neuropathic pain: a practical guide for the clinician. *CMAJ*. 2006; 175:265–275.

Grasso MG, Clemenzi A, Tonini A, et al. Pain in multiple sclerosis: a clinical and instrumental approach. *Mult Scler*. 2008;14(4):506–513.

Gray P. Pregabalin in the management of central neuropathic pain. *Expert Opin Pharmacther*. 2007;8(17): 3035–3041.

Hadjimichael O, Kerns RD, Rizzo MA, Cutter G, Vollmer T. Persistent pain and uncomfortable sensations in persons with multiple sclerosis. *Pain*. 2007;127(1–2): 35–41.

Hedley DW, Maroun JA, Espir LE. Evaluation of baclofen for spasticity in multiple sclerosis. *Postgrad Med*. 1975;51(599):615–618.

Hooge JP, Redekop WK. Trigeminal neuralgia in multiple sclerosis. *Neurology*. 1995;45(7):1294–1296.

Jensen PS, Rasmussen P, Reske-Nielsen E. Association of trigeminal neuralgia with multiple sclerosis: clinical and pathological features. *Acta Neurol Scand*. 1982; 65:182–185.

Kamen L, Henney HR, Runyan JD. A practical overview of tizanidine use for spasticity secondary to multiple sclerosis, stroke, and spinal cord injury. *Curr Med Res Opin*. 2008;24(2):425–439.

Kenner M, Menon U, Elliot DG. Multiple sclerosis as a painful disease. *Int Rev Neurobiol*. 2007;79:303–321.

Kerns RD, Kassirer M, Otis J. Pain in multiple sclerosis: a biopsychosocial perspective. *J Rehabil Res Dev*. 2002; 39(20):225–232.

Khan F, Pallant J. Chronic pain in multiple sclerosis: prevalence, characteristics, and impact on quality of life in an Australian community cohort. *J Pain*. 2007; 8(8):614–623.

Khan OA. Gabapentin relieves trigeminal neuralgia in multiple sclerosis patients. *Neurology*. 1998;51: 612–615.

Kroenke K, Krebs EE, Bair MJ. Pharmacotherapy of chronic pain: a synthesis of recommendations from systematic reviews. *Gen Hosp Psychiatry*. 2009;31(3): 206–219.

Langer-Gould A, Moses HH, Murray TJ. Strategies for managing the side effects of treatments for multiple sclerosis. *Neurology*. 2004; 63(11 suppl 5):S35–S41.

Lepore FE. The origin of pain in optic neuritis. *Arch Neurol*. 1991;48(7):748–749.

L'hermitte J, Bollack J, Nicolas M. Les douleurs a type de decharge electrique consecutives a la flexion cephalique dans la sclerose en plaques. *Revue Neurol*. 1924;31:56.

Lunardi G, Leandri M, Albano C, et al. Clinical effectiveness of lamotrigine and plasma levels in essential and symptomatic trigeminal neuralgia. *Neurology*. 1997; 48:1714–1717.

Miller H, Simpson CA, Yeats WK. Bladder dysfunction in multiple sclerosis. *Br Med J*. 1965;1:1265–1269.

Minagar A, Sheremata WA. Glossaopharyngeal neuralgia and MS. *Neurology*. 2000;54(6):1368–1370.

Moore RA, Straube S, Wiffen PJ, Derry S, McQuary HJ. Pregabalin for acute and chronic pain in adults. *Cochrane DB Syst Rev*. 2009;(3):CD007076.

Moulin DE, Foley KM, Ebers GC. Pain syndromes in multiple sclerosis. *Neurology*. 1988;38:1830–1834.

Moulin DE. Pain in multiple sclerosis. *Neurol Clin*. 1989;7(2):321–331.

Moulin DE. Neuropathic pain syndromes: pain in central and peripheral demyelinating disorders. *Neurol Clin*. 1998;16:890–897.

Moulin DE, Clark AJ, Gilron I, et al. Pharmacological management of chronic neuropathic pain: Consensus statement and guidelines from the Canadian Pain Society. *Pain Res Manag*. 2007;12(1):13–21.

Lynch ME, Watson CP. The pharmacotherapy of chronic pain: a review. *Pain Res Manag*. 2006;11(1): 11–38.

O'Connor AB, Schwid SR, Herrmann DN, Markman JD, Dworkin RH. Pain associated with multiple sclerosis: systematic review and proposed classification. *Pain*. 2008;137(1):96–111.

O'Malley PG, Jackson JL, Santoro J, Tomkins G, Balden E, Kroenke K. Antidepressant therapy for unexplained symptoms and symptom syndromes. *J Fam Pract*. 1999;48:980–990.

Oppenheim H. *Textbook of Nervous Diseases*. 5th ed. Vol 1. London: Bruce R Foulis; 1911.

Optic Neuropathy Study Group. The clinical profile of optic neuritis. Experience of the Optic Neuritis Treatment Trial. *Arch Ophth*. 1991;109:1673–1678.

Osterberg A, Boivie J, Thuomas K-A. Central pain in multiple sclerosis: prevalences, clinical characteristics and mechanisms. *Eur J Pain*. 2005;9:531–542.

Osterman PO, Westerberg CE. Paroxysmal attacks in multiple sclerosis. *Brain*. 1975;98:189–202.

Paty DW, Ebers GC. *Multiple Sclerosis*. Philadelphia: FA Davis Co; 1998.

Penn RD. Intrathecal baclofen for spasticity of spinal origin: seven years of experience. *J Neurosurg*. 1992; 77:236–240.

Pichiecchio A, Bergamaschi R, Tavazzi E, Romani A, Todeschini A, Bastianello S. Bilateral trigeminal enhancement on magnetic resonance imaging in a patient with multiple sclerosis and trigeminal neuralgia. *Mult Scler.* 2007;13(6):814–816.

Piwko C, Desjardins OB, Bereza BG, et al. Pain due to multiple sclerosis: analysis of the prevalence and economic burden in Canada. *Pain Res Manag.* 2007; 12(4):259–265.

Pollmann W, Feneberg W, Steinbrecher A, Haupts MR, Henze T. *Fortschr Neurol Psychiatr.* 2005;73(5): 268–285.

Pollmann W, Fineberg W. Current management of pain associated with multiple sclerosis. *CNS Drugs.* 2008; 22(4):291–324.

Putzki N, Pfriem A, Limmroth V, et al. Prevalence of migraine, tension-type headache and trigeminal neuralgia in multiple sclerosis. *Eur J Neurol.* 2009;16(2): 262–267.

Ramirez-Lassepas M, Tulloch JW, Quinones MR, et al. Acute radicular pain as a presenting symptom in multiple sclerosis. *Arch Neurol.* 1992;49:255–258.

Raskin J, Pritchett YL, Wang F, et al. A double blind, randomized multicenter trial comparing duloxetine with placebo in the management of diabetic peripheral neuropathic pain. *Pain Med.* 2005;6:346–356.

Ricther RW, Portenoy R, Sharma U, et al. Relief of painful diabetic peripheral neuropathy with pregabalin: a randomized placebo-controlled trial. *J Pain.* 2005;6: 253–260.

Rog DJ, Nurmikko TJ, Friede T, Young CA. Randomized controlled trial of cannabis based medicine in central pain in multiple sclerosis. *Neurology.* 2005;65(6): 812–819.

Rolak LA, Brown S. Headaches and multiple sclerosis: a clinical study and review of the literature. *J Neurol.* 1990;237(5):300–302.

Rossi S, Mataluni G, Codeca C, et al. Effects of levetiracetam on chronic pain in multiple sclerosis: results of a pilot, randomized, placebo-controlled study. *Eur J Neurol.* 2009;16(3):360–366.

Russo EB. Cannabinoids in the management of difficult to treat pain. *Ther Clin Risk Manag.* 2008;4(1):245–259.

Sabatowski R, Galvez R, Cherry DA, et al. Pregabalin reduces pain and improved sleep and mood disturbances in patients with postherpetic neuralgia: results of a randomized, placebo-controlled clinical trial. *Pain.* 2004;109:26–35.

Samkoff LM, Daras M, Tuchman AJ, Koppel BS. Amelioration of refractory dysesthetic limb pain in multiple sclerosis by gabapentin. *Neurology.* 1997;49: 305–306.

Satkunam LE. Rehabilitation medicine: 3. Management of adult spasticity. *CMAJ.* 2003;169(11):1173–1179.

Schreiber S. The antinociceptive properties of reboxetine in acute pain. *Eur Neuropsychopharmacol.* 2009; 19(10):735–739.

Schwartzman RJ, Gurusinghe C, Gracely E. Prevalence of complex regional pain syndrome in a cohort of multiple sclerosis patients. *Pain Phys.* 2008;11(2):133–136.

Serpell MG, Neuropathic Pain Study Group. Gabapentin in neuropathic pain syndromes: a randomized, double blind placebo controlled trial. *Pain.* 2002;99: 557–566.

Shibasaki H, McDonald WI, Kuroiwa Y. Racial modification of the clinical picture of multiple sclerosis: comparison between British and Japanese patients. *J Neurol Sci.* 1981;49:253–271.

Shibvasaki H, Kuroiwa Y. Painful tonic seizures in multiple sclerosis. *Arch Neurol.* 1974;30:47–51.

Siddall PJ, Cousins MJ, Otte A, Griesling T, Chambers R, Murphy TK. Pregabalin in central neuropathic pain associated with spinal cord injury: a placebo-controlled trial. *Neurology.* 2006;67(10):1792–1800.

Solaro C, Lunardi GL, Capello E, et al. An open label trial of gabapentin treatment of paroxysmal symptoms in multiple sclerosis patients. *Neurology.* 1998;51: P1714–P1717.

Solaro C, Restivo D, Mancardi GL, Tanganelli P. Oxcarbazepine for treating paroxysmal painful symptoms in multiple sclerosis: a pilot study. *Neurol Sci.* 2007;28(3):156–158.

Spillane JD. The treatment of trigeminal neuralgia: preliminary experience with "Tegretol". *Practitioner.* 1964; 192:72.

Svendsen KB, Jensen TS, Bach FW. Does the cannabinoids dronabinol reduce central pain in multiple sclerosis? Randomized double blind placebo controlled crossover trial. *B MJ.* 2004;329(7460):253.

Taylor RS. Epidemiology of refractory neuropathic pain. *Pain Pract.* 2006;6(1):22–26.

Thompson AJ. Multiple sclerosis: symptomatic management. *J Neurol.* 1996;243:559–565.

Twomey JA, Espir MLE. Paroxysmal symptoms as the first manifestations of multiple sclerosis. *J Neurol Neurosurg Psychiatry.* 1980;43:296–304.

Vacca G, Marano E, Brescia Morra V, et al. Multiple sclerosis and headache co-morbidity. A case-control study. *Neurol Sci.* 2007;28(3):133–135.

Vickrey BG, Shekelle P, Morton S, Clark K, Pathak M, Kamberg C. Prevention and management of urinary tract infections in paralyzed persons. *Evid Rep Technol Assess (Summ).* 1999;(6):1–3.

Wiffen PJ, Rees J. Lamotrigine for acute and chronic pain. *Cochrane DB Syst Rev.* 2007;(2):CD006044.

Zvartau-Hind M, Din NU, Gilani A, Lisak RP, Kahn OA. Topiramate relieves refractory trigeminal neuralgia in MS patients. *Neurology.* 2000;55(10):1587–1588.

Tiffany Braley and Alon Y. Avidan

In recent years, several sleep disorders have become recognized as common comorbid conditions among persons with multiple sclerosis (MS). Restless legs syndrome, chronic insomnia, sleep disordered breathing, certain parasomnias, and central nervous system (CNS) hypersomnia frequently impact the general health and quality of life in persons impacted by MS. Moreover, these conditions have been shown to contribute significantly to fatigue, one of the most common and debilitating symptoms of the disease, and one of the most important predictors of quality of life (QOL). Physicians caring for persons with MS should be aware of sleep disorders common to MS patients, as these conditions are largely diagnosable, treatable, and contribute significantly to quality of life.

In this chapter we will review the most common sleep disorders that affect persons with MS; discuss their definition, evaluation, and potential etiologies; and offer an approach to diagnosis and treatment. Figure 21–1 summarizes the etiology of sleep problems in MS based on both direct and indirect causes.

INSOMNIA

Definition/Epidemiology

Insomnia is a common sleep disorder characterized by persistent difficulty initiating or maintaining sleep despite the opportunity and circumstances for sleep, which leads to impairment in daytime functioning (American, 2005). The International Classification of Sleep Disorders (ICSD) defines chronic insomnia as insomnia lasting greater than one month. Insomnia is one of the most

common sleep disorders, affecting approximately 10% of the general population, yet it has a significantly higher prevalence in the MS population, approaching 40% (Tachibana et al., 1994). Chronic insomnia is classified as either primary (idiopathic) or comorbid if attributable to another psychiatric or medical condition, underlying sleep disorder, psychosocial cause, or medication effect (National Institutes of Health State of the Science Conference statement on Manifestations and Management of Chronic Insomnia in Adults, 2005; Benca, 2006). By virtue of several unique conditions that are common in MS—nocturia, stiffness, and pain—patients are at risk for several forms of comorbid insomnia (Fig. 21-1). Identification and treatment of insomnia is crucial, as poor sleep quality strongly correlates with decreased quality of life (National Institutes of Health State of the Science Conference statement on Manifestations and Management of Chronic Insomnia in Adults, 2005; Benca, 2006; Merlino et al., 2009).

Etiology

In persons with MS, insomnia is most frequently attributable to secondary or comorbid causes. Etiologies of primary insomnia such as paradoxical insomnia, idiopathic insomnia, and inadequate sleep hygiene will not be discussed in this chapter as they are beyond the scope of this discussion.

Neurogenic Bladder

Symptoms of neurogenic bladder, including urinary urgency and urge incontinence, affect approximately 75% of persons with MS (Amarenco et al., 1995) and are a common cause of chronic insomnia

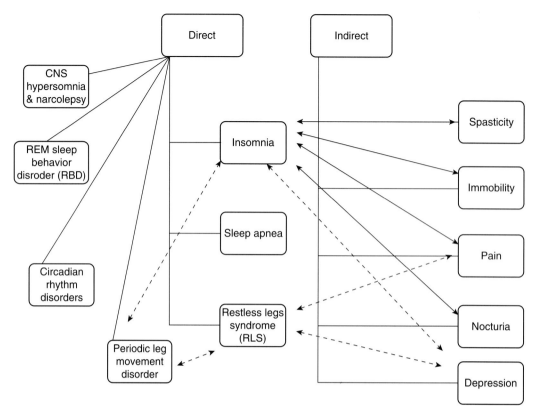

Figure 21-1 Summary of the etiology of sleep problems in multiple sclerosis based on direct and indirect causes. Solid line arrows demonstrate a causative effect, while double dotted line-arrows highlight bidirectional effects, which are discussed in the text. CNS, central nervous system.

in MS patients. Symptoms of neurogenic bladder contribute to prolonged sleep latency and nocturnal awakenings, which are associated with increased daytime fatigue (Leo, 1991). Patients who present with insomnia should be screened for symptoms of neurogenic bladder, with questions regarding frequency of nighttime bathroom trips, episodes of nocturia, and difficulties reinitiating sleep following these episodes.

Depression

Depression is frequently encountered in persons with MS, affecting between 25% and 50% of the MS population at some point during the disease course (Scott et al., 1996; Figved et al., 2005). Depression and insomnia share a common bidirectional relationship and overlapping neurobiology; untreated depression can cause insomnia, and

untreated insomnia can contribute to depression (Benca and Peterson, 2008). A separation of the two symptoms can be challenging, as MS patients are independently at risk for both depression and insomnia. Moreover, several selective serotonin reuptake inhibitors (SSRIs), while helpful for depressive symptoms, may worsen insomnia. Regardless of whether insomnia is a cause or consequence of depression, a multidisciplinary approach, with the addition of both cognitive behavioral therapy (CBT) and pharmacologic treatments is suggested.

Pain/Spasticity

Neuropathic pain and discomfort caused by lower-extremity spasticity experienced by the majority of persons with MS are major contributors to both sleep initiation and sleep maintenance insomnia

(Rae-Grant et al., 1999). Pain also has a strong influence on perception of sleep. Among MS subjects surveyed about conditions that impaired their sleep, a significantly higher number of subjects classified as "poor sleepers" (by the Pittsburgh Quality Sleep Index) reported pain due to MS compared to subjects who were "good sleepers" (Merlino et al., 2009). Not surprisingly, scores for each domain of the Short Form-36 (SF-36) quality of life self-assessment instrument were significantly lower in poor sleepers compared to good sleepers. This finding was especially true with the impact on physical domains of life quality (Lobentanz et al., 2004). At present, only a handful of studies that address quality-of-life issues in persons with MS address the impact of pain and sleep (Attarian, 2009). Because of pain's significant impact on sleep quality and quality of life, assessment of pain should be a routine part of the assessment of patients who complain of sleep disturbances. If pain or spasticity is endorsed, a special effort should be made to incorporate treatment for these symptoms into the insomnia treatment regimen.

parameters recommend an in-depth medical history, physical examination, and sleep history, which require knowledge of other primary sleep disorders, medications, and psychiatric disorders which can cause or contribute to insomnia (Chesson, Jr. et al., 2000). Sleep tests such as polysomnography (PSG) and multiple sleep latency tests (MSLTs) are not routinely indicated unless conditions such as obstructive sleep apnea or periodic leg movement disorder, which may contribute to insomnia, are suspected. While self-administered questionnaires or surveys may help to identify patients with insomnia, they have not been shown to differentiate subtypes or causes of insomnia (Chesson, Jr. et al., 2000). Nonetheless, it is often useful to encourage patients to keep a sleep log to provide the most accurate information about sleep onset, nighttime awakenings, and sleep duration. Persons with MS should also be queried about their sleep pattern and other comorbid conditions that can contribute to insomnia (see later discussion). Table 21-1 provides a sample sleep questionnaire to be used in persons with MS who complain of sleep disturbances.

Diagnosis/Clinical Presentation

As part of the diagnostic workup, the American Academy of Sleep Medicine (AASM) practice

Management

The management of insomnia in the setting of MS should be multifaceted. Due to the multitude

TABLE 21-1 Sleep Disorder Clinic Questionnaire

1. Do you have difficulties falling asleep or maintaining sleep?
2. How many hours do you sleep every night?
3. What is your sleep/wake schedule during the weekdays/weekends?
4. How long does it take you to "get going" after you get out of bed?
5. How long does it take you to fall asleep after deciding to go to sleep?
6. How many times do you wake up during a typical night?
7. Do you wake up frequently due to your urinary symptoms?
8. Do you wake up frequently due to spasticity or discomfort?
9. Do you wake up frequently due to pain?
10. Do you feel that you are excessively sleepy during the day?
11. Do you take naps during the day and if so at what time and for how long?
12. Do you snore loudly or stop breathing at night
13. Do you have creepy crawling or aching feelings in your legs during the day which get worse or start in the evenings or when trying to fall asleep?
14. Have you been told that you kick or twitch your arms or leg during sleep?
15. Have you ever been told that you seem to "act out your dreams" while sleeping? (punched or flailed arms in the air, shouted or screamed

of secondary causes that are common in MS, the physician must be aware of their potential contributions, and efforts should be made to treat these conditions either prior to or in tandem with first-line therapies for insomnia.

If primary insomnia is suspected, or symptoms of insomnia persist despite addressing secondary causes, guidelines for a variety of pharmacologic and nonpharmacologic treatments are available (NIH State-of-the-Science Conference Statement on Manifestations and Management of Chronic Insomnia in Adults, 2005). Many studies have demonstrated the long-term benefits of CBT, specifically for primary insomnia (Espie et al., 2001). This benefit is also translatable to the MS population (van Kessel et al., 2008), although the effects of CBT on secondary forms of insomnia have not been as well established. Common principles of CBT include stimulus control therapy (SCT), sleep restriction, relaxation therapy, cognitive therapy, and sleep hygiene education, which can be successfully administered by a variety of clinicians (Espie et al., 2001). A practical table highlighting behavioral interventions for insomnia is shown in Table 21-2.

Hypnotic management for insomnia consists of benzodiazepines, benzodiazepine agonists (zolpidem, zaleplon, *eszopiclone*), and a melatonin receptor agonist (ramelteon) (Table 21-3). These agents are among the most efficacious and extensively studied, although with the exception of zolpidem Extended Release (ER), *eszopiclone*, and ramelteon, trials regarding the effects of these agents beyond a month are lacking. When selecting hypnotic therapy, the drug's half-life should be considered, as short-acting agents (ramelteon, zolpidem, zaleplon) typically have more robust effects on sleep latency and less efficacy on sleep maintenance, while longer acting agents (*eszopiclone*) have better effects on total sleep time. If a patient endorses sleep onset and sleep maintenance insomnia, a drug with a longer half-life (*eszopiclone*) may be most appropriate.

Side effects and risks should be considered carefully before selecting a benzodiazepine or benzodiazepine agonist. Rebound insomnia following abrupt discontinuation of the drug may occur, especially with shorter acting agents. Several cases of anterograde amnesia, somnambulism (sleep walking), and sleep-related eating following the use of zolpidem have been reported (Roth et al., 1980; Canaday, 1996; Chiang and Krystal, 2008). Tolerance is also a concern among clinicians, as study periods examining the effects of these agents have generally been short, in some cases as few as 8–12 weeks (Perlis et al., 2004) and none

TABLE 21-2

Techniques	Target	Goal
Sleep Hygiene	Inadequate sleep hygiene (e.g irregular bed and wake time, excessive caffeine and alcohol before bedtime, excessive naps, watching TV in bed)	Encourage habits that promote sleep; provide rationale for subsequent instructions
Stimulus Control Therapy	Excessive time awake in bed, irregular sleep-wake schedules, hyperarousal and activities incompatible with sleep.	Strengthen bed and bedroom as sleep stimulus
Sleep Restriction		Improve sleep continuity by limiting time spent in bed awake
Relaxation		Reduce arousal and decrease anxiety (progressive muscular relaxation, transcendental meditation, yoga, biofeedback)
CognitiveTherapy	Unrealistic sleep expectations, misconceptions about sleep, anxiety associated with sleep anticipation and poor cognitive coping skills	Facilitate the development of more rational thoughts about sleep and the consequences of sleep loss.

TABLE 21-3

Agent	Dose (mg)	Onset of Action (min)	Half-life (hours)	Active Metabolites
Nonselective Benzodiazepines				
Triazolam(Halcion®)	0.125–0.25 (0.125)	15–30	2–5	No
Temazepam(Restoril®)	15–30 (7.5–15)	45–60	8–20	No
Estazolam(ProSom®)	1–2(0.5–1.0)	15–60	8–24	No
Flurazepam(Dalmane®)	15–30(7.5)	0.5–1 hr	47–100 including metabolites	Yes
Quazepam(Doral®)	7.5–15(7.5)	20–45	15–40 including metabolites	Yes
New Generation Hypnotics				
Zolpidem(Ambien®)	5–10	Short	2.5	None
Zolpidem-Extended Release(Ambien®-CR)	6.25–15.5	Short	2.8 h	None
Zaleplon(Sonata®)	5–10	Ultrashort	1	None
Eszopiclone(Lunesta®)	1–3	Intermediate	6	Yes
Melatonin Receptor Agonist				
Ramelteon (Rozerem®)	8	Short	1–2.6 Hours	Yes

greater than 24 weeks (Krystal et al., 2003; Chiang and Krystal, 2008). Regardless of which agent is selected, patients should be monitored closely for these symptoms.

An available melatonin agonist has also recently gained recognition as an effective treatment for insomnia. Ramelteon is a Food and Drug Administration (FDA) approved short-acting melatonin receptor agonist with affinity for melatonin MT_1 and MT_2 receptors that has been shown to improve sleep latency in patients with insomnia (Mayer et al., 2009). It is generally well tolerated with no known abuse potential, making it an attractive option for patients who have a history of benzodiazepine abuse.

MOTOR DISTURBANCES OF SLEEP

Definition/Epidemiology

Restless legs syndrome (RLS) and periodic limb movement disorder (PLMD) are common motor disorders of sleep that primarily affect the lower extremities (Hening et al., 2007; Yee et al., 2009). Although considered separate clinical entities, both conditions are relatively common, have the potential to cause disrupted sleep, share a similar pathogenesis, and have an increased prevalence among persons with MS (Deriu et al., 2009).

Restless legs syndrome is defined as a restlessness or uncomfortable sensation of the lower extremities that is exacerbated by rest and inactivity, has a tendency to occur in the evening or before bedtime, and is universally relieved with movement (Hening et al., 2007; Yee et al., 2009). Restless legs syndrome is a common sleep disorder, affecting approximately 10% of the general population (Rothdach et al., 2000) and is a known cause of sleep initiation insomnia (Chesson, Jr. et al., 2000). Restless legs syndrome is classified as idiopathic or primary if no other cause can be identified, or secondary, if caused by another comorbid medical condition known to increase vulnerability, such as MS, in which case the prevalence increases to 3–5 times that of the general population (Auger et al., 2005; Deriu et al., 2009).

Periodic limb movements of sleep (PLMS) consist of rhythmic, stereotyped movements of the lower extremities during sleep. While frequently associated with RLS, PLMS are a separate diagnosis and often exist independently. Like RLS, PLMS are a common cause of disrupted sleep and excessive daytime sleepiness, in which case their terminology is more appropriately revised to periodic limb movement disorder (PLMD). Both primary and secondary forms exist, with many of the secondary causes overlapping with those of RLS. Approximately 80% of patients with RLS also have PLMS (Montplaisir et al., 1997), yet this accounts for a relatively small proportion of PLMS patients and the exact incidence of PLMS in the general population is unknown.

Etiology

Genetic influences

Although the exact cause of primary or idiopathic RLS is yet to be elucidated, genetic factors are strongly implicated, especially in patients younger than 45 years old presenting with RLS complaints. Patients with symptoms of idiopathic RLS have greater than a 50% likelihood of having a first-degree relative with the condition (Walters et al, 1996), and multiple study groups have identified genetic loci associated with increased susceptibility (Winkelmann et al., 2007; Pichler et al., 2008). Despite these findings, however, little is known about the role of genetics in the pathogenesis of RLS.

Dopaminergic dysfunction

A central dopamine hypothesis has long been implicated in the pathogenesis of RLS and PLMD, despite the relative lack of evidence of dopaminergic dysfunction. Prior positron emission tomography (PET) and single photon emission computed tomography (SPECT) studies examining striatal dopamine-2 receptors have yielded conflicting results (Cervenka et al., 2006). Based on the rodent model, loss/dysfunction of dopaminergic neurons in the A11 region of the hypothalamus was postulated as a potential etiology, but a recent study of hypothalamic autopsy specimens from primary RLS patients does not support this hypothesis (Earley et al., 2009). Other authors have proposed dysfunction of downstream dopaminergic pathways, namely diencephalospinal and reticulospinal pathways (Clemens et al., 2006; Frauscher et al., 2007), that project to multiple areas in the spinal cord. Through dopaminergic transmission, these pathways are normally responsible for the suppression of sensory inputs and autonomic output and are susceptible to damage from a variety of pathologic processes. This hypothesis may explain the increased prevalence of RLS in certain neurologic conditions, including spinal cord injury and MS, especially if significant spinal cord involvement is present. In fact, a "symptomatic form" of RLS exists in MS and is associated with higher disability and cervical cord damage, representing a significant risk factor for RLS in MS patients (Manconi et al., 2008).

Deficiency of iron stores

As iron is a component of the enzyme tyrosine dehydroxylase (responsible for the rate-limiting step in dopamine synthesis), it seems intuitive that impaired iron metabolism has been implicated in the pathogenesis of RLS and contributes to its severity. This observation is supported clinically by lower serum and CSF ferritin levels in patients with idiopathic RLS (Earley et al., 2005) and low brain iron stores in RLS patients in MRI and autopsy studies (Allen et al., 2001; Connor et al., 2003). Because of the strong association between low iron stores and RLS, it is recommended that any patient who presents with idiopathic RLS should undergo testing of his or her ferritin level, and iron supplementation should be implemented for ferritin level less than 45 g/L.

Medication/substance effects

Certain medications used in the management of persons with MS, namely antiemetics and antipsychotic dopamine antagonists, are known to cause or worsen RLS. Antidepressants and antihistamines may also contribute to worsening symptoms. Patients should be questioned about the use of these medications and efforts should be made to taper these medications, if medically feasible, before considering treatment with other agents.

Presentation/Diagnosis

Restless legs syndrome

Patients presenting with RLS describe an uncomfortable sensation in their legs, which interferes with rest. Many descriptors have been used to define this sensation, including creeping, crawling, itching, burning, tightening, or tingling. Some patients will have trouble characterizing the symptoms beyond a description of discomfort or an urge to move (Allen, 2003), while others will describe this sensation as painful (Bassetti et al., 2001). Restless legs syndrome is a clinical diagnosis with four required criteria (Allen, 2003):

1. An urge to move the legs (or less often, the arms) is accompanied or caused by uncomfortable sensations.
2. The urge to move worsens at times of rest or inactivity.
3. The aforementioned symptoms are partially or totally relieved by movement.
4. The aforementioned symptoms are exacerbated or are solely present at night.

While the symptoms mentioned previously are necessary for diagnosis of RLS, in some instances, they may not be the patient's primary complaint. Restless legs syndrome is a frequent cause of insomnia. If insomnia is endorsed even in the absence of voluntary leg complaints, the patient should be asked about the presence of the four clinical features of RLS. In addition, a thorough medical evaluation including physical and laboratory studies screening for the most common causes (i.e., iron deficiency anemia) of RLS is recommended.

Lower-extremity spasticity is a common feature of MS that can interfere with sleep, and uncomfortable symptoms of lower-extremity spasticity (tightening, aching) may overlap with symptoms of RLS. Clinicians should bear this in mind when evaluating a patient for RLS. Although sometimes challenging, symptoms of RLS can be teased out with questions regarding their temporal course (Are symptoms solely or predominantly present at night?) and the presence/absence of relief with

movement. If the patient cannot provide clear answers to these questions, empiric treatment may also be diagnostic.

Periodic limb movements

Periodic limb movements in sleep (PLMS) consist of series of stereotyped lower-extremity movements that include flexion at the hip and knee, dorsiflexion of the foot, and extension of the big toe (triple flexion), which occur on an average every 20–40 seconds throughout the night (Fig. 21-3). Unlike RLS, patients with PLMD do not experience sensory symptoms or an urge to move, but instead report disturbed sleep, poor sleep quality, insomnia, or hypersomnia (sleepiness) secondary to arousals, which may occur secondary to periodic limb movements. A bed partner may also provide the history of limb movements.

Also unlike RLS, which is a clinical diagnosis, patients with suspected PLMD need to undergo polysomnography (PSG) to allow for leg movement recording and establish the diagnosis via surface EMG leads placed over the anterior tibialis muscles (see Fig. 21-2). This is particularly important in persons with MS, as triple flexion, a reflex associated with upper motor neuron lesions, can also occur involuntarily in MS. Although a diagnosis of PLMD is not synonymous with RLS, the presence of PLMD strongly supports a diagnosis of RLS. Table 21-4 lists a differential diagnosis of RLS.

Management

Conservative and pharmacologic treatments are available for the treatment of RLS and PLMD, and they can be considered alone or in combination. Conservative approaches are a reasonable first step, and they include the removal of various agents known to exacerbate these conditions. For primary RLS, this may include abstinence from substances such as alcohol, tobacco, and caffeine. An evaluation of the patient's medication list is also recommended, with reduction or discontinuation of medications that can cause or worsen RLS or PLMD (dopamine antagonists, lithium, selective serotonin reuptake inhibitors, tricyclic antidepressants). Iron deficiency should be supplemented, when appropriate.

TABLE 21-4 Differential Diagnosis of RLS

Restless Legs Syndrome	Awake symptom diagnosis made by clinical history, uncomfortable deep creepy crawling sensation brought on at time of inactivity or rest (sitting and lying) immediate relief either complete or partial with movement, symptomatic relief is persistent as long as movement continues, presence of circadian pattern.
PLMD	Sleep phenomenon, diagnosis formally made by sleep study, no sensory symptoms like an urge to move or parastheisas while awake. May patients have sleep disturbance and complaint of hypersomnia and insomnia. One must exclude other causes of periodic leg movements of sleep, including sleep disorder breathing. The condition may respond to benzodiazepines and dopaminergic agents.
Nocturnal leg cramps	Leg cramps or "Charlie horse cramps" are a common experience. Despite coming on at night and being relieved with stretching, cramps are experienced as a usually painful muscular contraction, unlike RLS sensations.
Neuropathic Pain	Sensory symptoms commonly reported as numbness, burning and pain, these descriptors are not as common in RLS. Although the sensory symptoms can increase at night, they usually present throughout the day, while complete and persistent relief is not obtained while walking or during sustained movement.
Arthritis lower limb	Discomfort centered more in joints, does not usually have prominent circadian pattern as seen in RLS.
Neuroleptic induced akathisia	Usually whole body sensation rather than centered only in limbs with no pronounced circadian pattern, less associated sensations, and often no relieve with movement. Should have history of specific medication exposure.
Triple flexion response	A spasm in which the thigh flexes toward the pelvis, the calf toward the thigh, and the foot toward the calf. While often a result of an involuntary reflex secondary to upper motor neuron lesions, it is also the characteristic movement seen in periodic limb movement disorder (PLMD).
Spasticity	An involuntary, velocity-dependent, increase in muscle tone secondary to central nervous system damage, that results in resistance to movement.

Modified from Lesage S, Hening WA. The restless legs syndrome and periodic limb movement disorder: a review of management.
Semin Neurol 2004;24(3):249–259

Pharmacologic treatment should be reserved for those who meet the established diagnostic criteria for RLS and PLMD. PLMD should be treated only if the patient endorses poor sleep quality or excessive daytime sleepiness secondary to the limb movements. Any patient receiving therapy for RLS or PLMD requires periodic follow-up throughout the course of therapy and should be monitored for adverse side effects, augmentation, and tolerance.

Treatments with dopaminergic agents are the most extensively studied and the most appropriate first-line therapy for most patients. The dopamine precursor levodopa, in combination with a decarboxylase inhibitor, has Class I evidence supporting its use in the treatment of RLS and PLMD (Chesson et al., 1999b). More recently, the advent of dopamine agonists, including pramipexole and ropinirole, have moved to the fore as first-line treatments and at this time are the only US Food and Drug Administration (FDA) approved medications for moderate-to-severe RLS (Littner et al., 2004). The effectiveness of other dopamine agonists is less well established. Side effects and risks of dopaminergic agents, including nausea, hypotension, hallucinations, and dyskinesias, should

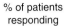

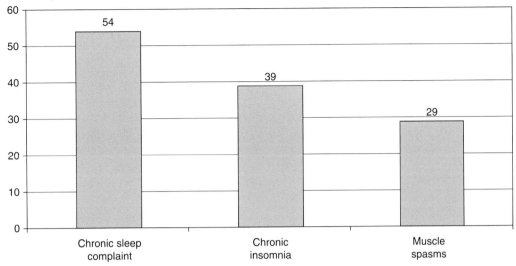

Figure 21-2 Prevalence of sleep disturbances in selected multiple sclerosis cohort (Figure adapted from Tachibana N, Howard RS, Hirsch NP, Miller DH, Moseley IF, Fish D. Sleep problems in multiple sclerosis. *Eur Neurol* . 1994;34(6):320–323.)

be discussed with the patient. The risk of compulsive behaviors, including pathologic gambling, has been reported with dopamine agonists and may not be appropriate for patients with a history of these behaviors (Evans and Butzkueven, 2007; Bostwick et al., 2009).

Augmentation, a phenomenon that involves worsening of RLS symptoms earlier in the day after an evening dose of medication, is associated with levodopa in 70% of patients, especially in doses exceeding 200 mg (Allen and Earley, 1996). If dopaminergic agents are inappropriate or poorly tolerated, other drug classes should be considered. Various anticonvulsants, including gabapentin and carbamazepine, have demonstrated efficacy and may be ideal choices for patients who also suffer from secondary RLS or suffer from other conditions such as neuropathic pain or seizures. Benzodiazepines have also demonstrated therapeutic effect, with clonazepam being the most extensively studied, although data supporting these agents are less robust and confounded by other benzodiazepine effects on sleep (Chesson, Jr.

et al., 1999a), including sedation and potential respiratory depression in older adults. Various opioid agents, including oxycodone and methadone, may also be of benefit in selected individuals, but the addiction potential and side effect profile associated with opioids should be strongly considered and may preclude their use. To date, no trials assessing the safety and efficacy of pharmacologic agents for the treatment of RLS in pregnant patients are available. Table 21-5 highlights the therapeutic options in patients with RLS.

PARASOMNIAS AND REM SLEEP BEHAVIOR DISORDER

Parasomnias constitute a heterogeneous group of abnormal motor, emotional, autonomic or verbal behaviors that occur during sleep or sleep–wake transition (Mahowald et al., 2004). Examples of key parasomnias include sleepwalking (somnambulism), nightmares, sleep terrors, hypnic jerks, confusional arousals, bruxism, and REM sleep behavioral disorder (RBD). For the purposes of

TABLE 21-5

Drug: class (generic/brand)	Dose	Potential side effects
Iron:		
Ferrous Sulfate	325 mg BID/TID with Vitamin-C 100–200mg Recommended for Ferritin<45 ug/L	GI side effects: Constipation
Dopamine Agonists:		
Pramipexole (Mirapex)* Ropinirole (Requip)*	0.125–1.5mg, 1–2 hours before symptoms. Start low and increase slowly. 0.5–4 mg 1–2 hours before symptoms. Start low and increase slowly.	Significant daytime sleepiness, sleep attaches, nausea, compulsive behaviors (compulsive hypersexuality, hallucinations,
Dopamine Precursors:		
Levodopa/Cardidopa (Sinemet)	25/200 mg: ½ tab–3 tabs 30 minutes before onset of symptoms	Augmentation, Rebound, Nausea, sleepiness, gastrointestinal disturbances
Anticonvulsants:		
Gabapentin (Nuerotin)	100–1800mg/day divided TID	Daytime sleepiness, nausea,
Benzodiazepines: Temazepam, Triazolam	Temazepam: Triazolam: 7.5–30mg 0.25–0.5	Drowsiness, dizziness, sedation, amnesia, ataxia, gastrointestinal symptoms
Benzodiazepine agonists: Zolpidem, Zaleplon	5–10mg 15–30 minutes before bedtime	
Opiates Darvocet (Darvoset-N) Darvon (Propozypen) Codeine	300mg/day 65–135 mg at bedtime 30mg	Nausea, vomiting, restlessness, constipation.Addiction, tolerance may be possible

*Only FDA indicated treatment for moderate-severe RLS as of July, 2009 (Adler, 1997; Ahmed, 2002; Akpinar, 1987; Albanese & Filippini, 2003; Allen & Earley, 1996; Hening, 2004; Hening, et al., 2004; Silber, Girish, & Izurieta, 2003)

Adler CH: Treatment of restless legs syndrome with gabapentin. Clinical Neuropharmacology 20:148–151, 1997.

Ahmed I: Ropinirole in restless leg syndrome Mo Med 99:500–501, 2002.

this chapter, we will describe those parasomnias that are clinically relevant to persons with MS, namely RBD. REM sleep behavioral disorder has rarely been reported as the first manifestation of MS, has the potential to mimic other disorders common in MS (other sleep disorders, epilepsy), and may be a consequence of medications used to treat concomitant conditions in MS patients.

Definition/Epidemiology

REM behavioral sleep disorder is characterized as a loss of motor inhibition during REM sleep, resulting in excessive and sometimes violent

nocturnal vocal or motor activity and dream enactment (Schenck and Mahowald, 2005; Mahowald et al., 2007). Identification of the condition is essential, as patients with RBD and their bed partners are at risk for potential injury related to the violent behaviors of the affected patient (Schenck et al., 1989; Comella et al., 1998). The prevalence of RBD is less than 1% of the general population (Ohayon, 1997). Both idiopathic and secondary forms exist. Idiopathic RBD comprises approximately 40% of all RBD patients and is most common in male patients age 50 years or older (Schenck et al., 1993). Secondary forms are most commonly associated with neurologic diseases

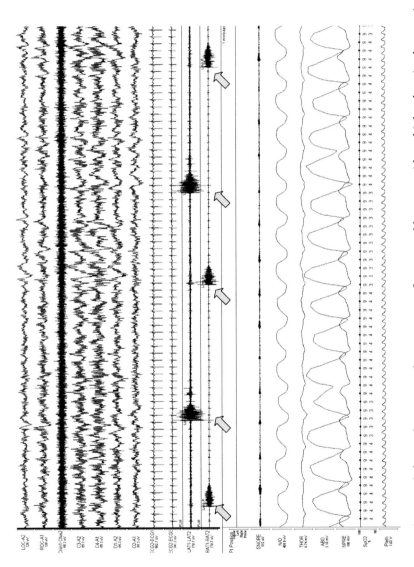

Figure 21-3 This is a 1-minute sleep epoch from a diagnostic polysomnogram of a 37-year-old woman with multiple sclerosis who experiences difficulties initiating sleep, excessive daytime sleepiness, and uncomfortable sensation in her legs associated with an irresistible urge to move her legs. Her husband reports that she has frequent night-time kicking and jerking movements, which disrupt his sleep. Illustrated in this figure is a succession of five periodic limb movements occurring in the right and left anterior tibialis muscles. According to the American Academy of Sleep Medicine, periodic leg movements are diagnosed when more than 15 leg movements per hour of sleep are captured. Four or more consecutive movements are required and the interval between movements is typically 20–40 seconds. The movements should appear at sequence of four or more separated by an interval of more than 5 and less than 90 seconds and have an amplitude of greater or equal to 25% of toe dorsiflexion during the calibration. Channels are as follows: Electrooculogram (left: LOC-A2, right: ROC-A1), chin EMG (Chin-Chin), EEG [Left central (C3-A1), right central (C4-A1), left occipital (O1-A2), right occipital (O2-A1)], electrocardiogram (ECG), limb EMG [left leg (LAT), right leg (RAT)], patient position, snoring (SNORE), nasal-oral airflow (N/O), respiratory effort [Thoracic (THOR), Abdominal (ABD)], nasal pressure (NPRE), and oxygen saturation (SpO2) and plethysmography channel.

that affect the extrapyramidal system or brainstem REM generators, including the synucleinopathies, tauopathies, narcolepsy, and MS (Fig. 21-3) (Schenck et al., 1993; Tippmann-Peikert et al., 2006). While the incidence of RBD in MS is not known, case reports have shown that in otherwise young and healthy individuals, RBD may be the first clinical manifestation of the disease (Plazzi and Montagna, 2002).

Etiology

The etiology of idiopathic RBD is still largely unknown. Genetic influences, specifically involving HLA class II genes, may play a role (Mahowald and Schenck, 1996). Interestingly, the incidence of RBD is increased in narcoleptic patients, lending further support to this hypothesis (Nightingale et al., 2005). Due to the disproportionate number of males affected by the condition, hormonal influences have also been proposed, yet several studies have found no association between hormonal levels and the incidence of RBD (Chou et al., 2007; Iranzo et al., 2007). Decreased dopamine innervation in the striatal regions has also been implicated as a potential contributor (Albin et al., 2000).

Secondary RBD is most often associated with neurodegenerative processes, structural brainstem lesions, or demyelination involving the dorsal mesopontine tegmentum or ventromedial medulla (Tippmann-Peikert et al., 2006) (Fig. 12-4). The most common neurologic diseases associated with RBD are the synucleinopathies, including Parkinson disease, Lewy body disease, and multisystem atrophy (Schenck et al., 1993; Olson et al., 2000), although any CNS disorder that affects REM generators may increase the risk, including MS (see MRI depicting a demyelinating lesion in the dorsal pons in Fig. 21-4A).

Clinicians should also be aware that it is not uncommon for RBD to precede neurodegenerative disease, and it is exceptionally rare in young adults and women. Thus, the presence of RBD in the unsuspected patient who does not fit the correct demographic predisposition should alert the clinician to investigate for secondary causes.

Secondary RBD may also be precipitated by medications frequently utilized in MS. Various selective serotonin reuptake inhibitors (SSRIs), selective norepinephrine reuptake inhibitors (SNRIs), and monoamine oxidase inhibitors (MAOIs) have all been implicated in RBD or REM without atonia, considered by some to be a form fruste of RBD (Louden et al., 1995; Schutte and Doghramji, 1996; Winkelman and James, 2004). Drug or alcohol abuse or withdrawal may also exacerbate RBD (Schenck et al., 1993). Physicians evaluating patients for suspected RBD should pay close attention to the patient's medication list and consider alternative medications if at all possible.

Presentation/Diagnosis

As per ICSD-II guidelines, a combination of clinical and polysomnographic criteria are required for a diagnosis of RBD (American, 2005). Clinical diagnostic criteria include movements of the body or limbs associated with dreaming and at least one of the following: potentially harmful sleep behavior, dreams that appear to be acted out, and sleep behavior that disrupts sleep continuity.

When evaluating a patient for possible RBD, it is also important to rule out other conditions that disproportionately affect persons with MS and may present with similar clinical findings. Complex partial seizures, which commonly occur at night and may be associated with fear or violent outbursts, should be ruled out with nocturnal EEG (Silvestri et al., 1989). Other sleep disorders associated with abnormal motor activity which can mimic RBD include sleep terrors and somnambulism (Schenck et al., 1989), arousals related to apneic events (Nalamalapu et al., 1996), and periodic limb movements (Schenck et al., 1993), highlighting the importance of polysomnogram.

Management

Before considering pharmacologic therapies, one should incorporate safety measures to avoid injurious behavior to the patient or the bed partner. This may involve sleeping in a sleeping bag on the floor to decrease fall risk, sleeping in separate beds/bedrooms for the bed partner's safety, and removing all items next to the bed that may be potentially hazardous (glass or sharp objects, heavy objects, etc.) The second step involves the avoidance of factors known to exacerbate RBD, such as caffeine, alcohol, or certain antidepressants.

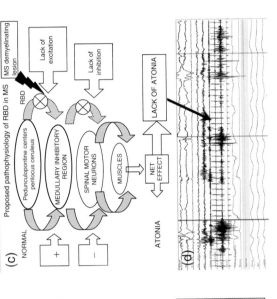

A, B: Demyelinating lesion in the patient's dorsal pons (A-sagital & B-coronal views) consistent with her demyelination lesion

C: Muscle atonia during REM sleep results from pontine-mediated perilocus ceruleus inhibition of motor activity. In RBD, the brainstem mechanisms generating muscle become disrupted.

D: Excessive limb muscle tone during REM sleep as reflected by abnormal electromyography (EMG) augmentation.

Normal REM sleep is reflected by EMG atonia which is not seen here.

Figure 21-4 Structural lesions associated with REM sleep behavioral disorder in a 51-year-old woman with multiple sclerosis whose husband described witnessing nightly sleep-related groaning, screaming, limb flailing, and violent thrashing. (Based on a case published in Tippmann-Peikert M, Boeve BF, Keegan, M. *Neurology.* 2006; 66(8):1277–1279.)

Pathophysiology of REM sleep behavior Disorder: Muscle atonia during REM sleep results from pontine-mediated perilocus ceruleus inhibition of motor activity. This pontine activity exerts an excitatory influence on medullary inhibitory centers (magnocellularis neurons) via the lateral tegmentoreticular tract. These neuronal groups, in turn, hyperpolarize the spinal motor neuron postsynaptic membranes via the ventrolateral reticulospinal tract. In REM sleep behavior disorder (RBD), the brainstem mechanisms generating muscle become disrupted. The pathophysiology of RBD in humans is based on the cat model. In the cat model, bilateral pontine lesions result in a persistent absence of REM atonia associated with prominent motor activity during REM sleep, similar to that observed in RBD in humans. The pathophysiology of the idiopathic form of RBD in humans is still not very well understood but may be related to reduction of striatal presynaptic dopamine transporters. (Modified from Avidan, AY. Sleep disorders in the elderly, primary care. *Clin Off Pract Sleep Dis.* 2005;32(2):536–587; and Tippmann-Peikert M, Boeve BF, Keegan, M. *Neurology.* 2006; 66(8):1277–1279.)

Pharmacologic therapies most commonly used to treat RBD include clonazepam, melatonin, dopamine agonists, and precursor agents and anticonvulsants (Ferini-Strambi and Zucconi, 2000; Takeuchi et al., 2001; Boeve et al., 2003; Fantini et al., 2003; Schmidt et al., 2006). Of these, clonazepam is probably the most widely used, and it is usually effective at relatively low doses of 0.25–0.5 mg administered before bedtime (Olson et al., 2000). If other comorbid conditions exist, another agent may be more appropriate, such as dopaminergic agents for patients with RLS, or an anticonvulsant for patients with seizures or neuropathic pain.

CENTRAL NERVOUS SYSTEM HYPERSOMNIA AND NARCOLEPSY

What Is the Difference between Sleepiness and Fatigue?

Even before moving into the specific discussion of hypersomnia (severe sleepiness) and narcolepsy, one needs to set the ground rules for distinguishing between seemingly simple terms, which are often used interchangeably, leading to confusion. Unlike "tiredness," "fatigue," and "weakness," "sleepiness" is associated with falling asleep or fighting sleep at inappropriate times. Fatigue is usually associated with other comorbid conditions such as MS, cardiopulmonary disease, endocrine disorders, viral illness, neuromuscular disease, and chronic fatigue syndrome and is usually not accompanied by episodes of inappropriate sleep unless disrupted sleep is part of the clinical picture (Aldrich, 1999).

Definition/Epidemiology

Narcolepsy is defined as a pentad of symptoms that include severe excessive daytime sleepiness (EDS), disturbed nocturnal sleep, cataplexy, hypnagogic hallucinations, and sleep paralysis; the latter three are abnormal manifestations of REM sleep intrusion into wakefulness (Mitler et al., 1990; Aldrich, 1999; Bassetti, 1999). The prevalence of narcolepsy in the general population is estimated to be between 0.03% and 0.07%; male to female prevalence is equal. The prevalence among persons with MS is unknown.

Etiology

Hypothalamic dysfunction

Recent evidence suggests that loss of hypocretin-1-secreting cells in the hypothalamus, possibly on an autoimmune basis, plays a pathogenetic role in the majority of cases (Kanbayashi et al., 2002; Mignot, 2004). Despite the substantial clinical similarities between narcolepsy without cataplexy and narcolepsy with cataplexy, some evidence suggests that the underlying pathophysiology of the two conditions is not identical. Cerebrospinal fluid (CSF) hypocretin-1 levels are most often normal in narcolepsy without cataplexy, whereas they are substantially decreased or undetectable when cataplexy is present (Kanbayashi et al., 2002). This suggests that the underlying cause or causes for narcolepsy without cataplexy may not involve loss of hypocretin-1-secreting hypothalamic neurons.

Genetic influences

Narcolepsy is associated with both human leukocyte antigen (HLA) DR2 and HLA DQ1 (Lin et al., 2001; Mignot et al., 2001; Mignot, 2005). DQB1*0602 is a more sensitive marker for narcolepsy and appears to be correlated with frequency and severity of cataplexy (Lin and Mignot, in press; Mignot et al., 2001). Although the HLA antigen may be important in the pathogenesis of narcolepsy, it is neither sufficient nor necessary for disease expression. The DR2 appears to occur almost as frequently in narcolepsy without cataplexy as it does in the narcolepsy-cataplexy syndrome (Mignot, 2005). At the same time, it is interesting to note that the DR2 histocompatibility antigen is simultaneously positive in both MS and narcolepsy patients, especially the DRB5*0101 allele (Younger et al., 1991; Fogdell et al., 1995). This may point to bidirectional communication pathways between the immune system and the CNS, influencing these two neurological disorders (Grosskopf et al., 1998), and the relationship may have an even more significant role for the narcolepsy- and

MS-associated HLA allele DQB1*0602 in schizo-phrenia subtypes (Grosskopf et al., 1998).

Clinical Presentation/Diagnosis

The ICSD II classifies conditions characterized by primary hypersomnolence into a single category entitled "Hypersomnias of central origin not due to a circadian rhythm disorder, sleep related breathing disorder, or other case of disturbed nocturnal sleep" (American, 2005). Familiarity with the five symptoms of narcolepsy is also essential. These symptoms and the subtypes of narcolepsy are reviewed later.

Excessive daytime sleepiness

Excessive daytime sleepiness (EDS) is the most common and initial symptom of narcolepsy. Nonetheless, clinicians should be aware that sudden sleep episodes or sleep attacks can occur with *any* cause of sleepiness, including sleep deprivation sleep apnea, idiopathic hypersomnia, and medication-related drowsiness (Bassetti, 1999).

Cataplexy

In Greek, *cataplexy* means "to strike down." It is characterized by a transient sudden loss of muscle tone, usually triggered by a strong emotional state. The loss of muscle tone may be partial, involving only a few muscle groups such as the face or neck, or complete, leading to full body collapse. Cataplexy is a defining feature of narcolepsy, and its presence is virtually diagnostic (Fry, 1987; Karitani et al., 1997; Aldrich, 1999; Bassetti, 1999; Silber, 2001; Olejniczak and Fisch, 2003).

Sleep paralysis

Sleep paralysis is characterized by an inability to move during sleep onset or upon awakening (Aldrich, 1999). It occurs in 25%–50% of patients with narcolepsy. Patients describe the sensation of a struggle to move that lasts for a few seconds or minutes during sleep onset or offset. The paralysis usually ends spontaneously or after mild sensory stimulation but sometimes continues even after vigorous attempts at arousal.

Hypnagogic and hypnopompic hallucinations

Hypnagogic (drowsiness preceding sleep) and hypnopompic (drowsiness preceding wakefulness) hallucinations occur in about 20%–40% of patients with narcolepsy. Visual dream-like hallucinations are the rule, although there may be auditory or tactile hallucinations.

Disrupted nocturnal sleep

Disrupted nocturnal sleep occurs in about 70%–80% of patients with narcolepsy. In some, it may be the prominent complaint, but it is not the major cause of daytime sleepiness. In addition to cataplexy, hypnagogic hallucinations, and sleep paralysis, which make up the narcolepsy tetrad, disrupted nocturnal sleep makes the "narcolepsy pentad."

Automatic behaviors

Automatic behaviors may be due to chronic sleepiness. These are amnesic episodes associated with semipurposeful activity that may occur in up to 8% of narcoleptics as well as patients with other sleep disorders.

Subtypes of narcolepsy

Important hypersomnias of relevance to the neurologists who treats MS patients include the following:

1. *Narcolepsy with cataplexy.* Narcolepsy with cataplexy is characterized by excessive daytime sleepiness (EDS) and cataplexy. Patients also have significant nocturnal sleep disruption.
2. *Narcolepsy without cataplexy.* Narcolepsy without cataplexy is similar to narcolepsy with cataplexy in most clinical respects except for the lack of definite cataplexy (American, 2005).
3. *Narcolepsy due to medical condition.* Narcolepsy with and without cataplexy is found in a number of genetic, medical, and neurological conditions. Structural lesions in the hypothalamic region, including tumors, sarcoidosis, and MS, may also cause secondary narcolepsy (Villablanca et al., 1976;

Aldrich and Naylor, 1989; Rao and Singhal, 1997; Wang et al., 1998; Vetrugno et al., 2009). Symptomatic narcolepsy has also been reported in several neurological disorders in the absence of demonstrable hypothalamic involvement, including acute disseminated encephalomyelitis, multiple system atrophy, and head injury (Melberg et al., 1995; Bruck and Broughton, 2004).

Management

Behavioral therapy

Patient and family education regarding proper sleep hygiene is an appropriate first step for patients with narcolepsy. The risks associated with sleepiness while driving and in the work place, and the role of medications, should be discussed. Patients should be encouraged to obtain adequate sleep, as sleep deprivation will aggravate symptoms. It is customary to recommend that patients take "power naps": One-to-three 20-minute naps per day can lead to improvement in alertness and psychomotor performance without exacerbating nocturnal sleep disruption. Although few studies have been conducted regarding the effects of naps in narcolepsy, many clinicians and patients believe that naps are helpful (nonpharmacologic and pharmacologic treatments are summarized in Table 21-6).

Pharmacologic treatments for excessive daytime sleepiness

A variety of pharmacologic therapies are available to increase wakefulness, vigilance, and performance, and decrease the sense of fatigue in patients with narcolepsy and excessive daytime sleepiness secondary to narcolepsy. Until recently, CNS stimulants were the mainstay of treatment, but these have largely been replaced by the wake promoting agents modafinil and armodafinil.

While its exact mechanism is not known, methylphenidate is a stimulant that presumably acts by blocking norepinephrine and dopamine reuptake into presynaptic neurons. It is FDA-indicated for attention-deficit/hyperactivity disorder (ADHD), but it has also been shown to improve objective and subjective sleepiness in patients with narcolepsy. Doses range from 30 to 60 mg/day, divided b.i.d or t.i.d. Side effects include nervousness, agitation, insomnia, akathisia, and headaches. Caution should be used in patients with a history of cardiac abnormalities. Methylphenidate should be avoided in patients with monoamine oxidase

TABLE 21-6

Condition	Nonpharmacologic	Pharmacologic
Narcolepsy	Prophylactic "power naps"	I. **Armodafinil, Modafinil,* Dextroamphetamine;* Mamphetamine;* Methylphenidate;* Sodium oxybate;***
		II. **Hypnotics (disturbed nighttime sleep),**
		III. **Antidepressants (cataplexy)**
Insufficient Sleep Syndrome	Increase total sleep time; e.g, naps	Not recommended
Obstructive Sleep Apnea	Positive pressure therapy, airway surgery	Armodafinil*, Modafinil* (for residual sleepiness with CPAP compliance or other standard therapy)
Shift Work Sleep Disorder	Naps, bright-light therapy, avoid a.m. sunlight, protected sleep environment	Armodafinil*, Modafinil,*Stimulants, caffeine, melatonin, hypnotics

* FDA-approved

inhibitors, such as isocarboxazid, phenelzine, selegiline, and tranylcypromine, as concomitant use may cause hypertensive crisis.

Dextroamphetamine is FDA approved for the treatment of ADHD and narcolepsy. Formulations include 5 and 10 mg tablets. Sustained and extended release capsules are also available. Dosing typically starts at 10 mg/day but may be gradually increased to a maximum dose of 60 mg/day, divided b.i.d or t.i.d. Contraindications are numerous but include advanced arteriosclerosis, symptomatic cardiovascular disease, moderate-to-severe hypertension, hyperthyroidism, history of drug abuse, glaucoma, or concomitant MAOI use. Side effects include hypertension, tachycardia, weight loss, headache, and agitation.

Modafinil (Provigil) and its R-enantiomer, armodafinil (Nuvigil), are wake-promoting agents approved by the FDA for managing sleepiness associated with narcolepsy, shift-work sleep disorder, and obstructive sleep apnea with residual excessive sleepiness despite optimal use of continuous positive airway pressure (CPAP). While the precise mechanism of action for both drugs is not fully characterized (Lankford, 2008), the proposed mechanism involves a central α_1-adrenergic agonistic effect at the level of the hypothalamus. Both drugs are generally well tolerated, but potential side effects include headaches, psychiatric disturbances, and gastrointestinal irritation. Modafinil and armodafinil are Schedule IV drugs with lower abuse potential relative to Schedule II or III drugs. For most patients with relatively mild sleepiness, a starting dose of modafinil at 100 mg every morning may be suggested, which can be slowly titrated up over several weeks to 200 mg every morning. Doses of 400 mg have been well tolerated, but there is no consistent evidence that this dose confers additional benefit beyond that of 200 mg/day. Lower doses should be used in hepatically impaired patients.

It should be noted that modafinil is not FDA approved for MS-related fatigue. Nonetheless, several studies have demonstrated improved fatigue, focused attention and dexterity, and enhanced motor cortex excitability at doses lower than those required for narcolepsy patients (Rammohan et al., 2002; Willoughby, 2002; Zifko et al., 2002; McAllister, 2003; Tellez and Montalban, 2004; Lange et al., 2009). Modafinil may also have a role in improving primary nocturnal enuresis in MS (Carrieri et al., 2007).

Treatments for cataplexy/REM sleep intrusions

Antidepressants are the mainstay of treatment for cataplexy and sleep paralysis. Current therapy focuses on symptom management through a variety of REM sleep–suppressing medications that are used off label, including tricyclic antidepressants (TCAs) and serotonin-selective reuptake inhibitors (SSRIs). Caution must be taken in discontinuing these medications, as an abrupt discontinuation may precipitate a marked increase in number and severity of attacks, the so-called rebound cataplexy. Another agent that may be considered is sodium oxybate, an endogenous metabolite of GABA that is currently approved for both the management of cataplexy and hypersomnia in narcolepsy. This drug has abuse potential and some CNS adverse events that may preclude its use.

SLEEP DISORDERED BREATHING

Sleep-disordered breathing (SDB) describes a group of disorders characterized by respiratory abnormalities during sleep. The most notable types of sleep-disordered breathing, obstructive sleep apnea (OSA) and central sleep apnea (CSA), will be reviewed here.

Definition/Epidemiology

Obstructive sleep apnea (OSA), the most ubiquitous type of sleep-disordered breathing, was first described in 1976 (Guilleminault et al., 1976). Its prevalence is estimated to be 4% among middle-aged men and 2% among middle-aged women (Young et al., 1993), although this risk may be higher among predisposed individuals (see section on "Etiology"). Obstructive sleep apnea is defined as an obstruction in the upper airway despite the subject's attempt to resume normal respiration (Peppard et al., 2000). The episodes, which by definition last for 10 seconds or longer, can be complete (apneas), or there may be a partial impairment in ventilation (hypopneas) despite continuous respiratory effort. Repeated arousals are required to re-establish sufficient muscular tone in the pharynx to reopen the upper airways and normalize oxygen levels. As a result, patients often have reduced sleep efficiency and quality, which is reflected by a decrease in slow-wave sleep and REM sleep.

In contrast to OSA, central sleep apnea (CSA) results from complete or partial impairment of airflow in the *absence* of a respiratory effort (Shochat and Pillar, 2003). This is typically due to impaired respiratory control at the level of the brain stem, namely the medullary reticular formation. While the prevalence of CSA is much less than that of OSA, patients with CNS disorders that affect the brain stem, including MS, may be at increased risk for this condition.

Etiology

Obstructive sleep apnea may occur at multiple levels of obstruction, including the nasopharynx, oropharynx, and hypopharynx. Predisposed individuals include patients with macroglossia, hypertrophy of the tonsils, or a long uvula (Shochat and Pillar, 2003).

In persons with MS, brainstem involvement is a risk factor for CSA and potential death during sleep. Several case reports of apneic events or sudden death associated with medullary lesions have been described (Auer et al., 1996). This suggests that even unilateral lesions of the medullary reticular formation may give rise to SDB, highlighting the need to assess all persons with MS with medullary and brainstem involvement for SDB (Table 21-1).

Clinical Presentation/Diagnosis

The diagnosis of sleep-disordered breathing begins with the clinical history and physical exam. The presence of obesity, thick neck, crowded oropahryngeal inlet, retrognathia, or micrognathia are common physical examination findings associated with OSA. Common symptoms include severe hypersomnolence, concentration problems, memory disturbances, nocturnal hypertension, nighttime arousals, confusion, and impairment in neuropsychological functioning. Some patients may experience potentially fatal cardiac arrhythmias in association with desaturation events. There is also a surge of sympathetic activity associated with elevation of blood pressure and tachycardia (Somers et al., 1995), which may increase cardiovascular morbidity with OSA (Narkiewicz and Somers, 1997; Morgan et al., 1998; Young et al., 2002). Obstructive sleep apnea is also an independent risk factor for the development of hypertension in adults, even after adjusting for age, sex, and body mass index (Lavie and Hoffstein, 2000).

In regard to MS, intractable hiccups may be a clinical sign to the presence of SDB, due to lesions in the tegmentum of the medulla oblongata, including the paramedian and lateral reticular formations (Funakawa et al., 1992, 1993).

To confirm the diagnosis, a full-night polysomnogram (PSG), the gold standard and study of choice for diagnosing OSA, should be performed. The presence of more than five apneas or hypopneas per hour of sleep (Young et al., 1993), despite continuous respiratory effort, is necessary for the diagnosis (see Fig. 21-2).

In central sleep apnea, the PSG demonstrates breathing cessation for 10 seconds or longer in the absence of respiratory effort and may be associated with frequent arousals from sleep, bradytachyarrhythmia, and arterial oxygen desaturation.

Management

Evidence suggests that treatment options for central sleep apnea (CSA) should be based on the underlying pathophysiology, and be tailored to address hypercapnic versus nonhypercapnic CSA. Although a discussion of the various forms of CSA and their etiologies are beyond the scope of this chapter, treatment may include weight loss, supplemental oxygen, and bi-level positive airway pressure (PAP; Eckert et al., 2007).

Management of obstructive sleep apnea may be divided into conservative and non-conservative (surgical) approaches. Conservative approaches include modification of behavioral factors such as weight loss, avoidance of alcohol, limiting the use of sedating compounds, and smoking cessation. The most commonly accepted conservative mode of therapy includes the use of positive pressure therapy in the form of nasal continuous positive airway pressure (nasal CPAP). For the purposes of this chapter, surgical approaches will not be discussed.

Positive pressure therapy, in the form of either continuous positive pressure therapy (CPAP) or bi-level PAP, should be considered as a first-line treatment option. Continuous positive pressure therapy is the most widely used treatment for obstructive sleep apnea and has been shown to improve the nocturnal oxygen saturation and quality of sleep in younger adults. Nasal CPAP consists of an air pressure–generating device (used at a predetermined level) that is applied over the nose (and sometimes the mouth) of the patient utilizing a securely fitting mask (Strollo Jr. et al., 1998). The positive air pressure acts as a pneumatic splint in maintaining upper airway patency while the patient is asleep (Quinnell and Smith, 2004).

Oral appliances (Fig. 21-3) work by repositioning the mandible in the anterior and inferior position, improving the upper airway space at the hypopharyngeal level. Oral appliances are considered by many as a useful conservative nonsurgical approach for the treatment of mild to moderate obstructive sleep apnea and for snoring, due to their portability, size, and low cost (Quinnell and Smith, 2004). They are also an attractive alternative for claustrophobic patients who are unable to tolerate CPAP.

CONCLUSION

While the treatment of MS and its symptoms can be challenging, physicians should be aware of the variable presentations of sleep disorders in persons with MS to facilitate early evaluation and treatment. As we continue to learn more about the impact of sleep and its influence on general health, we predict that these influences will be of even greater import in MS. An in-depth knowledge of these conditions will facilitate better patient care and lead to increased quality of life.

ACKNOWLEDGMENTS

Dr. Braley's contribution was supported (in part) by a Sylvia Lawry Physician Fellowship from the National Multiple Sclerosis Society.

REFERENCES

Albin RL, Koeppe RA, Chervin RD, et al. Decreased striatal dopaminergic innervation in REM sleep behavior disorder. Neurology. 2000;55:1410–1412.

Aldrich MS. Sleep Medicine. Vol. 53, Sleep Medicine. New York: Oxford University Press; 1999.

Aldrich MS, Naylor MW. Narcolepsy associated with lesions of the diencephalon. Neurology. 1989;39: 1505–1508.

Allen RP. Ambulatory activity monitoring. In: Chokroverty S, Hening WA, Walters AS, eds. Sleep and Movement Disorders. Philadelphia: Butterworth-Heinemann; 2003: 144–152.

Allen RP, Barker PB, Wehrl F, Song HK, Earley CJ. MRI measurement of brain iron in patients with restless legs syndrome. Neurology. 2001;56:263–265.

Allen RP, Earley CJ. Augmentation of the restless legs syndrome with carbidopa/levodopa. Sleep. 1996; 19:205–213.

Amarenco G, Kerdraon J, Denys P. Bladder and sphincter disorders in multiple sclerosis. Clinical, urodynamic and neurophysiological study of 225 cases [in French]. Rev Neurol (Paris). 1995;151:722–730.

American Academy of Sleep Medicine. ICSD— International Classification of Sleep Disorders, Second Edition: Diagnostic and Coding Manual. 2nd ed. Westchester, IL: American Academy of Sleep Medicine; 2005.

Attarian H. Importance of sleep in the quality of life of multiple sclerosis patients: a long under-recognized issue. Sleep Med. 2009;10:7–8.

Auer RN, Rowlands CG, Perry SF, et al. Multiple sclerosis with medullary plaques and fatal sleep apnea (Ondine's curse). Clin Neuropathol. 1996;15:101–105.

Auger C, Montplaisir J, Duquette P. Increased frequency of restless legs syndrome in a French-Canadian population with multiple sclerosis. Neurology. 2005;65: 1652–1653.

Bassetti C. Narcolepsy. Curr Treat Options Neurol. 1999;1:291–298.

Bassetti CL, Mauerhofer D, Gugger M, Mathis J, Hess CW. Restless legs syndrome: a clinical study of 55 patients. Eur Neurol. 2001;45:67–74.

Benca R. Insomnia. In: Avidan A, Zee PC, eds. Handbook of Sleep Medicine. Philadelphia: Lippincott Williams & Wilkins; 2006: 36–69.

Benca RM, Peterson MJ. Insomnia and depression. Sleep Med. 2008;9(suppl 1):S3–S9.

Boeve BF, Silber MH, Ferman TJ. Melatonin for treatment of REM sleep behavior disorder in neurologic disorders: results in 14 patients. Sleep Med. 2003;4: 281–284.

Bostwick JM, Hecksel KA, Stevens SR, et al. Frequency of new-onset pathologic compulsive gambling or hypersexuality after drug treatment of idiopathic Parkinson disease. Mayo Clin Proc. 2009;84:310–316.

Bruck D, Broughton RJ. Diagnostic ambiguities in a case of post-traumatic narcolepsy with cataplexy. Brain Inj. 2004;18:321–326.

Canaday BR. Amnesia possibly associated with zolpidem administration. *Pharmacotherapy.* 1996;16:687–689.

Carrieri PB, de Leva MF, Carrieri M, et al. Modafinil improves primary nocturnal enuresis in multiple sclerosis. *Eur J Neurol.* 2007;14:e1.

Cervenka S, Palhagen SE, Comley RA, et al. Support for dopaminergic hypoactivity in restless legs syndrome: a PET study on D2-receptor binding. *Brain.* 2006; 129:2017–2028.

Chesson A, Jr., Hartse K, Anderson WM, et al. Practice parameters for the evaluation of chronic insomnia. An American Academy of Sleep Medicine report. Standards of Practice Committee of the American Academy of Sleep Medicine. *Sleep.* 2000;23:237–241.

Chesson AL, Jr., Anderson WM, Littner M, et al. Practice parameters for the nonpharmacologic treatment of chronic insomnia. An American Academy of Sleep Medicine report. Standards of Practice Committee of the American Academy of Sleep Medicine. *Sleep.* 1999a; 22:1128–1133.

Chesson AL, Jr., Wise M, Davila D, et al. Practice parameters for the treatment of restless legs syndrome and periodic limb movement disorder. *Sleep.* 1999b; 22:961–968.

Chiang A, Krystal A. Report of two cases where sleep related eating behavior occurred with the extended-release formulation but not the immediate-release formulation of a sedative-hypnotic agent. *J Clin Sleep Med.* 2008;4:155–156.

Chou KL, Moro-De-Casillas ML, Amick MM, et al. Testosterone not associated with violent dreams or REM sleep behavior disorder in men with Parkinson's. *Mov Disord.* 2007;22:411–414.

Clemens S, Rye D, Hochman S. Restless legs syndrome: revisiting the dopamine hypothesis from the spinal cord perspective. *Neurology.* 2006;67:125–130.

Comella CL, Nardine TM, Diederich NJ, et al. Sleep-related violence, injury, and REM sleep behavior disorder in Parkinson's disease. *Neurology.* 1998;51:526–529.

Connor JR, Boyer PJ, Menzies SL, et al. Neuropathological examination suggests impaired brain iron acquisition in restless legs syndrome. *Neurology.* 2003;61:304–309.

Deriu M, Cossu G, Molari A, et al. Restless legs syndrome in multiple sclerosis: a case-control study. *Mov Disord.* 2009;24:697–701.

Earley CJ, Allen RP, Connor JR, Ferrucci L, Troncoso J. The dopaminergic neurons of the A11 system in RLS autopsy brains appear normal. *Sleep Med.* 2009; 10(10):1155–1157.

Earley CJ, Connor JR, Beard JL, Clardy SL, Allen RP. Ferritin levels in the cerebrospinal fluid and restless legs syndrome: effects of different clinical phenotypes. *Sleep.* 2005;28:1069–1075.

Eckert DJ, Jordan AS, Merchia P, Malhotra A. Central sleep apnea: Pathophysiology and treatment. *Chest.* 2007;131(2):595–607.

Espie CA, Inglis SJ, Tessier S, et al. The clinical effectiveness of cognitive behaviour therapy for chronic insomnia: implementation and evaluation of a sleep clinic in general medical practice. *Behav Res Ther.* 2001;39:45–60.

Evans AH, Butzkueven H. Dopamine agonist-induced pathological gambling in restless legs syndrome due to multiple sclerosis. *Mov Disord.* 2007;22:590–591.

Fantini ML, Gagnon JF, Filipini D, et al. The effects of pramipexole in REM sleep behavior disorder. *Neurology.* 2003;61:1418–1420.

Ferini-Strambi L, Zucconi M. REM sleep behavior disorder. *Clin Neurophysiol.* 2000;111(suppl 2):S136–S140.

Figved N, Klevan G, Myhr KM, et al. Neuropsychiatric symptoms in patients with multiple sclerosis. *Acta Psychiatr Scand.* 2005;112:463–468.

Fogdell A, Hillert J, Sachs C, et al. The multiple sclerosis- and narcolepsy-associated HLA class II haplotype includes the DRB5*0101 allele. *Tissue Antigens.* 1995; 46:333–336.

Frauscher B, Loscher W, Hogl B, Poewe W, Kofler, M. Auditory startle reaction is disinhibited in idiopathic restless legs syndrome. *Sleep.* 2007;30:489–493.

Fry JM. Sleep disorders. *Med Clin North Am.* 1987;71: 95–110.

Funakawa I, Hara K, Yasuda T, et al. Intractable hiccups and sleep apnea syndrome in multiple sclerosis: report of two cases. *Acta Neurol Scand.* 1993;88:401–405.

Funakawa I, Yasuda T, Terao A. A case of multiple sclerosis with intractable hiccups and sleep apnea syndrome [in Japanese]. *Rinsho Shinkeigaku.* 1992;32:733–738.

Grosskopf A, Muller N, Malo A, et al. Potential role for the narcolepsy- and multiple sclerosis-associated HLA allele DQB1*0602 in schizophrenia subtypes. *Schizophr Res.* 1998;30:187–189.

Guilleminault C, Tilkian A, Dement WC. The sleep apnea syndromes. *Annu Rev Med* 27. 1976.

Hening WA, Allen RP, Chaudhuri KR, et al. Clinical significance of RLS. *Mov Disord.* 2007;22(suppl 18): S395–S400.

Iranzo A, Santamaria J, Vilaseca I, de Osaba MJ. Absence of alterations in serum sex hormone levels in idiopathic REM sleep behavior disorder. *Sleep.* 2007;30: 803–806.

Kanbayashi T, Inoue Y, Chiba S, et al. CSF hypocretin-1 (orexin-A) concentrations in narcolepsy with and without cataplexy and idiopathic hypersomnia. *J Sleep Res.* 2002;11:91–93.

Karitani M, Gascon GG, Leonard HL, et al. Sleep disorders. *J Am Acad Child Adolesc Psychiatry.* 1997;36: 1161–1162.

Krystal AD, Walsh JK, Laska E, et al. Sustained efficacy of eszopiclone over 6 months of nightly treatment: results of a randomized, double-blind, placebo-controlled study in adults with chronic insomnia. *Sleep.* 2003; 26:793–799.

Lange R, Volkmer M, Heesen C, et al. Modafinil effects in multiple sclerosis patients with fatigue. *J Neurol.* 2009; 256:645–650.

Lankford DA. Armodafinil: a new treatment for excessive sleepiness. *Expert Opin Investig Drugs.* 2008;17: 565–573.

Lavie P HP, Hoffstein V. Obstructive sleep apnoea syndrome as a risk factor for hypertension: population study. *BMJ.* 2000;320:479–482.

Leo GJ. Sleep disturbances in multiple sclerosis. *Neurology.* 1991;41(suppl 1):320.

Lin L, Hungs M, Mignot E. Narcolepsy and the HLA region. *J Neuroimmunol.* 2001;117:9–20.

Lin L, Mignot E. HLA and narcolepsy: present status and relationship with familial history and hypocretin deficiency. In: Bassetti C, Billiard M, Mignot E, eds. *Narcolepsy and Hypersomnias of Central Origin.* New York: Marcel Dekker/Taylor & Francis Health Sciences, in press.

Littner MR, Kushida C, Anderson WM, et al. Practice parameters for the dopaminergic treatment of restless legs syndrome and periodic limb movement disorder. *Sleep.* 2004;27:557–559.

Lobentanz IS, Asenbaum S, Vass K, et al. Factors influencing quality of life in multiple sclerosis patients: disability, depressive mood, fatigue and sleep quality. *Acta Neurol Scand.* 2004;110:6–13.

Louden MB, Morehead MA, Schmidt HS. Activation by selegiline (Eldepryle) of REM sleep behavior disorder in parkinsonism. *WV Med J.* 1995;91:101.

Mahowald MW, Bornemann MC, Schenck CH. Parasomnias. *Semin Neurol.* 2004;24:283–292.

Mahowald MW, Schenck CH, Bornemann MA. Pathophysiologic mechanisms in REM sleep behavior disorder. *Curr Neurol Neurosci Rep.* 2007;7:167–172.

Manconi M, Rocca MA, Ferini-Strambi L, et al. Restless legs syndrome is a common finding in multiple sclerosis and correlates with cervical cord damage. *Mult Scler.* 2008;14:86–93.

Mayer G, Wang-Weigand S, Roth-Schechter B, Lehmann R, Staner C, Partinen M. Efficacy and safety of 6-month nightly ramelteon administration in adults with chronic primary insomnia. *Sleep.* 2009;32:351–360.

McAllister TW. The safety and efficacy of modafinil in multiple sclerosis-related fatigue. *Curr Psychiatry Rep.* 2003;5:367.

Melberg A, Hetta J, Dahl N, et al. Autosomal dominant cerebellar ataxia deafness and narcolepsy. *J Neurol Sci.* 1995;134:119–129.

Merlino G, Fratticci L, Lenchig C, et al. Prevalence of 'poor sleep' among patients with multiple sclerosis: an independent predictor of mental and physical status. *Sleep Med.* 2009;10:26–34.

Mignot E. Sleep, sleep disorders and hypocretin (orexin). *Sleep Med.* 2004;5(suppl 1):S2–S8.

Mignot E. Narcolepsy: pharmacology, pathophysiology and genetics. In: Kryger M, Roth T, Dement W, eds. *Principles and Practice of Sleep Medicine.* Philadelphia: Elsevier Saunders; 2005: 761–779.

Mignot E, Lin L, Rogers W, et al. Complex HLA-DR and -DQ interactions confer risk of narcolepsy-cataplexy in three ethnic groups. *Am J Hum Genet.* 2001;68:686–699.

Mitler MM, Hajdukovic R, Erman M, et al. Narcolepsy. *J Clin Neurophysiol.* 1990;7:93–118.

Montplaisir J, Boucher S, Poirier G, Lavigne G, Lapierre O, Lesperance P. Clinical, polysomnographic, and genetic characteristics of restless legs syndrome: a study of 133 patients diagnosed with new standard criteria. *Mov Disord.* 1997;12:61–65.

Morgan BJ, Dempsey JA, Pegelow DF, et al. Blood pressure perturbations caused by subclinical sleep-disordered breathing. *Sleep.* 1998;21:737–746.

Nalamalapu U, Goldberg R, DiPhillipo MA, Fry JM. Behaviors simulating REM behavior disorder in patients with severe obstructive sleep apnea. *Sleep Res.* 1996;25:311.

Narkiewicz K, Somers VK. The sympathetic nervous system and obstructive sleep apnea: implications for hypertension. *J Hypertens.* 1997;15:1613–1619.

National Institutes of Health State-of-the-Science Conference Statement on Manifestations and Management of Chronic Insomnia in Adults, June 13–15, 2005. Sleep. 2005;28:1049–1057.

Nightingale S, Orgill JC, Ebrahim IO, et al. The association between narcolepsy and REM behavior disorder (RBD). *Sleep Med.* 2005;6:253–258.

Ohayon MM. Prevalence of DSM-IV diagnostic criteria of insomnia: distinguishing insomnia related to mental disorders from sleep disorders. *J Psychiatr Res.* 1997;31:333–346.

Olejniczak PW, Fisch BJ. Sleep disorders. *Med Clin North Am.* 2003;87:803–833.

Olson EJ, Boeve BF, Silber MH. Rapid eye movement sleep behaviour disorder: demographic, clinical and laboratory findings in 93 cases. *Brain.* 2000;123:331–339.

Peppard PE, Young T, Palta M, et al. Longitudinal study of moderate weight change and sleep-disordered breathing. *JAMA.* 2000;284:3015–3021.

Perlis ML, McCall WV, Krystal AD, et al. Long-term, non-nightly administration of zolpidem in the treatment of patients with primary insomnia. *J Clin Psychiatry.* 2004;65:1128–1137.

Pichler I, Hicks AA, Pramstaller PP. Restless legs syndrome: an update on genetics and future perspectives. *Clin Genet.* 2008;73:297–305.

Plazzi G, Montagna P. Remitting REM sleep behavior disorder as the initial sign of multiple sclerosis. *Sleep Med.* 2002;3:437–439.

Quinnell TG, Smith IE. Obstructive sleep apnoea in the elderly: recognition and management considerations. *Drugs Aging.* 2004;21:307–322.

Rae-Grant AD, Eckert NJ, Bartz S, et al. Sensory symptoms of multiple sclerosis: a hidden reservoir of morbidity. *Mult Scler.* 1999;5:179–183.

Rammohan KW, Rosenberg JH, Lynn DJ, et al. Efficacy and safety of modafinil (Provigil) for the treatment of fatigue in multiple sclerosis: a two centre phase 2 study. *J Neurol Neurosurg Psychiatry.* 2002;72:179–183.

Rao DG, Singhal BS. Secondary narcolepsy in a case of multiple sclerosis. *J Assoc Physicians India.* 1997;45:321–322.

Roth T, Hartse KM, Saab PG, et al. The effects of flurazepam, lorazepam, and triazolam on sleep and memory. *Psychopharmacology (Berl).* 1980;70:231–237.

Rothdach AJ, Trenkwalder C, Haberstock J, et al. Prevalence and risk factors of RLS in an elderly population: the MEMO study. Memory and morbidity in Augsburg elderly. *Neurology.* 2000;54:1064–1068.

Schenck CH, Hurwitz TD, Mahowald MW. Symposium: normal and abnormal REM sleep regulation: REM sleep behaviour disorder: an update on a series of 96 patients and a review of the world literature. *J Sleep Res.* 1993;2:224–231.

Schenck CH, Mahowald MW. Rapid eye movement sleep parasomnias. *Neurol Clin.* 2005;23:1107–1126.

Schenck CH, Milner DM, Hurwitz TD, et al. Dissociative disorders presenting as somnambulism: polysomnographic, video and clinical documentation (8 cases). *Dissociation.* 1989;2:194–204.

Schmidt MH, Koshal VB, Schmidt HS. Use of pramipexole in REM sleep behavior disorder: results from a case series. *Sleep Med.* 2006;7:418–423.

Schutte S, Doghramji K. REM behavior disorder seen with venlafaxine (Effexor). *Sleep Res.* 1996;25:364.

Scott TF, Allen D, Price TR, McConnell H, Lang D. Characterization of major depression symptoms in multiple sclerosis patients. *J Neuropsychiatry Clin Neurosci.* 1996;8:318–23.

Shochat T, Pillar G. Sleep apnoea in the older adult: pathophysiology, epidemiology, consequences and management. *Drugs Aging.* 2003;20:551–560.

Silber MH. Sleep disorders. *Neurol Clin.* 2001;19:173–186.

Silvestri R, De Domenico P, Musolino R, et al. Nocturnal complex partial seizures precipitated by REM sleep. A case report. *Eur Neurol.* 1989;29:80–85.

Somers VK, Dyken ME, Clary MP, et al. Sympathetic neural mechanisms in obstructive sleep apnea. *J Clin Invest.* 1995;96:1897–1904.

Strollo PJ. Jr., Sanders M, Atwood CW. Positive pressure therapy. *Clin Chest Med.* 1998;19:55–68.

Tachibana N, Howard RS, Hirsch NP, et al. Sleep problems in multiple sclerosis. *Eur Neurol.* 1994;34:320–323.

Takeuchi N, Uchimura N, Hashizume Y, et al. Melatonin therapy for REM sleep behavior disorder. *Psychiatry Clin Neurosci.* 2001;55:267–269.

Tellez N, Montalban X. [Modafinil and fatigue in multiple sclerosis]. *Neurologia.* 2004;19:434–437.

Tippmann-Peikert M, Boeve BF, Keegan BM. REM sleep behavior disorder initiated by acute brainstem multiple sclerosis. *Neurology.* 2006;66:1277–1279.

van Kessel K, Moss-Morris R, Willoughby E, et al. A randomized controlled trial of cognitive behavior therapy for multiple sclerosis fatigue. *Psychosom Med.* 2008;70: 205–213.

Vetrugno R, Stecchi S, Plazzi G, et al. Narcolepsy-like syndrome in multiple sclerosis. *Sleep Med.* 2009;10: 389–391.

Villablanca JR, Marcus RJ, Olmstead CE. Effect of caudate nuclei or frontal cortex ablations in cats. II. Sleep-wakefulness, EEG, and motor activity. *Exp Neurol.* 1976;53:31–50.

Walters AS, Hickey K, Maltzman J, et al. A questionnaire study of 138 patients with restless legs syndrome: the 'Night-Walkers' survey. *Neurology* 1996;46: 92–95.

Wang CY, Kawashima H, Takami T, et al. A case of multiple sclerosis with initial symptoms of narcolepsy [in Japanese]. *No To Hattatsu.* 1998;30:300–306.

Willoughby E. Modafinil for fatigue in multiple sclerosis. *J Neurol Neurosurg Psychiatry.* 2002;72:150.

Winkelmann J, Schormair B, Lichtner P et al. Genome-wide association study of restless legs syndrome identifies common variants in three genomic regions. *Nat Genet.* 2007;39:1000–1006.

Winkelman JW, James L. Serotonergic antidepressants are associated with REM sleep without atonia. *Sleep.* 2004;27:317–321.

Yee B, Killick R, Wong K. Restless legs syndrome. *Aust Fam Physician.* 2009;38:296–300.

Young T, Palta M, Dempsey J, et al. The occurrence of sleep-disordered breathing among middle-aged adults. *N Engl J Med.* 1993;328:1230–1235.

Young T, Peppard PE, Gottlieb DJ. Epidemiology of obstructive sleep apnea: a population health perspective. *Am J Respir Crit Care Med.* 2002;165: 1217–1239.

Younger DS, Pedley TA, Thorpy MJ. Multiple sclerosis and narcolepsy: possible similar genetic susceptibility. *Neurology.* 1991;41:447–448.

Zifko UA, Rupp M, Schwarz S, et al. Modafinil in treatment of fatigue in multiple sclerosis. Results of an open-label study. *J Neurol.* 2002;249:983-987.

22 Pediatric Multiple Sclerosis

E. Ann Yeh, Tanuja Chitnis, Lauren B. Krupp, Jayne M. Ness, Dorothee E. Chabas, Nancy Kuntz, and Emmanuelle L. Waubant for the US Network of Pediatric MS Centers

In the past 5 years, there has been an increased interest and growth in knowledge about pediatric multiple sclerosis (MS), its treatment, pathogenesis, demographics, natural history, and magnetic resonance imaging (MRI) and laboratory features. In this chapter, we review the currently available literature on this disorder, including the most recent advances in research.

DEFINITIONS

According to consensus definitions of the International Pediatric MS Study Group (IPMSSG), pediatric MS may be diagnosed after two clinical episodes of central nervous system (CNS) demyelination that are separated by at least 30 days (dissemination in space and time). No lower age limit is specified. While in these definitions, the Barkhof adult brain MRI criteria can be used to meet the requirement for dissemination in space, these criteria have not been validated in children. The combination of an abnormal cerebrospinal fluid (CSF) and two lesions on MRI, of which one must be in the brain, can also meet the dissemination in space criteria; the CSF must show either two or more oligoclonal bands (OCBs) or an elevated IgG index. The MRI may also be used to satisfy criteria for dissemination in time following the initial clinical event, even in the absence of a new clinical demyelinating event; new T2-bright or gadolinium-enhancing foci must develop three or more months following the initial clinical event. Importantly in these operational definitions, an episode consistent with the clinical features of acute disseminated encephalomyelitis (ADEM) cannot be considered to be the first event of MS, although our experience in the past 4 years

is challenging this notion, as detailed below (see Fig. 22-1 for a diagnostic algorithm) (Krupp et al., 2007). It has become clear in recent years that clinical and radiographic features have limited ability to distinguish between ADEM and a first attack of MS at the time of initial presentation, emphasizing the need for accurate biomarkers to distinguish monophasic from recurrent conditions.

INCIDENCE AND PREVALENCE

Although the worldwide prevalence of pediatric MS is unknown, data are available from individual countries or MS centers. Several large series, including those from France and Belgium (Renoux et al., 2007), Boston (Chitnis et al., 2009), Italy (Ghezzi et al., 1997), and Canada (Boiko et al., 2002), have found prevalence rates of reported MS onset in childhood ranging from 2.2% to 4.4% of all MS cases. Age cutoffs in these studies were <18 years in the Boston study and <16 years in the Italian and Canadian studies. It is unclear whether the incidence of pediatric MS has increased in the past decades, as has been reported in adults.

DEMOGRAPHIC FEATURES

The male:female ratio of pediatric MS varies by age. Before age 6, the ratio of girls to boys is 0.8:1. It increases from age 6 to 10 to 1.6:1, to 2.1:1 for children over age 10, and 3:1 in adolescents (Banwell et al., 2007a).

While MS in adults is more common in white non-Hispanics, several studies have pointed out significant racial and ethnic variability in the pediatric population in North America. Using for race

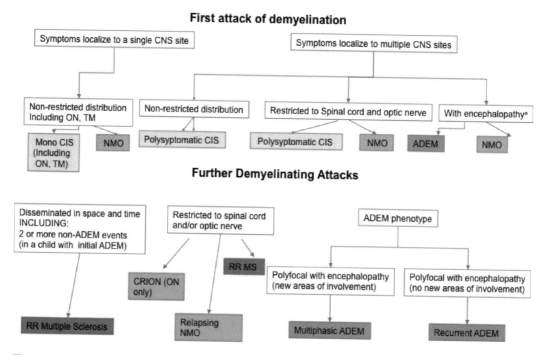

Figure 22-1 Diagnostic algorithm of pediatric-onset demyelinating disorders. ADEM, acute disseminated encephalomyelitis; CIS, clinically isolated syndrome; CNS, central nervous system; NMO, xx; ON, optic neuritis; RRMS, relapsing-remitting multiple sclerosis; TM, xx. (Figure revised from E. Waubant, with permission.)

(American Indian or Alaska Native, Asian, black or African American, Native Hawaiian or Other Pacific Islander, and white) and ethnicity ("Hispanic or Latino," and "Not Hispanic or Latino"; U.S. Office of Management and Budget, 1997), two pediatric MS centers in the United States have reported higher proportions of blacks/African Americans (7.4% vs. 4.3%; Chitnis et al., 2009) and Hispanic and first-generation Americans (Krupp et al., 2008) than in the adult MS population and, in one study, the general population. Finally, studies from a Canadian and a U.S. center showed that the pediatric cases were more likely to report Caribbean, Asian, or Middle-Eastern ancestry and less likely to report European ancestry (Kennedy et al., 2006; Krupp et al., 2008). The reasons behind this greater diversity in ethnicity, race, and ancestry in pediatric MS remains unclear, but it likely represents a combination of genetic and environmental influences, in addition to changing regional demographic factors affecting that age range in North America (i.e., increased influx of immigrants of non-European ancestry across North America in recent years).

PATHOPHYSIOLOGY/IMMUNOLOGY

There are limited data regarding the underlying immunopathophysiology of pediatric MS, as comprehensive studies have not been performed. In addition, there are no systematic studies comparing the immunopathophysiology of pediatric MS to adult MS, which would shed light on the similarities and differences between these two age groups. A recent study of a large cohort of children with CNS inflammatory demyelination, type I diabetes (T1D), and CNS injury demonstrated that children with CNS inflammatory demyelination, CNS injury, and T1D exhibited heightened peripheral T cell responses to a wide array of self-antigens. Children with autoimmune diseases and CNS injury also exhibited abnormal T cell responses against multiple cow-milk proteins (Banwell et al., 2008). A smaller study evaluating

T cell responses to myelin basic protein (MBP) and myelin oligodendrocyte glycoprotein (MOG) epitopes in adult and pediatric MS found similar responses predominantly to MBP 83–102, 139–153, 146–162, and MOG1–26, 38–60, and 63–87, in both groups to the same set of peptides (Correale and Tenembaum, 2006). Interestingly, responses to fetal-MBP were minimal, and similar in both groups. Using a tetramer approach, up to 20% of children with ADEM, but none with pediatric MS demonstrated elevations of anti-MOG antibodies (O'Connor et al., 2007).

Cerebrospinal fluid studies have demonstrated that children younger than age 11 exhibit a distinct cellular profile in comparison to their adolescent counterparts (Chabas et al., 2010). Younger children with their first MS event were more likely to lack OCB or elevated IgG index, and had a higher percentage of neutrophils in their CSF, suggesting a more prominent activation of the innate immune response as opposed to the typical activation of the adaptive response seen in older patients. The absence of neutrophils in the CSF was associated with an earlier second event.

Studies examining markers of axonal damage in the CSF found minimal changes in the majority of children with MS; however, a subgroup with prominent clinical symptoms at the time of CSF examination exhibited elevated levels of tau protein (Rostasy et al., 2005). The significance of this is unclear.

ENVIRONMENTAL RISK FACTORS FOR PEDIATRIC MULTIPLE SCLEROSIS SUSCEPTIBILITY

Environmental factors have been shown to play a pivotal role in adult MS susceptibility. These include the patient's place of residence (i.e., latitude), exposure to viruses, and more particularly Epstein-Barr virus (EBV), smoking, and vitamin D status.

Studying the role of viruses in the pediatric MS population provides a unique opportunity given the close temporal relationship between possible infection and MS onset, and the fact that exposure to those viruses is less in children than in adults. In a study comparing 137 European and American children with definite MS to age-matched controls, (Banwell et al., 2007b) seropositivity to cytomegalovirus (CMV), herpes simplex virus type 1 (HSV-1),

varicella zoster virus (VZV), and parvovirus B19 was similar in both groups. EBV seropositivity, however, was associated with an almost three times increased likelihood of MS. Similarly, Pohl et al. compared 147 patients with pediatric MS to controls and found seropositivity for EBV in more patients with pediatric MS than controls (99% vs. 72%, $p = 0.001$) (Pohl et al., 2006a).

Data from the US Pediatric MS Network confirm the substantial association between EBV and increased pediatric MS susceptibility. This association appears to be stronger for EBNA-1 than VCA and remains after adjusting for age and race (Waubant et al., 2009). Further supporting the specific role of EBNA-1 in pediatric MS susceptibility, EBNA-1 titers in positive pediatric MS patients are higher than titers in positive controls. Finally, patients' EBNA-1 humoral response is also more likely to target at least two additional regions compared to age-matched controls (James et al., 2009).

More recently, Mikaeloff et al. evaluated 137 children with MS and 1061 controls for clinical episodes of chicken pox. Seventy-seven percent of the MS population had a history of chicken pox, compared to 85% of the control population. The odds ratio was 0.58 (95% CI 0.36, 0.92), suggesting a possible protective effect of chicken pox that remains to be confirmed (Mikaeloff et al., 2009a).

In addition to studying the role of common viruses, the relationship of vaccinations, most recently the hepatitis B vaccine, to the subsequent development of pediatric-onset MS has been investigated. Mikaeloff et al. found that the risk of developing a first episode of childhood MS up to 3 years post vaccination in the French population was not increased (Mikaeloff et al., 2007a). However, these authors showed a trend for the Engerix B vaccine to increase the risk in the longer term. This needs to be confirmed in the future on larger cohorts. A second study by the same authors found no increase in the relapse rate after a first episode of CNS inflammatory demyelination in childhood when subsequently vaccinated against hepatitis B or tetanus. The risk of conversion to MS did not appear to increase, although the study was not powered to detect a small increase in risk (Mikaeloff et al., 2009b).

Interestingly, the same group evaluated the risk of childhood-onset MS as related to exposure to passive smoking (Mikaeloff et al., 2007b).

They compared 129 cases of pediatric MS in France with 1038 matched controls. The relative risk for a first episode of MS was found to be over twice that of the control population, and it was even higher for those with exposure of 10 years or more. Finally, the effect of vitamin D reported for adult MS susceptibility has not yet been confirmed in children, although the vast majority of pediatric patients seen at pediatric MS clinics have low serum levels of 25(OH) vitamin D_3 (Waubant et al., 2009). Further studies are required to explore the precise mechanisms leading from specific environmental exposures to disease onset.

CLINICAL PRESENTATION OF PEDIATRIC MULTIPLE SCLEROSIS

Over 25 retrospective and prospective studies with greater than 10 patients have described the clinical presentation of pediatric MS (Gall et al., 1958; Duquette et al., 1987; Boutin et al., 1988; Hanefeld et al., 1991; Sindern et al., 1992; Cole and Stuart, 1995; Guilhoto et al., 1995; Selcen et al., 1996; Ghezzi et al., 1997; Pinhas-Hamiel et al., 1998; Belopitova et al., 2001; Dale et al., 2000; Boiko et al., 2002; Ghezzi et al., 2002; Gusev et al., 2002; Simone et al., 2002; Brass et al., 2003; Ozakbas et al., 2003; Mikaeloff et al., 2004a; Shiraishi et al., 2005; Deryck et al., 2006; Etemadifar et al., 2007; Pohl et al., 2007; Stark et al., 2008; Alper et al., 2009; Atzori et al., 2009). Retrospective and prospective studies show considerable variability in the frequency of initial MS symptoms. A combined analysis of four prospective studies reveals 28% of patients presenting with cerebellar findings (range 12%–52%), significantly higher than in 21 retrospective studies (11%) ($p < 0.0001$). Similarly, sensory deficits were identified in 27% of patients in prospective studies but in only 15% of patients in the retrospective studies ($p < 0.0001$). Other neurologic signs such as motor deficits and optic neuritis were reported with equal frequency in both retrospective and prospective studies (27% with motor deficits; >20% with optic neuritis). Brainstem deficits were also identified at a similar rate (19% retrospective; 22% prospective).

Encephalopathy has been defined by the IPMSSG as comprising behavioral change, for example, confusion or excessive irritability or alteration in consciousness (e.g., coma or lethargy) (Krupp et al., 2007). Following operational definitions that require encephalopathy for the diagnosis of ADEM (Krupp et al., 2007), two small studies have suggested its presence may be somewhat useful in distinguishing a first episode of MS from ADEM (Dale et al., 2007; Alper et al., 2009). However, increasingly, data suggest that encephalopathy may also occur with a first episode of MS or neuromyelitis optica, especially in younger patients (Dale et al., 2000; Tenembaum et al., 2002; Banwell et al., 2007b; Chabas et al., 2008; McKeon et al., 2008). Thus, rather than being disease specific (i.e., MS versus ADEM), the presence of encephalopathy may be related to immaturity of the brain or the immune system in younger patients.

Mental status has not been consistently described in either retrospective or prospective studies and is sometimes not discussed at all. Encephalopathy was reported in a subset of studies (only 8/21 retrospective studies accounting for 46% of retrospective patients; 2 of 4 prospective studies with 60% of patients). Criteria for altered mental status or encephalopathy, if described at all, were not used consistently across studies. Despite these limitations, 16% of prospectively analyzed patients (29/180) were described as having encephalopathy, which was significantly higher than in the subset of retrospective patients (8.7%; 62 of 712 patients; $p < 0.0001$). These differences may be due to recall bias or heightened awareness of evaluating mental status during demyelinating episodes, although validated criteria for encephalopathy are still lacking.

DIAGNOSTIC TESTING

Diagnostic testing for pediatric MS includes serum and CSF evaluation, visual evoked potentials (VEPs), and MRI.

CSF Analysis

As noted above, the CSF profile in childhood-onset MS may vary by age. The IgG index has been found to be elevated in 68% of adolescents with MS (>11 years), but in 35% of younger children (<11 years) (Chabas et al., 2010). Younger children have more neutrophils in the CSF than older children. These features tend to be age dependent rather than dependent on disease duration. This distinct CSF IgG and cellular profile in younger children tends to vanish on repeat CSF analysis (mean 19 months after initial analysis), suggesting a transient immunological phenomenon associated with disease onset.

Although one study reports OCB to be present in the CSF of up to 92% of children with MS (Pohl et al., 2004), this may be laboratory, disease duration, and age dependent. Another study also found OCB to be less frequent in younger children (43% versus 63% in adolescents) (Chabas et al., 2010). By contrast, in ADEM, 0%–29% of cases were found to have OCB (Dale et al., 2000; Tenembaum et al., 2002; Hynson et al., 2001; Pohl et al., 2004). Within the French KIDMUS cohort, 94% of children with positive OCB (69/72) went on to develop MS, although the timing of the lumbar puncture was not provided. Only 40% of established MS patients in this study had OCB, suggesting that this test has a low sensitivity but high specificity for the development of MS when present at disease onset (Mikaeloff et al., 2004a).

Visual Testing

Approximately one-third of children who go on to have a diagnosis of MS experience optic neuritis as an initial presenting symptom (Simone et al., 2002; Mikaeloff et al., 2004b). An even higher proportion of children with MS may experience subclinical abnormalities of the visual pathway (Pohl et al., 2006b). The limited ability of standard Snellen charts to distinguish subtle visual dysfunction is well documented in the adult MS population (Frohman et al., 2006). Low-contrast letter acuity charts (LCLA, Sloan charts) have been shown to provide a sensitive and reliable assessment of visual acuity in the pediatric MS population (Yeh et al., 2009).

Other tests such as VEP (or pattern reversal visual evoked potentials [PRVEPs]) have been shown to be of diagnostic utility in childhood MS, with almost half of such patients showing increased visual latency, which revealed a second focus of demyelination prior to a second clinical attack (Pohl et al., 2006b).

More recently, optical coherence tomography (OCT), used for patients with glaucoma, has been applied to pediatric patients with MS. This procedure uses near infrared light to quantify the thickness of the retinal nerve fiber layer (RNFL) (which contains only nonmyelinated axons). It has been shown to provide a sensitive evaluation of the RNFL thickness in this population, a correlate of optic atrophy (Yeh et al., 2009). Taken together, VEP, OCT, and LCLA testing can provide objective evidence of previous inflammatory insult to the optic nerve in the pediatric population with MS. They may help to establish a diagnosis of MS and may also be used for disease monitoring on follow-up.

MAGNETIC RESONANCE IMAGING

In the past, limited data have suggested that pediatric MS patients may not meet adult MS MRI criteria (Hahn et al., 2004). In a small study, patients with pediatric MS were reported to have fewer brain MRI T2-bright foci and more frequent tumefactive MS lesions than reported in adults with MS (Chabas et al., 2008). However, more recent data collected at disease onset have shown that children with MS may have a higher lesion burden on their initial brain MRI scan than adults, especially in the brain stem and cerebellum (Waubant and Chabas, 2009). This is of concern, as both higher lesion burden and brainstem and cerebellar involvement have been reported to be associated with a worse outcome in adults.

It is intriguing that younger children with MS (age <11 years) may present with atypical MRI features, rendering diagnosis challenging, and possibly delaying the initiation of preventative therapies (Chabas et al., 2008). Brain lesions in these children are typically large, with poorly defined borders and are frequently confluent at disease onset (Fig. 22-2). Such T2-bright foci in younger children may vanish on repeat scans, unlike that seen in teenagers or adults. This suggests that disease processes in the developing brain, including immune response, may be different from those in older patients (Chabas et al., 2008).

Several studies have evaluated the utility of MRI in the diagnosis of MS. One study suggested that the presence of well-defined periventricular and corpus callosum lesions may be specific but very insensitive predictors of MS after a first CNS demyelinating event in childhood (KIDMUS

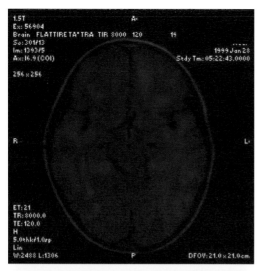

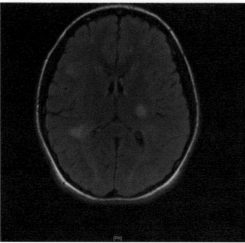

Figure 22-2 Brain magnetic resonance image (MRI) of a young child with multiple sclerosis (*top*) and an adolescent with multiple sclerosis (*bottom*). Note the large, poorly defined lesions in the MRI of the younger child.

criteria) (Mikaeloff et al., 2004b). More recent studies have confirmed these general findings and have found that the presence of any of the Barkhof criteria for MS as well as lesions that are perpendicular to the corpus callosum and small or well defined may be effective in differentiating children with MS from those with a monophasic disease at the time of disease presentation (Neuteboom et al., 2008). Another small study using some of the same patients as the

aforementioned one reported that a combination of two of the following criteria may distinguish a first attack of pediatric MS from ADEM (Callen et al., 2008): *(1)* presence of T1-black holes; *(2)* presence of two or more periventricular lesions; and *(3)* absence of diffuse bilateral lesions. Importantly, this study failed to analyze the presence of gadolinium-enhancing foci that may also appear dark on T1-weighted imaging. While advanced imaging techniques have not been evaluated in assessing future risk of MS in children yet, the use of standard MRI techniques to diagnose MS early in young patients must be refined.

PATHOLOGY

Although pathology may lead to a definitive MS diagnosis, biopsies are rarely performed in these children due to concerns regarding potential morbidity from the procedure. Biopsies are usually performed on patients with atypical clinical or radiological presentations. There are no studies describing pathological differences between adult and pediatric MS.

CLINICAL AND DEMOGRAPHIC PREDICTORS OF THE RISK TO DEVELOP MULTIPLE SCLEROSIS AFTER AN INITIAL DEMYELINATING EVENT

At present, outside of MRI features, no clear prognostic factors at the time of presentation determine whether a child with an acute demyelinating event will develop MS. Clinical studies have been hampered in part by the lack of consistent definitions used across publications, and the small numbers of subjects at any one site. In available studies, the risk of developing MS after ADEM has been reported to be between 0% and 29% in studies from Argentina (Tenembaum et al., 2002), San Diego (Leake et al., 2004), and France (Mikaeloff et al., 2004a, 2004b). When "change in mental status" was as a qualifying criterion for ADEM, 18% of children were found to subsequently develop MS in a French collaborative study (Mikaeloff et al., 2007c).

Over half of the children with an initial demyelinating event followed by the KIDMUS group in France developed a second attack during a mean follow-up period of 5.4 years (Mikaeloff et al., 2004a).

Positive predictive factors for the development of MS were age at onset 10 years or older or optic nerve involvement. A lower risk of developing MS was found in patients with mental status change at presentation.

PEDIATRIC MULTIPLE SCLEROSIS: CLINICAL COURSE

The initial clinical course in most patients with childhood-onset MS is relapsing-remitting, with remission of neurological symptoms followed by relapse rather than progressive neurological disability in 85.7% to 100% of cases (Duquette et al., 1987; Boiko et al., 2002; Renoux et al., 2007). After several days or weeks, patients recover partially or fully from their exacerbations and remain clinically stable until they develop their next MS relapse. During the relapsing-remitting phase, disability can occur as the result of incomplete recovery from relapses. In some cases, patients later develop a more insidious progression of disability with or without superimposed exacerbations. This phase of the disease is called secondary progressive.

Relapses

The annualized relapse rate in pediatric-onset MS has been estimated to be between 0.38 to 0.87 for the whole relapsing-remitting period in the few studies with mean disease duration of 10 years or more (Sindern et al., 1992; Boiko et al., 2002; Ghezzi et al., 2002). A prospective study of patients with MS seen at a large MS center showed that patients with an onset before 18 years had a higher relapse rate during the first few years of their disease than adults seen at the same institution (Gorman et al., 2009). The quality of recovery after subsequent relapses during the relapsing-remitting phase has been reported to be good, at least in the very early stages.

Evolution to the Secondary Progressive Phase

The proportion of pediatric-onset MS patients reported as reaching the secondary progressive phase is highly variable from one study to the other, largely because of variability in follow-up from study to study (Cole et al., 1995; Boiko et al.,

2002; Simone et al., 2002; Renoux et al., 2007). The median time between onset of the disease (first neurological episode) and conversion to secondary progression is therefore more informative. The estimated median time from onset of MS to the secondary progressive phase has been reported to be between 16 and 28 years in pediatric-onset MS compared to 7 to 19 years for adult-onset MS patients. However, patients with childhood-onset MS are younger when reaching this stage (median age 31–41 years compared to 37.5–52 years in adult-onset MS).

Time to Irreversible Disability and Limited Ambulation

Although the rate of disability progression varies from individual to individual regardless of the age at onset, the estimated median time from MS onset to use of unilateral device to ambulate has been reported to be between 28 and 29 years compared to 18 years for the adult group (Duquette et al., 1987; Cole et al., 1995; Ghezzi et al., 1997; Boiko et al., 2002; Renoux et al., 2007).)[5,67] Although it takes approximately 10 more years to patients with childhood-onset MS to reach irreversible limitation of ambulation than in patients with adult-onset MS, patients with childhood-onset MS reach these disability scores at a younger age (i.e., at the time they start a family and are entering the workforce). The impact of the use of disease-modifying therapies for MS on delaying the development of the secondary progressive phase in pediatric-onset MS has yet to be studied.

COGNITIVE AND PSYCHOSOCIAL OUTCOMES

Preliminary data focusing specifically on cognitive outcomes in pediatric MS have been published. Studies from two North American centers (Stony Brook, NY and Toronto, Canada) describing 37 and 10 patients, respectively, suggest significant cognitive impairment in a large proportion of patients. In the larger study, impairments were found in over one-third of patients (attention, memory, and confrontation naming) with strong correlations with EDSS, number of relapses, and total disease duration; these were found after a relatively short disease duration of 19 months on average. Depression was noted to be present in half of the cases.

Similarly, the 10 children with an EDSS of 1.5 or less evaluated by the Toronto group were found to have deficits in executive function, processing speed, or working memory (Banwell et al., 2005; MacAllister et al., 2005, 2007; Amato et al., 2008). Both of these studies are limited in that they lacked controls, did not provide longitudinal data, and, finally, testing was not performed systematically after a given disease duration (e.g., 1 year). Preliminary data suggesting progressive cognitive decline were published in a small longitudinal study of 12 patients (MacAllister et al., 2007). Again, this was a small study that lacked controls.

More recently, a larger, multi-institutional cross-sectional Italian study evaluating 66 children with RR MS and 57 healthy controls was published (Amato et al., 2008). After an average disease duration of 3 years, almost one-third of patients met criteria for significant cognitive impairment. Neither disease duration nor number of relapses was found to be of significance when comparing MS children with cognitive impairment with those who were not impaired. Strikingly, almost three-fourths of children with MS in this study reported fatigue, although unlike the earlier U.S. study, only 6% reported depression. Over half of the children reported that MS had negative effects on their everyday life and school.

The functional impact of cognitive impairment in children with MS is not clearly documented in these studies, but one might postulate that these impairments would translate to an increased need for school-based interventions and accommodations. Certainly, cognitive decline, disability level, together with progressive course were found to influence social and work-related function in adults with early onset MS (Amato et al., 1995). Importantly, several of the studies noted previously showed variably increased rate of depression, fatigue, as well as negative effects on school and everyday life. This highlights the need for multidisciplinary care with attention to school-related accommodations and close attention to the emotional well-being of this patient population.

One study has reported on health-related quality of life in children with CIS or early MS (Mowry et. al. 2008). Although mean disease duration in this cohort of 51 patients was short (2.3 +/− 1.8 years) and disability low (median EDSS 1.5), patients had significant reductions in their health-related quality-of-life scores, emphasizing the dramatic consequences of early MS on the quality of life in children.

One recent longitudinal multicenter study in Italy has emphasized the worrisome rate of worsening of cognitive deficits (70% of the pediatric MS patients worsened) over a relatively short period of time (2 years), although most patients were on disease-modifying therapies for MS and remained otherwise clinically relatively stable (Amato et al., 2009). Further longitudinal studies including controls may help to elucidate whether progressive deterioration in cognitive function correlates with disease duration, and further, whether this corresponds to decline in social functioning, as one might expect. Finally, as a clear correlation between disease duration and cognitive impairment was not found in these earlier studies, evaluation of neuropsychological outcomes with respect to MRI measures of atrophy may provide more insight into factors affecting functional outcome.

DISEASE -MODIFYING THERAPIES IN PEDIATRIC MULTIPLE SCLEROSIS

Although four first-line disease-modifying therapies—glatiramer acetate, intramuscular (IM) and subcutaneous (SC) interferon beta-1a, and SC interferon beta-1b— have been approved for treatment of relapsing-remitting MS in the adult population, data regarding these therapies in children are limited. At present, most treatment decisions are based in part on treatment studies performed in adults. The relatively small number of patients with pediatric MS presents practical barriers to performing double-blind, randomized controlled trials on first-line DMT in this population. Indeed, no such trials evaluating the efficacy of agents approved for adult MS or new agents have been performed in pediatric-onset MS. Use of DMT may vary from country to country because of issues including, but not limited to, variations in insurance coverage and rate of patient follow-up.

Interferon Beta

The clinical benefit of interferon beta therapy in relapsing-remitting MS may be mediated via several mechanisms, including the inhibition of pro-inflammatory cytokines, induction of anti-inflammatory mediators, reduction of lymphocyte migration, and inhibition of autoreactive T cells (IFNB MS Study Group, 1993; Jacobs et al., 1996). In adult MS, studies have demonstrated an approximately 30% reduction in exacerbation rate compared to placebo for periods of 2–3 years (PRISMS Study Group, 1998).

Two retrospective analyses evaluating the effect of interferon on relapse rate in children have been published. An open-label study published by an Italian cooperative group has suggested a reduction in annualized relapse rate (1.9 to 0.4) in 52 children on interferon beta-1a. Limitations of this study include the lack of untreated controls and its retrospective and nonrandomized nature, introducing the possibility of patient selection bias, and the relatively small number of patients included. Further, the standard deviation of the initial annualized relapse rate and that in follow-up overlap (1.9 ± 1.1 and 0.4 ± 0.5), suggesting the possibility that the actual effect of the medication compared to pretreatment may be moderate.

Some of these issues were addressed in a recent study published by the KIDSEP group. This retrospective, nonrandomized comparative cohort study evaluated the timing of first attack after initiation of interferon beta in 24 patients in a cohort of 197 pediatric MS patients. The risk of first attack was reduced in children on interferon at 1 year (HR 0.31, 95% CI 0.13–0.72) and 2 years (HR 0.40, 95% CI 0.40, 0.2–0.83). The HR after 4 years of treatment was 0.57 (95% CI 0.30–1.10). It is unclear whether these data at 4 years suggest a decreased benefit of interferon therapy or whether it is related to attrition of the number of patients followed until then. As expected with such a small sample size, no difference in EDSS progression was found.

Retrospective case series suggest that interferon beta-1a and -1b are safe and well tolerated in this population at the same doses as those used in adults (Mikaeloff et al., 2001; Pohl et al., 2005; Banwell et al., 2006; Bykova et al., 2006). Reported side effects include flu-like symptoms (35%–65%), leucopenia (8%–27%), thrombopenia (16%), anemia (12%), and transient elevation in transaminases (21%–33%) (Mikaeloff et al., 2001; Pohl et al., 2005; Banwell et al., 2006; Tenembaum and Segura, 2006). Injection site reactions (>2/3), abscesses (6%), and injection site necrosis (6%)

may occur in children taking the SC formulations (Pohl et al., 2005).

Dosing of interferon therapy has not been established in pediatric MS. However, retrospective studies have described titration schedules following adult protocols, that is, gradual titration to 30 μg once weekly for IM interferon beta-1a, and 22 μg TIW or 44 μg TIW for SC interferon beta-1a. Children over the age of 10 appear to be able to tolerate full doses of interferon beta, though decreased tolerance may exist in the younger population (Banwell et al., 2006). In the U.S. Pediatric MS Network series of children with MS receiving therapy (mean follow-up 3.5 years, $n = 264$), of the children started on interferon beta-1a IM therapy, 42/97 (42%) required change to another therapy; 24 due to breakthrough disease and 18 due to side effects or compliance. Of those who were initially started on interferon beta-1a SC therapy, 21/74 (28%) required a change to another therapy; 10 due to breakthrough disease and 11 due to side effects/compliance. Of the 31 started on interferon beta-1b SC, 15/31 (48%) required a change to another therapy, 10 due to breakthrough disease and 5 due to side effects or compliance (Yeh et al., 2009a).

Little information regarding neutralizing antibodies to interferon in this population is available, although one small study has suggested that positive neutralizing antibodies may be less commonly seen in pediatric MS than in the adult population (Yeh et al., 2009c). This remains to be confirmed.

Glatiramer Acetate

Glatiramer acetate (GA, Copaxone) is the acetate salt of a mixture of synthetic polypeptides composed of L-alanine, L-glutamic acid, L-lysine, and L-tyrosine. It is designed to mimic human myelin basic protein and is postulated to induce myelin-specific response of suppressor T-lymphocytes, inhibit specific effector T-lymphocytes, and act via an effect on antigen-presenting cells (Dhib-Jalbut, 2002). In adult relapsing-remitting MS patients, a 29% reduction of the number of relapses in the treated group versus placebo has been found over a period of 2 years (Johnson et al., 1995). One small retrospective study describing the use of glatiramer acetate in seven children with MS suggested that the medication is well tolerated

(Kornek et al., 2003). In the U.S. Pediatric MS Network series of 56 children with MS who were initially started on this medication, 12/58 (21%) required change to another therapy; 9 due to breakthrough disease and 3 due to side effects over a mean follow-up of 3.5 years (Yeh et al., 2009a).

Second-Line Agents

First-line treatment failure is a concern in both adult and pediatric MS. It is widely accepted that currently available first-line disease-modifying therapies are only partially effective, resulting in a reduction in relapse rate of approximately 30% in the adult population (Coyle, 2008). Treatment failure may arise because of unacceptable side effects or the presence of an unacceptable level of breakthrough disease (either in severity or frequency), continued presence of gadolinium-enhancing lesions on MRI, or progression of disability despite adherence to medication. The biologic mechanisms behind poor response to therapy have not been elucidated, but they may be due to heterogeneity of disease processes between individuals due to genetic, immunological, or environmental variability.

Compliance and side effects are key issues in treatment of children with MS, as daily to weekly injections of medication are required and are frequently associated with unpleasant side effects. Fifteen percent of children followed at the six centers participating in the U.S. Network of Pediatric MS Centers of Excellence changed therapies due to compliance issues or side effects (Yeh et al., 2009a).

The definition of treatment failure is challenging. It has undergone considerable debate among those treating adult- and pediatric-onset MS. Consensus criteria for the adult MS population, proposed by Cohen et al. (2004), include the presence of >1 relapse/yr, no decrease in relapse rate, incomplete recovery from relapses/accumulation of disability, new brainstem/spinal cord lesions on MRI, poly-regional disease, or worsening motor or cognitive impairment. In general, these criteria are reserved for those who have been on therapy for at least 6 months (Cohen et al., 2004).

Consensus definitions of breakthrough disease in the pediatric MS population are not available.

However, at present, many practitioners adhere to the guidelines described earlier that are used for the adult population. Approximately one-fourth of children with MS experience breakthrough disease, although poorly defined, prompting a switch to a second therapy an average of 1.5 years after starting a first-line therapy (Yeh et al., 2009a).

The use of second-line agents, including cyclophosphamide, mitoxantrone, mycophenolate mofetil, daclizumab, rituximab, and natalizumab, has been described in retrospective case series/reports with limited follow-up (Huppke et al., 2008; Borriello et al., 2009; Yeh et al., 2009a, 2009b). Due to the retrospective, open-label nature of the studies, conclusions regarding the efficacy and safety of these agents cannot be drawn. A retrospective study of cyclophosphamide use in 17 children with MS suggested a temporary reduction in relapses and disease progression. However, use was associated with secondary bladder cancer in one case, and amenorrhea and infertility in several patients (Makhani et al., 2009). Further studies evaluating the short- and long-term safety as well as the efficacy of these agents are needed. Randomized placebo-controlled trials of these agents are unlikely for ethical reasons.

CONCLUSION AND FUTURE DIRECTIONS

Pediatric MS represents a relatively rare, but important entity as it provides a new window into disease processes related to MS. Studies have suggested great variability in presenting symptoms, laboratory, and imaging features between children with pre- versus postpubertal disease. Given the distinct features that characterize onset prior to puberty, the possible contribution of hormonal influences and maturation of the immune and central nervous systems on pediatric MS deserve further study.

Although no disease-modifying therapies have been approved by the FDA for the treatment of children with MS, currently available first-line therapies for adults appear to be safe and well tolerated in this population. Further studies are required to assess the safety and efficacy of second-line treatments in children with MS.

Validation of studies reviewed in this chapter as well as studies to define additional risk factors, clinical features, and biomarkers are needed to further improve our ability for early recognition of acquired CNS demyelinating diseases in children. Newer imaging modalities such as diffusion tensor imaging, magnetization transfer ratios, and volumetric analysis will likely play a future role to further elucidate biological processes involved in disease pathogenesis in pediatric MS.

ACKNOWLEDGMENTS

The National Multiple Sclerosis Society provided funding for the six pediatric MS centers that participated in drafting this chapter.

The authors deny any conflict of interest with the data reported in the present manuscript.

REFERENCES

Alper G, Heyman R, Wang L. Multiple sclerosis and acute disseminated encephalomyelitis diagnosed in children after long-term follow-up: comparison of presenting features. *Dev Med Child Neurol.* 2009;51: 480–486.

Amato MP, Goretti B, Ghezzi A, et al. Cognitive and psychosocial features of childhood and juvenile MS. *Neurology.* 2008;70:1891–1897.

Amato M, Gordetti B, Ghezzi A, et al. Cognitive and psychosocial features of childhood and juvenile MS: a reappraisal after 2 years. *Neurology.* 2009;72:A97.

Amato MP, Ponziani G, Pracucci G, Bracco L, Siracusa G, Amaducci L. Cognitive impairment in early-onset multiple sclerosis. Pattern, predictors, and impact on everyday life in a 4-year follow-up. *Arch Neurol.* 1995; 52:168–172.

Amato MP, Ponziani G, Siracusa G, Sorbi S. Cognitive dysfunction in early-onset multiple sclerosis: a reappraisal after 10 years. *Arch Neurol.* 2001;58:1602–1606.

Atzori M, Battistella PA, Perini P, et al. Clinical and diagnostic aspects of multiple sclerosis and acute monophasic encephalomyelitis in pediatric patients: a single centre prospective study. *Multiple Scler.* 2009;15:363–370 (2009).

Banwell BL, Anderson PE. The cognitive burden of multiple sclerosis in children. *Neurology.* 2005;64: 891–894.

Banwell B, Bar-Or A, Cheung R, et al. Abnormal T-cell reactivities in childhood inflammatory demyelinating disease and type 1 diabetes. *Ann Neurol.* 2008;63: 98–111.

Banwell B, Ghezzi A, Bar-Or A, Mikaeloff Y, Tardieu M. Multiple sclerosis in children: clinical diagnosis, therapeutic strategies, and future directions. *Lancet Neurol.* 2007a;6:887–902.

Banwell B, Kennedy J, Sadovnick D, et al. Incidence of acquired demyelination of the CNS in Canadian children. *Neurology.* 2009;72:232–239.

Banwell B, Krupp L, Kennedy J, et al. Clinical features and viral serologies in children with multiple sclerosis: a multinational observational study. *Lancet Neurol.* 2007b; 6:773–781.

Banwell B, Reder AT, Krupp L, et al. Safety and tolerability of interferon beta-1b in pediatric multiple sclerosis. *Neurology.* 2006;66:472–476.

Belman A, Chabas D, Chitnis T, et al. Clinical spectrum of disorders masquerading as pediatric multiple sclerosis [abstract]. *Ann Neurol.* 2007;62:A15–A20.

Belopitova L, Guergueltcheva PV, Bojinova V. Definite and suspected multiple sclerosis in children: long-term follow-up and magnetic resonance imaging findings. *J Child Neurol.* 2001;16:317–324.

Boiko A, Vorobeychik G, Paty D, Devonshire V, Sadovnick D. Early onset multiple sclerosis: a longitudinal study. *Neurology.* 2002;59:1006–1010.

Borriello G, Prosperini L, Luchetti A, Pozzilli C. Natalizumab treatment in pediatric multiple sclerosis: a case report. *Eur J Paediatr Neurol.* 2009;13:67–71.

Boster AL, Endress CF, Hreha SA, Caon C, Perumal JS, Khan OA. Pediatric-onset multiple sclerosis in african-american black and European-origin white patients. *Pediatr Neurol.* 2009;40:31–33.

Boutin B, Esquivel E, Mayer M, Chaumet S, Ponsot G, Arthuis M. Multiple sclerosis in children: report of clinical and paraclinical features of 19 cases. *Neuropediatrics.* 1988;19:118–123.

Brass SD, Caramanos Z, Santos C, Dilenge ME, Lapierre Y, Rosenblatt B. Multiple sclerosis vs acute disseminated encephalomyelitis in childhood. *Pediatr Neurol.* 2003;29:227–231.

Bykova OV, Kuzenkova LM, Maslova OI. The use of beta-interferon-1b in children and adolescents with multiple sclerosis [in Russian]. *Zhurnal nevrologii i psikhiatrii imeni S.S.* 2006;106:29–33.

Callen DJ, Shroff MM, Branson HM, et al. Role of MRI in the differentiation of ADEM from MS in children. *Neurology.* 2008;72:968–973.

Chabas D, Castillo-Trivino T, Mowry EM, Strober JB, Glenn OA, Waubant E. Vanishing MS T2-bright lesions before puberty: a distinct MRI phenotype? *Neurology.* 2008;71:1090–1093.

Chabas D, Ness J, Belman A, et al. Younger children with pediatric MS have a distinct CSF inflammatory profile at disease onset. *Neurology.* 2010;74(5):399–405.

Chiaravalloti ND, DeLuca J. Cognitive impairment in multiple sclerosis. *Lancet Neurol.* 2008;7:1139–1151.

Chitnis T, Glanz B, Jaffin S, Healy B. Demographics of pediatric-onset multiple sclerosis in an MS center population from the Northeastern United States. *Mult Scler.* 2009;15:627–631.

Cole GF, Auchterlonie LA, Best PV. Very early onset multiple sclerosis. *Dev Med Child Neurol.* 1995;37:667–672.

Cole GF, Stuart CA. A long perspective on childhood multiple sclerosis. *Dev Med Child Neurol.* 1995;37: 661–666.

Cohen BA, Khan O, Jeffery DR, et al. Identifying and treating patients with suboptimal responses. *Neurology.* 2004;63:S33–S40.

Correale J, Tenembaum SN. Myelin basic protein and myelin oligodendrocyte glycoprotein T-cell repertoire in childhood and juvenile multiple sclerosis. *Mult Scler.* 2006;12:412–420.

Coyle PK. Switching algorithms: from one immunomodulatory agent to another. *J Neurol.* 2008;255(suppl 1): 44–50.

Dale RC, de Sousa C, Chong WK, Cox TC, Harding B, Neville BG. Acute disseminated encephalomyelitis, multiphasic disseminated encephalomyelitis and multiple sclerosis in children. *Brain.* 2000;123(pt 12): 2407–2422.

Dale RC, Pillai SC. Early relapse risk after a first CNS inflammatory demyelination episode: examining international consensus definitions. *Dev Med Child Neurol.* 2007;49:887–893.

Deryck O, Ketelaer P, Dubois B. Clinical characteristics and long term prognosis in early onset multiple sclerosis. *J Neurol.* 2006;253:720–723.

Dhib-Jalbut S. Sustained immunological effects of Glatiramer acetate in patients with multiple sclerosis treated for over 6 years. *J Neurol Sci.* 2002;201: 71–77.

Duquette P, Murray TJ, Pleines J, et al. Multiple sclerosis in childhood: clinical profile in 125 patients. *J Pediat.* 1987;111:359–363.

Etemadifar M, Nasr-Esfahani AH, Khodabandehlou R, Maghzi AH. Childhood-onset multiple sclerosis: report of 82 patients from Isfahan, Iran. *Arch Iran Med.* 2007;10:152–156.

Frohman E, Costello F, Zivadinov R, et al. Optical coherence tomography in multiple sclerosis. *Lancet Neurol.* 2006;5:853–863.

Gall JC, Jr., Hayles AB, Siekert RG, Keith HM. Multiple sclerosis in children; a clinical study of 40 cases with onset in childhood. *Pediatrics.* 1958; 21:703–709.

Ghezzi A, Amato MP, Capobianco M, et al. Treatment of early-onset multiple sclerosis with intramuscular interferonbeta-1a: long-term results. *Neurol Sci.* 2007; 28:127–132.

Ghezzi A, Deplano V, Faroni J, et al. Multiple sclerosis in childhood: clinical features of 149 cases. *Mult Scler.* 1997;3:43–46.

Ghezzi A, Pozzilli C, Liguori M, et al. Prospective study of multiple sclerosis with early onset. *Mult Scler.* 2002; 8:115–118.

Gorman MP, Healy BC, Polgar-Turcsanyi M, Chitnis T. Increased relapse rate in pediatric-onset compared with adult-onset multiple sclerosis. *Arch Neurol.* 2009; 66:54–59.

Guilhoto LM, Osório CA, Machado LR, et al. Pediatric multiple sclerosis report of 14 cases. *Brain Dev.* 1995; 17:9–12.

Gusev E, Boiko A, Bikova O, et al. The natural history of early onset multiple sclerosis: comparison of data from Moscow and Vancouver. *Clin Neurol Neurosurg.* 2002;104:203–207.

Hahn CD, Shroff MM, Blaser SI, Banwell BL. MRI criteria for multiple sclerosis: Evaluation in a pediatric cohort. *Neurology.* 2004;62:806–808.

Hanefeld F, Bauer HJ, Christen HJ, Kruse B, Bruhn H, Frahm J. Multiple sclerosis in childhood: report of 15 cases. *Brain Dev.* 1991;13:410–416.

Huppke P, Stark W, Zürcher C, Huppke B, Brück W, Gärtner J. Natalizumab use in pediatric multiple sclerosis. *Arch Neurol.* 2008;65:1655-1658.

Hynson JL, Kornberg AJ, Coleman LT, Shield L, Harvey AS, Kean MJ. Clinical and neuroradiologic features of acute disseminated encephalomyelitis in children. *Neurology.* 2001;56:1308–1312.

IFNB Multiple Sclerosis Study Group. Interferon beta-1b is effective in relapsing-remitting multiple sclerosis. I Clinical results of a multicenter, randomized, double blind, placebo-controlled trial. *Neurology.* 1993;43: 655–661.

Jacobs L, Cookfair D, Rudick R, et al. Intramuscular interferon beta-1a for disease progression in relapsing multiple sclerosis. *Ann Neurol.* 1996;39:285–294.

James J, Anderson J, Chabas D, Strober J, Waubant E. Pediatric-onset multiple sclerosis patient sera recognize unique regions of Epstein-Barr nuclear antigen 1 compared to matched controls [abstract]. *Multiple Scler.* 2009;15: 1406.

Johnson K, Brooks B, Cohen J, et al. Copolymer 1 reduces relapse rate and improves disability in relapsing-remitting multiple sclerosis: results of a phase III multicenter, double-blind, placebo-controlled trial. *Neurology.* 1995;45:1268–1276.

Kennedy J, O'Connor P, Sadovnick AD, Perara M, Yee I, Banwell B. Age at onset of multiple sclerosis may be influenced by place of residence during childhood rather than ancestry. *Neuroepidemiology.* 2006;26: 162–167.

Kornek B, Bernert G, Balassy C, Geldner J, Prayer D, Feucht M. Glatiramer acetate treatment in patients with childhood and juvenile onset multiple sclerosis. *Neuropediatrics.* 2003;34:120–126.

Krupp LB, Banwell B, Tenembaum S. Consensus definitions proposed for pediatric multiple sclerosis and related disorders. *Neurology.* 2007;68:S7–S12.

Krupp LB, McLinskey N, Troell R, et al. Racial and ethnic findings in pediatric MS: an update. *Neurology.* 2008; 70:A135.

Leake JA, Albani S, Kao AS, et al. Acute disseminated encephalomyelitis in childhood: epidemiologic, clinical and laboratory features. *Pediatr Infect Dis J.* 2004; 23:756–764.

MacAllister WS, Boyd JR, Holland NJ, Milazzo MC, Krupp LB, International Pediatric MS Study Group. Cognitive functioning in children and adolescents with multiple sclerosis. *Neurology.* 2005;64:1422–1425.

MacAllister WS, Christodoulou C, Milazzo M, Krupp LB. Longitudinal neuropsychological assessment in pediatric multiple sclerosis. *Dev Neuropsychol.* 2007;32: 625–644.

Makhani N, Gorman MP, Branson HM, Stazzone L, Banwell BL, Chitnis T. Cyclophosphamide therapy in pediatric multiple sclerosis. *Neurology.* 2009;72: 2076–2082.

McKeon A, Lennon VA, Lotze T, et al. CNS aquaporin-4 autoimmunity in children. *Neurology.* 2008;71: 93–100.

Mikaeloff Y, Adamsbaum C, Husson B, et al. MRI prognostic factors for relapse after acute CNS inflammatory demyelination in childhood. *Brain.* 2004b;127: 1942–1947.

Mikaeloff Y, Caridade G, Assi S, Tardieu M, Suissa S. Hepatitis B vaccine and risk of relapse after a first childhood episode of CNS inflammatory demyelination. *Brain.* 2007a;130:1105–1110.

Mikaeloff Y, Caridade G, Husson B, Suissa S, Tardieu M. Acute disseminated encephalomyelitis cohort study: prognostic factors for relapse. *Eur J Paediatr Neurol.* 2007c;11:90–95.

Mikaeloff Y, Caridade G, Suissa S, Tardieu M. Clinically observed chickenpox and the risk of childhood-onset multiple sclerosis. *Am J Epidemiol.* 2009a;169: 1260–1266.

Mikaeloff Y, Caridade G, Suissa S, Tardieu M. Hepatitis B vaccine and the risk of CNS inflammatory demyelination in childhood. *Neurology.* 2009b;72:873–880.

Mikaeloff Y, Caridade G, Tardieu M, Suissa S. Parental smoking at home and the risk of childhood-onset multiple sclerosis in children. *Brain.* 2007b;130: 2589–2595.

Mikaeloff Y, Caridade G, Tardieu M, Suissa S. Effectiveness of early beta interferon on the first attack after confirmed multiple sclerosis: a comparative cohort study. *Eur J Paediatr Neurol.* 2008;12:205–209.

Mikaeloff Y, Moreau T, Debouverie M, et al. Interferon-beta treatment in patients with childhood-onset multiple sclerosis. *J Pediatr.* 2001;139:443–446.

Mikaeloff Y, Suissa S, Vallee L, et al. First episode of acute CNS inflammatory demyelination in childhood: prognostic factors for multiple sclerosis and disability. *J Pediatr.* 2004a;144:246–252.

Mowry E, et al. Health-related quality of life is reduced in children with early multiple sclerosis. *Mult Scler.* 2008;14:S147.

Neuteboom RF, Boon M, Catsman Berrevoets CE, et al. Prognostic factors after a first attack of inflammatory CNS demyelination in children. *Neurology.* 2008;71:967–973.

O'Connor KC, McLaughlin KA, De Jager PL, et al. Self-antigen tetramers discriminate between myelin autoantibodies to native or denatured protein. *Nat Med.* 2007;13:211–217.

Ozakbas S, Idiman E, Baklan B, Yulug B. Childhood and juvenile onset multiple sclerosis: clinical and paraclinical features. *Brain Dev.* 2003;25:233–236.

Pinhas-Hamiel O, Barak Y, Siev-Ner I, Achiron A. Juvenile multiple sclerosis: clinical features and prognostic characteristics. *J Pediatr.* 1998;132:735–737.

Pohl D, Hennemuth I, von Kries R, Hanefeld F. Paediatric multiple sclerosis and acute disseminated encephalomyelitis in Germany: results of a nationwide survey. *Eur J Pediatr.* 2007;166:405–412.

Pohl D, Krone B, Rostasy K, et al. High seroprevalence of Epstein-Barr virus in children with multiple sclerosis. *Neurology.* 2006a;67:2063–2065.

Pohl D, Rostasy K, Gartner J, Hanefeld F. Treatment of early onset multiple sclerosis with subcutaneous interferon beta-1a. *Neurology.* 2005;64:888–890.

Pohl D, Rostasy K, Reiber H, Hanefeld F. CSF characteristics in early-onset multiple sclerosis. *Neurology.* 2004;63:1966–1967.

Pohl D, Rostasy K, Treiber-Held S, Brockmann K, Gärtner J, Hanefeld F. Pediatric multiple sclerosis: detection of clinically silent lesions by multimodal evoked potentials. *J Pediatr.* 2006b;149:125–127.

PRISMS Study Group. Randomized double-blind placebo-controlled study of interferon β-1a in relapsing/remitting multiple sclerosis. *Lancet Neurol.* 1998;352: 1498–1504.

Renoux C, Vukusic S, Mikaeloff Y, et al. Natural history of multiple sclerosis with childhood onset. *N Engl J Med.* 2007;356:2603–2613.

Rostasy K, Without E, Pohl D, et al. Tau, phospho-tau, and S-100B in the cerebrospinal fluid of children with multiple sclerosis. *J Child Neurol.* 2005;20:822–825.

Selcen D, Anlar B, Renda Y. Multiple sclerosis in childhood: report of 16 cases. *Eur Neurol.* 1996;36: 79–84.

Shiraishi K, Higuchi Y, Ozawa K, Hao Q, Saida T. Clinical course and prognosis of 27 patients with childhood onset multiple sclerosis in Japan. *Brain Dev.* 2005; 27:224–227.

Simone IL, Carrara D, Tortorella C, et al. Course and prognosis in early-onset MS: comparison with adult-onset forms. *Neurology.* 2002;59:1922–1928.

Sindern E, Haas J, Stark E, Wurster U. Early onset MS under the age of 16: clinical and paraclinical features. *Acta Neurol Scand.* 1992;86:280–284.

Stark W, Huppke P, Gartner J. Paediatric multiple sclerosis: the experience of the German Centre for Multiple Sclerosis in Childhood and Adolescence. *J Neurol.* 2008;255(suppl 6):119–122.

Tenembaum S, Chamoles N, Fejerman N. Acute disseminated encephalomyelitis: a long-term follow-up study of 84 pediatric patients. *Neurology.* 2002;59:1224–1231.

Tenembaum SN, Segura MJ. Interferon beta-1a treatment in childhood and juvenile-onset multiple sclerosis. *Neurology.* 2006;67:511–513.

U.S. Office of Management and Budget. *Standards for Maintaining, Collecting, and Presenting Federal Data on Race and Ethnicity. OMB Statistical Directive 15 - New.* As Adopted October 30, 1997.

Waubant E, Centers The US Network of Pediatric MS Centers, Mowry E, James J. Remote EBV, CMV, and HSV-1 and -2 infection status in children with pediatric-onset MS and age-matched healthy controls [abstract]. *ACTRIMS* Taken from *Multiple Scler.* 2009;15: 1403.

Waubant E, Chabas D. Pediatric multiple sclerosis. *Curr Treat Options Neurol.* 2009;11:203–210.

Waubant E, Chabas D, Stroer J, et al. Vitamin D levels in children with pediatric-onset MS and controls [abstract]. *Multiple Sclerosis.* 2009;15:1403.

Yeh E, Heim R, Karpinski M, Ray J, Weinstock-Guttman B. Neutralizing antibodies to interferon in children with MS on interferon treatment. Annals of Neurology. 2009;(66):A19–25.

Yeh E, Weinstock-Guttman B, Lincoff N, et al. Retinal nerve fiber thickness in inflammatory demyelinating diseases of childhood onset. *Mult* Scler. 2009;15: 802–810.

Yeh E, Krupp L, Ness, J, et al. Breakthrough disease in pediatric MS patients: a pediatric network experience. *Annual Meeting of the American Academy of Neurology.* Seattle, WA, 2009. Neurology 72 (Suppl).

Yeh E, et al. Use of natalizumab in pediatric MS: A collaborative network study. Neurology 2010, 74 (Suppl 2): A100.

Part 5 **Therapeutics**

23 | Immunomodulatory Agents for Relapsing-Remitting Multiple Sclerosis

Lawrence M. Samkoff

The treatment of relapsing-remitting multiple sclerosis (RRMS) has greatly expanded since the first MS-specific immunomodulatory agent was introduced in 1993. There are currently six approved disease-modifying therapies (DMTs) available for the treatment of RRMS, including interferon beta-1b (Betaseron), intramuscular interferon beta-1a (Avonex), subcutaneous interferon beta-1a (Rebif), glatiramer acetate (Copaxone), natalizumab (Tysabri), and mitoxantrone (Novantrone). Each of these DMTs has been studied in randomized placebo-controlled trials, with evidence-based data supporting their use (Goodin, 2008).

Neurologists caring for patients with RRMS must choose a DMT on the basis of numerous variables, including the clinical course of the disease, class of agent, dosage and frequency of administration, potential adverse effects, and patient preference. Some of the decision making can be made based upon results of clinical trials; however, there is only limited information available regarding valid comparisons among the established DMTs (Goodin, 2008).

This chapter will present an overview of five of the six FDA-approved DMTs for RRMS, including interferon beta-1b, two formulations of interferon beta-1a, glatiramer acetate, and natalizumab (see Table 23-1). Mitoxantrone will be discussed in another section of this book. The role of these DMTs in patients with clinically isolated demyelinating syndromes (CISs), arguably the earliest clinical manifestation of RRMS, and secondary progressive multiple sclerosis (SPMS) will also be discussed. Recently completed comparative studies between agents will also be reviewed.

GENERAL CONSIDERATIONS

Multiple sclerosis (MS) is a chronic immune-mediated disease of the central nervous system (CNS), characterized pathologically by inflammation, demyelination (involving both white and gray matter), and axonal injury (Trapp et al., 1998; Stadelman et al., 2008). Eighty-five percent of patients with MS present with a relapsing-remitting course (Vollmer, 2007). Relapses of MS are associated with neurologic disability, functional impairment, and psychosocial disruption, all of which impact upon quality of life (Coyle and Johnson, 2007). Approximately 50% of individuals with RRMS develop SPMS, with slowly accruing disability, within 10 years of disease onset (Weinshenker et al., 2009). One-half of patients with RRMS will require an aid for ambulation from 15 to 23 years after disease onset (Weinshenker et al., 2009). The relationship between relapse rate and long-term disability remains controversial. However, favorable prognostic factors in early RRMS include monosymptomatic onset, complete recovery during remission, longer duration between first and second relapse, and low frequency of relapses (Vukusic and Confavreux, 2007).

GOALS OF DISEASE-MODIFYING THERAPY IN RELAPSING-REMITTING MULTIPLE SCLEROSIS

Relapsing-remitting multiple sclerosis is primarily an inflammatory disease of CNS myelin, characterized by periodic relapses followed by complete or incomplete recovery, and separated by variable

TABLE 23-1 Disease-Modifying Agents in Multiple Sclerosis

Agent	Dosing	Multiple Sclerosis Type	Common Adverse Effects	Monitoring
Betaseron (β interferon-1b)	250 mcg SQ every other day	RRMS CIS SPMS	Flu-like symptoms Leukopenia Elevated liver enzymes Thyroid dysfunction ?depression	CBC, LFT q 3 months during first year, then q 6 months thereafter. Thyroid function tests q 3–6 months during first year, then yearly thereafter.
Avonex (β interferon-1a)	30 mcg IM weekly	RRMS CIS	Flu-like symptoms Leukopenia Elevated liver enzymes Thyroid dysfunction	CBC, LFT q 3 months during first year, then q 6 months thereafter. Thyroid function tests q 3–6 months during first year, then yearly thereafter.
Rebif (β interferon-1a)	44 mcg SQ tiw	RRMS SPMS	Flu-like symptoms Leukopenia Elevated liver enzymes Thyroid dysfunction	CBC, LFT q 3 months during first year, then q 6 months thereafter. Thyroid function tests q 3–6 months during first year, then yearly thereafter.
Copaxone (glatiramer acetate)	20 mg SQ qd	RRMS CIS	Injection-site reactions Lipoatrophy Post-injection vasomotor syndrome	None
Tysabri (natalizumab)	300 mg IV q 4 weeks	RRMS	Hypersensitivity reactions Infusion reactions (headache, rigors) Progressive multifocal leukoencephalopathy Hepatic failure (rare)	LFT q 3 months

CIS, clinically isolated syndrome; RRMS, relapsing-remitting multiple sclerosis; SPMS, secondary progressive multiple sclerosis.

intervals of clinical remission (Vollmer, 2007; Coyle, 2008). However, Trapp et al. (1998) demonstrated pathologic evidence of irreversible axonal transsection in early relapsing disease in addition to inflammation and demyelination. Although the precise relationship between inflammation and neurodegeneration in MS is uncertain, it is postulated that early control of the inflammatory component of MS may also mitigate axonal degeneration (Coyle, 2008). This hypothesis is in part supported by magnetic resonance imaging (MRI)-based studies

in patients with RRMS of intramuscular interferon beta-1a (Filippi, 2001) and glatiramer acetate (Rudick et al., 1999), which respectively demonstrated reduced progression of whole-brain atrophy and T1-hypointensities, MRI correlates of axonal degeneration in RRMS (Bakshi et al., 2008), over 9 months to 2 years.

None of FDA-approved MS immunomodulatory medications are curative; they are at best partially effective. In separate studies employing differing methodologies, they have all been demonstrated to reduce relapse rate, limit disability progression, and control disease-associated MRI activity in short-term trials; however, their efficacy in reducing long-term disability remains unproven (IFNB MS Study Group, 1993; Johnson et al., 1995; Jacobs et al., 1996; PRISMS Study Group, 1998; Polman et al., 2006; Coyle, 2008).

There is broad consensus that treatment with DMTs should be initiated early in the course of RRMS, as advocated by consensus statements of both the National Multiple Sclerosis Society and the American Academy of Neurology (Goodin et al., 2002; National Clinical Advisory Board, 2007). It is widely held that the DMTs are more effective during the early inflammatory phase of RRMS and less potent as the disease transitions into a neurodegenerative process (Bermel and Rudick, 2007; Coyle, 2008).

DISEASE-MODIFYING THERAPIES IN RELAPSING-REMITTING MULTIPLE SCLEROSIS

Interferon Beta

There are three formulations of interferon beta (IFNβ) approved for the treatment of RRMS: subcutaneous IFNβ-1b, intramuscular IFNβ-1a, and subcutaneous IFNβ-1a. It is postulated that the benefits of IFNβ in RRMS are modulated primarily through an anti-inflammatory mechanism of action (Bermel and Rudick, 2007). Potential immunomodulatory effects of IFNβ in RRMS include downregulation of proinflammatory cytokines such as IFNγ, reduced expression of major histocompatibility antigens, and decreasing transmigration of T-lymphocytes across the blood–brain barrier (Bermel and Rudick, 2007).

Subcutaneous inteferon beta-1b in
relapsing-remitting multiple sclerosis

IFNβ-1b, a nonglycosylated recombinant product derived from *Escherichia coli*, differs from natural IFNβ by a single amino acid substitution. In a 2-year multicenter, double-blind, placebo-controlled study of 372 patients with RRMS and Expanded Disability Status Scale (EDSS) score 0 to 5.5, 8 million international units (MIU) IFNβ-1b

administered subcutaneously (SC) every other day decreased annual relapse rate 32% from 1.27 to 0.84 ($p = 0.0001$) (IFNB MS Study Group, 1993). A lower dose of IFNβ-1b, 1.6 MIU, was also significantly effective compared to placebo, but less so. Patients in the high-dose arm of the study had less severe relapses and were more likely to be relapse-free during the study. There was benefit on cranial MRI activity reflected by significant reductions in both lesion burden and activity in patients treated with eight MIU IFNβ-1b compared to placebo at the end of 3 years (Paty et al., 1993). The placebo group had a mean increase in lesion load of 17.1%, whereas the IFNβ-1b group had a mean reduction of 6.2% ($p = 0.002$). In a 5-year analysis of the original patient cohort, the benefits of IFNβ-1b on relapse rate were maintained (IFNB MS Study Group, 1995). Although fewer patients on IFNβ-1b had confirmed EDSS progression after 5 years, this difference was not significant.

Intramuscular interferon beta-1a in
relapsing-remitting multiple sclerosis

IFNβ-1a (IM) is a naturally sequenced glycosylated recombinant mammalian product. In a randomized, placebo-controlled, double-blinded study of 301 patients with RRMS and EDSS 1.0 to 3.5, weekly IM IFNβ-1a (IM) 30 µg weekly significantly slowed disability progression, defined as a 1.0-point increase on the EDSS persisting for at least 6 months, over 104 weeks (Jacobs et al., 1996). Disability progression occurred in 34.9% of the placebo group and in 21.9% of IFNβ-1a (IM) recipients ($p = 0.02$), representing a 37% reduction. The annual relapse rate for all patients studied was 0.82 in the placebo group and 0.62 in the IFNβ-1a (IM) group (18% reduction, $p = 0.04$). In 170 patients followed for at least 104 weeks, IFNβ-1a (IM) reduced relapse rate by 32% ($p = 0.002$). Patients treated with IFNβ-1a (IM) had significantly reduced number and volume of gadolinium-enhancing (GdE) lesions at 12 and 24 months. There was a trend to reduced T2-hyperintense lesion load after 2 years in the IFNβ-1a (IM) group (−13.2% versus −6.5%), but the difference was not significant. Significantly fewer patients treated with IFNβ-1a (IM) progressed to EDSS levels of 4.0 and 6.0 over 2 years (Rudick et al., 1997).

Post-hoc MRI analysis of brain parenchymal fraction demonstrated that patients treated with IFNβ-1a (IM) had reduced progression of brain atrophy compared to placebo during the second year of the study ($p = 0.03$) (Rudick et al., 1999).

Interferon beta-1a by subcutaneous injection in relapsing-remitting multiple sclerosis

In a 2-year multinational RCT (PRISMS) of 560 patients with RRMS and EDSS 0–5.0, IFNβ-1a (SC) 22 and 44 μg three times per week reduced relapse rate over 1 year by 27% and 2 years by 33% (PRISMS Study Group, 1998). Both doses prolonged time to first relapse, and patients in both treatment groups were significantly more likely to be relapse-free compared to the placebo group. Time to sustained disability was significantly prolonged ($p < 0.05$) in both treatment groups compared to placebo. However, in patients with high baseline EDSS (>3.5), a significant benefit in time to sustained progression was seen only in the 44 μg group. Accumulation of disability was also less in the IFNβ-1a (SC) groups compared with placebo. Benefit on MRI lesion activity and T2-burden of disease was demonstrated for both active treatment arms. A modest dose effect favoring the 44 μg group was seen for some clinical parameters, including relapse rate and relapse severity, but the difference was greater for MRI measures.

In a 2-year blinded extension study of the original study (PRISMS-4), patients initially treated with placebo were re-randomized to receive IFNβ-1a (SC) 22 or 44 μg (crossover groups), while patients on active treatment continued on their originally assigned dosages (PRISMS Study Group, 2001). Patients treated for 4 years with IFNβ-1a at 22 μg and 44 μg tiw had relapse rates of 0.80 and 0.72; patients in the crossover group (i.e., on IFNβ-1a treatment for only 2 years) had a relapse rate of 1.02, a significant reduction from the prior placebo period. There was a significant reduction ($p < 0.001$) in exacerbation rate in patients treated with IFNβ-1a for 4 years compared with those treated for 2 years. Time to confirmed disability progression was significantly prolonged in patients in the 44 μg group (42.1 months) compared with the crossover (24.2 months) groups ($p = 0.047$). The difference in disability accumulation between the 44 μg and 22 μg groups and between the 22 μg and crossover groups did not reach statistical significance. There was, however, a significant decrease in MRI activity in patients treated for 4 years compared with 2 years, with a dose effect.

The results of the PRISMS-4 trial confirmed ongoing efficacy of high-dose IFNβ-1a in reducing relapse rate, disability progression, and MRI activity in patients with RRMS. Furthermore, it appeared that delaying treatment adversely affected these same parameters, as patients in the crossover groups fared significantly worse on clinical and MRI measures of disease activity (PRISMS Study Group, 2001; Schwid and Bever, 2001). Kappos et al. have reported partially blinded long-term follow-up at 8 years on 68% of the original PRISMS cohort (Kappos et al., 2006b). Patients originally randomized to treatment with subcutaneous IFNβ-1a 44 μg tiw showed lower EDSS progression, relapse rate, and T2 lesion burden compared to patients whose treatment was delayed. The results of this study support the long-term safety of subcutaneous IFNβ-1a but are potentially limited by selection bias.

Adverse effects of interferon beta

Administration of IFNβ can be associated with a number of adverse effects. A flu-like syndrome, which includes fever, chills, myalgias, fatigue, and headache occurs in up to 50%–75% of patients treated with IFNβ (Langer-Gould et al., 2004; Bermel and Rudick, 2007). This reaction typically begins within 6 hours of injection and may last up to 24 hours. Administration of IFNβ at bedtime may reduce daytime symptoms. These symptoms commonly abate within the first 3 months of therapy and may be avoided and relieved by acetaminophen and nonsteroidal anti-inflammatory drugs (NSAIDs), given both preinjection and postinjection (Langer-Gould et al., 2004). Low-dose prednisone (10 mg) may be given on the day of injection if NSAIDs are ineffective in preventing or ameliorating flu-like symptoms (Langer-Gould et al., 2004). Pentoxifylline (800 mg bid) has also reported to be effective (Rieckmann et al., 1996). Alternatively, to reduce side effects, IFNβ may be initiated at one-quarter to one-half the recommended dose and then gradually titrated to full dosage over 3–4 weeks (Bermel and Rudick, 2007).

Injection-site reactions are common in patients treated with subcutaneous IFNβ, typically including mild local erythema, bruising, and pain (Bermel and Rudick, 2007). However, more severe reactions, including infection and, rarely, skin necrosis, have also been reported (Galetta and Markowitz, 2005). In most cases, modification of injection technique and rotation of injection sites will ameliorate untoward skin effects (Bermel and Rudick, 2007). Occurrence of skin necrosis rarely warrants surgical consultation and withdrawal of IFNβ (Langer-Gould et al., 2004).

The association between IFNβ and depression has not been completely established and depressive symptoms such as anhedonia, insomnia, and hopelessness are common in the MS population (Langer-Gould et al., 2004). In the pivotal IFNβ-1b trial (IFNB MS Study Group, 1993, 1995) depression and suicide attempts occurred more frequently in treated patients, although the difference in attempted suicide was not statistically significant between the IFNβ-1b and placebo groups. None of the IFNβ-1a studies demonstrated an increased risk of suicide in treated patients (Jacobs et al., 1996; PRISMS Study Group, 1998). Prior to initiating therapy with IFNβ patients should be prescreened for depression. Depression that develops while on IFNβ can be managed with antidepressant medication and psychotherapy, but cessation of IFNβ is recommended until psychiatric symptoms are controlled (Langer-Gould et al., 2004).

The most commonly reported laboratory abnormalities with IFNβ are leukopenia, lymphopenia, neutropenia, and elevated liver enzymes (Langer-Gould et al., 2004; Galetta and Markowitz, 2005; Bermel and Rudick, 2007). These are usually mild and asymptomatic. Leukopenia may persist unchanged during treatment with IFNβ but warrants discontinuation if persistently below 3000. In a 6-year retrospective study, Tremlett and Oger (2004) reported that normal liver function returned in 74% of patients who were maintained on IFNβ therapy despite developing grade 1 or grade 2 aminotransferase elevation. However, fulminant liver failure requiring liver transplantation has been described in a patient treated with IFNβ-1a (Yoshida et al., 2001). Less commonly, autoimmune hypothyroidism or hyperthyroidism have been associated with IFNβ treatment (Schwid et al., 1997; Monzani et al., 2000; Kriesler et al., 2003).

Clinical thyroid dysfunction is rarer than laboratory thyroid dysfunction. The risk of thyroid disease appears to be greatest during the first year of therapy (Monzani et al., 2000).

It is recommended that complete blood count and liver profile be obtained prior to initiating therapy with IFNβ and monitored during the first 12 months of treatment and as required, with at least yearly assessment thereafter (Langer-Gould et al., 2004). Thyroid functions should also be obtain pretreatment and monitored during the first year of IFNβ and then thereafter when clinical suspicion of thyroid disease develops (Monzani et al., 2000).

Interferon beta neutralizing antibodies

The treatment of relapsing MS with IFNβ-1a and IFNβ-1b is associated with formation of neutralizing antibodies (NAb) directed against IFN (Giovannoni and Goodman, 2005), occurring in 22% to 38% of patients in the randomized pivotal clinical trials (IFNB MS Study Group, 1996; Jacobs et al., 1996; PRISMS Study Group, 1998). On both clinical and MRI measures, the efficacy of IFNβ can be reduced in NAb-positive patients treated with IFNβ-1a and IFNβ-1b (Giovannoni and Goodman, 2005).

In the pivotal IFNβ-1b trial, 38% of patients treated with 8 MIU sc qod had detectable NAb by the third year of the study (IFNB MS Study Group, 1996). Positivity of NAb was defined as two consecutive serum samples (3 months apart) demonstrating the presence of NAb using an established bioassay. Exacerbation rates at 18 months in NAb-positive (NAb+) patients were two-fold higher ($p < 0.001$) than in NAb-negative (NAb−) patients; MRI activity was also increased in the NAb+ group compared with the NAb− arm, although the difference was not statistically significant ($p = 0.067$).

In the PRISMS trial (PRISMS Study Group, 1998, 2001), persistent NAb+ were found in 23.7% and 14.3% of patients treated with IFNβ-1a 22 μg sc tiw and 44 μg sc tiw, respectively, for 4 years. There were no effects of NAbs on clinical and MRI disease activity seen during the first 2 years of the study (PRISMS Study Group, 1998). However, over 4 years, NAb+ patients in both treatment groups had higher exacerbation rates, which was significantly greater in years 3 and 4 of the study

(0.82 vs. 0.51, $p = 0.004$). MRI disease activity was also increased in NAb+ patients; median number of T2 active lesions in the 44 μg group was 0.3 for NAb− patients and 1.4 for NAb+ patients. The impact of Nab seropositivity was examined in a re-analysis of the PRISMS data (Rudick et al., 1998). Patients who were interval-positive for NAbs at the end each 6-period during the 4-year study had significantly reduced benefit on multiple measures of relapse and MRI activity compared to NAb− patients. Similarly, there was a significant benefit on time to confirmed progression in NAb− patients compared to NAb+ patients.

In the controlled trial of IFNβ-1a 30 μg IM weekly, 22% of patients tested NAb+ at week 104 (Jacobs et al., 1996). Using a two-step assay, Rudick et al. (1998) subsequently analyzed the incidence and significance of NAb in patients from the phase III trial and participants from an open-label study of IFNβ-1a. Nab status did not correlate with measures of clinical efficacy (disability progression, relapse rate) in the phase III group treated with IFNβ-1a for 2 years, although in vivo biologic activity of IFN was reduced in the NAb-positive group. On cranial MRI at week 104, however, NAb+ patients (titer ≥ 20) had more gadolinium-enhancing lesions than those who were NAb−. The difference did not reach statistical significance (1.6 vs. 0.6 lesions; $p = 0.062$). In the open-label study, 6% of IFNβ-naïve patients ($n = 84$) treated with IFNβ-1a for 24 months developed NAbs. In the majority of subjects, NAbs were detected after 9 months of therapy. In patients who previously received IFNβ-1b ($n = 118$), the percentage of Nab positivity to IFNβ-1a at study entry correlated with duration of prior treatment; approximately 25% of patients treated with IFNβ-1b for over 12 months had NAb directed against IFNβ-1a.

The European Interferon Beta-1a IM Dose-Comparison Study compared the efficacy of once weekly IFNβ-1a at dosages of 30 μg and 60 μg for up to 4 years in patients with RRMS (Kappos et al., 2005). Although there was no significant difference on clinical and MRI measures, the proportion of patients who developed NAbs in the high-dose group was significantly higher than those in the low-dose group (4.8% vs. 1.8%, $p = 0.02$). Mean time to NAb+ status was 14.5 ± 6.2 months. NAb+ patients had significantly higher relapse rates from months 12 to 48 ($p = 0.04$) and mean change

in EDSS over 48 months ($p = 0.01$). Magnetic resonance imaging measures of disease activity were also significantly greater in the NAb+ group. Although NAb+ patients were more likely to have sustained disability progression over 48 months, time to 3-month sustained disability was not significantly different in NAb+ and NAb− groups.

Finally, a prospective study of NAbs in patients treated with IFNβ was conducted through the Danish MS Treatment Register (Soelber Sorensen et al., 2005). In this study, an antiviral neutralization assay was used to measure NAbs from 6 to 78 months in 455 patients with RRMS who had been treated with IFNβ for at least 24 months. The authors found that 52.2% of patients were persistently NAb− and 40.9% became definitely NAb+, the latter defined as patients who had at least two consecutive positive samples. Fluctuating NAb status was detected in 6.8% of patients. Patients treated with intramuscular IFNβ-1a were more likely to be persistently NAb− compared with treatment with subcutaneous IFNβ-1a or IFNβ-1b ($p < 0.0001$); there was no difference between IFNβ-1a and IFNβ-1b NAb status. Patients who remained NAb− after 24 months rarely converted to NAb+. The majority of patients who were NAb+ from 12 to 30 months after start of therapy remained NAb+, although reversion to NAb− occurred in 33% of patients, more commonly with treatment with subcutaneous IFNβ-1b compared with subcutaneous IFNβ-1a ($p = 0.0154$).

The European Federation of Neurological Societies (EFNS) recommends testing for NAbs on all patients treated with IFNβ at 12 and 24 months on therapy (Level A). Patients who remain NAb− at 24 months do not require further testing (Level B). Patients who are NAb+ require repeat testing at 3–6 month intervals, and the EFNS recommends stopping IFNβ in patients with high titers of NAbs at repeated measurements (Level A) (Sorensen et al., 2005).

The Therapeutics and Technology Assessment Subcommittee of The American Academy of Neurology (AAN) has also reviewed the data concerning the impact of IFNβ NAbs in the treatment of RRMS (Goodin et al., 2007). The AAN also concludes that treatment with IFNβ is associated with the production of NAbs (Level A), with probable reduction of clinical and radiologic therapeutic efficacy of IFNβ in patients with persistently elevated titers (Level B). Intramuscular weekly IFNβ-1a is less immunogenic than multiple-dosed weekly subcutaneous IFNβ-1a or IFNβ-1b (Level A). Because NAbs can disappear in some patients on continued treatment with IFNβ, the AAN does not provide specific recommendations on timing or frequency of testing for NAbs; the cutoff titer above which treatment might be stopped is uncertain and left to the discretion of the treating physician.

Taken together, it seems reasonable that patients treated with IFNβ who have significant breakthrough clinical or radiologic disease activity should undergo serologic testing for NAbs; those patients with sustained high titers of NAbs should be considered for alternative therapy.

Glatiramer Acetate in Relapsing-Remitting Multiple Sclerosis

Glatiramer acetate (GA) is a complex mixture of random synthetic polypeptides consisting of four amino acids, L-glutamate, L-lysine, L-alanine, and L-tyrosine. Glatiramer acetate was originally developed as an analog of myelin basic protein and was found to modify or suppress experimental autoimmune encephalomyelitis, an animal model of MS (Farina et al., 2005). Clinical studies of GA in the treatment of MS were based on these early findings. Bornstein et al. (1987) demonstrated that GA reduced relapses in RRMS in a pilot study of 50 patients. Subsequently, Johnson et al. (1995) reported clinical benefits of GA in a randomized, multicenter, placebo-controlled trial of 251 patients with RRMS (EDSS 0 to 5.0). Patients administered 20 mg GA SC daily had a 2-year relapse reduction of 29% compared to placebo (p = 0.007). Relapse rate reduction was more pronounced in patients with entry EDSS 0–2.0. At the end of the study, significantly more patients in the GA arm had improved EDSS, while patients in the placebo arm were more likely to have increased EDSS. Trends in percentage of relapse-free patients and median time to first relapse favored GA, although these differences were not significant. In a double-blind extension study with average additional follow-up of 5.5 months, GA continued to favorably impact upon relapse rate and disability progression (Johnson et al., 1998). In an 8-year open-label extension study involving 142 patients

from the original cohort, a significantly larger percentage of patients treated with GA for the entire length of the study had stable or improved neurologic disability based on the EDSS compared to the group whose treatment was delayed by 30 months (65.3% versus 50.4%, p = 0.0263; Johnson et al., 1995), suggesting that earlier initiation of treatment with GA resulted in better clinical outcomes. Annualized relapse rate declined to 0.2 in both groups. In a long-term, prospective, open-label analysis of 232 patients from the pivotal randomized study, patients who received continuous GA (n = 108) had less accumulation of disability compared with patients who stopped GA for any reason (n = 50) at a follow-up visit at 10 years. Long-term safety of GA was also substantiated (Ford et al., 2006). The significance of this study is limited due to selection bias and unknown outcomes of over half of the patients in the withdrawn cohort.

Beneficial effects of GA on disease activity determined by cranial MRI were confirmed in a separate RCT (Comi et al., 2001b). Two hundred thirty-nine patients with RRMS were randomized to receive either daily GA 20 mg or placebo by daily SC injection and underwent monthly cranial MRI and clinical evaluation for 9 months. The primary outcome measure was the cumulative number of GdE lesions, which was reduced 29% in the GA-treated patients (p = 0.003). Glatiramer acetate was also associated with significant differences in development of new GdE lesions, new T2-hyperintense lesions, and total T2-hyperintense lesion volume during the study period. Treatment differences emerged at 6 months, suggesting a delayed mechanism of action of GA.

Finally, the safety and efficacy of double-dose GA (40 mg daily) compared to the currently approved 20 mg formulation was addressed in a 9-month randomized, double-blind trial of 90 patients with RRMS (n = 46 and 44, respectively) (Cohen et al., 2007). Patients receiving 40 mg GA had reduced cranial MRI lesion activity as measured by gadolinium enhancement, the primary endpoint, at months 7, 8, and 9, although the difference did not reach statistical significance (p = 0.09). There was a significant difference favoring the 40 mg group in secondary clinical endpoints, time to first relapse (p = 0.018) and proportion of relapse-free subjects (p = 0.037).

Injection site reactions and post-injection vasomotor response were more common in the high-dose cohort. The authors concluded that the 40 mg GA daily dose may be more effective than the currently approved 20 mg dosage. The results of this study require confirmation with a larger phase III investigation.

The mechanism of action of GA in RRMS remains speculative. Recent studies suggest that GA promotes an anti-inflammatory Th2 shift of T cells in the peripheral circulation, which may be mediated through an inhibitory effect on antigen-presenting cells (Farina et al., 2005). A neuroprotective effect of GA has been postulated but not proven (Farina et al., 2005).

Adverse effects of glatiramer acetate

In general, GA is well tolerated. The most common adverse effect is an injection-site reaction, consisting of mild erythema, induration, pruritis, or tenderness (Ford et al., 2006). Lipoatrophy, dimpling of the skin caused by loss of subcutaneous fat with repeated injections in the same location, sometimes occurs (Edgar et al., 2004). The significance of this adverse effect primarily is cosmetic, but it can be disfiguring and irreversible (Edgar et al., 2004). Erythema nodosum related to GA treatment has also been reported (Thouvenot et al., 2007).

Administration of GA is also associated with a postinjection systemic reaction, characterized by variable combinations of flushing, diaphoresis, chest tightness, dyspnea, palpitations, and anxiety, beginning within minutes after injection and resolving spontaneously in 30 seconds to 30 minutes (Johnson et al., 1995; Ford et al., 2006). This systemic reaction is sporadic and unpredictable. It was reported at least once in 15% of patients in the pivotal studies (Johnson et al., 1995). Typically it occurs once in a given patient, but it occasionally occurs repeatedly. The etiology remains uncertain. It does not appear to be a hypersensitivity reaction, and there have been no reports of cardiopulmonary compromise (Ford et al., 2006). Nevertheless, patients should be advised of this potential reaction prior to commencing treatment with GA.

Finally, GA is not associated with abnormalities of blood counts or liver studies, and laboratory monitoring is not required (Ford et al., 2006). In summary, GA often is better tolerated than IFNβ.

This advantage is offset for some patients by its requirement for more frequent injections.

Natalizumab

Natalizumab (Tysabri) is a recombinant humanized monoclonal antibody that binds to the α_4-subunit of $\alpha_4\beta_1$-integrin that is expressed on activated T-lymphocytes. By blocking the interaction of $\alpha_4\beta_1$-integrin with the vascular cell adhesion molecule 1 (VCAM-1) ligand on endothelial cells, natalizumab blocks adhesion and transmigration of activated T-lymphocytes across the blood–brain barrier, reducing the inflammatory component in the MS plaque (Ropper, 2006).

In a double-blind, placebo-controlled phase II study, Miller et al. (2003). found that intravenous natalizumab given at doses of 3 mg/kg and 6 mg/kg every 4 weeks for 6 months reduced accumulation of new lesions on cranial MRI (0.7 vs. 9.6 [$p < 0.001$] and 1.1 vs. 9.6 [$p < 0.001$], respectively), which was the primary outcome of the study. Treated patients had fewer relapses compared to the placebo group, 19% for both natalizumab groups versus 38 % for placebo ($p < 0.02$), a secondary endpoint for the study. The encouraging results of this study led to two phase III randomized, placebo-controlled investigations of natalizumab in RRMS (Polman et al., 2006; Rudick et al., 2006). In each study, the primary outcome was the annualized relapse rate at 1 year. Prespecified secondary endpoints at 1 year in both studies included the proportion of relapse-free subjects, reduction of new or enlarging T2-hyperintense cranial MRI lesions, and the number of GdE lesions.

The AFFIRM study (Polman et al., 2006) randomized 942 patients previously untreated with IFNβ or GA to 300 mg natalizumab ($n = 627$) or placebo ($n = 315$) IV every 4 weeks up to 28 months. Natalizumab reduced the annualized relapse rate compared to placebo by 68% (0.26 vs. 0.81, $p < 0.0001$) at year 1 and by 59% at year 2 (0.23 vs. 0.73, $p < 0.001$). The risk of sustained EDSS progression over 2 years was reduced by 42% ($p < 0.001$). T2-hyperintense brain MRI lesions that were new or enlarged at 2 years versus baseline were reduced by 83% in the natalizumab group compared with placebo ($p < 0.001$). The mean number of GdE lesions was reduced by 92% at years 1 and 2 in the treated group ($p < 0.001$).

The SENTINEL study (Rudick et al., 2006) recruited 1171 patients with RRMS who had experienced one or more relapses in the previous year despite treatment with IFNβ-1a (IM). All patients continued IFNβ-1a (IM) 30 μg weekly and were randomized to receive either 300 mg natalizumab ($n = 589$) or placebo ($n = 582$) IV every 4 weeks as add-on therapy for 116 weeks. Subjects in the natalizumab arm had an annualized relapse rate over 2 years of 0.34 versus 0.75 in the placebo group, representing a 55% relative reduction ($p < 0.001$). Combination therapy resulted in a 24% reduction in the relative risk of sustained EDSS progression over 2 years (hazard ratio 0.76, $p = 0.02$). The number of new or enlarging T2-hypertense lesions over 2 years was reduced from 5.4 with IFNβ-1a (IM) alone to 0.9 with combination therapy (83% reduction, $p < 0.001$). GdE lesions at 2 years were reduced 89% in the combination group compared to the control group ($p < 0.001$).

Natalizumab and progressive multifocal leukoencephalopathy

In February, 2005, 3 months after natalizumab first received FDA approval for treatment of RRMS, the drug was withdrawn from the market, when three cases of progressive multifocal leukoencephalopathy (PML) were reported in natalizumab-treated patients who participated clinical trials in MS (2 patients) and Crohn disease (1 patient) (Kleinschmidt-DeMasters and Tyler, 2005; Langer-Gould et al., 2005; VanAssche et al., 2005).

The two RRMS patients who contracted PML were treated with both natalizumab and interferon-β-1a as part of the SENTINEL combination therapy trial (Kleinschmidt-DeMasters and Tyler, 2005; Langer-Gould et al., 2005). One patient was a 46-year-old woman with RRMS who died from autopsy-confirmed PML after she received 37 doses of natalizumab (300 mg intravenously every 4 weeks) while continuing to receive weekly intramuscular interferon-β-1a (30 μg), which had been initiated 26 months earlier for RRMS (Kleinschmidt-DeMasters and Tyler, 2005). The second patient, a 44-year-old man with RRMS, was diagnosed with biopsy-proven PML after administration of 28 infusions of natalizumab at 4-week intervals;

weekly intramuscular interferon-β-1a had been started 4 years prior to entering the clinical trial with natalizumab. Treatment with intravenous cytarabine was associated with some neurologic improvement 3 months after natalizumab was discontinued (Langer-Gould et al., 2005). The third patient was a 60-year-old man with Crohn disease who had received a total of eight infusions of natalizumab monotherapy during a clinical trial (three monthly infusions) and open-label extension study (five infusions at 4-week intervals) over a period of 17 months (VanAssche et al., 2005). He had also received azathioprine and infliximab for Crohn disease prior to treatment with natalizumab. In this case, originally diagnosed as a grade 3 astrocytoma by brain biopsy, the diagnosis of PML was made 3 years postmortem. Retrospective analysis of frozen serum samples from this patient detected increasing titers of JC virus DNA by polymerase-chain reaction assay over a 2-month interval prior to presentation with PML.

Subsequent to these reports, Yousry et al. (2006) evaluated 3116 of 3417 (91%) of subjects who participated in clinical trials of natalizumab, for either MS or Crohn disease, with a mean exposure of 17.6 months. No additional cases of PML were diagnosed. The authors concluded that the risk of PML was approximately 1 in 1000 patients treated with natalizumab for a mean of 17.6 months.

Natalizumab was reapproved by the FDA as monotherapy for relapsing MS in 2006, with a black box warning about PML (Rasnohoff, 2007). Prescription and administration of natalizumab are restricted to certified providers, pharmacies, and infusion centers under the TOUCH system, which requires mandatory education, monitoring, and reporting. As of January 21, 2010, postmarketing surveillance had identified 31 confirmed cases of PML in 66,000 MS patients receiving natalizumab monotherapy from 12 to 36 months (FDA Safety Communication, February 5, 2010). Of these 31 cases, 10 patients were from the US and there have been 8 deaths. No cases of PML have been reported in patients receiving less than 12 infusions of natalizumab. The overall worldwide cumulative risk of PML in patients who have received at least 24 infusions is 1.3 per 1000 patients.

Progressive multifocal leukoencephalopathy is a typically fatal opportunistic infection of CNS oligodendrocytes caused by reactivation of latent

JC polymavirus infection (Berger and Korlanik, 2001). It is primarily seen in disorders associated with severely impaired cell-mediated immunity, including acquired immunodeficiency syndrome (AIDS) leukemia, and organ transplantation. After infection in immunocompetent hosts, JC virus remains quiescent in kidney tissue and is often detected in urine (Berger and Koralnik, 2001). Infection of CNS is likely established via hematogenous dissemination of virus across the blood–brain barrier (Berger and Koralnik, 2001). It is plausible that inhibition of leukocyte trafficking into the CNS by natalizumab was responsible in part or whole for development of PML (Berger and Koralnik, 2001). It is uncertain what, if any, role interferon-β-1a contributed in the patients with MS. Equally unknown is whether prospective monitoring of serum JC viral load in patients treated with natalizumab or similar agents could prevent development of PML (Berger and Koralnik, 2005).

Clinical manifestations of PML include progressive hemiparesis, hemianopia and cortical blindness, and behavioral disturbances (Ransohoff, 2007). Typical characteristics of MS exacerbations, such as acute onset of symptoms, involvement of the optic nerve or spinal cord, and steroid responsiveness are not usually associated with PML. Suspicion of PML in natalizumab-treated individuals should prompt immediate cessation of therapy, followed by MRI imaging, CSF testing for JC virus by PCR, and if necessary, brain biopsy. There is no established therapy for PML other than immune reconstitution. However, Khatri et al. (2009) recently reported the effects of plasma exchange (PLEX) on 12 patients receiving natalizumab. Patients received three 1.5-volume PLEX treatments over 5 or 8 days. PLEX accelerated natalizumab clearance (mean serum concentration reduction of 92% after 1 week), and at natalizumab concentrations below 1 µg/ml, desaturation of α4-integrin was seen; transmigration of leukocytes across an in vitro blood–brain barrier improved after PLEX. The authors concluded that PLEX may be a useful modality to restore immunity in natalizumab-treated patients.

Other adverse effects of natalizumab

In clinical trials of natalizumab (Polman et al., 2006; Rudick et al., 2006; Rudick and Panzara, 2008) the most commonly reported adverse events associated with treatment were hypersensitivity reactions, infusion-related events, and infection. Hypersensitivity reactions warranting discontinuation of natalizumab treatment, including urticaria, pruritus, anaphylaxis, and anaphylactoid syndrome occurred in 4% of natalizumab subjects in the AFFIRM study and 1.9% of patients receiving natalizumab-IFNβ-1a combination therapy in the SENTINEL study (Polman et al., 2006; Rudick et al., 2006). In AFFIRM, the incidence of anaphylaxis/anaphylactoid reactions was 0.8% (Polman et al., 2006). There were no reports of anaphylaxis/anaphylactoid syndrome in SENTINEL (Rudick et al., 2006). Natalizumab treatment should be discontinued in any patient who develops a hypersensitivity reaction. Other reported infusion-related adverse events, defined as symptoms occurring within 2 hours of study drug administration, occurred in 24% of natalizumab-treated subjects and 18%–20% of placebo patients in the AFFIRM and SENTINEL studies; these consisted of headache, flushing, erythema, rigors, nausea, fatigue, and dizziness. Urinary and respiratory tract infections also occurred more frequently in the natalizumab group compared with the placebo group (2.1% vs. 1.3%).

Two patients receiving natalizumab who developed melanoma were recently reported, suggesting caution treating with natalizumab in patients with a personal or family history of melanoma or those with atypical nevi (Mullen et al., 2008). Fulminant hepatic failure associated with natalizumab has also been reported in postmarketing surveillance (Tysabri, 2006). Elevated transaminases and bilirubin have occurred as early as 6 days after the first dose. Clinical or laboratory evidence of hepatic injury should be monitored regularly in natalizumab-treated patients, and when detected, natalizumab should be discontinued.

Natalizumab antibodies

In both the AFFIRM and SENTINEL studies, persistent antibodies against natalizumab, defined as having detectable antibodies (≥ 0.5 µg/ml) in serum samples measured at least 6 weeks apart, were observed in 6% of patients (Calabresi et al., 2007). Transiently positive antibodies occurred in 3% of patients; the majority of subjects (91%) were persistently antibody-negative. Of all patients who developed antibodies, 88% showed detectable titers at 12 weeks. Detectable antibodies occurred in 9% of patients at week 24 and in 2% by week 36. One patient who was transiently antibody-positive at week 60 reverted to antibody-negative at week 72. Fifty-three percent of persistently antibody-positive patients reverted to antibody-negative by the end of the 2-year studies.

Compared with antibody-negative patients, persistently positive subjects demonstrated loss of clinical efficacy after 6 months of treatment on measures of annualized relapse rate and MRI activity in both AFFIRM and SENTINEL; effect on sustained disability was significantly reduced by antibody-seropositivity in the AFFIRM study only. The incidence of infusion-related adverse events, including hypersensitivity and allergic reactions, were significantly higher in persistently positive patients compared to antibody-negative patients (76% vs. 20% in AFFIRM; 79% vs. 19% in SENTINEL). Given the findings of AFFIRM and SENTINEL, natalizumab-treated patients who experience continued MS clinical relapses or persistent infusion-related events after 6 months should be tested for antibodies against natalizumab.

Recommendations on natalizumab treatment in relapsing-remitting multiple sclerosis

The results of the AFFIRM and SENTINEL trials were recently reviewed by the Therapeutics and Technology Assessment Subcommittee of the American Academy of Neurology (Goodin et al., 2008). The authors conclude that based on level A evidence, natalizumab reduces clinical and MRI disease activity and disease severity in RRMS, including beneficial effects on relapse rate, sustained EDSS disability progression, gadolinium-enhancement, new and enlarging T2-lesions, and T2-hyperintense and T1-hypotensive lesion burden. However, the relative efficacy of natalizumab compared with other disease-modifying agents based on number needed to treat analysis is unknown. There is evidence that natalizumab increases the risk of PML in combination with intramuscular IFNβ-1a (level A) and as monotherapy (level C).

The authors recommend that due to the increased risk of PML, natalizumab should be prescribed to selected patients with RRMS whose disease fails to respond to first-line agents, who are intolerant to these medications, or whose initial course of illness is particularly aggressive. Natalizumab should not be used in combination with IFNβ or other immunosuppressant; its use in combination with other disease-modifying agents should be reserved for appropriately controlled clinical trials.

CHOOSING DISEASE-MODIFYING AGENTS FOR RELAPSING-REMITTING MULTIPLE SCLEROSIS

Neurologists treating patients with RRMS can now choose from a variety of agents that have proven efficacy in relapse reduction, disability progression, and MRI lesion activity from short-term randomized, placebo-controlled trials. None of the short-term pivotal studies provide information on long-term benefits of agents now being used to manage RRMS, which is a chronic disease. Methodological differences among the pivotal studies make cross-trial comparisons difficult and misleading (Goodin, 2008). A recent meta-analysis by Goodin (2008) using relative risk and number needed to treat analyses produced several discrepancies regarding relative efficacies among the approved agents for RRMS, confirming that only prospectively designed head-to-head trials can address these issues.

Dosage of IFNβ in Relapsing-Remitting Multiple Sclerosis

Dosing of IFNβ has been addressed in several studies. In the pivotal trial of subcutaneous IFNβ-1b there was a benefit to high-dose IFNβ-1b compared to intermediate-dose IFNβ-1b on both clinical and MRI measures (IFNB MS Study Group, 1993; Paty et al., 1993). A 48-week, MRI-based, randomized, double-blind trial comparing once-weekly subcutaneous IFNβ-1a 22 μg, 44 μg, or placebo demonstrated a dose-dependent reduction in the median number of combined active lesions measured by MRI at 24 weeks (29% for 22 μg; 53% for 44 μg); however, treatment effect was statistically significant only for high-dose IFNβ-1a compared with placebo (Once the Weekly, 1999). T2 new lesion count at 48 weeks was significantly lower in both the 22 μg and 44 μg arms; MRI burden of disease at 48 weeks was increased in the placebo group but decreased in both IFNβ-1a groups. Interestingly, there was no significant difference in secondary outcomes of relapse rate or percentage of patients relapse-free at 48 weeks, although there was a trend favoring high-dose IFNβ-1a compared with placebo and low-dose IFNβ-1a. A double blind, parallel-group, 34-center European Interferon Beta-1a Dose-Comparison Study (n = 802) using IFNβ-1a (Avonex) in doses of 30 μg or 60 μg IM once weekly for up to 4 years showed no significant dose effect on sustained disability progression (primary endpoint), relapse rate, or MRI lesion activity (Clanet et al., 2002). To date, no studies have compared weekly versus more frequently administered intramuscular IFNβ-1a.

Head- to-Head Comparative Trials of IFNβ Formulations

The Independent Comparison of Interferon Study (INCOMIN) was a 2-year prospective investigation conducted in multiple MS centers in Italy (Durelli et al., 2002). In this open-label study, 188 consecutive patients with RRMS were randomly selected to receive either intramuscular IFNβ-1a (30 μg weekly) or subcutaneous IFNβ-1b (250 μg every other day) for 2 years. Clinical (unblinded) and MRI (blinded) outcomes were evaluated after 6, 12, and 24 months. The primary clinical outcome was the percentage of patients who were relapse free. At the end of 2 years, 51% of patients in the IFNβ-1b group were relapse free, compared with 36% of patients receiving IFNβ-1a (p = 0.03); the relative risk of relapse in the IFNβ-1b group was 0.76 compared with the IFNβ-1a cohort. Significant differences in proportion relapse free were observed only after 6 months but thereafter increased in favor of IFNβ-1b. Blinded evaluation of MRI parameters of active disease, determined by the absence of new proton density/T2 lesions after 24 months of therapy, favored treatment with IFNβ-1b over IFNβ-1a (55% vs. 26%, respectively; p<0.001), consistent with clinical findings. Common adverse effect of IFNβ (flu-like symptoms, fatigue, elevated liver enzymes) were similar in both groups; however, injection site reactions and neutralizing antibodies were seen more frequently in the IFNβ-1b cohort.

The results of the INCOMIN study have been criticized on several factors (Bermel and Rudick, 2007).

Patients in the IFNβ-1a group had more active MRI disease prior to study entry; IFNβ-1a patients were older and duration of disease was longer in this group; and, finally, both patients and examiners were unblinded to treatment. The latter criticism was somewhat mitigated by blinded MRI results favoring IFNβ-1b.

Panitch et al. (2002) reported the results of a 48-week prospective, randomized, single-blinded trial comparing therapy with IFNβ-1a at two different doses and methods of administration. The Evidence of Interferon Dose Response European-North American Comparative Efficacy (EVIDENCE) Study enrolled 677 patients with RRMS, who were randomized to treatment with either IFNβ-1a (Rebif) 44 μg subcutaneously (SC) three times weekly (tiw) or IFNβ-1a (Avonex) 30 μg intramuscular (IM) weekly for 48 months. Although examiners were blinded to treatment, patients were aware of study agent. Clinical evaluations were performed every 12 weeks and all patients had screening brain MRI with and without gadolinium and every 4 weeks thereafter, with a final unenhanced scan at 48 weeks. The primary endpoint was proportion of patients who were relapse free at 24 weeks, with MRI active lesion count a secondary outcome. At the end of 24 weeks, the proportion of patients relapse free were 74.9% and 63.3% in the 44 μg tiw group and the 30 μg weekly group, respectively (odds ratio 1.9, p = 0.009). At 48 weeks, the benefit on proportion of patients remaining relapse free in the 44 μg tiw group compared to the 30 μg IM group (62% vs. 52%, odds ratio 1.5, p < 0.009) favored the 44 μg tiw group, but the effect was attenuated. Nevertheless, the proportion of patients with active lesions on brain MRI was significantly lower in the 44 μg tiw group compared with the 30 μg weekly group at 24 and 48 weeks. Adverse effects, including injection site reactions, elevated liver enzymes, and leucopenia, were more common in the high-dose IFNβ-1a group. Neutralizing antibodies were detected in titers of >1:20 in 25% of the high-dose SC group compared to 3% in the once weekly IM group.

Schwid et al. (2005) reported the results of an extension of the EVIDENCE trial, in which subjects who had been initially randomized to receive IM weekly IFNβ-1a switched to SC IFNβ-1a 44 μg tiw. Posttransition relapse rate and MRI activity were analyzed. Of the original IM cohort 223 subjects

(73%) chose to switch to SC IFNβ-1a 44 μg tiw and 272 SC subjects (91%) continued on SC IFNβ-1a for a mean of 32 weeks. The posttransition annualized relapse rate decreased from 0.64 to 0.32 for patients changing from IFNβ-1a IM to IFNβ-1a SC ($p < 0.001$) and from 0.46 to 0.34 for patients continuing IFNβ-1a SC ($p = 0.03$), representing a relapse reduction of 26% in the ongoing SC group and 50% relapse reduction in the initial IM group, a difference that was modestly significant ($p = 0.047$). Patients converting to SC IFNβ-1a had a significantly greater reduction ($p = 0.02$) in posttransition active MRI lesions on T2-weighted scans than those who continued the SC dose regimen. These results do not address long-term differences in efficacy between low-dose IM IFNβ-1a and high-dose SC IFNβ-1a.

The EVIDENCE study has been criticized for several methodological shortcomings, including its relatively short duration, its unblinded patient cohort, and its use of different products with multiple variants (route of administration, dose frequency, and total dose) (Kieburtz and McDermott, 2002). It is unclear whether the primary outcome of the study, proportion of patients relapse free over 24 weeks, has any relationship to long-term disability progression.

The Prospective and Retrospective Long-Term Observational Study of Avonex and Rebif (PROOF; Minagara et al., 2008) was designed to compare the relative efficacy and tolerability of low-dose IM IFNβ-1a (30 μg weekly) and high-dose SC IFNβ-1b (44 μg tiw) in patients with RRMS for up to 5 years. Because of low enrollment, the study was terminated earlier than planned. Patients in the low-dose group ($n = 69$) and high-dose group ($n = 67$) were studied retrospectively from 12 to 24 months up to time of enrollment and prospectively for 6 months after enrollment (total time studied 18 to 30 months). After controlling for baseline EDSS, there were no statistically significant differences between the treatment groups in prospective measures of disability progression, relapse rates, or MRI lesion activity. Neutralizing antibodies occurred more frequently in SC IFNβ-1a patients than IM IFNβ-1b patients (19% vs. 0%), but there was no statistical difference in proportion with sustained disability progression between NAb+ and NAb− patients. Adverse events were similar in each group. The results of the PROOF study are limited by its mixed retrospective-prospective design and low sample size (Boster and Racke, 2009).

It is important to note that short-term differences in efficacy of high-dose, high-frequency subcutaneous IFNβ-1a or 1b compared with low-dose intramuscular IFNβ-1a may be mitigated in the long-term by development of NAbs (Bermel et al., 2007).

Head- to-Head Comparative Trials of IFNβ and Glatiramer Acetate

Two recently completed industry-sponsored trials have compared the relative efficacy of IFNβ and GA in patients with RRMS (Mikol et al., 2008; O'Connor et al., 2008).

The Rebif versus Glatiramer Acetate in Relapsing MS Disease (REGARD) study randomized 764 patients with RRMS diagnosed by the McDonald criteria and who had at least one relapse in the previous 12 months, to receive either open-label subcutaneous IFNβ-1a 44 μg tiw ($n = 386$) or GA 20 mg daily ($n = 378$) for 96 weeks (Mikol et al., 2008). A subpopulation of 460 subjects had serial MRI scans to assess T2-weighted and gadolinium-enhancing lesion number and volume. After 96 weeks, there was no significant difference between treatment groups in the primary endpoint of time to first relapse. Kaplan-Meier analysis revealed no delayed onset of action for GA, as was noted previously (Comi et al., 2001b). No differences were found on secondary clinical endpoints of relapse rate, proportion of patients remaining relapse free, and disability progression. With regard to MRI measures, the only significant difference was in the number of gadolinium-enhancing lesions, which favored IFNβ-1a. No new safety issues regarding either agent were found. Flu-like symptoms and elevated liver enzymes were more frequent in the IFNβ-1a group and injection site reactions and postinjection vasomotor syndrome were more common in the GA group. Notably, the on-trial relapse rates in both treatment groups were lower than expected, which may have limited the ability to detect a clinically meaningful difference between the treatment groups (Goodin, 2008; Mikol et al., 2008).

The Betaferon/Betaseron Efficacy Yielding Outcomes of a New Dose (BEYOND) study has been published in abstract form (O'Connor et al., 2008). In this trial 2244 patients with RRMS with EDSS scores ≤ 5.0 were randomized (2:2:1 ratio) to receive subcutaneous IFN-1b 500 μg (n = 899) or 250 μg (n = 897) every other day, or GA 20 mg daily (n = 448) for ≥ 104 weeks. No difference in the primary outcome of relapse risk was found among treatment groups. Annualized relapse rate in each treatment arm decreased by nearly 80% compared to the prestudy rate. Secondary outcomes of relapse activity, sustained disability, and most MRI measures were similar in each group. The cumulative number of T2 lesions and relative increase in T2 lesion volume were greater in GA subjects compared with patients in both IFNβ-1b subgroups. No unexpected adverse drug effects were noted. The authors concluded that the currently FDA-approved dosage of subcutaneous IFNβ-1b of 250 μg every other day was optimal. The long-term significance of discordant results in clinical and MRI endpoints of disease activity and severity for IFNβ-1b and GA is unclear.

Summary: Disease-Modifying Agents in Relapsing-Remitting Multiple Sclerosis

On the basis of available data from head-to-head studies and cross-trial analysis, it appears that high-dose subcutaneous IFNβ (1a or 1b) is more effective than low-dose intramuscular IFNβ-1a on short-term clinical and MRI measures of RRMS disease activity, and subcutaneous IFNβ and GA have similar clinical efficacies (Goodin, 2008). Long-term differences among these agents have not been established.

In general, patients with low disease activity can probably be treated with any of the first-line agents for RRMS. Natalizumab should be reserved for patients who either fail first-line therapy or are intolerant to first-line agents. Patients treated with low-dose intramuscular IFNβ-1a who have breakthrough disease activity can be switched to high-dose IFNβ, GA, or natalizumab.

DISEASE-MODIFYING THERAPIES IN CLINICALLY ISOLATED SYNDROMES

Patients with a first isolated demyelinating event (e.g., optic neuritis, partial transverse myelitis, or brainstem-cerebellar syndrome) are at high risk to develop clinically definite multiple sclerosis

(CDMS) within 3 to 10 years (Optic Neuritis Study Group, 1997; O'Riordan et al., 1998; Brex et al., 2002). O'Riordan et al. (1998) found that 83% of patients who presented with a clinically isolated syndrome (CIS) of the optic nerve, brainstem, or spinal cord, and an abnormal T2-weighted brain MRI, developed CDMS after 10 years. The number of MRI lesions on initial exam correlated with EDSS and disease severity at 10-year follow-up. At a mean follow-up of 14 years, 88% of patients with abnormal initial MRI had CDMS (Brex et al., 2002). In another study of 156 patients presenting with CIS, the number of lesions detected on baseline cranial MRI correlated with both the risk of converting to CDMS and disability status at 5 years (Tintore et al., 2006). Furthermore, Tintore et al. reported that the presence of cerebrospinal fluid (CSF) oligoclonal bands in patients with CIS independently doubled the risk of a experiencing a second demyelinating event during a mean follow-up of 50 months (Tintore et al., 2008).

Thus, patients with CIS in whom cranial MRI demonstrates lesion dissemination consistent with MS based on the Barkhof criteria (Barkhof et al., 1997) and in whom other possible diagnoses have been excluded are often considered to be in the earliest clinical stage of MS, in which therapeutic intervention may be particularly beneficial (Coyle, 2008). Several studies have addressed the efficacy of MS disease-modifying agents in patients with CIS who are at high risk to develop CDMS.

Intramuscular Interferon Beta-1a in Clinically Isolated Syndromes

In the CHAMPS study (Jacobs et al., 2000), 383 patients with an acute isolated demyelinating event (e.g., unilateral optic neuritis, partial transverse myelitis, or brainstem-cerebellar syndrome), no prior neurologic or visual symptoms, and two or more white matter lesions on cranial MRI were assigned to receive treatment with 30 μg IFNβ-1a IM weekly or placebo. All patients were given a 14-day course of intravenous and oral steroids. The primary outcome was development of CDMS; serial unenhanced T2 and gadolinium-enhanced T1 MRI findings were also analyzed. The 3-year study was terminated after a preplanned interim analysis. The projected 3-year Kaplan-Meier cumulative probability of developing CDMS was

35% in the IFNβ-1a group and 50% in the placebo group (relative risk 0.56, $p < 0.002$); thus, patients treated with IFNβ-1a had a significantly lower risk (44%) of 3-year conversion to CDMS. Patients in the IFNβ-1a group also had significant reductions in MRI lesion load and fewer new, enlarging, or gadolinium-enhancing lesions at 18 months. In a 5-year open-label extension of the CHAMPS study involving 100 patients originally randomized to treatment (immediate treatment group) and 103 patients originally assigned to placebo (delayed treatment group), the cumulative probability to develop CDMS was significantly lower, albeit modestly, in the immediate treatment cohort (36 ± 9 vs. 49 ± 10%, $p < 0.03$) (CHAMPIONS Study Group, 2006). No significant difference between the two groups at 5 years on neurologic disability as measured by EDSS or on MRI parameters of disease activity and severity, including number of new or enlarging T2-lesions, change in T2-lesion volume, or gadolinium-enhancing lesions.

Subcutaneous Interferon Beta-1a in Clinically Isolated Syndrome

A randomized, double-blind trial (ETOMS) of subcutaneous IFNβ-1a in CIS was conducted in Europe by Comi et al. (2001a). In this study, 308 patients with a first demyelinating event, either unifocal or multifocal, and a brain MRI demonstrating three or more white matter lesions typical of MS, were administered 22 μg IFNβ-1a subcutaneously once weekly or placebo for 2 years. Fewer patients in the IFNβ-1a arm compared with the placebo group (34% vs. 45%, respectively; $p = 0.047$) converted to CDMS at the end of 2 years. The time at which 30% of patients developed CDMS was 569 days in the IFNβ-1a group and 252 days in the placebo group ($p = 0.034$). There was also a modest but significant reduction in relapse rate favoring treatment with IFNβ-1a (0.33; placebo 0.43; $p = 0.045$). The number of new lesions and lesion load on MRI were significantly lower in the IFNβ-1a group.

Subcutaneous Interferon Beta-1b in Clinically Isolated Syndrome

In a 2-year randomized, double-blind, placebo-controlled study of 438 patients with a first clinical demyelinating event and at least two clinically silent brain lesions, subcutaneous interferon beta-1b (IFNβ-1b) at a dosage of 250 μg every other day significantly delayed conversion to definite MS compared to placebo (Kappos et al., 2006a). Conversion to CDMS by the Poser criteria (McDonald et al., 1983) was significantly reduced in the IFNβ-1b cohort compared to placebo (28% vs. 45%, $p < 0.0001$). Two-year probability of conversion to MS by the McDonald criteria (McDonald et al., 2001) was reduced in the treated group compared to placebo (69% vs.85%, $p < 0.00001$). Patients treated with IFNβ-1b had significantly reduced cranial MRI activity as well, including cumulative number of combined active lesions, and cumulative number of newly gadolinium-enhancing lesions or new T2 lesions. Eighty-nine percent of patients ($n = 418$) who completed the initial randomized phase of the study were then entered into an open-label follow-up study of IFNβ-1b, which analyzed the effect of early versus delayed treatment with IFNβ-1b after diagnosis of CDMS or after 2 years in the study (Kappos et al., 2007). Primary outcomes in this intention-to-treat analysis were time to diagnose CDMS, time to confirmed sustained disability progression by EDSS, and score on a patient-assessed functional scale. After 3 years, there was a significant difference in conversion to CDMS in the two groups favoring the early treatment cohort (37% vs. 51%), with a risk reduction of CDMS of 41% (early vs. delayed treatment, $p = 0.0011$). Over 3 years disability progression was 16% in the early treatment group and 24% in the delayed treatment group, representing a 40% reduced risk ($p = 0.022$) in the early treatment group. The authors concluded that early treatment with IFNβ-1b of patients with CIS reduced sustained EDSS disability after 3 years.

Glatiramer Acetate in Clinically Isolated Syndromes

The PRECISE study randomized 481 patients with monosymptomatic CIS and brain MRI with at least two T2-lesions to either GA 20 mg/day or placebo (Comi and Filippi, 2008). A preplanned interim analysis of this 3-year study, presented at the American Academy of Neurology Annual Meeting in 2008, showed that GA significantly reduced conversion to CDMS compared to placebo (25% vs. 43%, risk reduction 45%, $p < 0.0001$) (Comi and Filippi, 2008). Further analysis of the results of this study, including effects on MRI activity, awaits publication in peer-reviewed literature.

Treatment of Clinically Isolated Syndromes

All patients with CIS require vigilant clinical, laboratory, and imaging monitoring to establish a diagnosis of CDMS. However, based upon the evidence from randomized controlled studies, patients who present with CIS typical of MS and who are judged to be at high risk to convert to CDMS based on findings on MRI and CSF examination, and in whom alternative diagnoses have been excluded, can be considered for treatment with one of the first-line MS immunomodulators (Coyle et al., 2008). Treatment should be withheld from patients with atypical clinical presentations and neuroimaging pending definitive diagnosis. Whether therapeutic intervention at the time of CIS confers additional protection against long-term disability remains uncertain.

DISEASE-MODIFY THERAPIES IN SECONDARY PROGRESSIVE MS

Natural history studies have shown that after 10 years, approximately 50% of patients with RRMS transition into SPMS, with gradually accruing disability with or without superimposing relapses (Weinshenker et al., 1989; Bermel and Rudick, 2007). The pathogenesis of SPMS is characterized by a shift from the inflammatory features of RRMS to neurodegeneration, which is less amenable to the current immunomodulatory therapies (Bermel and Rudick, 2007).

The efficacy of IFNβ in SPMS has been evaluated in several clinical trials, all of which had sustained disability progression as the primary outcome. Neither GA nor natalizumab has been studied in the SPMS population.

Subcutaneous IFNβ-1b in Secondary Progressive Multiple Sclerosis

The European IFNβ-1b trial randomized 718 patients with SPMS to receive IFNβ-1b 8 million IU subcutaneously or placebo every other day for up to 3 years (European Study Group, 1998). There was a significant delay in time to sustained

progression (726 days vs. 549 days, $p < 0.008$) favoring the IFNβ-1b cohort. Sustained disability progression was reduced by 21.7% in the treated group compared to placebo over mean follow-up of 2.5 years (49.7% vs. 38.9%, $p = 0.0048$).

The North American IFNβ-1b trial in SPMS enrolled 939 patients randomized to receive either IFNβ-1b (250 μg or 160 μg/m²) or placebo subcutaneously every other day (Panitch et al., 2004). There was no significant difference in time to confirmed disability progression between the treated and placebo groups. However, patients in the IFNβ-1b group had significantly reduced secondary outcomes of relapse rate and MRI lesion activity compared to placebo.

Post hoc meta-analysis of the European and North American SPMS studies addressed the discrepancy in their results regarding the primary outcome of sustained EDSS progression (Kappos et al., 2004). The authors found that the patients in the European cohort were in an earlier phase of SPMS, with more active inflammatory disease (greater number of relapses and MRI activity) prior to enrollment. Pooled analysis demonstrated a modest risk reduction of 20% ($p = 0.008$) in confirmed disability progression in the IFNβ-1b group compared to placebo. It was concluded that SPMS patients with rapid disability progression or ongoing relapses may derive benefit from IFNβ-1b.

Subcutaneous IFNβ-1a in Secondary Progressive Multiple Sclerosis

The efficacy of subcutaneous IFNβ-1a in SPMS was investigated in a multicenter trial of 618 patients randomized to receive IFNβ-1a 22 μg, 44 μg, or placebo three times weekly for 3 years (Li et al., 2001; Secondary Progressive Efficacy Clinical Trial, 2001). There was no significant treatment effect on disability progression, but there was a modest but significant reduction of relapse rate in the treated cohort compared to the placebo group (0.50 per year vs. 0.71 per year, $p < 0.001$). A trend toward decreased disability progression favoring treatment was seen in patients who experienced pre-study relapses and in women. There was a significant benefit with treatment on multiple measures of MRI lesion activity, particularly in patients with relapses in the 2 years before the study.

Intramuscular IFNβ-1a in Secondary Progressive Multiple Sclerosis

Intramuscular IFNβ-1a was evaluated in 436 patients with SPMS and EDSS score 3.5 to 6.5, who were randomized to receive either IFNβ-1a 60 µg or placebo weekly for 2 years (Cohen et al., 2002). The primary outcome measure was baseline to 24-month change in the MS functional composite (MSFC), which is a combined score in tests of ambulation (timed 25-foot walk), upper extremity function (9-hole peg test [9HPT]), and cognition (paced auditory serial addition test [PASAT]). Median MSFC Z-score progression was reduced by 40.4% in the treated cohort compared to placebo (−0.096 vs. −0.161, $p = 0.033$), which was mainly attributed to effects on 9HPT and PASAT. There was no effect on change in EDSS. There were benefits favoring treatment on multiple secondary measures, including relapse rates (33% reduction, $p = 0.008$), quality of life, and active MRI lesions.

IFNβ in Secondary Progressive Multiple Sclerosis: Summary

Multiple formulations of IFNβ have demonstrated efficacy in reducing relapses and MRI activity in SPMS, albeit with only a modest effect on disability progression. Treatment appears to be most efficacious in SPMS patients in the early phase of their disease or who continue to have superimposed relapses and active MRI lesions (gadolinium enhancement). Both subcutaneous IFNβ-1a and IFNβ-1b at the standard doses for RRMS have received FDA approval for the treatment of relapsing SPMS.

PRIMARY PROGRESSIVE MULTIPLE SCLEROSIS

Patients with PPMS encompass 10%–15% of the MS population and present with slowly progressive neurologic impairment at disease onset, without superimposed relapses (Wolinsky et al., 2007). Most patients with PPMS present with spinal cord involvement, with insidiously progressive spastic paraparesis that eventually also affects the upper extremities. The female:male ratio in PPMS is 1:1, unlike that in RRMS.

The efficacy of GA in PPMS was studied in a large multicenter, randomized, placebo-controlled trial of 943 patients (Wolinsky et al., 2007). The primary endpoint was time to sustained 3-month disability. The 3-year trial was stopped after an interim analysis revealed no significant treatment effect of GA compared with placebo. There were benefits favoring GA on some MRI parameters and post hoc analysis demonstrated a modest treatment benefit of GA compared with placebo for males ($p = 0.0193$).

There have been no similarly large trials in PPMS for any of the interferons or natalizumab. Small pilot trials of intramuscular interferon beta 1a (Leary et al., 2003) and subcutaneous interferon beta 1b (Montalban, 2004) did not demonstrate an effect on disease progression in patient with PPMS.

More recently, a large RCT of rituximab versus placebo in over 400 PPMS patients (OLYMPUS) failed to show a statistically significant effect on disease progression (Hawker et al., 2009). It is likely that definitive treatments for PPMS will not be available until the pathophysiology has been more clearly elucidated.

REFERENCES

Bakshi R, Neema M, Healy BC, et al. Predicting clinical progression in multiple sclerosis with the magnetic resonance disease severity scale. *Arch Neurol.* 2008;65:1449–1453.

Barkhof F, Filippi M, Miller DH, et al. Comparison of MRI criteria at first presentation to predict conversion to clinically definite multiple sclerosis. *Brain.* 1997; 120:2059–2069.

Berger JR, Koralnik IJ. Progressive multifocal leukoencephalopathy and natalizumab—unforeseen consequences. *N Engl J Med.* 2005;353:414–416.

Bermel RA, Rudick R. Interferon-β treatment for multiple sclerosis. *Neurotherapeutics.* 2007;4:633–646.

Bornstein MB, Miller A, Slagle S, et al. A pilot trial of Cop-1 in exacerbating-remitting multiple sclerosis. *N Engl J Med.* 1987;317:408–414.

Boster A, Racke MK. Pharmacotherapy of multiple sclerosis: the PROOF trial. *Expert Opin Pharmacother.* 2009; 10:1235–1237.

Brex PA, Ciccarelli O, O'Riordan JI, Sailer M, Thompson AJ, Miller DH. A longitudinal study of abnormalities on MRI and disability from multiple sclerosis. *N Engl J Med.* 2002;346:158–164.

Calabresi PA, Giovannoni G, Confavreux C, et al. The incidence and significance of anti-natalizumab antibodies: results from AFFIRM and SENTINEL. *Neurology.* 2007; 69(14):1391–1403.

CHAMPIONS Study Group. IM interferon β-1a delays definite multiple sclerosis five years after a first demyelinating event. *Neurology.* 2006;66:678–684.

Clanet M, Radue EW, Kappos L, et al. A randomized, double-blind, dose-comparison study of weekly interferon b-1a (Avonex) in relapsing MS. *Neurology.* 2002;59: 1507–1517.

Comi G, Filippi M. Treatment with glatiramer acetate delays conversion to clinically definite multiple sclerosis (CDMS) in patients with clinically isolated syndromes (CIS). Abstract (LBS.003). Taken from a paper presented at: 60th Annual Meeting of the American Academy of Neurology; 2008; Chicago, IL. Available at: http://www.aan.com/globals/axon/assets/4088.pdf.Accessed March 1, 2010.

Comi G, Filippi M, Barkhof F, Early Treatment of Multiple Sclerosis Study Group. Effect of early interferon treatment on conversion to definite multiple sclerosis: a randomised study. *Lancet.* 2001a;357:1576–1582.

Comi G, Filippi M, Wolinsky JS, European/Canadian Glatiramer Acetate Study Group. European/Canadian multicenter, double-blind, randomized, placebo-controlled study of the effects of glatiramer acetate on magnetic resonance imaging-measured disease activity and burden in patients with relapsing multiple sclerosis. *Ann Neurol.* 2001b;49:290–297.

Cohen JA, Cutter GR, Fischer JS, et al. Benefit of interferon beta-1a on MSFC progression in secondary progressive MS. *Neurology.* 2002;59:679–687.

Cohen JA, Rovaris M, Goodman AD, et al. Randomized, double-blind, dose-comparison study of glatiramer acetate in relapsing-remitting MS. *Neurology.* 2007; 68:939–944.

Coyle PK. Early treatment of multiple sclerosis to prevent neurologic damage. *Neurology.* 2008;71(suppl 3):S3–S7.

Coyle PK, Johnson KP. Relapses matter: the costs & consequences of multiple sclerosis relapses. *J Neurol Sci.* 2007;256:S1–S4.

Durelli L, Verdun E, Barbero P, Independent Comparison of Interferon (INCOMIN) Trial Study Group. Every-other-day interferon beta-1b versus once-weekly interferon beta-1a for multiple sclerosis: results of a 2-year prospective randomized multicenter study (INCOMIN). *Lancet.* 2002;359:1453–1460.

Edgar CM, Brunet DG, Fenton P, et al. Lipoatrophy in patients with multiple sclerosis on glatiramer acetate. *Can J Neurol Sci.* 2004;31:58–63.

European Study Group on Interferon β-1b in Secondary Progressive MS. Placebo-controlled multicenter randomised trial of interferon β-1b in treatment of secondary progressive multiple sclerosis. *Lancet.* 1998; 352:1491–1497.

FDA Safety Communication: Risk of Progressive Multifocal Leukoencephalopathy (PML) with the use of Tysabri (natalizumab). February 5, 2010. Available at:http://www.fda.gov/Drugs/DrugSafety/Postmarket DrugSafetyInformationforPatientsandProviders/ ucm199872.htm. Accessed 4/5/2010.

Farina C, Weber MS, Meinl E, Wekerle H, Hohlfeld R. Glatiramer acetate in multiple sclerosis:update on potential mechanisms of action. *Lancet Neurol.* 2005;4: 567–575.

Filippi M, Rovaris M, Rocca MA et al. Glatiramer acetate reduces the proportion of new MS lesions evolving into "black holes." *Neurology.* 2001;57:731–733.

Ford CC, Johnson KP, Liak RP, et al. A prospectivr open-label study of glatiramer acetate: over a decade of continuous use in multiple sclerosis patients. *Multiple Sclerosis.* 2006;12:309–320.

Francis GS, Rice GPA, Alsop JC, et al. Interferon β-1a in MS. Results following development of neutralizing antibodies in PRISMS. Neurology. 2005;65:48–55.

Galetta SL, Markowitz C. US FDA-approved disease-modifying therapies for multiple sclerosis: review of adverse effects profiles. *CNS Drugs.* 2005;19:239–252.

Giovannoni G, Goodman A. Neutralizing anti-IFNβ antibodies. How much more evidence do we need to use them in practice? *Neurology.* 2005;65:6–8.

Goodin DS. Disease-modifying therapy in multiple sclerosis: update and clinical implications. *Neurology.* 2008; 71(suppl 3):S8–S13.

Goodin DS, Cohen BA, O'Connor P, Kappos L, Stevens JC, Therapeutics and Technology Assessment Subcommittee of the American Academy of Neurology. Assessment: the use of natalizumab (tysabri) for the treatment of multiple sclerosis (an evidence-based review): report of the Therapeutics and Technology Assessment Subcommittee of the American Academy of Neurology. *Neurology.* 2008;71(10): 766–773.

Goodin DS, Frohman EM, Garmany GP, et al. Disease modifying therapies in multiple sclerosis: report of the Therapeutics and Technology Assessment Subcommittee of the American Academy of Neurology and the MS Council for Clinical Practice Guidelines. *Neurology.* 2002;58:169–178.

Goodin DS, Frohman EM, Hurwitz B, et al. Neutralizing antibodies to interferon beta: assessment of their clinical and radiographic impact: an evidence report. *Neurology.* 2007;68:977–984.

Hawker K, O'Connor P, Freedman M et al. Rituximab in patients with PPMS: results of a randomized double blind, placebo controlled multi center trial. *Ann. Neurol.* 2009;66:460–471.

IFNB Multiple Sclerosis Study Group. Interferon beta-1b is effective in relapsing-remitting multiple sclerosis. I. Clinical results of a multicenter, randomized, double blind, placebo-controlled trial. *Neurology.* 1993;43: 655–661.

IFNB Multiple Sclerosis Study Group and the University of British Columbia MS/MRI Analysis Group. Interferon beta-1b in the treatment of multiple sclerosis: final outcome of the randomized controlled trial. *Neurology.* 1995;45:1277–1285.

IFNB Multiple Sclerosis Study Group, University of British Columbia MS/MRI Analysis Group. Neutralizing antibodies during treatment of multiple sclerosis with interferon beta-1b: experience during the first three years. *Neurology.* 1996;47:889–894.

Jacobs LD, Beck RW, Simon JH et al. Intramuscular interferon beta-1a therapy initiating during a first demyelinating event in multiple sclerosis. *N Engl J Med.* 2000; 343:898–904.

Jacobs LD, Cookfair DI, Rudick RA et al. Intramuscular interferon beta-1a for disease progression in relapsing multiple sclerosis. *Ann Neurol.* 1996;39: 285–294.

Johnson KP, Brooks RR, Cohen JA, et al. Copolymer 1 reduces relapse rate and improves disability in relapsing-remitting multiple sclerosis: results of a phase III multicenter, double-blind, placebo-controlled trial. *Neurology.* 1995;45:1268–1278.

Johnson KP, Brooks BR, Cohen JA, et al. Extended use of glatiramer acetate (Copaxone) is well tolerated and maintains its clinical effect on multiple sclerosis relapse rate and degree of disability. *Neurology.* 1998;50: 701–708.

Kappos L, Clanet M, Sandberg-Wollheim M, et al. Neutralizing antibodies and efficacy of interferon β-1a. A 4-year controlled study. *Neurology.* 2005;65: 40–47.

Kappos L, Freedman MS, Polman, et al. Effect of early versus delayed interferon beta-1b treatment on diability after a first clinical event suggestive of multiple sclerosis: a 3-year follow-up analysis of the BENEFIT study. *Lancet.* 2007;370:389–397.

Kappos L, Polman CH, Freedman MS, et al. Treatment with interferon beta-1b delays conversion to clinically definite and McDonald MS in patients with clinically isolated syndromes. *Neurology.* 2006a;67:1242–1249.

Kappos L, Traboulsee A, Constantinescu C, et al. Long-term subcutaneous interferon beta-1a therapy in patients with relapsing-remitting MS. *Neurology.* 2006b;67: 944–953.

Kappos L, Weinshenker B, Pozzilli C, et al. Interferon beta-1b in secondary progressive MS: a combined analysis of the two trials. *Neurology.* 2004;63:1779–1787.

Khatri BO, Man S, Giovannoni G, et al. Effect of plasma exchange in accelerating natalizumab clearance and restoring leukocyte function. *Neurology.* 2009;72: 402–409.

Kieburtz, K, McDermott, M. Needed in MS: evidence, not EVIDENCE. *Neurology.* 2002;59:1482–1483.

Kleinschmidt-DeMasters BK, Tyler KL. Progressive multifocal leukoencephalopathy complicating treatment with natalizumab and interferon-beta-1a for multiple sclerosis. *N Engl J Med.* 2005;353:369–374.

Kreisler A, deSeze J, Stojkovic T. Multiple sclerosis, interferon beta, and clinical thyroid dysfunction. *Acta Neurol Scand.* 2003;107:154–157.

Langer-Gould A, Atlas SW, Bollen AW, Pelletier D. Progressive multifocal leukoencephalopathy in a patient treated with natalizumab. *N Engl J Med.* 2005; 353:375–381.

Langer-Gould A, Moses HH, Murray TJ. Strategies for manaing the side effects of treatments for multiple sclerosis. *Neurology.* 2004;63:S35–S41.

Leary S, Miller D, Stevenson V et al. Interferon beta 1a in PPMS: an exploratory, randomized, controlled trial. *Neurology.* 2003;60:44–51.

Li DK, Zhao GJ, Paty DW, University of British Columbia MS/MRI Analysis Research Group. The SPECTRIMS Study Group. Randomized controlled trial of interferon-beta-1a in secondary progressive MS: MRI results. *Neurology.* 2001;56:1505–1513.

McDonald WI, Compton A, Edan G. Recommended diagnostic criteria for multiple sclerosis: guidelines from the International Panel on the diagnosis of multiple sclerosis. *Ann Neurol.* 2001;50:121–127.

Medical News Today. Incidence of PML with tysabri in multiple sclerosis lower than previously thought. 2009. Available at: http://www.medicalnewstoday.com/articles/149354.php. Accessed March 1, 2010.

Mikol DD, Barkhof F, Chang P, et al. Comparison of subcutaneous interferon beta-1a with glatiramer acetate in patients with relapsing multiple sclerosis (the REbif vs glatiramer acetate in relapsing MS disease [REGARD] study): a multicentre, randomised, parallel, open-label trial. *Lancet Neurol.* 2008;7: 903–914.

Miller DH, Khan O, Sheremata W, et al. A controlled trial of natalizumab for relapsing multiple sclerosis. *N Engl J Med.* 2003;348:15–23.

Minagara A, Murray TJ, PROOF Study Investigators. Efficacy and tolerability of intramuscular interferon beta-1a compared with subcutaneous interferon beta-1a in relapsing MS: results from PROOF. *Curr Med Res Opin.* 2008;24:1049–1055.

Montalban X. Overview of European pilot study of interferon beta 11b in PPMS. *Mult. Scler.* 2004;10 (suppl 1) S62–64.

Monzani F, Caraccio M, Casolaro A, et al. Long-term interferon beta 1b therapy for MS: is routine thyroid assessment always useful? *Neurology.* 2000;55:549–552.

Mullen JT, Vartanian TK, Atkins MB. Melanoma complicating treatment with natalizumab for multiple sclerosis. *N Engl J Med.* 2008;358:647–648.

National Clinical Advisory Board of the National Multiple Sclerosis Society. Disease Management Consensus Statement 2007. Available at: http://www.nationalmssociety.org/for-professionals/healthcare-professionals/publications/expert-opinion-papers/download.aspx?id=8. Accessed March 1, 2010.

O'Connor P, Aronson B, Comi G, et al. Interferon beta-1b 500 mcg, interferon beta-1b 250 mcg and glatiramer acetate: primary outcomes of the Betaferon/Betaseron Efficacy Yielding Outcome of a New Dose (BEYOND) study. Abstract (LBS.004). Taken from a paper presented at: 60th Annual Meeting of the American Academy of Neurology; 2008; Chicago, IL. Available at: http://www.aan.com/globals/axon/assets/4088.pdf. Accessed March 1, 2010.

Once the Weekly Interferon for MS Study Group (OWIMS). Evidence of interferon b-1a dose response in relapsing-remitting MS. The OWIMS study. *Neurology.* 1999;53:679–686.

Optic Neuritis Study Group. The 5-year risk of MS after optic neuritis: experience of the optic neuritis treatment trial. *Neurology.* 1997;49:1406–1413.

O'Riordan JI, Thomson AJ, Kingsley DPE, et al. The prognostic value of brain MRI in clinically isolated syndromes of the CN: a 10-year follow-up. *Brain.* 1998; 121:495–503.

Panitch H, Goodin DS, Francis G, et al. Randomized, comparative study of interferon-β-1a treatment regimens in MS: the EVIDENCE trial. *Neurology.* 2002; 59:1496–1506.

Panitch H, Miller A, Paty D, Weinshenker B, North American Study Group on Interferon beta-1b in Secondary Progressive MS. Interferon beta-1b in secondary progressive MS: results from a 3-year controlled study. *Neurology.* 2004;63:1788–1795.

Paty DW, Li DKB, UBC MS/MRI Study Group, IFNB Multiple Sclerosis Study Group. Interferon beta-1b is effective in relapsing-remitting multiple sclerosis. II. MRI analysis results of a multicenter, randomized, double-blind, placebo-controlled study. *Neurology.* 1993;43:662–667.

Polman CH, O'Connor PW, Hardova E, et al. A randomized, placebo-controlled trial of natalizumab for relapsing multiple sclerosis. *N Engl J Med.* 2006;354: 899–910.

Poser CM, Paty DW, Scheinberg L, et al. New diagnostic criteria for multiple sclerosis: guidelines for research protocols. *Ann Neurol.* 1983;13:227–231.

PRISMS (Prevention of Relapses and Disability by Interferon-β-1a Subcutaneously in Multiple Sclerosis) Study Group. Randomised double-blind placebo-controlled study of interferon beta-1a in relapsing-remitting multiple sclerosis. *Lancet.* 1998;352: 1498–1504.

PRISMS Study Group and the University of British Columbia MS/MRI Analysis Group. PRISMS-4: long-term efficacy of interferon-β-1a in relapsing MS. *Neurology.* 2001;56:1628–1636.

Ransohoff RM. Natalizumab for multiple sclerosis. *N Engl J Med.* 2007;356:2622–2629.

Rieckmann P, Weber F, Günther A, Poser S. The phosphodiesterase inhibitor pentoxifylline reduces early side effects of interferon-β1b treatment in patients with multiple sclerosis. *Neurology.* 1996;46:604.

Ropper A. Selective treatment of multiple sclerosis. *N Engl J Med.* 2006;354:965–967.

Rudick RA, Fisher E, Lee J-C et al. Use of the *Brain* parenchymal function to measure whole brain atrophy in relapsing-remitting MS. *Neurology.* 1999;53: 1698–1704.

Rudick RA, Goodkin DE, Jacobs LD et al. Impact of interferon beta-1a on neurologic disability in relapsing multiple sclerosis. *Neurology.* 1997;49:358–363.

Rudick RA, Panzara MA. Natalizumab for the treatment of relapsing multiple sclerosis. *Biologics.* 2008;2: 189–199.

Rudick RA, Simonian NA, Alam JA, et al. Incidence and significance of neutralizing antibodies to interferon beta-1a in multiple sclerosis. *Neurology.* 1998;50(5): 1266–1272.

Rudick RA, Stuart WH, Calabresi PA, et al. Natalizumab plus interferon beta-1a for relapsing multiple sclerosis. *N Engl J Med.* 2006;354(9):911–923.

Schwid SR, Bever CT. The cost of delaying treatment in multiple sclerosis. What is lost is not regained. Neurology. 2001;56:1620.

Schwid SR, Thorpe J, Sharief M, et al. Enhanced benefit of increasing interferon beta-1a dose and frequency in relapsing multiple sclerosis. The EVIDENCE study. *Arch Neurol.* 2005;62:785–792.

Schwid SR, Goodman AD, Mattson DH. Autoimmune hyperthyroidism in patients with multiple sclerosis treated with interferon beta-1b. *Arch Neurol.* 1997;54: 1169–1190.

Secondary Progressive Efficacy Clinical Trial of Recombinant Interferon-beta-1a in MS (SPECTRIMS) Study Group. Randomized controlled trial of interferon- beta-1a in secondary progressive MS: clinical results. *Neurology.* 2001;56:1496–1504.

Soelber Sorensen P, Koch-Henriksen N, Ross C, et al. Appearance and disappearance of neutralizing antibodies during interferon-beta therapy. *Neurology.* 2005; 65:33–39.

Sorensen PS, Deisenhammer F, Duda P, et al. Guidelines on use on anti IFNβ antibody measurements in multiple sclerosis: report of an EFNS task force on IFNβ antibodies in multiple sclerosis. *Euro J Neurology.* 2005;12:817–827.

Stadelmann C, Albert M, Wegner C, Brück W. Cortical pathology in multiple sclerosis. *Curr Opin Neurol.* 2008;21:229–234.

Thouvenot E, Hillaire-Buys D, Bos-Thompson MA, et al. Erythema nodosum and glatiramer acetate treatment in relapsing-remitting multiple sclerosis. *Mult Scler.* 2007;13:941–944.

Tintoré M, Rovira A, Río J, et al. Baseline MRI predicts future attacks and disability in clinically isolated syndrome. *Neurology.* 2006;67:968–972.

Tintore M, Rovira A, Rio J, et al. Do oligoclonal bands add information to MRI in first attacks of multiple sclerosis? *Neurology.* 2008;70:1079–1083.

Trapp BD, Peterson J, Ransohoff RM, et al. Axonal transection in the lesions of multiple sclerosis. *N Engl J Med.* 1998;338:278–285.

Tremlett HL, Oger J. Elevated aminotransferases during treatment with interferon beta for multiple sclerosis: actions and outcomes. *Mult Scler.* 2004;10:298–301.

Tysabri Package Insert. Cambridge, MA: Biogen-Idec; 2006.

VanAssche GV, Van Ranst M, Sciot R, et al. Progressive multifocal leukoencephalopathy after natalizumab therapy for Crohn's disease. *N Engl J Med.* 2005; 353:362–368.

Vollmer T. The natural history of relapses in multiple sclerosis. *J Neurol Sci.* 2007;256:S5–S13.

Vukusic S, Confavreux C. Natural history of multiple sclerosis: risk factors and prognostic indicators. *Curr Opin Neurol.* 2007;20:269–274.

Weinshenker BG, Bass GPA, Rice J, et al. The natural history of multiple sclerosis: a geographically based study. I. Clinical course and disability. *Brain.* 1989; 112:133–146.

Wolinsky JS, Natayana PA, O'Connor P, et al. Glatiramer acetate in primary progressive multiple sclerosis: results of a multinational, multicenter, double-blind, placebo-controlled trial. *Ann Neurol.* 2007;61:14–24.

Yoshida EM, Rasmussen SL, Steinbrecher UP, et al. Fulminant liver failure during interferon beta therapy of multiple sclerosis. *Neurology.* 2001;56:1416.

Yousry TA, Major EO, Ryschkewitsch C, et al. Evaluation of patients treated with natalizumab for progressive multifocal leukoencephalopathy. *N Engl J Med.* 2006; 354:924–933.

There have now been over two decades of trial and clinical experience with immunomodulating therapy for persons with multiple sclerosis (MS). In general, these agents are safe and effective for the majority of patients who take them. Additionally, they have been demonstrated to have a favorable impact on relapses, magnetic resonance imaging (MRI) markers of disease activity, and progression of disability, primarily for the relapsing-remitting form of the disease. However, when patients fail to respond to, or cannot tolerate, the first-line agents that are approved for MS (i.e., beta-interferon and glatiramer acetate), other immunomodulating and immunosuppressive strategies may need to be employed.

The use of natalizumab in this regard has been discussed in the chapter on immunomodulating therapies (see Chapter 23). This chapter will discuss immunosuppressive agents that (with the exception of mitoxantrone) are used off label to treat refractory relapsing or progressive MS. Treatment of acute exacerbations will also be discussed, as well as several new immunomodulating/immunosuppressive agents that, as of this writing, are in large clinical trials.

TREATMENT OF ACUTE RELAPSES

It is estimated that 85% of persons with MS will begin with the relapsing-remitting form of the disease and as such will experience periodic relapses or exacerbations. These are usually defined as the appearance of new neurologic signs or symptoms or worsening of a previously stable neurologic deficit, which lasts at least 24 hours (Thrower, 2009). If there is a known precipitant such as infection or rise in body temperature,

then the episode is referred to as a "pseudoexacerbation" and tends to resolve with cooling or treating the underlying cause.

Patients commonly ask whether trauma can precipitate an exacerbation. One large study examined 170 persons with MS who sustained 1407 episodes of physical trauma (e.g., automobile accident, surgery, fracture, etc.) over an 8-year period and found no association between the occurrence of physical trauma and risk of exacerbation, except for electrical injury. There was in fact a significant negative correlation between exacerbation rate and the first 3 months following surgery or fracture (Sibley et al., 1991). A review by the therapeutics subcommittee of the American Academy of Neurology found no correlation between physical trauma and onset of MS or MS exacerbation but concluded that it was possible that antecedent psychological stress might be correlated with MS onset or attack. The authors cautioned that there were insufficient data for the latter (Goodin et al., 1999). Stress is self-reported by many patients to worsen symptoms, and in some studies, the occurrence of stressful life events was reported to be temporally correlated with increased risk of exacerbation (Ackerman et al., 2002; Buljevac et al., 2003).

Another area of concern for patients is vaccination. A large randomized trial of influenza vaccine versus placebo in persons with MS did not reveal any difference in relapse rate or disease progression between the two groups (Miller et al., 1997). Subsequent studies have reported that vaccination with hepatitis B, varicella, tetanus, or bacillus calmette guerin (BCG) does not cause exacerbations and may safely be given to patients with MS (Confavreaux et al., 2001; Rutschmann et al., 2002).

The National MS Society recommendations state that persons with MS should avoid vaccination with live attenuated vaccine, particularly if they are receiving immunosuppressant therapy (NMSS, August 2009).

Whether to treat an acute relapse is usually determined by the impact the episode has on the patient's ability to function. Results from studies such as the Optic Neuritis Treatment Trial indicate that treatment of an acute relapse will hasten recovery, without providing long-term benefit (Brusaferri and Candelise, 2000; Thrower, 2009). An expert opinion paper from the National MS Society regarding steroid treatment of acute relapses recommends that relapses with a significant effect on a patient's ability to function be treated "as quickly as possible"(Panitch et al 2008)

CORTICOSTEROIDS

First-line treatment for an acute relapse is usually 500–1000 g/day of intravenous methyl prednisolone, administered for 3–5 days (Thrower, 2009). A brief oral prednisone taper is not mandatory, and one large review has reported that patients treated with intravenous steroids plus an oral taper had no better outcome at 3, 6, and 12 months after relapse than a group that did not receive the taper after intravenous treatment (Perumal et al., 2008). High-dose oral steroids have been demonstrated in several studies to be comparable to intravenous methyl prednisolone in terms of bioavailability, tolerability, and efficacy (Barnes et al., 1997; Morrow et al., 2004; Burton et al., 2009). Prednisone, methylprednisolone, and dexamethasone are commonly used oral preparations.

Side effects of steroids commonly include gastritis, insomnia, irritability and mood changes, flushing, hypertension, and acne. Rare adverse events may be thrombophlebitis and psychosis. Transient elevations in blood glucose also occur, but they resolve with cessation of therapy. Adjuvant medications that are commonly prescribed to ameliorate these side effects may include proton pump inhibitors, H2 blockers and/or antacids, and benzodiazepines or hypnotics to help with the sleep and mood disturbances. Persons with MS and diabetes may have to be hospitalized during steroid therapy for appropriate monitoring of blood glucose and administration of insulin as needed.

A few studies have examined the utility of pulse corticosteroids in preventing relapses and disability. Zivadinov et al. (2001) randomized 88 patients with relapsing-remitting (RR) MS to receive either 1 g/day for 5 days intravenous methylprednisolone (IVMP) plus oral taper every 4 months for 3 years, then every 6 months for 2 years, or IVMP therapy just for relapses. After 5 years follow-up, there was a significant reduction (32%) in the risk of sustained disability in the regularly treated IVMP group, and slowing of the rate of whole-brain atrophy. Goodkin et al. (1998) randomized 108 patients with secondary progressive (SP) MS to either high-dose (1500 mg IVMP) or low-dose (30 mg IVMP) pulse therapy every 2 months over 2 years and demonstrated a trend to delay in onset of sustained progression in the high-dose group.

There are also studies that have investigated the use of pulse steroids as add-on therapy to standard immunomodulators to prevent relapses. The ACT trial, which added every other month pulses of methyl prednisolone to Avonex showed a trend toward decreased relapses in the combination therapy group (Cohen et al., 2009a). The NORMIMS study randomized 66 patients to combination therapy with Rebif plus methyl prednisolone 1000 mg/month versus 64 patients on beta-interferon plus placebo. The reduction of risk of annual relapse was reduced 68% in the combination therapy group compared to those taking interferon plus placebo (Sorensen et al., 2009). A report of pulse steroid therapy added to glatiramer acetate (GA) treated 89 persons with RRMS and active MRI lesions with GA plus 1 g/month methyl prednisolone for 6 months, followed by GA alone. Compared to baseline, there was a 65% drop in gadolinium-enhancing lesions over the first 6 months, which was sustained in the second 6-month (GA only) period (DeStefano et al., 2008).

Summary

High-dose oral or intravenous corticosteroids are appropriate to treat acute relapses of MS that impact function. They will hasten short-term recovery, but there are no data to substantiate long-term benefit in terms of degree of recovery from acute relapse. Additionally, repeated pulse steroids alone or in combination with immunomodulating therapy may decrease relapse rate and disability.

INTRAVENOUS IMMUNOGLOBULIN

For persons who cannot tolerate or who do not respond to steroids, there are other off-label alternatives for treating acute exacerbations. Intravenous immunoglobulin (IVIG) is often used as a second-line therapy for treating acute relapses, but according to the EFNS guideline on treatment of MS relapses, there are insufficient data to formally recommended IVIG for this purpose (Sellebjerg et al., 2005). In the Treatment of Acute Relapse in MS (TARIMS) study, 76 patients with relapsing-remitting or relapsing progressive MS who were in an acute relapse were randomized to receive IVIG 1 g/kg or placebo, which was administered 24 hours before receiving methylprednisolone, 1 g/day for 3 days. There were no significant differences in neurologic deficit at 12 weeks between the two groups, and no significant differences in relapse-free patients between the two groups at 6 months (Sorensen et al., 2004).

A small double-blind study that randomized 68 patients with acute optic neuritis to receive either IVIG 0.4 mg/kg or placebo demonstrated no significant difference in recovery between the two groups at 6 months (Roed et al., 2005). In contrast, an open-label study treated 47 patients with corticosteroid refractory optic neuritis with either IVIG or more corticosteroids; 78% of the IVIG-treated patients recovered near-normal visual acuity, compared to only 12.5% of the corticosteroid treated patients (Tselis et al., 2008).

In addition to its use as an agent for treating acute relapses, IVIG has also been studied with regard to its efficacy in preventing relapses. Several randomized controlled trials have reported mixed results in evaluating this agent for this purpose.

The Austrian Immunoglobulin in MS Study (AIMS) randomized 148 patents with RRMS to either placebo (saline) or IVIG 0.15–2.0 mg/kg monthly for 2 years (Fazekas et al., 1997). The primary outcome measure, change in EDSS, was significantly different in favor of the IVIG-treated group, which also demonstrated a significant reduction in the annual relapse rate compared to placebo. Achiron et al. (1998) administered a 2 gm/kg loading dose of IVIG and then 0.4 mg/kg every two months for 2 years or placebo, to a total of 40 patients. This study demonstrated a significant

reduction in annual relapse rate and proportion of relapse free patients in the IVIG treated group (Achiron et al., 1998). Sorensen et al. (1998) utilized a crossover design in which 26 patients received either IVIG 1 g/kg or placebo for two consecutive days/months during two 6-month treatment periods. The primary outcome measure, occurrence of gadolinium (Gd)-enhancing lesions, showed a significant reduction in the number of new lesions and total Gd+ lesions for the IVIG treatment period. There was a trend toward reduction of relapses and number of relapse-free patients in the IVIG-treated subjects (Sorensen et al., 1998). Lewanska et al. (2002) examined two different doses of IVIG (0.4 mg/kg/month vs. 0.2 mg/kg/month) in 49 patients and reported a trend to lower annualized relapse rate in both treatment groups compared to placebo. Additionally, there was a significant reduction in the cumulative number of Gd+ lesions, new T2-weighted lesions, and total T2 lesion volume in both IVIG treatment groups (Lewanska et al., 2002). Subsequent smaller studies that examined the effect of IVIG on MRI parameters also reported positive effects of IVIG (Kocer et al., 2004). A large retrospective study of over 100 patients who had received IVIG reported a 69% reduction in annualized relapse rate compared to the pre-IVIG treatment period (Hass et al., 2005).

One study has examined the use of IVIG in clinically isolated syndrome (Achiron et al., 2004a). In that study 91 patients with an initial demyelinating event were randomized to receive either 5 days of IVIG (0.4 g/kg) followed by single doses of 0.4 g/kg every 6 weeks for 1 year, or saline placebo. IVIG reduced the probability of the patients fulfilling the criteria for clinically definite MS (i.e., having a second attack) by 48%. The volume and number of T2-weighted lesions on MRI was also significantly lower in the IVIG groups compared to placebo, but the mean number of Gd+ lesions was not significantly different.

In contrast to the aforementioned reports, a recent large double-blind randomized trial (PRIVIG: Prevention of Relapses with IVIG) compared two doses of a new IVIG preparation, IVIG-C 10%, to albumin placebo in persons with RRMS. Forty-four subjects received 0.2 g/kg, 42 subjects received 0.4 g/kg, and 42 subjects received 0.1% albumin monthly for 48 weeks. There was no difference in the primary outcome measure, percentage of relapse-free patients, between either treatment group and placebo (Fazekas et al., 2008). A secondary outcome measure, MRI lesion activity, also was no different between the two groups.

A few studies have investigated the use of IVIG as a remyelinating agent to reverse fixed neurologic deficits. These trials have been negative for both clinical and paraclinical outcome measures (Dudesek and Zettl, 2006). Additionally, a large double-blind randomized trial of monthly IVIG at 1 g/kg for 2 years versus albumin placebo in persons with secondary progressive MS (ESIMS; Hommes et al., 2004) failed to show a difference between IVIG and placebo-treated patients in terms of the primary outcome measure, change in EDSS. There was also no effect on relapse rate or T2-weighted lesion load.

In light of the heterogeneity of the results of the above reports, it is of interest to note an analysis done by Hommes et al. (2009). They compared 15 randomized double-blind placebo trials of IVIG in MS and separated them into those which had a saline, dextrose, or vehicle control, and those which used albumin for the placebo group. In their review, 6 out of 7 studies with saline or dextrose as a control showed a positive treatment effect of IVIG, compared to 0 of 8 studies with albumin as the control substance. The authors cite neuroprotective effects of albumin that have been reported in the stroke literature, and they suggest that a large randomized, double-blind trial using saline versus IVIG for RRMS is warranted.

The use of IVIG in mothers with MS to prevent postpartum relapses is described in the chapter on gender and reproductive issues (Chapter 17). IVIG may be considered for this purpose in individual patients who are most at risk for postpartum relapse (i.e., those with active disease prior to pregnancy and who do not wish to take standard disease-modifying agents, e.g., because they wish to breastfeed).

Side effects of IVIG may include headache, fever, and myalgia. Rare serious side effects that have been reported include myocardial infarction, renal injury, and aseptic meningitis (Sapir et al., 2005). Additionally, patients who are IgA deficient may have an allergic reaction to IgA-containing IVIG preparations, and so it is prudent to determine IgA levels in patients before administration of IVIG.

Summary

There are conflicting data for the efficacy of IVIG as an agent to treat acute MS relapses and as a prophylactic immunomodulatory agent. It may be appropriate as an off-label second-line agent for these purposes for some patients who cannot tolerate or who have not responded to steroids or conventional disease-modifying therapy.

PLASMA EXCHANGE

Another second-line treatment modality for persons with exacerbations who do not respond to or who cannot tolerate steroids is plasma exchange (PLEX). A small randomized controlled trial conducted by Weinshenker et al. (1999) randomized 22 patients with acute central nervous system (CNS) demyelinating disease (12 with MS) who had not responded to IV corticosteroid treatment to PLEX or sham pheresis. Improvement was reported in 42% of the PLEX-treated patients compared to only 6% of controls. A subsequent retrospective study of 59 patients with acute episodes of CNS demyelination who had received treatment with PLEX found improvement in 44% of the subjects (Keegan et al., 2002). In that study, male sex, preserved reflexes, and early initiation of treatment were the variables that tended to be associated with recovery. The EFNS guidelines list PLEX as a second-line treatment for acute exacerbations in those persons who do not respond to corticosteroid therapy.

PLEX may be administered every other day for 5–7 treatments, and it is usually done in the inpatient setting but is also feasible for outpatient administration. Potential side effects of PLEX include infection, metabolic acidosis, hypocalcemia, or increased risk of bleeding due to depletion of coagulation factors (Tumani, 2008).

ONGOING DISEASE ACTIVITY

Despite treatment with standard immunomodulating therapy, some persons with MS may continue to have numerous relapses, increasing lesion burden and inflammation on MRI, and/or clinically progressive disease. In these cases, switching immunomodulatory agents, treatment with natalizumab, or treatment with immunosuppressive agents may be the appropriate next step.

There are no definitive guidelines for when to modify therapy. Some parameters to consider in making this decision are frequency of relapses (e.g., more than one clinically significant exacerbation in a 6–12 month period), incomplete degree of recovery from relapses, continued enlarging and/or enhancing lesion activity on MRI, or continuing progression of disease as manifest by deterioration in neurologic exam and/or functional capacity. It is important to ascertain that recurring relapses are not due to pseudorelapses (i.e., caused by heat or infection) and that the patient has been adherent to therapy (Markowitz, 2009).

For patients who are on low-dose interferon, switching to higher dose interferon may be helpful. Patients on high-dose interferon may benefit from a change to glatiramer, particularly if they have persistent high titres of neutralizing antibodies to beta-interferon (Cook, S, et al. 2008). Patients who are having continued disease activity on glatiramer may do better on interferon. Alternatively, patients with relapsing disease who are not responding to interferon or glatiramer may be appropriate candidates for natalizumab.

If a change in first-line disease-modifying agents does not reduce relapses or progression, other agents may need to be used. This section will discuss immunosuppressive therapies, as well as combination regimens.

Mitoxantrone

Mitoxantrone (Novantrone) is currently the only immunosuppressive agent with an FDA indication for the treatment of MS. It is an analog of compounds that were developed as textile dyes; it is a deep blue solution, which may cause a bluish stain to patient's sclera and/or fingernails.

Chemically, mitoxantrone is an anthracenedione that intercalates into DNA and interferes with enzymatic DNA repair mechanisms. Immunologically, it inhibits proliferation of T cells, B cells, and macrophages and decreases secretion of Th1 cytokines such as tumor necrosis factor, interleukin 2, and gamma interferon (Boster et al., 2008).

Mitoxantrone tends to distribute in deep tissues with slow release into blood, and it has been estimated that immunocompetent cells may be exposed to mitoxantrone for at least 4 weeks (Fox, 2006).

However, concentrations have been detected in tissues for over 6 months after administration (Scott and Figett, 2004). It is primarily cleared through biliary excretion, and thus clearance can be impaired in patients with hepatic dysfunction.

Mitoxantrone was approved by the FDA in 2000 for the treatment of secondary progressive MS (SPMS), progressive relapsing MS (PRMS), and/or worsening relapsing-remitting MS (RRMS), based on reports of several small placebo-controlled trials indicating that mitoxantrone was well tolerated and had a favorable effect on clinical and MRI parameters. The pivotal phase III multicenter trial, MIMS (mitoxantrone in MS), was published in 2002 (Hartung et al., 2002). In this study, 194 patients with "worsening/active" RRMS, PRMS, or SPMS were randomized to either placebo, mitoxantrone ($5 \ mg/m^2$), or mitoxantrone ($12 \ mg/m^2$) every 3 months for 2 years. The primary outcome measure was a composite analysis of variables, including change in EDSS, time to first relapse, number of relapses, change in ambulation index, and change in a neurologic rating scale. The patients treated with the mitoxantrone $12 \ mg/m^2$ dose did significantly better than placebo-treated patients on all variables, including 68% decrease in relapse rate and 64% reduction in progression of disability as defined by change by >1 EDSS point. This positive effect was also sustained for at least 12 months after cessation of treatment, as measured by change from baseline in EDSS, ambulation index, and the Standardized Neurological Status scale.

Mitoxantrone has also been used as add-on therapy to standard immunomodulators in patients with active RRMS. Jeffrey et al. (2005) reported decrease in relapse rate by 64% and decrease in Gd+ lesions in 10 such patients with the addition of mitoxantrone to beta-interferon. Ramtahal et al. (2006) reported a series of 27 RR patients, who had active disease despite treatment with beta-interferon or glatiramer, or who were treatment naïve. These patients received 3–6 monthly does of mitoxantrone (variable dosing) and then were treated with glatiramer acetate (GA), followed by "booster" doses of mitoxantrone every 3 months. This regimen produced significant decrease in relapse rate and stabilization or improvement in EDSS in 25 of the 27 patients, with sustained benefit at 3 years of follow-up. A somewhat larger study by Vollmer et al. (2008) randomized 40 patients with relapsing-remitting MS to receive either GA alone, or three doses of mitoxantrone (12 mg/m²/month) followed by GA for a total treatment time of 15 months. The mitoxantrone plus GA group showed an 89% reduction in Gd enhancing lesions at months 6 and 9 and a 70% reduction in Gd-enhancing lesions at months 12–15 compared to the GA monotherapy group (Vollmer et al., 2008).

Mitoxantrone has also been used as "induction" therapy. One example of this is a large open-label trial in France that treated 100 patients with active RRMS with mitoxantrone 20 mg/month plus 1 g methyl prednisolone for 6 months. Fifty-seven of these patents then received maintenance therapy with either immunomodulatory or oral immunosuppressive agents. In the first 12 months after beginning treatment, annualized relapse rate was decreased by 91%, with 76% of patients being free of relapses, and 89% reduction in MR activity. Median time to first relapse was almost 3 years. Sixty percent of patients improved by at least 1 EDSS point, and this improvement in disability was sustained for up to 4 years (Le Page et al., 2006).

The primary risks of therapy with mitoxantrone are cardiac and neoplastic. Mitoxantrone has been reported to be associated with significant cardiotoxicity, including cardiomyopathy, reduced left ventricular ejection fraction (LVEF), and congestive heart failure. While this generally occurs above the recommended maximal lifetime dose of 140 mg/m², it may also occur at lower doses. It is recommended that baseline LVEF be determined and then performed before each dose of mitoxantrone, and that patients with LVEF <50% not receive mitoxantrone therapy. Decreased LVEF may continue even after cessation of mitoxantrone therapy (Fox, 2006),and newer guidelines suggest monitoring of cardiac function after cessation of mitoxantrone therapy (FDA July 29, 2008) The other potentially serious side effect of mitoxantrone is treatment-related leukemia (TRL). The risk of TRL has been estimated at 0.07%–0.25% for patients who received mitoxantrone as monotherapy (Ghalie et al., 2002; Fox, 2006). However, a recent review reported that this may be higher. Ellis and Boggild (2009) examined reports that contained a total of over 5400 patients who had received mitoxantrone in study protocols and found an incidence of TRL

of 0.30%. The mean dose of mitoxantrone received by all patients was 74 mg/m², but 80% of the TRL cases occurred in patients who had received >60 mg/m². This suggests that the risk of TRL is dose related and more likely to occur at cumulative doses >60 mg/m². Other side effects associated with mitoxantrone include nausea, vomiting, alopecia, urinary tract infection, leukopaenia, and hepatic enzyme elevation.

Mitoxantrone has also been associated with decreased sperm count, menstrual irregularities, and amenorrhea, which in a small percentage of patients may be permanent. The risks of amenorrhea are directly correlated with patient age over 40 and increasing dose of mitoxantrone (Cocco et al., 2008). One report has suggested that concomitant administration of estrogen/progesterone during mitoxantrone treatment may reduce this risk (Cocco et al., 2008).

Summary

Mitoxantrone is the only immunosuppressant currently FDA approved to treat worsening and progressive forms of MS. It has been demonstrated to significantly reduce relapse rate and slow progression of disability. Serious potential dose-limiting side effects include cardiotoxicity, treatment-related leukemia, and infertility. The report of the AAN Therapeutics and Technology Assessment Subcommittee of the American Academy of Neurology (AAN) has the following suggestions for use of mitoxantrone in persons with MS (Goodin et al., 2003):

- Evidence from clinical trials supports the probable beneficial effect of mitoxantrone on reducing relapse rate and disease progression, but its use should be "reserved for patients with rapidly advancing disease who have failed other therapies."
- Mitoxantrone should be administered by physicians"experienced in use of chemotherapeutic agents" with close monitoring of hepatic, renal, and cardiac parameters.

Cyclophosphamide

Cyclophosphamide (Cytoxan) is an immunosuppressive alkylating agent that suppresses rapidly dividing cells, such as T and B cells. It also has been demonstrated to produce a Th1-Th2 cytokine shift (Boster et al., 2008). It is indicated to treat several types of malignancies such as some leukemias and lymphomas, multiple myeloma, some solid tumors, and certain types of pediatric nephritic syndrome.

Open-label reports of the efficacy of cyclophosphamide in treating patients with MS date back to 1966 (Aimard et al., 1966). The first randomized controlled trial was published in 1983 (Hauser et al., 1983). Fifty-eight patients were randomized to either intravenous cyclophosphamide (400–500 mg/day for 10–14 days) plus ACTH, ACTH alone, or ACTH plus plasma exchange and oral cyclophosphamide (2 mg/kg/day). Eighty percent of the IV cyclophosphamide group was stable or improved at 12 months, compared to 50% of the plasmapheresis group and 20% of the ACTH-only patients. Subsequently, two large randomized trials showed conflicting results. In the Northeast Cooperative MS Treatment Group study, 256 patients with progressive MS were randomized to receive one of two induction regimens of cyclophosphamide and ACTH, with or without subsequent booster doses of cyclophosphamide every other month for 2 years (Weiner et al., 1993). There was no difference between the two induction regimens, but patients who had received booster doses of cyclophosphamide had significantly delayed time to progression (sustained progression on EDSS by at least 1 point) compared to those patients who had not received booster doses. This effect was more robust in younger patients; 40% of patients ages 18–40 were improved or stable at 30 months compared to 14% of patients older than 40.

In contrast, the Canadian Cooperative MS group randomized 168 patients with progressive MS to receive either cyclophosphamide plus prednisone, cyclophosphamide plus alternate day prednisone and plasampheresis, or oral placebo and sham pheresis. There was no difference in the primary endpoint, time to sustained progression on EDSS by at least 1 point, among the three different treatment groups (Canadian Cooperative Trial, 2001). A recent Cochrane review that compared four RCTs of cyclophosphamide administered either alone or in combination with ACTH or steroids found no effect of cyclophosphamide in preventing sustained disability progression (La Mantia et al., 2007).

Open-label trials of cyclophosphamide have reported more favorable results. These trials have generally involved variable numbers (e.g., 5–490) of patients and different cyclophosphamide regimens (500–1500 mg/m^2) but have reported stabilization and or improvement in disability as measured on EDSS, and also improvement in MRI parameters (Boster et al., 2008). Across these studies, patients who were more likely to respond were younger and had more inflammatory disease (Gauthier and Weiner, 2005).

More recently, high-dose (200 mg/kg) cyclophosphamide has been studied in two small open-label trials (Gladstone et al., 2006; Krishman et al., 2008). Gladstone et al. (2006) reported 12 patients with active RR or SP MS who were treated with 200 mg/kg cyclophosphamide over 4 days. At a median follow-up of 15 months (range 6–24 months), no patient had increase in EDSS by more than 1 point; 5/12 patients had decrease by 1 or more EDSS points. Only two patients showed a single enhancing MRI lesion in 24 months of follow-up. Treatment was well tolerated with no serious adverse events.

Krishman et al. (2008) treated nine patients with active RRMS with similar high-dose regimen (50 mg/kg/day for 4 days) and had a 23-month follow-up period. There was statistically significant reduction in disability as measured by EDSS and 81% reduction in enhancing lesions seen on MRI compared to pretreatment scans. There were no serious adverse events.

Two open-label comparison trials of cyclophosphamide versus mitoxantrone in secondary progressive (Perini et al., 2006) and secondary progressive and relapsing-remitting MS patients (Zipoli et al., 2008) showed comparable efficacy in reducing disability progression and relapse rate, and similar reduction in MRI activity, with similar tolerability in both treatment groups. Cyclophosphamide has also been used in combination with beta-interferon in patients with RR MS who were not responding to beta-interferon alone. The addition of cyclophosphamide to beta-interferon produced significant reduction in relapse rate and gadolinium-enhancing lesion activity on MRI (Patti et al., 2004; Smith et al., 2005).

Side effects of cyclophosphamide include nausea, vomiting, alopecia, leukopaenia, and infection. Similarly to what has been reported for mitoxantrone, the risk of permament amenorrhea appears to be dose and age related. Bladder toxicity (hemorrhagic cystitis) may be minimized by administration of concomitant mesna and copious hydration. Risk of malignancy is dose related, and it appears to be highest when total lifetime doses exceed 80–100 g (Gauthier and Weiner, 2005).

Summary

Cyclophosphamide may be used off label to treat active relapsing and progressive forms of MS. There is no consensus that this agent is definitively beneficial for this purpose, but it may benefit individual patients, particularly those who are younger and who have more relapsing (inflammatory) aspects to their disease.

Azathioprine

Azathioprine (Imuran) is a purine analog of the immunosuppressant 6-mercaptopurine. It is indicated to treat active rheumatoid arthritis and in renal transplant medicine, and it has been used off label in the treatment of MS for several decades. The first and largest double-blind, placebo-controlled randomized trial of azathioprine treated 354 patients with either relapsing-remitting or secondary progressive MS, who were randomized to either azathioprine 2.5 mg/kg/day or placebo. There was a trend toward slowing of progression as measured on EDSS in favor of azathioprine (British and Dutch MS Azathioprine Trial Group, 1988). Review of several subsequent double-blind, randomized controlled trials reported that azathioprine reduced relapse rate compared to placebo (Yudkin et al., 1991). A Cochrane review that looked at five randomized controlled trials comprising 698 patients reported the following. Azathioprine reduced the number of patients who had relapses at up to 3 years of follow-up. A smaller number of patients (87) were examined for effect on disease progression, and azathioprine significantly reduced the number of patients who progressed at up to 3 years of follow-up (Cassetta et al., 2007).

Studies that have examined the efficacy of azathioprine in combination with beta-interferon have yielded mixed results. A few small, open-label studies have reported that a combination of azathioprine in combination with either beta-interferon 1a or 1b produced significant decreases in MRI activity, relapse rate, and progression on EDSS (Gold, 2008). In contrast, a double-blind randomized placebo-controlled study that compared azathioprine plus beta-interferon 1a IM (Avonex), versus azathioprine plus Avonex plus alternate day prednisone, versus Avonex alone showed no difference in annualized relapse rate, MRI activity, or EDSS score at 2 and 5 year follow-up (Havrdova et al., 2009).

Azathioprine is generally well tolerated, with the most frequent side effects being gastrointestinal (e.g., nausea, abdominal pain, diarrhea) and headache. Anemia, leucopenia, and hepatic enzyme elevation are also common. Pancreatitis has been reported very rarely. The risk of cancer is dose related; it is said to be greatest with treatment duration greater than 10 years and cumulative dose greater than 600 g (Casetta et al., 2007).

Mycophenolate Mofetil and Methotrexate

Mycophenlate mofetil (CellCept) is an oral immunosuppressant used in transplant medicine and in the treatment of some autoimmune diseases. It is a purine synthesis inhibitor and thus inhibits proliferation of activated T cells, B cells, and macrophages.

Small open-label trials as monotherapy or add-on therapy have reported stabilization and/or improvement in persons with relapsing-remitting and progressive forms of MS (Ahrens et al., 2001; Frohman et al., 2004; Vermesch et al., 2007), but to date there are no completed randomized, double-blind, placebo-controlled studies.

Side effects of mycophenolate mofetil are similar to azathioprine. Additionally, cases of pure red cell aplasia secondary to mycophenolate mofetil have been reported (Engelen et al., 2003).

Methotrexate is an immunosuppressive agent that has been widely used to treat rheumatoid arthritis. A double-blind placebo-controlled study of low-dose (7.5 mg/week) methotrexate in patients with progressive MS demonstrated some benefit on upper-extremity function, but no effect on sustaining ambulatory ability (Goodkin et al., 1995). An open-label add-on study treated 15 patients with weekly beta-interferon 1a (Avonex) plus methotrexate (20 mg/week) because they were having disease activity on Avonex alone, and reported a 44% decrease in Gd+ lesions with a trend toward decreased relapses (Calabresi et al., 2002).

Summary

Oral immunosuppressive agents may be used as monotherapy or added on to standard immuno-modulating agents to reduce relapses and disease progression, but there are limited data to support these uses. They have the advantage of being easy to administer and are generally well tolerated. Table 24-1 summarizes some commonly used immunosuppressant treatments.

Hemopoetic Stem Cell Transplantation

Bone marrow ablation followed by autologous hemopoetic stem cell transplantation (AHSCT) in persons with MS was first reported in 1997 (Fassas et al., 1997) and has subsequently been used in over 400 MS patients worldwide. These trials have primarily been comprised of patients with progressive disease and more severe disability, but patients with relapsing disease have also been treated. According to Kraft et al. (2009), the patients who have been the best responders to this therapy are those with active relapsing disease and EDSS ≤ 5.5.

In 2002 Fassas and colleagues reported results of a multicenter open-label trial of AHSCT in 85 persons with progressive MS. In that study, the median age was 39, median disease duration was 7 years, and median EDSS was 6.5. After AHSCT, there was progression-free survival at 3 years in 74% of patients. There were seven deaths, or approximately 9% mortality. Subsequently, Saccardi and colleague (2006) reported a review

TABLE 24-1 Immunosuppressant Agents Used in Treating Multiple Sclerosis

Agent	Route	Dose Range	Side Effects	Comment
Azathioprine∗	Oral	2.0–2.5 mg/kg	Nausea, headache, leukopaenia, hepatic enzyme elevation, malignancy	Has been used as monotherapy or in combination with DMAs
Cyclophosphamide∗	IV, Oral	500–1500 mg/m² or 200 mg/kg	Nausea, vomiting, leukopaenia, hemorrhagic cystitis, malignancy, infertility	Different regimens include use as induction, with subsequent "booster" doses
Methotrexate∗	Oral	7.5–20 mg/week	Nausea, leukopaenia, hepatic enzyme elevation	
Mitoxantrone	IV	8–12 mg/m² up to max lifetime dose 140 mg/m²	Nausea, vomiting, leukopaenia, hepatic enzyme elevation, cardiotoxicity, infertility, leukemia	Has also been used as "induction" therapy prior to treatment with DMAs
Mycophenolate mofetil∗	Oral	1.5–2.0 g/day	Nausea, leukopaenia, hepatic enzyme elevation, red cell aplasia, infection, malignancy	Has also been used in treatment of neuromyelitis optica∗∗

∗ Off-label use in multiple sclerosis.

∗∗ Jacob et al., 2009.

DMAs, disease-modifying agents.

of the experience of the European Group for Blood & Marrow transplantation (EBMT) in treating 178 persons with progressive MS. In that study, there was improvement and/or stabilization in 63% of patients at median follow-up of 4 years. Mortality was 5.3% and was associated with regimens containing busulphan.

More recently, AHSCT has been used in patients with earlier, relapsing-remitting disease. Fagius and colleagues treated nine persons with aggressive relapsing-remitting MS, with median age 27, median disease duration about 6 years, and median EDSS of 7.0. After AHSCT, at median follow-up at 29 months, median EDSS was 2, and there was 1 relapse in 289 patient months (Fagius et al., 2009).

A larger study was recently reported by Burt et al. (2009). Twenty-one persons with RRMS were treated with AHCT. The median age was 33, duration of disease was 5 years, and median EDSS was 3.1 (range 2.0–5.5). All had been treated with at least one standard immunomodulating agent, and all had to have had at least two relapses or one clinical relapse and a gadolinium-enhancing lesion on MRI on a separate occasion. The conditioning regimen was cyclophosphamide (200 mg/kg) with either alemtuzumab or rabbit anti-thymocyte globulin, which did not produce complete bone marrow ablation. There were no deaths post transplant, and there were three infections and two cases of immune thrombocytopaenic purpura that resolved.

At mean 37 months follow-up, all patients were free from progression, and 16 were relapse free. Additionally, all patients had follow-up EDSS scores equal to or better than baseline EDSS. Mean EDSS scores were improved by 1.7 points. Improvements were also seen in parameters such as the 25-foot timed walk, and the PASAT, a test of cognition.

In contrast to these reports of clinical improvement, one study reported autopsy results on five patients who had undergone AHSCT (Metz et al., 2007). Brain tissues of these patients showed evidence of active demyelination and axonal damage despite therapy. Another report cited accelerated brain atrophy in nine persons with MS who had undergone AHSCT, and the authors suggested that chemotherapy-related neurotoxicity may be responsible (Chen et al., 2006).

Summary

At the time of this writing there are on going multicenter trials of AHSCT for persons with MS. This therapy has been reported to stabilize patients with progressive disease, and it also has been shown to reduce relapses and produce improvement in disability in patients with active relapsing-remitting disease. It is an aggressive treatment option and the optimal time and type of patient in whom to implement this intervention remain to be definitively determined.

As has been stated previously, definitive guidelines for identifying patients who are suboptimal responders to treatment with first-line immunomodulating therapies are not currently available. Furthermore, the data from clinical trials of other immunomodulatory/immunosuppressive agents are heterogeneous with regard to efficacy, and at this time there are few guidelines to identify which patients are most appropriate and most likely to benefit from these agents. Figure 24-1 describes one approach to the patient with active or progressive disease.

AGENTS IN TRIAL

The standard immunomodulating agents only reduce relapses by about one-third, although they are well tolerated. While immunosuppressive agents have been demonstrated to have efficacy in reducing relapses and slowing progression in patients who are not optimally responding to standard immunomodulators, they have many undesirable side effects. Is there an appropriate risk/benefit ratio in applying these agents? The answer is not clear, in part because there is not clear consensus on whether relapses contribute to long-term disability (Confavreaux et al., 2000; Lublin, 2007).

Lublin reported that 70% of a sample of 224 persons with relapsing-remitting MS demonstrated sustained deficit after an exacerbation, as measured by change in EDSS, at least 30 days after the episode, and about 36% of a subset of 63 patients had sustained deficit an average of 6 months after onset of an exacerbation (Lublin, 2007). His conclusion was that relapses do contribute to sustained disability, in contrast to another study, which did not find an association between relapses and

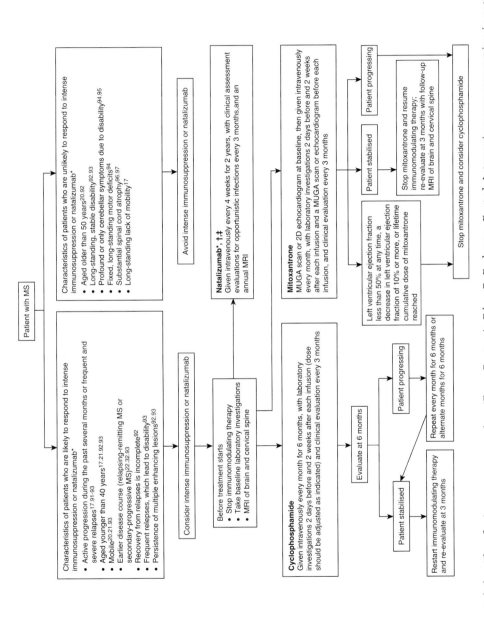

Figure 24-1 Suggested algorithm for immunosuppression. (From Boster A, Edan G, Frohman, E, et al. Intense immunosuppression in patients with rapidly worsening MS: treatment guidelines for the clinician. *Lancet Neurol.* 2008;7:173–183, with permission from Elsevier.)

long-term progression (Confavreaux et al., 2000). Nonetheless, exacerbations do have a significant impact upon persons with MS in terms of lost days at work or school, inability to care for children, increased health-care expenses, and disruption of usual daily activities.

Clearly, agents that are more effective, safer, and better tolerated need to be available. There are numerous agents in trials, several of which are likely to develop into the next generation of disease-modifying agents for MS. These drugs have different, and in some cases more specific, mechanisms of action than the current immunomodulators. It is hoped that these emerging therapies will be more effective and better tolerated than current therapies, and possibly even neuroprotective. Currently, there are phase III trials in progress of several agents that have had promising results in phase II studies.

Oral Agents

Fingolimod

Fingolimod (FTY-20) is a structural analog of the sphinsosine-1-phosphate receptor (S-1-P), an integral membrane component, which is highly expressed in lymphoid cells and also the CNS (Kappos et al., 2006). Fingolimod prevents egress of lymphocytes from lymphoid tissue and thus produces a profound decrease in circulating lymphocytes. However, memory T and B cell function and lymphocyte activation are not affected, so there is less of a general immunosuppressive effect. Fingolimod has also been shown to modulate T regulatory cell function and to downregulate pro-inflammatory cytokines (Sawicka et al., 2005; Wolf et al., 2009). Fingolimod also crosses the blood–brain barrier and has been reported to modulate oligodendrocyte processes that may have implications for remyelination (Miron et al., 2008).

The large phase II trial reported by Kappos et al. (2006) randomized 281 persons with RRMS (mean EDSS 2.6) to placebo, low-dose (1.25 g) or high-dose (5 mg) of fingolimod daily, for 6 months. At 6 months, the fingolimod-treated patients had significantly reduced gadolinium-enhancing lesions and decreased annualized relapse rate. In the 2-year extension phase, combining patients who continued on therapy and placebo patients

who were switched to fingolimod, 173 patients received open-label treatment. In the extension phase, at 24 months, the annualized relapse rate was reduced from 0.77 to 0.20, with gadolinium-enhancing and new T2 lesions reduced by approximately 90% (O'Connor et al., 2009). The most common adverse events were dyspnea, diarrhea, nasopharygitis, and headache. Serious adverse events included posterior reversible encephalopathy syndrome (PRES), bradycardia, and infections.

Most recently, the results of the large phase lll placebo controlled trial(FREEDOMS) of two doses of fingolimod were reported (Kappos et al (2010). Over 1000 patients who had been randomized to either fingolomod 0.5 or 1.25 mg/day or placebo completed this two year study. Relapse rates were reduced by 54% for the lower dose, and 60% for the higher dose, with significant reductions in gadolinium enhancing lesions, and brain atrophy for the treated groups. Adverse events were similar to those in the phase ll study (vide supra), and also included elevated hepatic enzyme levels and dose related macular edema.

The results of the trial assessing injectable interferon versus FTY-20 oral in RRMS (TRANSFORMS) was also recently reported.(Cohen et al 2010) This study investigated fingolimod at 0.5 mg or 1.25 mg versus IM beta-interferon 1a (Avonex). Approximately 1300 patients with RRMS (mean EDSS 2.2) wererandomized. Annualized relapse rate was 52% lower in patient on 0.5 mg fingolimod, and 38% lower in patients on 1.25 mg fingolimod. There was no difference in time to disability progression between fingolimod and beta-interferon treated groups.Adverse events in the fingolimod-treated patients included seven cases of skin cancers and two fatal herpetic infections (Cohen et al., 2010). An FDA advisory panel recommended approval of fingolimod in June 2010. Further action is currently pending.

Cladribine

The immunosuppressant cladribine is a purine analog that acts by leading to apoptosis of lymphocytes and producing lymphocyte depletion, preferentially affecting CD4+ cells. It is FDA approved to treat hairy cell leukemia. Small placebo-controlled trials of intravenous cladribine in the 1990s demonstrated some efficacy in RRMS (Cohen, 2009). Recently, a 2-year, double-blind placebo-controlled crossover trial of parenteral cladribine randomized 84 patients with RRMS to seven 5-day courses of IV cladribine at 5 mg/kg versus placebo for 1 year, with crossover of treatment in year 2. Relapse rates were lower during cladribine treatment, and patients required fewer courses of steroids while on cladribine (Stelmasiak et al., 2009). More recently, oral preparations of cladribine have been tested in clinical trials of persons with RRMS.

The CLARITY (Cladribine Tablets Treating MS Orally) study enrolled approximately 1300 persons with RRMS to receive either high-dose (5.25 mg/kg) (or low-dose (3.5 mg/kg)() oral cladribine or placebo for 96 weeks. Results reported that 80% of cladribine-treated patients were relapse free compared with 61% of patients on placebo, and that annualized relapse rate was reduced by 55% to 58% in cladribine-treated patients compared to placebo. Serious events that occurred more frequently in the cladribine treated groups included five cancers and 20 cases of herpes zoster. (Giovannoni et al., 2010). Two placebo-controlled trials in progress at the time of this writing are the ONWARD trial, a phase II study that is investigating the efficacy of oral cladribine added to beta-interferon, and the ORACLE study, which is a phase III trial investigating the efficacy of oral cladribine in delaying time to conversion to clinically definite MS in patients with a clinically isolated syndrome who are at high risk for converting.

Side effects of oral cladribine include lymphopenia, infection, and bone marrow suppression.

Fumaric Acid (BG-12)

Fumaric acid esters have been used for decades in Germany to treat psoriasis. They are thought to exercise immunomodulatory effects by inducing a Th1 to Th2 cytokine shift, downregulating adhesion molecules and VCAM expression, and stimulating apoptosis in activated T cells (Cohen, 2009). After efficacy was demonstrated in small uncontrolled trials, a phase II double-blind placebo-controlled trial was implemented. Over 250 persons with RRMS were randomized to placebo, or one of three doses of oral dimethyl fumarate. At the highest dose, 720 mg/day, there was a 69% reduction in Gd-enhancing lesions compared to placebo, and a 48% reduction in new T2 lesions. A 32% reduction in relapses in the fumarate-treated

group compared to placebo was not statistically significant. Side effects included flushing, nausea, diarrhea, headache and fatigue, and transient elevation of hepatic enzymes. Some patients experienced severe pruritis, which necessitated discontinuation of drug (Kappos et al., 2008). Larger phase III trials (DEFINE, oral fumarate vs. placebo) and CONFIRM (fumarate vs. placebo vs. glatiramer acetate) are in progress.

Laquinomod

Laquinomod is an oral immunosuppressant that has anti-inflammatory and immunomodulatory actions, the latter including a Th2 cytokine shift (Zou et al., 2002). A phase II trial, which randomized 209 patients to either 0.3 mg/day or 0.1 mg/day laquinomod, or placebo, showed statistically significant reduction (44%) in cumulative active MRI lesions at 6 months, in patients who completed the protocol on the higher dose (Polman et al., 2005), with no benefit demonstrated for the 0.1 mg/day dose.

A subsequent study comparing over 300 patients randomized to 0.6 mg/day, 0.3 mg/day, or placebo, demonstrated significant reduction (40%) in mean cumulative Gd-enhancing lesions at up to 36 weeks for the 0.6 mg/day dose (Comi et al., 2008). The higher dose was well tolerated, with primary adverse events being dose-dependant elevation of hepatic enzymes. Larger phase III trials, comparing laquinomod versus placebo, and laquinomod versus placebo and intramuscular interferon beta, are in progress.

Teriflunomide

Teriflunomide is a lymphocyte antiproliferative agent that is the active metabolite of lefluomide, a drug used to treat rheumatoid arthritis. A double-blind placebo-controlled trial of 179 persons with RRMS or SPMS who were randomized to one of two doses of teriflunomide or placebo showed significant reductions in active and new lesions on MRI for both doses of teriflunomide compared to placebo, with a trend toward reductions in relapses (O'Connor et al., 2006). Adverse events included nasophargygitis, alopecia, nausea and diarrhea, hepatic dysfunction, and myelosuppression. Additionally, teriflunomide is potentially teratogenic and may persist at levels that could present harm to a developing fetus for up to 2 years after discontinuation of therapy (Cohen, 2009). Phase II and III trials comparing teriflunomide versuss placebo, and teriflunomide in combination with beta-interferon and glatri-amer acetate, are in progress.

Other oral agents that have demonstrated some efficacy and tolerability in small pilot or phase II studies in patients with RRMS include minocy-cline, statins, and tesirolimus (Cohen, 2009). Larger trials are needed to determine whether these agents will be in fact be useful in the treat-ment of persons with MS.

A novel oral agent that is being considered for trial is helminth eggs. Epidemiologic studies sug-gest that helminth infection is associated with lower rates of some autoimmune diseases, includ-ing asthma, colitis, and diabetes (Elliott et al., 2007). This is thought to be in part due to a helm-inth-induced Th2 cytokine shift. Helminth infec-tion has been shown to abrogate the animal model of MS, experimental autoimmune encephalitis (La Flamme et al., 2003,Gruden-Movsesjian et al 2008). A small pilot study of administration of oral helminth egg suspension to five treatment-naïve patients with RRMS for 3 months did not identify any safety concerns, and it may permit larger trials of this biologic agent (Fleming et al., 2009).

Monoclonal Antibodies

Monoclonal antibody technology has enabled the development of more specific therapies to treat MS. This section will discuss the monoclonal agents that have shown efficacy in treating MS in phase II controlled studies.

Rituximab

Rituximab (Rituxan) is a chimeric monoclonal antibody directed against the CD 20 antigen on the surface of B cells. It produces a rapid and sus-tained depletion of circulating mature B cells, without affecting plasma cells. Thus, the potential benefit of rituximab in treating MS may be more related to loss of antigen-presenting cells and/or decreased production of inflammatory stimulat-ing factors by B cells, rather than lower antibody titres (Cohen, 2009). Rituximab is currently FDA

approved to treat non-Hodgkin lymphoma and severe forms of rheumatoid arthritis, but it is also used off label to treat other autoimmune diseases such as lupus, and it has also shown some efficacy in treating neuromyelitis optica (Jacob et al., 2008).

A multicenter, phase II randomized double-blind placebo-controlled trial of rituximab randomized 104 persons with RRMS to either rituximab, 1000 mg given on days 1 and 15, or placebo (Hauser et al., 2008). Eligible patients have to have had a relapse in the preceding year, and EDSS 0–5. There was a statistically significant decrease in the primary outcome measure, mean number of Gd + lesions in the treated group at up to 24 weeks (91% reduction), and also approxi-mately twice as many relapse-free patients in the treated group compared to placebo at 24 and 48 weeks, which was significant. There was greater than 95% B cell depletion in the rituximab group that persisted for approximately 6 months, with partial reconstitution thereafter. To date, severe complications associated with this B cell lymphope-nia, such as opportunistic infections or PML, have not been reported in the MS population, although there are reports of PML in patients treated with rituximab for lupus (Carson et al., 2009).

The usual side effects seen with rituximab infu-sions were headache, nausea, fever, and pruritits. Fatal infusion reactions have been reported in patients treated with rituximab for non-MS condi-tions. Additionally, because rituximab is a chima-eric (murine/human) antibody, 25% of patients in the phase II trial developed antibodies. Further trials are in progress using a humanized anti CD-20 monoclonal antibody (ocrelizumab), which should obviate this problem.

Alemtuzumab

Alemtuzumab (Campath) is a humanized anti-body directed against the CD-52 receptor. This is present on a number of immune cells, including T and B cells, natural killer cells, and macrophages, as well as spermatozoa (Cohen, 2009). It produces depletion of T cells that may last up to 16 months, and B cell depletion for 3–6 months (Coles et al., 1999). It is FDA approved to treat B cell leukemia.

A small open-label trial of alemtuzumab in 58 persons with RR or SP MS who had active disease were administered 20 mg/day of alemtuzumab for five doses. At mean follow-up of 29 months the relapse rate had decreased in the RRMS patients by 91%. At 6 months, there was stabilization or improvement in EDSS in 21 out of 22 patients. However, the SP patients continued to show ongoing cerebral atrophy and accumulation of disability as measured by change in EDSS (Coles et al., 2006).

A larger, double-blind placebo-controlled trial of alemuzumab enrolled 334 treatment naïve persons with RR MS with EDSS ≤3 and disease duration ≤3 years to receive either Rebif at standard doses versus high-dose (24 mg/day) or low-dose (12 mg/day) alemtuzumab, for 5 days at months 0, 3, and 12. At 2 years, up to 90% of alemtuzumab-treated patients were relapse free compared to 60% of interferon-treated patients. Benefit for both doses of alemtuzumab was also demonstrated for disability as measured by EDSS scores and T2 lesion volume (Coles et al., 2008).

Side effects associated with alemtuzumab include infusion reactions and fever, malaise, and headache. There are reports of 23% and 30% incidence of Graves disease in alemtuzumab treated patients (Coles et al., 1999) and approximately a 3% incidence of immune thrombocytopaenic purpura in the phase II alemtuzumab versus Rebif trial, with one fatality. Opportunistic infections and PML have been reported in patients receiving alemtuzumab for lymphoproliferative disorders (Martin et al., 2006). Phase III trials comparing alemtuzumab versus beta-interferon are currently in progress.

Daclizumab

Daclizumab (Zenapax) is a humanized monoclonal antibody directed against the CD25 (p55alpha) subunit of the IL-2 receptor on activated T cells. It has been shown to exert an immunomodulatory effect by increasing CD 56 natural killer cells, which regulate numbers of activated T cells (Bielekova et al., 2006). It is indicated for use in transplant medicine.

Small open-label studies of daclizumab as monotherapy (Rose et al., 2007) and as add-on therapy (Bielokova et al., 2004, 2009) in patients with active disease despite treatment with beta-interferon was shown to favorably impact relapse rate and gadolinium-enhancing lesions on MRI.

CHOICE (Kaufman et al., 2008), a randomized double-blind placebo-controlled phase II study of daclizumab, involved 230 patients with RRMS who were experiencing active disease despite treatment with beta-interferon. Participants continued to take beta-interferon, and in addition, were randomized to either high-dose daclizumab (2 mg/kg every 2 weeks), low-dose (1 mg/kg daclizumab every 2 weeks, or placebo). The high-dose daclizumab group showed a 72% reduction in new gadolinium-enhancing lesions at 6 months, compared to placebo, with a trend in the low-dose group. There was a nonsignificant reduction in relapses. Adverse events included fatigue, nausea and diarrhea, hepatic enzyme elevation, and nonopportunistic infections. A multicenter phase II trial comparing daclizumab as monotherapy versus placebo is currently in progress.

Other

Given that MS is widely held to be an immune-mediated disease, therapies that would promote immune tolerance would appear to be a potentially beneficial strategy. One example of this is BHT-3009, a DNA plasmid vaccine that codes for myelin basic protein. A phase II trial conducted by Garren and colleagues randomized 289 patients with RR MS to receive intramuscular injections of 0.5 mg of BHT 3009, 1.5 mg, or placebo over 44 weeks. Between weeks 24 and 48, gadolinium-enhancing lesions were reduced 50% in the 0.5 mg BHT-3009 treated patients ($n = 104$), although this effect did not reach significance ($p = 0.07$). There were no serious adverse events and the vaccine was in general well tolerated.

MBP8298 (dirucotide) is a peptide that is antigenically similar to human myelin. It has been shown to induce immunologic tolerance and suppression of myelin basic protein reactive clones (Warren et al., 2006). In a small ($n = 32$) double-blind placebo-controlled study of patients with progressive MS, MBP8298 was administered intravenously every 6 months for 24 months. There was no difference in disability in the overall study group compared to placebo at 24 months, but in a subgroup of patients who were HLA haplotype DR2 or DR 4 positive, time to progression was significantly prolonged, compared to placebo-treated patients (Warren et al., 2006). Based on these encouraging results, several multicenter trials (MAESTRO 01, 02, 03) studying MBP8298 in RR and SP patients with these genetic markers were initiated. The trial, which randomized 218 patients with RR MS, 154 of whom were HLA+, did not show a benefit of dirucotide on relapse rate compared to placebo. The trial in patients with SP MS also was negative and did not show delayed progression in patients on dirucotide compared to placebo (NMSS July,2009). Further trials have been discontinued at the time of this writing.

T cell vaccination

It was demonstrated almost 30 years ago that immunizing mice with T cells directed against myelin basic protein antigens could prevent the development of EAE (Ben-Nun et al., 1981). This approach is thought to promote immune regulation of pathogenic myelin reactive T cells by stimulating normal immune surveillance mechanisms with attenuated antigen-specific T cells. The vaccines are prepared specifically for an individual patient by stimulating blood or CSF lymphocytes with antigen (e.g., MBP) and then clonally expanding the desired cell lines. The cells are irradiated to prevent proliferation and are then injected back into the patient.

Several small open-label clinical trials have reported that this approach, using attenuated T cells reactive against myelin antigens, can produce stabilization or improvement in clinical outcome measures such as relapse rate, and paraclincal measures such as MRI lesion activity (Zhang et al., 2002; Achiron et al., 2004a). Most recently, preliminary results of a trial of a trivalent T cell vaccine(Tovaxin), which contains attenuated T cells which are reactive against myelin basic protein (MBP), proteolipid protein (PLP), and myelin oligodendrocyte glycoprotein (MOG), has been reported. A small open-label study treated 16 patients with RR or SP MS with Tovaxin, given at weeks 0, 4, 12, and 20, with follow-up for 52 weeks. At week 53, there was an 85% reduction in relapses compared to baseline, with a trend toward improvement in EDSS (Loftus, 2009). A phase IIb study, TERMS (Tovaxin for Early Relapsing MS), treated 100 patients with Tovaxin and 50 with placebo. Patients received injections of Tovaxin or placebo at weeks

0,4, 8, 12, and 24. No serious adverse events have been reported to date, and analysis is ongoing at the time of this writing.

REFERENCES

Achiron A, Gabbay U, Gilad R, et al. Intravenous immunoglobulin treatment in MS: effect on relapses. *Neurology.* 1998;50:398–402.

Achiron A, Kishner I, Sarova-Pinhas I, et al. Intravenous immunoglobulin following the first demyelinating event suggestive of MS: a randomized, double blind, placebo controlled trial. *Arch Neurol.* 2004;61: 1515–1520.

Achiron A, Lavie G, Kishner I, et al. T cell vaccination in MS relapsing remitting nonresponder patients. *Clin Immunol.* 2004a;113(2):155–160.

Ackerman K, Heyman R, Rubin B, et al. Stressful life events precede exacerbations of MS. *Psychosom Med.* 2002;64(6):916–920.

Ahrens N, Salama A, Haas J. Mycophenolate mofetil in the treatment of refractory MS. *J Neurol.* 2001; 248:713–714.

Aimard G, Girard P, Roveau J. MS and the autoimmunization process. Treatment by antimitotics. *Lyon Med.* 1966;215:345–352.

Barnes D, Hughes R, Morris R, et al. Randomized trial of oral and intravenous methyl prednisolone in acute relapses on MS. *Lancet.* 1997;349:902–906.

Ben-Nun A, Wekrele H, Cohen I. Vaccination against autoimmune encephalomyelitis with T lymphocyte line cells reactive against myelin basic protein. *Nature.* 1981;292:60–61.

Bielekova B, Catalfano M, Reichert-Scrivner S, et al. Regulatory CD56(bright) natural killer cells mediate immunomodulatory effects of IL-2 alpha targeted therapy (daclizumab) in MS. *Proc Nat Acad Sci USA.* 2006;103:5941–5946.

Bielekova B, Howrd T, Packer A, et al. Effect of anti CD25 antibody daclizumab in the inhibition and stabilization of disease progression in MS. *Arch Neurol.* 2009; 66(4):483–489.

Bielekova B Richert N, Howard T, et al. Humanized anti CD25 (daclizumab) inhibits disease activity in MS patients failing to respond to interferon beta. *Proc Nat Acad Sci USA.* 2004;101:8705–8708.

Boster A, Edan G, Frohman E, et al. Intense immunosuppression in patients with rapidly worsening MS: treatment guidelines for the clinician. *Lancet Neurol.* 2008; 7:173–183.

British and Dutch MS Azathioprine Trial Group. Double masked trial of azathioprine in MS. *Lancet.* 1988;2(8604): 179–183.

Brusaferri F, Candelise L. Steroids for MS and optic neuritis: A meta analysis of randomized controlled trials. *J Neurol.* 2000;247:435–442.

Buljevac D, Hop W, Reedecker W, et al. Self reported stressful life events and exacerbations in MS. *BMJ.* 2003;327:646.

Burt R, Cohen B, Stefosky D, et al. Autologous non-myeloablative haemopoietic stem cell transplantation in relapsing remitting MS: a phase l/ll study. *Lancet Neurol*. 2009;8244–253.

Burton J, O'Connor P, Hohol M, Beyene J. Oral vs. intravenous steroids for treatment of relapses in MS. *Cochrane DB Sys Rev*. 2009;3:CD006921.

Calabresi P, Wilterdink J, Rogg J, Mills P, Webb A, Whartenby K. An open label trial of combination therapy with interferon beta 1-a and oral methotrexate in MS. *Neurology*. 2002;58(2):314–317.

Canadian Cooperative Trial of cyclophosphamide and plasma exchange in progressive MS. *Lancet*. 1991;337:441–446.

Carson K, Evens A, Richey E, et al. Progressive multifocal leukoencephalopathy in HIV negative patients: a report of 57 cases from the Research on Adverse Drug Events and Reports Project. *Blood*. 2009;113(20):4834–4840.

Casetta I, Iuliano G, Fillipini G. Azathioprine for MS. Cochrane DB Sys Rev 2007;4: CD003982 DOI: 10.1002/14651858 CD003982.pub2.

Chen J, Eng, M, Collins D, et al. Brain atrophy after immunoablation and stem cell transplantation in MS. *Neurology*. 2006;66:1935–1937.

Cocco E, Sardu C, Gallo P, et al. Frequency and risk factors of mitoxantrone induced amenorrhea in MS: the FEMIMS study. *Mult Scler*. 2008;14:1225–1233.

Cohen JA. Emerging therapies for relapsing MS. *Arch Neurol*. 2009;66(7):821–828.

Cohen J, Imrey P, Calabresi P, Edwards K, Eickenhorst T, Felton W, III. Results of the Avonex® Combination Trial (ACT) in relapsing remitting MS. *Neurology*. 2009a;72(6):535–541.

Cohen J, Barkhof F, Comi G, et al. Oral fingolimod or imtramuscular interferon for relapsing remitting MS. *NEJM*. (2010);362(5):402–415.

Coles A, Compston D, Selmaj K, et al. Alemtuzumab vs. interferon beta 1-a in early MS. *N Engl J Med*. 2008;359(17):1786–1801.

Coles A, Cox A, Le Page E, et al. The window of therapeutic opportunity in MS: evidence from monoclonal antibody therapy. *J Neurol*. 2006;253:98–108.

Coles A, Wing M, Smith S, et al. Pulsed monoclonal antibody treatment and autoimmune thyroid disease in MS. *Lancet*. 1999;354:1691–1695.

Comi G, Pulizzi A, Rovaris M, et al. Effect of lacquiimod on MRI monitored disease activity in patients with relapsing remitting MS: a multicentre, randomized, double blind, placebo controlled phase llb study. *Lancet*. 2008;371:2085–2092.

Confavreaux C, Suissa S, Saddier P, Bourdes V, Vukusic S. Vaccinations and the risk of relapse in MS. *N Engl J Med*. 2001;344:319–326.

Confavreaux, C, Vukusic S, Moreau T, Adeleine P. Relapses and progression of disability in MS. *N Engl J Med*. 2000;343:1430–1438.

Cook, S, Coyle P, Cross A et al and the Changing Therapy Consensus Statement Taskforce, National Clinical Advisory Board of the National MS Society 2008

http://www.nationalmssociety.org/for-professionals/healthcare-professionals/publications/expert-opinion-papers/download.aspx?id=129

DeStefano N, Fillipi M, Hawkins C 9011 Study group. Short term combination of glatiramer acetate with intravenous steroids preceding treatment with glatiramer acetate alone measured by MRI disease activity in patients with relapsing remitting MS. *J Neurol. Sci*. 2008; 266(1–2):44–50.

Dudesek A, Zettl U. Intravenous immunoglobulins as therapeutic options in the treatment of MS. *J Neurol*. 2006;253(suppl 5):V50–V58.

Elliott, D, Summers R, Weinstock J. Helminths as governors of immune mediated inflammation. *Int J Parasitol*. 2007;37(5):457–464.

Ellis R, Boggild M. Therapy related acute leukemia with mitoxantrone: what is the risk and can we minimize it? *Mult Scler*. 2009;15:505–508.

Engelen W, Verpooten G, Van der Planken M, Helbert M, Bosmans J, DeBroe M. Four cases of red blood cell aplasia in associartion with the use of mycophenolate mofetil in renal transplant patients. *Clin. Nephrol*. 2003;60(2):119–124.

Fagius J, Lundgren J, Oberg G. Early highly aggressive MS successfully treated by haemopoietic stem cell transplantation. *Mult Scler*. 2009;15(2):229–237.

Fassas A, Anagnostopoulos A, Kazis A, et al. Peripheral blood stem cell transplantation in the treatment of progressive MS: first results of a pilot study. *Bone Marrow Transplant*. 1997;20:631–638.

Fazekas F, Deisenhammer F, Strasser-Fuxhs S, Nahler G, Mamoli B. Randomized placebo controlled trial of monthly intravenous immunoglobulin therapy in relapsing remitting MS. Austrian Immunoglobulin in MS Study Group. *Lancet*. 1997;349:589–593.

Fazekas F, Lublin F, Freedman M, et al. The PRIVIG study group and the UBC MS/MRI research group. Intravenous immunoglobulin in relapsing remitting MS. A dose finding trial. *Neurology*. 2008;71(4):265–271.

FDA July, 2008 http://www.fda.gov/Safety/MedWatch/SafetyInformation/SafetyAlertsforHuman Medical Products/ucm092708.htm accessed April 4, 2010).

Fleming J, Lee J, Luzzio C, Carrithers M, Field A, Fabry Z. A Phase 1 trial of probiotic helminth ova in relapsing remitting MS. *Neurology*. 2009;72(suppl 3): A358.

Fox E. Management of worsening MS with mitoxantrone: a review. *Clin Ther*. 2006;28(4):461–474.

Frohman E, Brannon K, Racke M, Hawker K. Mycophenolate mofetil in MS. *Clin Neuropharmacol*. 2004;27(2):80–83.

Garren H, Robinson W, Krasulova E, et al. Phase 2 trial of a DNA vaccine encoding myelin basic protein for MS. *Ann Neurol*. 2008;63:611–620.

Gauthier S & Weiner H. Cyclophosphamide therapy for MS. *Int MS J*. 2005;12:52–58.

Ghalie R, Mauch E, Edan G, et al. A study of therapy related acute leukemia after mitoxantrone therapy for MS. *Mult Scler*. 2002;8(5):441–445.

Giovannoni G, Comi G, Cook S, etal. A placebo controlled trial of oral cladribine for relapsing MS. *NEJM*. (2010);362(5):456–458.

Gladstone D, Zamkoff K, Krupp L, et al. High dose cyclophosphamide for moderate to severe refractory MS. *Arch Neurol*. 2006;63:1388–1393.

Gold R. Combination therapies in MS. *J Neurol*. 2008;255(suppl1):51–60.

Goodin D, Arnason B, Coyle P, Frohman E, Paty D. The use of mitoxantrone (Novantrone®) for the treatment of MS. Report of the Therapeutics and Technology Assessment Subcommittee of the AAN. *Neurology*. 2003;61:1332–1338.

Goodin D, Ebers G, Johnson K, Rodriguez M, Sibley W, Wollinsky J. The relationship of MS to physical trauma and psychologic stress: report of the Therapeutics and Technology Subcommittee of the AAN. *Neurology*. 1999;52(9):1737–1745.

Goodkin D, Kinkel R, Weinstock –Guttman B, et al. A phase ll study of IV methylprednisolone in secondary progressive MS. *Neurology*. 1998;51:239–245.

Goodkin D, Rudick R, Vanderbrug-Medendorp S, et al. Low dose (7.5 mg) oral methotrexate reduces the rate of progression in chronic progressive MS. *Ann Neurol*. 1995;37(1):30–40.

Gruden-Movsesjian A, Mostarica-Stojkovic M, Stosic-Grujicic S, Milic M, Sofronic-Milosavljevic L. Trichinella spiralis: modulation of experimental autoimmune encephalitis in DA rats. *Exp. Parasitol*. (2008); 18(4):641–647.

Hartung H, Gonsette R, Konig N, et al. Mitoxanrone in progressive MS: a placebo controlled double blind, randomized multi-center trial. *Lancet*. 2002;360:2018–2025.

Hass J, Mass-Enriquez M, Hartung H. Intravenous immunoglobulins in the treatment of relapsing remitting MS-results of a retrospective multicenter observational study over five years. *Mult Scler*. 2005;11: 562–567.

Hauser S, Dawson D, Lehrich R, et al. Intensive immunosuppression in progressive MS. A randomized three arm study of high dose intravenous cyclophosphamide, plasma exchange and ACTH. *N Engl J Med*. 1983;43: 173–180.

Hauser S, Waubant E, Arnold D, et al. HERMES Trial Group: B cell depletion with rituximab in relapsing remitting MS. *N Engl J Med*. 2008;358:676–688.

Havrdova E, Zivadinov R, Krasensky J, et al. Randomized study of interferon beta 1a, low dose azathioprine and low dose corticosteroids in MS. *Mult Scler*. 2009 May 22; Epub ahead of print.

Hommes O, Haas J, Soelberg-Sorenson P, Friedrichs M. IVIG trials in MS. Is albumin a placebo? *J Neurol*. 2009;256:268–270.

Hommes O, Sorensen P, Fazekas F, et al. Intravenous immunoglobulin in secondary progressive MS: randomized placebo controlled trial. *Lancet*. 2004;364(9440): 11149–11156.

Jacob A, Matiello M, Weinshenker B, et al. Treatment of neuromyelitis optica with mycophenolate mofetil: retrospective analysis of 24 patients. *Arch Neurol*. 2009;66(9):1128–1133.

Jacob A, Weinshenker B, Violich I, et al. Treatment of neuromyelitis optica with rituximab: retrospective analysis of 25 patients. *Arch Neurol*. 2008;65:1443–1448.

Jeffery D, Chapuri N, Durden D, et al. A pilot trial of combination therapy with mitoxantrone and interferon beta 1-b using monthly gadolinium enhanced MRI. *Mult Scler*. 2005;11:296–301.

Kappos L, Antel J, Comi G, et al. Oral fingolimod (FTY-20) for relapsing MS. *N Engl J Med*. 2006;355(11):1088–1091.

Kappos L, Gold R, Miller D, et al. BG-12 Phase llb study investigators. Efficacy and safety of oral fumarate in patients with relapsing remitting MS: a multicenter, randomized double blind placebo controlled phase llb study. *Lancet*. 2008;372(9648):1463–1472.

Kappos L, Radue E, O'Connor P et al. A placebo controlled trial of oral fingolimod in relapsing <S. *NEJM*. (2010); 362(5):456–458.

Kaufman M, Wynn D, Montalban X, Wang M, Fong A. A phase 2, randomized, double blinded placebo controlled multicenter study of subcutaneous daclizumab, a humanized anti CD25 monoclonal antibody in patients with active relapsing forms of MS: week 44 results. *Neurology*. 2008;70(suppl 1):A220.

Keegan M, Pineda A, McClelland R, Daily C, Rodriquez M, Weinshenker B. PEX for severe attacks of CNS demyelination: predictors of response. *Neurology*. 2002;58(1):143–146.

Kocer B, Yildirim-Gurel S, Tali E, Izkec C, Isik S. The role of qualitative and quantitative MRI assessment of MS lesions in evaluating the efficacy of intravenous immunoglobulin G. *Neuroradiology*. 2004;46:287–290.

Kraft G, Wundes A, Nash R. Stem cell transplantation in patient with MS in the HALT trial. *MSQR*. 2009; 28(2):7–10.

Krishman C, Kaplin A, Brodsky R, et al. Reduction of disease activity and disability with high dose cyclophosphamide in patients with aggressive MS. *Arch Neurol*. 2008;65(8):1044–1051.

LaFlamme A, Ruddenklau K, Backstrom B. Schistosomiasis decreases central nervous system inflammation and alters the progression of experimental auto immune encephalomyelitis. *Infect Immun*. 2003;71(9):4996–5004.

La Mantia L, Milanese C, Mascoli N, D"Amico R, Weinstock –Guttman B. Cyclophosphamide for MS. *Cochrane DB Sys Rev*. 2007;1: CD 002819.

Le Page E, Leray E, Taurin G, Coustans M, Chaperon J Edan G. Mitoxantrone as induction therapy in aggressive relapsing remitting MS: a descriptive analysis of 100 consecutive patients. *Rev Neurol (Paris)*. 2006; 162(92):185–194.

Lewanska M, Siger-Zajel M, Selmaj K. No difference in efficacy of two different doses of intravenous immunoglobulin in MS: clinical & MRI assessment. *Eur J Neurol*. 2002;9:565–572.

Loftus B, Newsom B, Montgomery M, et al. Autologous attenuated T cell vaccine (Tovaxin®) dose escalation in MS relapsing remitting and secondary progressive patients non-responsive to approved immunomodulatory therapies. *Clin Immunol*. 2009;131:202–215.

Lublin F. The incomplete nature of MS relapse resolution. *J Neurol Sci*. 2007;256:S14–S18.

Markowitz C. Inadequate responders: identification and treatment modification. *Johns Hopkins Adv Stud Med.* 2009;9(2):53–59.

Martin S, Marty F, Fumara K, et al. Infectious complications associated with alemtuzumab use for lymphoproliferative disorders. *Clin Infec Dis.* 2006;43:16–24.

Metz I, Luchinetti C, Openshaw H, et al. Autologous haematopoetic stem cell transplantation fails to stop demyelination and neurodegeneration in MS. *Brain.* (2007);130(5):1254–62.

Miller A, Morgante L, Buchwald L, et al. A multicentre, randomized, double blind placebo controlled trial of influenza immunization in MS. *Neurology.* 1997;49(5): 1474–1475.

Miron V, Jung C, Kim H, et al. FTY-20 modulates human oligodendrocyte progenitor process extension and survival. *Ann Neurol.* 2008;63:61–71.

Morrow S, Stoian C, Dmitrovic J, Chan S Metz L. The bioavailabiity of IV methyl prednisolone and oral prednisone in MS. *Neurology.* 2004;63:1079–1080.

National MS Society,2009 8/18/2009 http://www.national-mssociety.org/living-with-multiple-sclerosis/healthy-living/vaccinations/index.aspx accessed April4, 2010.

National MS Society News Release July 20, 2009 http://www.nationalmssociety.org/news/news-detail/index.aspx?nid=1854 accessed April4, 2010.

O'Connor P, Comi G, Montalban X, et al. Oral fingolimod in MS: Two year results of a phase ll extension study. *Neurology.* 2009;72(1):73–79.

O'Connor P, Li D, Freedman M, et al. A phase ll study of the safety and efficacy of teriflunomide in MS with relapses. *Neurology.* 2006;66:894–900.

Panitch H, Cohen J, Cross A et al. and the Corticosteroid use in MS Task Force, National Clinical Advisory Board of the National MS Society. Recommendations regarding corticosteroids in the management of MS. Expert Opinion Paper. 2008; http://www.nationalmssociety.org/for-professionals/healthcare-professionals/publications/expert-opinio-papers/download.aspx?id=553

Patti F, Reggio E, Palermo F, et al. Stabilization of rapidly worsening MS for 36 months in patients treated with interferon beta plus cyclophosphamide followed by interferon beta. *J Neurol.* 2004;251:1502–1506.

Perini P, Calabrese M, Tiberio M, Ranzato F, BAttistin L, Gallo P. Mitoxantrone vs. cyclophosphamide in secondary progressive MS: a comparative study. *J Neurol.* 2006;253:1034–1040.

Perumal J, Caon C, Hreha R, Tselis A, Lisak R, Khan O. Oral prednisone taper following intravenous steroids fails to improve disability or recover from relapses in MS. *Eur J Neurol.* 2008;15(7):677–680.

Polman C, Barkhof F, Sandberg-Wolheim M, et al. Treatment with laquinomod reduces development of active MRI lesions in relapsing MS. *Neurology.* 2005; 64:840–846.

Ramtahal J, Jacob A, Das K, Boggild M. Sequential maintenance treatment with glatiramer acetate after mitoxantroneissafeandcanlimitexposuretoimmunosuppression in very active, relapsing remitting MS. *J Neurol.* 2006; 253:1160–1164.

Roed H, Langkile A, Sellebjerg F, et al. A double blind randomized, placebo controlled trial of intravenous immunoglobulin treatment in acute optic neuritis. *Neurology.* 2005;64:804–810.

Rose J, Burns J, Bjorklund J, et al. Daclizumab phase ll trial in relapsing and remitting MS: MRI and clinical results. *Neurology.* 2007;69(8):785–789.

Rutschmann O, McCrory D, Matachar D, Immunization Panel of the MS Council for Clinical Practice Guidelines. Immunization and MS: a summary of published evidence and research. *Neurology.* 2002; 59(12):1837–1843.

Saccardi R, Kozak T, Bocelli-Tyndall C, et al. Autologous stem cell transplantation for progressive MS: update of the European Group for Blood and Marrow Transplantation autoimmune diseases working party database. *Mult Scler.* 2006;12:814–823.

Sapir T, Blank M, Shoenfeld. Immunomodulatory effects of intravenous immunoglobulins as a treatment for autoimmune diseases, cancer and recurrent pregnancy loss. *Ann NY Acad Sci.* 2005;1051:743–778.

Sawicka E, DuBois G, Jarai G, et al. The sphingosine-1-phosphate receptor agonist FTY-20 differentially affects the sequestration of CD4+/CD25+ T regulatory cells and enhances their functional activity. *J Immunol.* 2005;176:7973–7978.

Sellebjerg F, Barnes D, Fillipini G, et al. EFNS guideline on treatment of MS relapses: report of an EFNS task force on treatment of MS relapses. *Eur J Neurol.* 2005; 12:939–946.

Scott L, Figett D. Mitoxanrone: a review of its use in MS. *CNS Drugs.* 2004;18(6):379–396.

Sibley W, Bamford C, Clark K, Smith M, Laguna J. A prospective study of physical trauma in MS. *J Neurol Neurosurg Psychiatry.* 1991;54(7):584–589.

Smith D, Weinstock-Guttman B, Cohen J, et al. A randomized blinded trial of combination therapy with cyclophosphamide in patients with active MS on interferon beta. *Mult Scler.* 2005;11:573–582.

Sorensen P, Haas J, Sellebjerg F, Olssen T, Ravnborg M, TARIMS study Group. IV immunoglobulins as add on treatment to methyl prednisolone for acute relapses in MS. *Neurology.* 2004;63:2028–2033.

Sorensen P, Mellgren S, Svenningsson A, et al. NORdic trial of oral methyl prednisolone as add on therapy to interferon beta 1-a for treatment of relapsing remitting MS (NORMIMS study): a randomized placebo controlled trial. *Lancet Neurol.* 2009;8(6):519–529.

Sorensen P, Wanschler B, Jensen C, et al. Intravenous immunoglobulin G reduces MRI activity in relapsing remitting MS. *Neurology.* 1998;50:1273–1281.

Stelmasiak Z, Solski J, Nowicki J, Jakubowska B, Ryba M, Grieb P. Effect of parenteral cladribine on relapse rates in patients with relapsing forms of MS: results of a 2 year, double blind, placebo controlled crossover study. *Mult Scler.* 2009;15:767–770.

Thrower, B. Relapse management in MS. *Neurologist.* 2009;15(1):1–5.

Tselis A, Perumal J, Caon C, et al. Treatment of corticosteroid refractory optic neuritis in MS patients with intravenous immunoglobulin. *Eur J Neurol.* 2008;15(11):1163–1167.

Tumani H. Corticosteroids and plasma exchange in MS. *J Neurol.* 2008;255(suppl 6):36–42.

Vermesch P, Wauquier N, Michellin E, et al. Combination of IFN beta (Avonex®) and mycophenolate mofetil (Cellcept®) in MS. *Eur J Neurol.* 2007;14(1):85–89.

Vollmer T, Panitch H, Bar-Or A, et al. Glatiramer acetate after induction therapy with mitoxantrone in relapsing remitting MS. *Mult Scler.* 2008;14(5):663–670.

Warren K, Ctaz I, Ferenczi L, Krantz M. Intravenous synthetic peptide MBP 8298 delayed disease progression in an HLA class ll defined cohort of patients with progressive MS: results of a 24 month double blind placebo controlled clinical trial and 5 years of follow up treatment. *Eur J Neurol.* 2006;12:887–895.

Weiner H, Mackin G, Orav E, et al. Intermittant cyclophosphamide pulse therapy in progressive MS: final report of the Northeast Cooperative MS Treatment Group. *Neurology.* 1993;43:910–918.

Weinshenker B, O'Brien P, Petterson T, Noseworthy J, Luccinetti C, Dodick D. A randomized trial of plasma exchange in acute central nervous system inflammatory demyelinating disease. *Ann Neurol.* 1999;46:878–886.

Wolf A, Eller K, Zeiser R, et al. The sphingosine receptor agonist FTY-20 potently inhibits regulatory T cell proliferation in vitro and in vivo. *J Immunol.* 2009;183(6):3751–3760.

Yudkin P, Ellison G, Ghezzi A, et al. Overview of azathioprine treatment in MS. *Lancet.* 1991;338:1051–1055.

Zhang J, Rivera V, Tejada-Simon M, et al. T cell vaccination in MS: results of a preliminary clinical trial. *J Neurol.* 2002;249:212–218.

Zipoli V, Portaccio E, Hakiki B, Siracusa G, Sorbi S, Amato M. Intravenous mitoxantrone and cyclophosphamide as second line therapy in MS: an open label comparative study of efficacy and safety. *J Neurol Sci.* 2008;266(1–2):25–30.

Zivadinov R, Rudick R, De Masi R, et al. Effects of IV methylprednisolone on brain atrophy in relapsing remitting MS. *Neurology.* 2001;57:1239–1247.

Zou I, Abbas N, Volkmann I, et al. Suppression of experimental autoimmune neuritis by ABR-215062 is associated with altered Th1/Th2 balance and inhibited migration of inflammatory cells into the peripheral nerve tissue. *Neuropharmacology.* 2002;42:731–739.

25 Complementary and Alternative Medicine in Multiple Sclerosis

Allen C. Bowling

Many multiple sclerosis (MS) patients use complementary and alternative medicine (CAM). However, health professionals may have limited knowledge about CAM therapies and may not even know which CAM therapies are being utilized by patients who are under their care. These CAM therapies may be beneficial or harmful and may interact with conventional MS medications. Thus, quality of care may be improved if clinicians have the skills and knowledge to provide unbiased, evidence-based CAM information to patients and, when appropriate, to guide patients away from harmful or ineffective therapies and toward low-risk, possibly effective therapies.

This chapter provides information to practicing clinicians so that they will be able to guide and inform their MS patients about CAM. General background information about CAM is presented. In addition, there is a review of basic safety and efficacy information about CAM therapies that are likely to be encountered in day-to-day interactions with MS patients. This chapter is *not* intended to be an extensive evaluation of all of the available MS-relevant CAM therapies or to provide an in-depth analysis of CAM clinical studies; reviews with broader scopes and more detailed analyses may be found elsewhere (Bowling and Stewart, 2003, 2004; Stewart and Bowling, 2005; Polman et al., 2006; Bowling, 2007).

TERMINOLOGY

There are many different terms and definitions in the area of unconventional medicine. *Unconventional medicine* usually refers to forms of medicine that are not generally available in hospitals or widely taught in medical schools (Eisenberg et al., 1998).

The terms *complementary* and *alternative* refer to the ways in which these unconventional medical practices are used. *Complementary* indicates that they are used *in conjunction with* conventional medicine, while *alternative* means that they are used *instead of* conventional medicine. The term that is inclusive of both approaches is *complementary and alternative medicine*, or *CAM*. *Integrative medicine* is the combined use of conventional and unconventional medicine.

CONVENTIONAL AND UNCONVENTIONAL MEDICINE

Over the past decade, there have been remarkable advances in understanding, diagnosing, and treating MS. While MS treatment options were limited in the past, there are now many conventional medical therapies for modifying the disease course and alleviating symptoms.

Despite the significant advances, conventional treatment options for MS have limitations. Disease-modifying and symptomatic therapies may only be partially effective or may produce side effects. Additionally, proven therapies may be limited or nonexistent, especially for progressive forms of MS and for specific symptoms, such as weakness, incoordination, and gait disorders.

Due to the limitations of conventional medicine, as well as other reasons, many MS patients are interested in, and use, CAM. In studies in the United States (Berkman et al., 1999; Nayak et al., 2003; Shinto et al., 2006) as well as Canada (Page et al., 2003), Australia (Hooper et al., 2001), and Europe (Stenager et al., 1995; Apel et al., 2006), one-half to three-fourths of those with MS report using some form of CAM. In the United States,

40%–50% of the general population use some form of CAM (Eisenberg et al., 1998; Barnes et al., 2004). Among MS patients (Berkman et al., 1999), as well as the general population (Eisenberg et al., 1998), the majority of those who use CAM do so in combination with conventional medicine.

MULTIPLE SCLEROSIS-RELEVANT COMPLEMENTARY AND ALTERNATIVE MEDICINE THERAPIES

The remainder of this chapter provides evidence-based information about MS-relevant CAM therapies. This review will consider therapies that are relatively popular or have undergone MS-relevant investigation.

Acupuncture and Traditional Chinese Medicine

Acupuncture is one component of the ancient multimodal therapeutic approach known as traditional Chinese medicine (TCM). Other TCM components include herbs, nutrition, exercise, stress reduction, and massage (Bowling, 2007).

Efficacy

Studies of TCM in MS are limited. Trials of acupuncture for treating symptoms in MS patients are too limited to provide definitive information (Spoerel et al., 1974; Smith and Rabinowitz, 1986; Bowling, 2007; Donnelan and Shanley, 2008). In other conditions, acupuncture appears to relieve pain as well as nausea and vomiting (NIH Consensus Development Panel on Acupuncture, 1998; Bowling, 2007). There are no rigorous studies of Chinese herbs in MS (Bowling, 2007).

Safety

Acupuncture is generally well tolerated when performed by a well-trained practitioner (Bowling, 2007). In contrast, Chinese herbal medicine is of unknown safety in many medical conditions, including MS. Immune system activation, a theoretical risk for worsening MS or antagonizing the therapeutic effects of immune-modulating MS medications, may be caused by multiple Chinese herbs, including Asian ginseng, astragalus, and maitake and reishi mushrooms (Bowling and Stewart, 2004).

Conclusion

Acupuncture is a component of TCM that is low risk and moderately expensive. It is not well studied in MS, but, based on studies in other conditions, it may alleviate pain. In contrast, Chinese herbal therapy, which is also a component of TCM, is moderately expensive and has theoretical risks and unknown efficacy in MS.

Bee Venom Therapy

Bee venom therapy (BVT) is a form of *apitherapy*, which refers to the use of bees or bee products to treat medical conditions. In BVT, bees are placed on specific body parts with tweezers (Bowling, 2007).

Efficacy

The highest quality clinical trial of BVT in MS was conducted in the Netherlands in 2004 (Wesselius et al., 2005). This randomized crossover study of 26 patients with relapsing-remitting or secondary-progressive MS found that BVT did not produce any beneficial effects with measures of magnetic resonance imaging (MRI) lesions, attack frequency, neurological disability, fatigue, and overall quality of life.

Safety

Bee venom therapy is generally well tolerated (Castro et al., 2008)). Very rarely, bee stings cause anaphylaxis. Bee stings around the eye, which are sometimes claimed to relieve MS-related visual problems, should actually be avoided because they may cause optic neuritis (Song and Wray, 1991).

Conclusion

Bee venom therapy is a low–moderate cost, generally safe therapy that has not been shown to produce therapeutic effects in MS.

Chiropractic Medicine

Chiropractic medicine is one of the most popular types of CAM in the United States. Chiropractors believe that subluxations, which are misalignments of the vertebrae, cause muscle and organ dysfunction by exerting abnormal pressure on the nerves that travel from the spinal cord to muscles and organs (Bowling, 2007).

Efficacy

There are no well-designed studies that demonstrate that spinal manipulation (or other chiropractic methods) improves the disease course or symptoms of MS patients (Elster, 2004; Bowling, 2007). In studies of variable quality, it has been shown that spinal manipulation may decrease low back pain (Ernst, 2002; Hurwitz et al., 2002), a condition to which MS patients may be prone. There are not any rigorous studies that demonstrate that chiropractic treatment is effective for neck pain or headache (Smith et al., 2003).

Safety

Chiropractic treatment is generally well tolerated. A rare but serious complication of neck manipulation is stroke due to vertebral artery dissection (Smith et al., 2003). Very rarely, low back manipulation may cause cauda equina syndrome (Ernst, 2002; Bowling, 2007). Manipulation should be avoided by pregnant women, patients who take anticoagulant medications, and patients with spine fractures, spine trauma, significant disc herniations, cancers or infections of bone, severe osteoporosis, and severe arthritis (Bowling, 2007).

Conclusion

There are no well-designed studies that demonstrate that chiropractic spinal manipulation alters the disease course of MS or alleviates MS-specific symptoms. For low back pain, spinal manipulation is generally well tolerated and may be effective. In contrast, for other conditions, it has not been demonstrated to be effective. For neck pain, spinal manipulation may rarely cause strokes.

Cooling Therapy

Cooling is a CAM therapy that is unique to MS. Small increases in body temperature (0.5°C) may worsen MS symptoms. Likewise, small decreases in body temperature may improve symptoms (Guthrie and Nelson, 1995; Bowling, 2007).

Thus, for MS patients, various cooling methods have been developed. These methods range from simple strategies, such as drinking cold liquids and/or staying in air-conditioned areas, to complex methods, such as wearing specially designed cooling garments (Bowling, 2007).

Efficacy

Several small studies of variable quality have reported that cooling garments produce alleviate MS symptoms, especially fatigue (Bowling, 2007). There is one rigorous clinical trial of cooling in MS (NASA/MS Cooling Study Group, 2003). This randomized, controlled, blinded study found that, by objective measures, cooling was associated with mildly improved visual function and walking. On the basis of subjective measures, cooling improved fatigue, cognition, and strength. Cooling may be more effective in those who are known to be heat sensitive.

Safety

Cooling is usually usually well tolerated. The garments may be cumbersome. There may be a feeling of discomfort when cooling begins. Rarely, MS patients have a paradoxical sensitivity to cold; for those patients, cooling may actually worsen symptoms (Bowling, 2007).

Conclusion

Cooling is a low-risk, relatively inexpensive therapy that may relieve multiple MS symptoms, especially fatigue.

Dental Amalgam Removal

Dental amalgam removal has been claimed to treat MS. It has been proposed that amalgam causes MS or worsens MS by electrical currents generated by mercury, by allergic reactions to mercury, or by the slow release of solid mercury or mercury vapors (Bowling, 2007).

Efficacy

Although there are anecdotal reports of MS patients who have experienced beneficial effects with amalgam removal, there is no convincing clinical evidence that mercury causes MS or that removal of dental amalgam improves the course of MS (NIH Conference Assessment, 1992; Casetta et al., 2001; Bowling, 2007).

Safety

Amalgam removal is generally well tolerated. It may rarely damage tooth structure or injure nerves. Shortly after amalgam removal, there may actually be an *increase* in blood mercury levels (Eley and Cox, 1993; Ekstrand et al., 1998).

Conclusion

Amalgam removal is a moderately expensive, generally safe procedure that has not been demonstrated to produce symptomatic or disease-modifying effects in MS.

Dietary Supplements: Antioxidants

Free radical-induced oxidative damage has been implicated in the pathogenesis of myelin and axonal injury in MS. Thus, it is claimed that antioxidants may be beneficial for MS (Bowling and Stewart, 2003; Van Meeteren et al., 2005).

Efficacy

Specific studies of antioxidants in MS, especially clinical trials, are limited. In the animal model of MS, multiple antioxidant compounds have produced therapeutic effects (Marracci et al., 2002; Scott et al., 2002). Small, short-term MS clinical trials with various antioxidant regimens, including inosine (Spitsin et al., 2001), alpha-lipoic acid (Yadav et al., 2005), and a combination of selenium and vitamins C and E (Mai et al., 1990) indicate that these approaches are well tolerated. The studies thus far have not been powered adequately to determine efficacy.

Safety

Many antioxidant compounds activate immune cells, including T cells and macrophages (Bowling and Stewart, 2003, 2004). Consequently, these compounds pose theoretical risks for MS patients. However, as noted, the limited clinical trials to date indicate that antioxidants are generally well tolerated and have not produced adverse effects in MS patients.

Conclusion

Antioxidants are inexpensive and could, on the basis of theoretical and experimental evidence, have a therapeutic effect in MS. However, definitive clinical trials in MS have not been reported and there are theoretical risks associated with antioxidant use in MS. Further studies, which are currently underway, should provide more definitive information about the safety and efficacy of antioxidants in MS.

Dietary Supplements: Cranberry

Patients with MS are prone to bladder dysfunction, including urinary tract infections (UTIs). Cranberry may prevent UTIs through a novel mechanism of action in which constituents of the herb inhibit bacterial adhesion to uroepithelial cells (Raz et al., 2004; Bowling, 2007).

Efficacy

Multiple studies indicate that cranberry may be effective for *preventing* UTIs, especially in women with normal bladder function (Linsenmeyer et al., 2004; Waites et al., 2004; Hess et al., 2008; Jepson and Craig, 2008). There is not evidence to support the use of cranberry for *treating* UTIs. Importantly, MS patients may experience neurological decline (known as a *pseudoexacerbation*) in the setting of UTIs. Thus, clinicians should be vigilant for UTIs among MS patients, and, for those who are found to have UTIs, antibiotics (not cranberry) should be used promptly.

Safety

Cranberry is usually well tolerated. It may increase the anticoagulant effect of warfarin (Coumadin) (Suvarna, 2003). Long-term use may increase the risk of developing kidney stones (Jellin et al., 2008).

Conclusion

Cranberry is a low-risk, generally well-tolerated therapy that may *prevent* UTIs. It should not be used to *treat* UTIs.

Dietary Supplements: Echinacea and Other "Immune-Stimulating" Supplements

Some lay books on alternative medicine state erroneously that, since MS is an immune disease, MS patients should take echinacea and other dietary supplements that are known to activate T cells and macrophages (Bowling et al., 2000). This is misleading and potentially dangerous information.

Efficacy

Studies of immune system activation by dietary supplements are generally restricted to in vitro or animal model studies. Thus, the concerns with these supplements are theoretical risks. Commonly used herbs that have been shown to activate T cells or macrophages include echinacea, alfalfa, ashwagandha (*Withania somnifera*), Asian ginseng, astragalus, cat's claw, garlic, maitake mushroom, mistletoe, shiitake mushroom, Siberian ginseng, and stinging nettle (Bowling and Stewart, 2004). Other supplements with "immune-stimulating" effects include melatonin, zinc, and antioxidant vitamins and minerals (Bowling and Stewart, 2004) (see section on "Dietary Supplements: Antioxidants").

Safety

As noted, immune-stimulating supplements pose theoretical risks for MS patients. In addition, echinacea may increase the hepatotoxicity of medications, which include some MS medications such as methotrexate and interferons (Bowling and Stewart, 2004; Jellin et al., 2008).

Conclusion

There is no documented therapeutic effect for echinacea and other immune-stimulating supplements in MS. In fact, these compounds, which are of low–moderate cost, pose theoretical risks to those with MS.

Dietary Supplements: Ginkgo Biloba

Ginkgo biloba, an extract derived from the leaf of the *Ginkgo biloba* tree, could have disease-modifying as well as symptomatic effects in MS. Ginkgo exerts anti-inflammatory and antioxidant effects (Bowling and Stewart, 2003; Bowling, 2007).

Efficacy

In the animal model of MS, some, but not all, studies indicate that ginkgo decreases disease severity (Bowling and Stewart, 2003). In MS patients, ginkgo does not appear to be effective for treating attacks (Brochet et al., 1995). In small clinical studies in MS, ginkgo improved cognition (Lovera et al., 2007) and fatigue (Johnson et al., 2006).

Safety

Ginkgo is usually well tolerated. It has anticoagulant effects and may rarely provoke seizures (Bowling and Stewart, 2007; Jellin et al., 2008). Thus, it should be avoided or used with caution by those with seizure disorders and those who have coagulopathies, take antiplatelet or anticoagulant medication, or are undergoing surgery. It may also cause dizziness, rashes, headaches, nausea, vomiting, diarrhea, and flatulence (Bowling and Stewart, 2004; Jellin et al., 2008).

Conclusion

Ginkgo is an inexpensive, generally well-tolerated therapy that, in limited MS clinical studies, has improved fatigue and cognitive dysfunction. Further studies are needed to determine definitively the safety and efficacy of ginkgo in MS.

Dietary Supplements: Kava Kava

Anxiety is a relatively common MS symptom. Kava kava, an anti-anxiety herb derived from the root of the kava plant, contains compounds that, like benzodiazepines, interact with gamma-aminobutyric acid (GABA) receptors (Bowling and Stewart, 2004; Jellin et al., 2008).

Efficacy

Several clinical trials indicate that kava kava may be an effective therapy for mild anxiety (Russo, 2001).

Safety

Kava kava was previously thought to be a generally safe herb. However, since 2001, kava kava use has been associated with more than 50 cases of liver toxicity, some of which have led to death or liver transplantation (Clouatre, 2004; Jellin et al., 2008). Due to toxicity concerns, kava kava is banned in Europe and Canada. Kava kava is available in the United States.

Conclusion

Kava kava is inexpensive and may be effective for mild anxiety. However, it should not be used because of possible severe liver toxicity.

Dietary Supplements: St. John's Wort

St. John's wort has been used for more than 2000 years to treat depression (Bowling, 2007; Jellin et al., 2008), a relatively common MS symptom.

Efficacy

St. John's wort appears to be effective for mild–moderate depression. There is no evidence that it is effective for severe depression (Werneke et al., 2004; Jellin et al., 2008).

Safety

St. John's wort is generally well tolerated. It may cause fatigue and photosensitivity (Bowling and Stewart, 2004; Jellin et al., 2008). Also, since it induces cytochrome P-450 enzymes, St. John's wort may alter levels of many medications, including anticonvulsants, warfarin (Coumadin), antidepressants, and oral contraceptives (Izzo, 2004; Jellin et al., 2008).

Conclusion

St. John's wort is an inexpensive, generally safe, herbal therapy that may be effective for mild–moderate

depression. It may interact with prescription medications.

Dietary Supplements: Valerian

Valerian has been used as an herbal therapy for more than 1000 years. It is generally used for insomnia, a condition to which MS patients are prone (Bowling, 2007; Jellin et al., 2008).

Efficacy

Several studies of variable quality indicate that valerian may be effective for insomnia (Mischoulon and Rosenbaum, 2002). It is sometimes claimed to be effective for anxiety, depression, and spasticity, but it has not been rigorously evaluated for these conditions.

Safety

Valerian is usually well tolerated. It may cause sedation (Bowling and Stewart, 2004; Jellin et al., 2008).

Conclusion

Valerian is inexpensive and generally well tolerated. It may be effective for insomnia.

Dietary Supplements: Vitamin B12

It is sometimes claimed that vitamin B12 supplements are effective for treating MS.

Efficacy

There is no convincing evidence that vitamin B12 supplements provide clinically significant therapeutic effects to MS patients generally (Kira et al., 1994; Loder et al., 2002; Wade et al., 2002; Bowling, 2007) A small fraction of MS patients have vitamin B12 deficiency (Goodkin et al., 1994); for these patients, vitamin B12 supplementation is needed.

Safety

Vitamin B12 supplements are generally well tolerated. Rarely, they may cause rashes, itching, and diarrhea (Jellin et al., 2008).

Conclusion

Vitamin B12 supplements are inexpensive and generally safe. For MS patients with normal vitamin B12 levels, vitamin B12 supplements do not provide any definite beneficial effect. For MS patients with low vitamin B12 levels, oral or intramuscular vitamin B12 supplementation is recommended.

Dietary Supplements: Vitamin D

Two aspects of vitamin D biochemistry are relevant to MS. First, in terms of symptomatic effects, vitamin D is important for maintaining bone density and MS patients are at risk for developing osteopenia and osteoporosis (Weinstock-Guttman et al., 2004). Also, vitamin D has important immunomodulatory effects and thus could have a disease-modifying effect in MS (Smolders et al., 2008).

Efficacy

Several studies indicate that low vitamin D levels and low vitamin D intake are associated with increased risk for developing MS (Munger et al., 2004, 2006). Definitive studies, especially well-designed trials, of vitamin D supplementation as a preventive strategy or disease-modifying treatment in MS have not been reported (Fleming et al., 2000; Wingerchuk et al., 2005).

Safety

High doses of vitamin D may cause fatigue, abdominal cramps, nausea, vomiting, renal damage, hypertension, and multiple other side effects. The tolerable upper intake level (UL) of vitamin D is 2000 international units (IU) daily. The adequate intake (AI) of vitamin D is 200 to 600 IU daily (Bowling and Stewart, 2004; Jellin et al., 2008).

Conclusion

Vitamin D is a low-cost, generally safe therapy that should be considered in MS patients who are at risk for low bone density or who are known to have decreased bone density. Vitamin D could have preventive and disease-modifying effects in MS, but additional studies are needed in this area.

Diets: The Swank Diet and Other Polyunsaturated Fatty Acid-Enriched Diets

Dietary approaches are among the most popular CAM therapies used by MS patients. Scientific, epidemiologic, animal model, and clinical trial studies provide suggestive evidence for MS disease-modifying effects of diets that are low in saturated fats and high in polyunsaturated fatty acids (PUFAs). Polyunsaturated fatty acids include omega- and omega-s fatty acids (Stewart and Bowling, 2005; Bowling, 2007).

Efficacy

A broad-based dietary approach that is low in saturated fat and high in PUFAs was developed by Swank and Dugan. This diet, which is known as the "Swank diet," was reported to produce therapeutic effects in MS. However, the significance of these findings is not known because the trial was not controlled, blinded, or randomized (Swank, 1970; Swank and Dugan, 1990; Stewart and Bowling, 2005).

More rigorous trials have evaluated supplementation with specific PUFAs. For omega-6 supplementation, there have been three randomized controlled trials (Millar et al., 1973; Bates et al., 1978; Paty, 1983). Two of these trials reported a statistically significant decrease in attack severity and duration. The available data from all three trials were later pooled, reanalyzed, and found to show therapeutic effects on disability progression in those with mild MS at the start of the trial (Dworkin et al., 1984).

Limited studies have evaluated omega-3 supplementation. The most rigorous study to date, a large, randomized, double-blind, controlled trial, did not find a statistically significant treatment effect (Bates et al., 1989). However, for disability progression, there was a trend that favored the treatment group ($p < 0.07$). In another small randomized trial of omega-3 fatty acid supplements in combination with glatiramer acetate or interferons, there was a trend for improved physical and emotional functioning in those taking omega-3 fatty acids (Weinstock-Guttman et al., 2005).

Safety

Omega-3 and omega-6 supplements are usually well tolerated. In the United States, the Food and Drug Administration (FDA) has classified fish oil, a rich source of omega-3 fatty acids, as "generally regarded as safe." The long-term safety of supplementation with other omega-3 fatty acids and all omega-6 fatty acids is not known. Omega-6 fatty acids may raise triglyceride levels and may rarely provoke seizures. Some omega-3 and omega-6 fatty acids may have mild anticoagulant effects. Since supplementation with PUFAs (omega-3 or omega-6) may cause vitamin E deficiency, supplementation with modest doses of vitamin E may be indicated (Stewart and Bowling, 2005; Jellin et al., 2008).

Conclusion

Polyunsaturated fatty acid–enriched diets are inexpensive and generally well tolerated. These dietary strategies have produced suggestive results in MS clinical trials. Further studies are needed to determine whether these strategies are definitely effective in MS. These diets should not be used *instead of* conventional disease-modifying medications. The safety and effectiveness of these diets in combination with disease-modifying medications (interferons, glatiramer acetate, mitoxantrone, and natalizumab) have not been rigorously studied.

Guided Imagery

Guided imagery is a relaxation method in which an individual creates mental images that produce relaxation and may have specific effects on the mind and the body. Guided imagery may be used in combination with other relaxation methods, such as progressive muscle relaxation (Bowling, 2007).

Efficacy

One small study in MS ($n = 33$) found that guided imagery reduced anxiety but had no effect on depression or many other MS symptoms (Maguire, 1996). Limited studies of guided imagery in other conditions have found possible therapeutic effects on anxiety, depression, pain, and insomnia (Bowling, 2007).

Safety

Guided imagery is generally well tolerated. Relaxation may provoke spasticity. Guided imagery may cause fear of losing control, anxiety, and disturbing thoughts, especially in those with psychiatric conditions (Bowling, 2007).

Conclusion

Guided imagery is inexpensive, and generally well tolerated. It may decrease anxiety and several other MS-associated symptoms.

Hyperbaric Oxygen

Hyperbaric oxygen (HBO) has been claimed to be an effective treatment for MS as well as many other diseases. Hyperbaric oxygen is a recognized medical therapy, but only for a limited number of specific conditions, including burns, severe infections, decompression sickness, carbon monoxide poisoning, and radiation-induced tissue injury (Bowling, 2007).

Efficacy

One study in the 1980s reported that HBO was an effective therapy for MS (Fischer et al., 1983). However, multiple subsequent studies did not generally find significant therapeutic effects. Two independent reviews of the various HBO trials in MS concluded that HBO did not produce consistent therapeutic effects and that HBO should not be used to treat MS (Kleijnen and Knipschild, 1995; Bennett and Heard, 2004).

Safety

Hyperbaric oxygen is usually well tolerated. It may cause mild visual symptoms. Rare side effects include seizures, pressure injury to the ear, cataracts, and pneumothorax (Bowling, 2007).

Conclusion

Hyperbaric oxygen is expensive, associated with rare, but serious side effects, and does not produce any consistent therapeutic effects in MS.

Low-Dose Naltrexone

In MS, it is claimed that low doses of oral naltrexone, an opiate antagonist, relieve symptoms, prevent attacks, and slow disability progression. It has been proposed that low-dose naltrexone (LDN) is therapeutic for MS due to partial opiate agonist, excitotoxic, or antioxidant mechanisms (Bowling, 2007; Gironi et al., 2008).

Efficacy

Although there are many anecdotal reports about the benefits of LDN in MS, published studies of this therapy are limited. In the animal model of MS, two preliminary studies found that LDN decreased immune cell activation, nervous system inflammation, and disease severity (Rahn et al., 2008a, 2008b). The preliminary report of an 8-week study of 80 people with relapsing or progressive MS found that LDN did not affect physical functioning but did improve pain and mental health (Cree et al., 2008). An open-label, 6-month study of LDN in 40 people with primary progressive MS found that LDN was generally well tolerated (Gironi et al., 2008). Although this study was designed primarily to assess safety, it did have some efficacy outcome measures and found that LDN was associated with improvement in spasticity, worsening of pain, and had no effect on depression, fatigue, or overall quality of life.

Safety

In the limited studies in MS, LDN has generally been well tolerated. In the study of primary progressive MS, one patient had neurological worsening (Gironi et al., 2008).

Conclusion

Recent studies indicate that LDN, which is of moderate expense, may be well tolerated and produce beneficial effects in MS. However, these studies are preliminary and limited. Further studies are needed to be certain about the safety and efficacy of this therapy in MS.

Marijuana (Cannabis)

In studies of the possible therapeutic relevance of marijuana to MS, the pharmacology has been intriguing and animal as well as human studies have produced suggestive results. Marijuana, also known as cannabis, contains chemicals known as cannabinoids (CBs), which include tetrahydrocannabinol (THC). Cannabinoids suppress excessive neuronal activity and thus could theoretically relieve some MS symptoms, such as pain and spasticity. In addition, through immune-modulating and neuroprotective actions, CBs could have disease-modifying effects in MS (Bowling, 2003, 2006).

Efficacy

Cannabinoids have symptomatic and disease-modifying effects in the animal model of MS. A large, rigorous clinical trial of marijuana in MS found that CBs produce subjective, but not objective, evidence for symptomatic relief (Zajicek et al., 2003). A 12-month follow-up to this trial found that THC had a small treatment effect on spasticity and a possible effect on disability (Zajicek et al., 2005). In several studies of variable quality, an orally administered form of cannabis (*Sativex*) relieved multiple MS symptoms, including pain, spasticity, and sleeping difficulties (Barnes, 2006).

Safety

Marijuana has many possible adverse effects. It may cause sedation, increased risk of seizures, nausea, vomiting, impaired driving, incoordination, poor pregnancy outcomes, decreased lung function, and increased risk of cancer of the head, neck, and lung (Bowling and Stewart, 2004; Bowling, 2007).

Conclusion

Scientific and clinical studies indicate that marijuana may have symptomatic and disease-modifying effects in MS. Importantly, however, these findings are not definitive. In addition, marijuana may produce significant side effects and is illegal in many countries. Further studies of marijuana in MS are needed. Toward that end, a large study of cannabis (the *CUPID* study) in progressive MS is underway in the United Kingdom.

Massage

Massage is one of the oldest medical therapies. It is a form of bodywork in which soft tissue is manipulated with traction and pressure (Bowling, 2007).

Efficacy

Few studies have formally evaluated the effects of massage therapy in people with MS. In the largest study to date, 24 people with MS were assigned to receive either "standard medical care" or standard medical care in combination with twice-weekly, in-home, massage therapy (Hernandez-Reif et al., 1998). Over the course of the 5-week study, the treatment group exhibited improvement in anxiety, depression, self-esteem, body image, social functioning, and "image of disease progression." More rigorous studies of massage in MS are needed.

Safety

Massage is usually well tolerated. Mild side effects include headache, lethargy, and muscle pain. Rarely, massage may cause more serious side effects, including bone fractures and hepatic bleeding. Massage should be avoided or used with caution by pregnant women and by those with thrombosis, burns, skin infections, open wounds, bone fractures, osteoporosis, cancer, and heart disease (Bowling, 2007).

Conclusion

Massage is a low–moderate cost therapy that is generally well tolerated and has produced promising results in one small MS study. Further studies must be done to determine whether massage is definitely effective for treating MS symptoms.

Tai Chi

Tai chi is a martial art that has been practiced for centuries in China. It has undergone limited investigation in MS (Bowling, 2007).

Efficacy

Small, nonblinded studies of tai chi in MS have produced suggestive beneficial effects on spasticity, walking, and social and emotional functioning (Husted et al., 1999; Mills and Allen, 2000).

Safety

Tai chi is usually well tolerated. There is a risk of falling. It may cause mild side effects, such as strained muscles and joints. Tai chi may be modified for those with disabilities. It should be avoided or used with caution by those with severe osteoporosis, acute low back pain, significant joint injuries, or bone fractures (Bowling, 2007).

Conclusion

Tai chi is low–moderate cost and is generally well tolerated. It has produced improvement in multiple symptoms in limited MS studies. Larger and more rigorous studies of tai chi in MS are needed.

Yoga

Yoga was developed in India thousands of years ago. It is widely practiced yet has undergone limited clinical investigation (Bowling, 2007).

Efficacy

In MS, one well-designed, controlled trial found that, relative to controls, those who practiced yoga or did conventional exercise had significantly less fatigue (Oken et al., 2004).

Safety

Yoga is generally safe. It may be modified for people with disabilities. Difficult postures or vigorous exercise should be avoided or done with caution by pregnant women and those with fatigue, heat sensitivity, gait instability, or significant lung, heart, or bone conditions (Bowling, 2007).

Conclusion

Yoga is a low-cost, generally safe therapy that may decrease fatigue in MS. Further studies of yoga in MS are needed.

CONCLUSION

Using CAM for a complex disease such as MS requires thoughtful consideration. Within the context of MS, some CAM therapies are possibly beneficial, while others are unstudied, ineffective, or potentially harmful. Conventional health providers may play an important role in the care of MS patients by differentiating CAM therapies that may have a reasonable efficacy-safety profile from those that are ineffective, unstudied, or unsafe.

REFERENCES

Apel A, Greim B, Konig N, Zettl UK. Frequency of current utilisation of complementary and alternative medicine by patients with multiple sclerosis. *J Neurol.* 2006; 253:1331–1336.

Barnes MP. Sativex: clinical efficacy and tolerability in the treatment of symptoms of multiple sclerosis and neuropathic pain. *Expert Opin Pharmacother.* 2006;7:607–615.

Barnes PM, Powell-Griner E, McFann K, Nahin RL. Complementary and alternative medicine use among adults: United States, 2002. *Adv Data.* 2004;343: 1–20.

Bates D, Cartlidge N, French J, et al. A double-blind controlled trial of long chain n-3 polyunsaturated fatty acids in the treatment of multiple sclerosis. *J Neurol Neurosurg Psychiatry.* 1989;52:18–22.

Bates D, Fawcett P, Shaw D, Weightman D. Polyunsaturated fatty acids in treatment of acute remitting multiple sclerosis. *Brit Med J.* 1978;2:1390–1391.

Bennett M, Heard R. Hyperbaric oxygen therapy for multiple sclerosis. *Cochrane DB Sys Rev.* 2004;1: CD003057.

Berkman C, Pignotti M, Cavallo P, Holland NJ. Use of alternative treatments by people with multiple sclerosis. *Neurorehabil Neural Repair.* 1999;13:243–254.

Bowling AC. Worthless weed or pot of gold? *Int J MS Care.* 2003;5:138, 166.

Bowling AC. Cannabinoids in MS—are we any closer to knowing how best to use them? *Mult Scler.* 2006; 12:523–525.

Bowling AC. Complementary and Alternative Medicine and Multiple Sclerosis. New York: Demos Medical Publishing; 2007.

Bowling AC, Ibrahim R, Stewart TM. Alternative medicine and multiple sclerosis: an objective review from an American perspective. *Int J MS Care.* 2000;2:14–21.

Bowling AC, Stewart TM. Current complementary and alternative therapies of multiple sclerosis. *Curr Treat Options Neurol.* 2003;5:55–68.

Bowling AC, Stewart TM. Dietary Supplements and Multiple Sclerosis: A Health Professional's Guide. New York: Demos Medical Publishing; 2004.

Brochet B, Guinot P, Orgogozo J, Confavreux C, Rumbach L, Lavergne V. Double-blind, placebo controlled, multicentre study of ginkgolide B in treatment of acute exacerbations for multiple sclerosis. The Ginkgolide Study Group in multiple sclerosis. *J Neurol Neurosurg Psychiatry.* 1995;58:360–362.

Casetta I, Invernizzi M, Granieri E. Multiple sclerosis and dental amalgam: case control study in Ferrara, Italy. *Neuroepidemiology.* 2001;20:134–137.

Castro HJ, Mendez-Lnocencio JI, Omidvar B, et al. A phase I study of the safety of honeybee venom extract as a possible treatment for patients with progressive forms of multiple sclerosis. *Allergy Asthma Proc.* 2008;26:470–476.

Clouatre DL. Kava kava: examining new reports of toxicity. *Toxicol Lett.* 2004;150:85–96.

Cree BA, Goodin DS, Ross M, Kornyeyeva E. Low dose naltrexone improves quality of life in patients with multiple sclerosis: a randomized, masked, placebo-controlled trial. *Mult Scler.* 2008;14:S295.

Donnelan CP, Shanley J. Comparison of the effect of two types of acupuncture on quality of life in secondary progressive multiple sclerosis: a preliminary single-blind randomized controlled trial. *Clin Rehabil.* 2008; 22:195–205.

Dworkin R, Bates D, Millar J, Paty DW. Linoleic acid and multiple sclerosis: a reanalysis of three double-blind trials. *Neurology.* 1984;34:1441–1445.

Eisenberg D, Davis R, Ettner S, et al. Trends in alternative medicine use in the United States, 1990–1997. *JAMA.* 1998;280:1569–1575.

Ekstrand J, Bjorkman L, Edlund C, Sandborgh-Englund G. Toxicological aspects on the release and systemic uptake of mercury from dental amalgam. *Eur J Oral Sci.* 1998;106:678–686.

Eley BM, Cox SW. The release, absorption, and possible health effects of mercury from dental amalgam: a review of recent findings. *Brit Dental J.* 1993;175:355–362.

Elster E. Eighty-one patients with multiple sclerosis and Parkinson's disease undergoing upper cervical chiropractic care to correct vertebral subluxation: a retrospective analysis. *J Vertebral Sublux Res.* 2004;23:1–9.

Ernst E. Chiropractic care: attempting a risk-benefit analysis. *Am J Public Health.* 2002;92:1603–1604.

Fischer BH, Marks M, Reich T. Hyperbaric oxygen treatment of multiple sclerosis. A randomized, placebo-controlled, double-blind study. *New Eng J Med.* 1983; 308:181–186.

Fleming JO, Hummel AL, Beinlich BR, et al. Vitamin D treatment of relapsing-remitting multiple sclerosis (RRMS): a MRI-based pilot study. *Neurology.* 2000; 54:A338.

Gironi M, Martinelli-Boneschi F, Sacerdote P, et al. A pilot trial of low-dose naltrexone in primary progressive multiple sclerosis. *Mult Scler.* 2008;14:1076–1083.

Goodkin D, Jacobsen D, Galvez N, Daughtry M, Secic M, Green R. Serum cobalamin deficiency is uncommon in multiple sclerosis. *Arch Neurol.* 1994;51:1110–1114.

Guthrie TC, Nelson DA. Influence of temperature changes on multiple sclerosis: critical review of mechanisms and research potential. *J Neurol Sci.* 1995;29:1–8.

Hernandez-Reif M, Field T, Field T, et al. Multiple sclerosis patients benefit from massage therapy. *J Bodywork Movement Ther.* 1998;2:168–174.

Hess MJ, Hess PE, Sullivan MR, Nee M, Yalla SV. Evaluation of cranberry tablets for the prevention of urinary tract infections in spinal cord injured patients with neurogenic bladder. *Spinal Cord.* 2008;46: 622–626.

Hooper KD, Pender MP, Webb PM. Use of traditional and complementary medical care by patients with multiple sclerosis in South-East Queensland. *Int J MS Care.* 2001;3:13–28.

Hurwitz IL, Morganstern H, Harber P, et al. A randomized trial of medical care with and without physical therapy and chiropractic care with and without physical modalities for patients with low back pain: 6-month follow-up outcomes from the UCLA back pain study. *Spine.* 2002;27:2193–2204.

Husted C, Pham L, Hekking A. Improving quality of life for people with chronic conditions: the example of t'ai chi and multiple sclerosis. *Altern Ther Health Med.* 1999; 5:70–74.

Izzo AA. Drug interactions with St. John's wort (Hypericum perforatum): review of the clinical evidence. *Int J Clin Pharmacol Ther.* 2004;42:139–148.

Jellin JM, Gregory PJ, Batz F, Bonakdar R. *Pharmacist's Letter/Prescriber's Letter Natural Medicines Comprehensive Database.* 8th ed. Stockton, CA: Therapeutic Research Faculty; 2008.

Jepson RG, Craig JC. Cranberries for preventing urinary tract infections. *Cochrane DB Sys Rev.* 2008;CD001321.

Johnson SK, Diamond BJ, Rausch S, Kaufman M, Shiflett SC, Graves L. The effect of Ginkgo biloba on functional measure in multiple sclerosis: a pilot randomized controlled trial. *Explore (NY).* 2006;2:19–24.

Kira J, Tobimatus S, Goto I. Vitamin B12 metabolism and massive-dose methyl vitamin B12 therapy in Japanese patients with multiple sclerosis. *Int Med.* 1994;33: 82–86.

Kleijnen J, Knipschild P. Hyberbaric oxygen for multiple sclerosis: review of controlled trials. *Acta Neurol Scand.* 1995;91:330–334.

Linsenmeyer T, Harrison B, Oakley A, Kirshblum S, Stock JA, Millis SR. Evaluation of cranberry supplement for reduction of urinary tract infections in individuals with neurogenic bladders secondary to spinal cord injury. A prospective, double blinded, placebo-controlled, crossover study. *J Spinal Cord Med.* 2004;27:29–34.

Loder C, Allawi J, Horrobin DF. Treatment of multiple sclerosis with lofepramine, L-phenylalanine, and vitamin B-12: mechanism of action and clinical importance: roles of the locus coeruleus and central noradrenergic systems. *Med Hyp.* 2002;59:594–602.

Lovera J, Bagert B, Smoot K, et al. Ginkgo biloba for the improvement of cognitive performance in multiple sclerosis: a randomized, placebo-controlled trial. *Mult Scler.* 2007;13:376–85.

Maguire BL. The effects of imagery on attitudes and moods in multiple sclerosis patients. *Altern Ther Health Med.* 1996;2:75–79.

Mai J, Sorenson P, Hansen J. High dose antioxidant supplementation to MS patients: effects on glutathione peroxidase, clinical safety, and absorption of selenium. *Biol Trace Elem Res.* 1990;24:109–117.

Marracci GH, Jones RE, McKeon GP, Bourdette DN. Alpha lipoic acid inhibits T cell migration into the spinal cord and suppresses and treats experimental autoimmune encephalomyelitis. *J Neuroimmunol.* 2002;131:104–114.

Millar J, Zilkha K, Langman M, et al. Double-blind trial of linoleate supplementation of the diet in multiple sclerosis. *Brit Med J.* 1973;1:765–768.

Mills M, Allen J. Mindfulness of movement as a coping strategy in multiple sclerosis. A pilot study. *Gen Hosp Psychiatry.* 2000;22:425–431.

Mischoulon D, Rosenbaum JF. *Natural Medications for Psychiatric Disorders: Considering the Alternatives.* Philadelphia, PA: Lippincott Williams Wilkins; 2002: 132–146.

Munger KL, Levin LI, Hollis BW, Howard NS, Ascherio A. Serum 25-hydroxyvitamin D levels and risk of multiple sclerosis. *JAMA.* 2006;296:2832–2838.

Munger KL, Zhang, SM, O'Reilly E, et al. Vitamin D intake and incidence of multiple sclerosis. *Neurology.* 2004;62:60–65.

NASA/MS Cooling Study Group. A randomized controlled study of the acute and chronic effects of cooling therapy for MS. *Neurology.* 2003;60:1955–1960.

Nayak S, Matheis RJ, Schoenberger NE, Shiflett SC. Use of unconventional therapies by individuals with multiple sclerosis. *Clin Rehabil.* 2003;17:181–191.

NIH Conference Assessment. Effects and side-effects of dental restorative materials. *Adv Dental Res.* 1992;6: 1–144.

NIH Consensus Development Panel on Acupuncture. *JAMA.* 1998;280:1518–1524.

Oken BS, Kishiyama S, Zajdel D, et al. Randomized controlled trial of yoga and exercise in multiple sclerosis. *Neurology.* 2004;62:2058–2064.

Page SA, Verhoef MJ, Stebbins RA, Metz LM, Levy JC. The use of complementary and alternative therapies by people with multiple sclerosis. *Chronic Dis Canada.* 2003;24:75–79.

Paty D. Double-blind trial of linoleic acid in multiple sclerosis. *Arch Neurol.* 1983;40:693–694.

Polman CH, Thompson AJ, Murray TJ, Bowling AC, Noseworthy JH. *Multiple Sclerosis: The Guide to Treatment and Management.* New York: Demos Medical Publishing; 2006.

Rahn KA, Bonneau RH, Turel AP, Thomas GA, McLaughlin PJ, Zagon IS. Opioid growth factor (OGF) and low dose naltrexone (LDN) inhibit immunological responses associated with EAE. *Mult Scler.* 2008a; 14:S234.

Rahn KA, McLaughlin PJ, Bonneau RH, Turel AP, Thomas GA, Zagon IS. Low-dose naltrexone (LDN) prevents development or delays onset and severity of experimental autoimmune encephalomyelitis in mice. *Mult Scler.* 2008b;14:S84–S85.

Raz R, Chazan B, Dan M. Cranberry juice and urinary tract infection. *Clin Infect Dis.* 2001;38:1413–1419.

Russo E. *Handbook of Psychotropic Herbs: A Scientific Analysis of Herbal Remedies for Psychiatric Conditions.* New York: Haworth Herbal Press; 2001.

Scott GS, Spitsin SV, Kean RB, Mikheeva T, Koprowski H, Hooper DC. Therapeutic intervention in experimental allergic encephalomyelitis by administration of uric acid precursors. *Proc Natl Acad Sci USA.* 2002; 99:16303–16308.

Shinto L, Yadav V, Morris C, Lapidus JA, Senders A, Bourdette D. Demographic and health-related factors associated with complementary and alternative medicine (CAM) use in multiple sclerosis. *Mult Scler.* 2006;12: 94–100.

Smith MO, Rabinowitz N. Acupuncture treatment of multiple sclerosis: two detailed clinical presentations. *Am J Acupuncture.* 1986;14:143–146.

Smith WS, Johnston SC, Skalabrin EJ, et al. Spinal manipulative therapy is an independent risk factor for vertebral artery dissection. *Neurology.* 2003;60:1424–1428.

Smolders J, Damoiseaux J, Menheere P. Vitamin D as an immune modulator in multiple sclerosis, a review. *J Neuroimmunol.* 2008;194:7–17.

Song H-S, Wray SH. Bee sting optic neuritis. *J Clin Neuro-Ophthalmol.* 1991;11:1145–1149.

Spitsin S, Hooper DC, Leist T, Streletz LJ, Mikheeva T, Koprowski H. Inactivation of peroxynitrite in multiple sclerosis patients after oral administration of inosine may suggest possible approaches to therapy of the disease. *Mult Scler.* 2001;7:313–319.

Spoerel WE, Paty DW, Kertesz A, Leung CY. Acupuncture and multiple sclerosis. *CMA Journal.* 1974;110:751.

Stenager E, Stenager EN, Knudsen L, Jensen K. The use of non-medical/alternative treatment in multiple sclerosis: a 5 year follow-up study. *Acta Neurol Belg.* 1995; 95:18–22.

Stewart TM, Bowling AC. Polyunsaturated fatty acid supplementation in MS. *Int MS J.* 2005;12:88–93.

Suvarna R. Possible interaction between warfarin and cranberry juice. *Brit Med J.* 2003;327:1454.

Swank R. Multiple sclerosis: twenty years on low fat diet. *Arch Neurol.* 1970;23:460–474.

Swank R, Dugan B. Effect of low saturated fat diet in early and late cases of multiple sclerosis. *Lancet.* 1990; 336:37–39.

Van Meeteren ME, Teunissen CE, Dijkstra A, Van Tol EA. Antioxidants and polyunsaturated fatty acids in multiple sclerosis. *Eur J Clin Nutr.* 2005;59:1347–1361.

Wade DT, Young CA, Chaudhuri KR, Davidson DLW. A randomized placebo controlled exploratory study of vitamin B-12, lofepramine, and L-phenylalanine (the "Cari Loder regime") in the treatment of multiple sclerosis. *J Neurol Neurosurg Psychiatry.* 2002;73: 246–249.

Waites KB, Canupp KC, Armstrong S, DeVivo MJ. Effect of cranberry extract on bacteriuria and pyuria in persons with neurogenic bladder secondary to spinal cord injury. *J Spinal Cord Med.* 2004;27:35–40.

Weinstock-Guttman B, Baier M, Park Y, et al. Low fat dietary intervention with omega-3 fatty acid supplementation in multiple sclerosis patients. *Prostaglandins Leukot Essent Fatty Acids.* 2005;73:92–404.

Weinstock-Guttman B, Gallagher E, Baier M, et al. Risk of bone loss in men with multiple sclerosis. *Mult Scler.* 2004;10:170–175.

Werneke U, Horn O, Taylor DM. How effective is St. John's wort? The evidence revisited. *J Clin Psychiatry.* 2004;65:611–617.

Wesselius T, Heersema DJ, Mostert JP, et al. A randomized crossover study of bee sting therapy for multiple sclerosis. *Neurology.* 2005;65:1764–1768.

Wingerchuk DM, Lesaux J, Rice GPA, Kremenchutzky M, Ebers GC. A pilot study of oral calcitriol (1,25-dihydroxyvitamin D3) for relapsing-remitting multiple sclerosis. *J Neurol Neurosurg Psychiatry.* 2005;76: 1294–1296.

Yadav V, Marracci G, Lovera J, et al. Lipoic acid in multiple sclerosis: a pilot study. *Mult Scler.* 2005;11:159–165.

Zajicek J, Fox P, Sanders H, et al. Cannabinoids for treatment of spasticity and other symptoms related to multiple sclerosis (CAMS study): multicentre randomized placebo-controlled trial. *Lancet.* 2003;362: 1517–1526.

Zajicek J, Sanders HP, Wright DE, et al. Cannabinoids in multiple sclerosis (CAMS) study: safety and efficacy data for 12 months follow-up. *J Neurol Neurosurg Psychiatry.* 2005;76:1664–1669.

Part 6 **Psychosocial Issues**

Living with Multiple Sclerosis: The Psychosocial Challenges for Patients and Their Families

Rosalind C. Kalb

Multiple sclerosis (MS) is a chronic disease characterized by variability and unpredictability, as well as change and loss. From the onset of the first puzzling symptoms, it tests people's ability to adapt, cope, and problem solve. This chapter provides an overview of the psychosocial challenges confronting individuals and families at different stages of the illness, the most common reactions to those challenges, and the recommended interventions to help people maintain their quality of life throughout the disease course. The discussion will focus first on the MS patient and then address the issues confronting family members, with a particular emphasis on couples, children of a parent who has MS, and caregivers. Resources to help facilitate conversations with patients and family members on a range of challenging topics are provided at the end of the chapter.

"BECOMING" A PERSON WITH MULTIPLE SCLEROSIS

Paralleling the diagnostic process—which can take a shorter or longer time, depending on the person's history, symptoms and signs, and test results—is a process of adaptation and adjustment that can also take variable amounts of time. The word "acceptance" is notably missing from this discussion. Expecting someone to "accept" a major life change—particularly an ongoing change that might be compared to a perpetual earthquake shaking the ground underfoot—seems unrealistic. The more reasonable and attainable goal for people diagnosed with MS is to find a way to adapt to its presence, making space for it in one's life without giving it more space or attention than it actually needs.

Prior to the diagnosis, each person has spent a lifetime creating a self-image that incorporates all that makes him or her unique. With the words, "You have multiple sclerosis," the person needs to figure out where this new piece of information is going to fit into that self-image, and into daily life (Kalb, 2008). Clinical experience tells us that some people simply refuse to acknowledge the information for awhile, denying the truth of these life-changing words until symptoms or disease progression force acceptance of their new reality. At the other extreme, are those who grab onto the role of "MS patient" with an intensity and enthusiasm that baffles clinicians and family members alike—turning the diagnosis into a new, full-time occupation and preoccupation. For the vast majority, however, there is a more gradual adaptation that involves grieving over the loss of the old self and beginning slowly to incorporate the realities of a chronic, progressive disease into everyday life (Kalb et al., 2007; Kalb, 2008).

The role of grieving has not received much attention in the MS literature. As Ahlström's (2007) work in chronic illness has demonstrated, however, chronic sorrow is a common accompaniment to the losses people often experience, particularly related to "loss of bodily function," "loss of relationship," "loss of autonomous life," "loss of the life imagined," and "loss of identity." To the extent that clinicians recognize and acknowledge the intensity of this *normal, expectable* reaction to the real or at least threatened losses related to MS (as distinguished from the major depression and other mood disorders discussed in Chapter 19) we can help our patients come to terms with this new part of themselves—while also providing medical, rehabilitative, and psychosocial interventions to ensure that the disease impacts other aspects of their lives as little as possible.

COMMON EMOTIONAL REACTIONS OVER THE DISEASE COURSE

In addition to the grieving that ebbs and flows with the changes and losses imposed by the disease, patients commonly experience feelings of anxiety, anger, and guilt.

Anxiety

Anxiety is more common than depression in the MS population (Feinstein et al., 1999; Zorzon et al., 2001), particularly in the early period following the diagnosis (Janssens et al., 2006). In spite of its higher prevalence, however, anxiety has received much less attention in the literature than depression. It has been found to be more common in women than men and in people who are depressed and socially isolated (Korostil and Feinstein, 2007). Anxiety has also been shown to be a stronger predictor of excessive alcohol consumption than depression (Quesnel and Feinstein, 2004).

From the clinical perspective, MS-related anxiety seems to result primarily from the variability and unpredictability of the disease; not knowing how one is going to feel, or how one's body is going to function from one day or week to the next, threatens a person's sense of control and confidence. Patients express anxiety about their ability to manage day to day ("Will I be able to function at work today…make it to the bathroom on time…drive my child to her soccer game…get dinner on the table?") as well as worrying about what the future will bring ("Will I be able to walk…work…support my family…have children…live independently…?").

Experience suggests that patients' anxieties about the near and distant future can be effectively addressed by helping them problem solve around specific issues or concerns for which they can take some concrete action rather than focusing on the more global, overwhelming fear of the unpredictable future. To the extent that they are able to put in place strategies and resources to deal with potential problems or losses, they feel more prepared and less vulnerable in the face of uncertainty.

Thus, for example, a patient whose worries about loss of bladder control have led to absence from work, social isolation, and chronic worry might be encouraged to:

- Discuss symptoms and concerns with her MS physician or nurse
- Visit the National MS Society Web site for publications about bladder management
- Talk to her employer about getting office space closer to the bathroom
- Raise the subject in a support group or online chat to hear how others have handled this kind of problem

A patient who is anxious about his ability to remain in his current job may be encouraged to:

- Consult with an occupational therapist about ways to utilize assistive technology and modify his work space to conserve energy and maximize productivity
- Talk to a vocational counselor about other career options that he might begin to train for now
- Meet with a financial planner to discuss ways to optimize the family's financial security

As patients identify strategies and resources to manage each problem or concern, their anxiety diminishes, leaving them feeling more in control and more confident in their ability to deal with whatever the next set of challenges might be. Medication is always an option if these behavioral interventions are ineffective, but the behavioral interventions offer patients the opportunity to increase their feelings of confidence and mastery in the face of significant challenges.

Anger

Anger is a normal response to feeling frustrated and out of control. As MS-related losses take their toll on a person's abilities, activities, and roles, he or she is likely to feel increasingly resentful about the unfairness of it all. Clinicians have two primary challenges in dealing with their patients' anger. The first is to distinguish accurately between normal, expectable anger or frustration and the irritability that is so common in people with MS who are depressed (Minden et al., 1987). When irritability is the result of depression, it can be relieved by prompt diagnosis and treatment of the underlying mood disorder. The second is to help patients channel the angry feelings in productive ways. When the energy consumed by simmering anger can be put toward constructive problem solving, people feel more comfortable and more in control. Since family members, and caregivers in particular, are likely to be experiencing very similar feelings of anger and resentment, helping patients and families to acknowledge, communicate, and problem solve around the issues leading to greatest frustration could help reduce the incidence of abuse in the MS population.

Guilt

Although guilt has received little attention in the MS literature, it is a feeling commonly expressed by people who worry about being unable to contribute fully at home or at work. They talk about letting others down; not pulling their weight; not fulfilling their obligations. Their anger may also be a source of guilt, particularly if they have been taking their anger out on an undeserving spouse, child, or colleague, or experiencing anger at God for their MS. Clinicians can address this guilt by offering optimal symptom management; helping people identify tools and strategies that enhance mobility, comfort, and productivity; and encouraging their patients to work with family members and colleagues to swap tasks and responsibilities in ways that take MS-related impairments into account while ensuring an equitable balance in the relationship.

EARLY MULTIPLE SCLEROSIS

Several issues confront any person with a recent diagnosis of MS or a clinically isolated syndrome (CIS) that may evolve into MS. The most significant among them include initiating the coping process; choosing among treatment options; making disclosure decisions; and dealing with invisible symptoms.

Initiating the Coping Process

The coping process begins when the onset of puzzling neurologic symptoms sets in motion the quest for answers. People need to identify and

engage the appropriate health professionals, inform themselves about MS, make important decisions about their care, and begin to create a support system. The patients who seem to deal most successfully with these initial challenges of MS have been found to exhibit a *problem-focused* rather than an *emotion-focused* style of coping (Pakenham, 1999; McCabe et al., 2004; Dennison et al., 2009; Goretti et al., 2009). They tackle each challenge as a problem to be solved rather than a fate to be either denied or simply endured, taking steps to locate and implement the resources that will help them be successful.

Clinicians can support and facilitate a problem-focused approach in several ways: patients who see MS as a war to be won ("I'll beat this disease…I won't let this disease get to me") are prone to feelings of guilt and self-blame when and if the disease progresses in spite of their best efforts. By reminding them that MS is a chronic, often progressive disease (i.e., a war that we don't yet know how to win), and encouraging them to approach MS instead as a series of individual challenges to be met (e.g., treating symptoms, initiating a disease-modifying therapy, maximizing employment options, enhancing wellness, making sound life-planning decisions), the health-care team can promote effective problem solving. Engaging patients in collaborative decisions about treatment, pointing them toward reliable resources in the community, and being available to address questions and concerns through the disease course are additional strategies that promote a problem-focused approach.

Making Disclosure Decisions

Unfortunately, most people begin disclosing information about their symptoms or diagnosis before taking time to consider the ramifications of doing so. A person who has been given a diagnosis of MS or CIS, or has been experiencing puzzling symptoms for weeks or months, may look for support from friends, relatives, or colleagues at work, without realizing that once health information has been given out, it can never be taken back. In the absence of a clear, preemptive message from the doctor or nurse about the importance of thoughtful disclosure decisions, many people disclose sooner and regret it later—particularly if their early symptoms totally remit (Kalb et al., 2007).

Health professionals can assist their patients by mentioning the disclosure issue during the first visit, providing brochures about the pros and cons of disclosure from voluntary MS advocacy groups, and referring people to *Disclosing MS on the Job: A Tool to Help You Consider Your Options* on the National MS Society Web site (http://www. nationalMSsociety.org/DisclosureTool). For more information about disclosure in the workplace, see Chapter 27.

Initiating Treatment

Prior to the advent of the first FDA-approved disease-modifying therapy in 1993, people diagnosed with MS had very limited treatment options. The fortunate patients were treated by physicians who recognized the importance of a clear and prompt diagnosis, active relapse and symptom management, and the availability of psychosocial support. Far too many, however, received what Dr. Labe Scheinberg referred to as the "Diagnose and Adios" model of MS care. With no cure to offer, many physicians simply sent patients home to fend for themselves.

Today, MS patients are fortunate to have an array of treatment options available to them; the challenges arise around deciding when to begin immunomodulatory therapy and which medication to choose, particularly since none of the approved medications is a cure or designed to make people feel better, each has its own side effect profile and associated risks, and all are only partially effective (Karussis et al., 2006; Wingerchuk, 2008).

Most MS experts agree that treatment with a disease-modifying therapy should be considered as early as possible in the disease course, when these medications have been shown to be most effective (Frohman et al., 2006; National MS Society, 2007). And patients diagnosed with a CIS and lesions on magnetic resonance imaging (MRI) that are consistent with MS may be prescribed treatment to delay the diagnosis of MS (Thrower, 2007). For patients whose initial symptoms have resolved, and who may be eager to delay thinking about the realities of MS as long as possible, the recommendation to begin an injectable medication flies in the face of their emotional defenses.

People will differ significantly in their readiness to initiate treatment—particularly with a medication that may make them feel worse than the disease it is meant to treat (Holland et al., 2001a,b).

With those patients who express a readiness to begin, some physicians take the time to discuss the first-line treatment options (interferon-beta and glatiramer acetate) and recommend the medication that they think is most appropriate, most likely to be covered by insurance, and most in line with the person's lifestyle. Others simply send the patient home with several instructional videos and tell the person to decide. While there are some MS patients who are comfortable with this level of autonomy in medical decision making, most experience a variety of concerns about the decision process: "Which medication is the most effective....Which one is best for me....What if I choose the wrong one...?"

Clearly, the increased number of treatment options—while welcomed by health professionals and patients alike—has led to anxiety on the part of patients who want to make the best possible choices. Clinicians can help reduce this anxiety— and promote long-term adherence—by educating patients about the importance of early treatment, assessing patient readiness (Holland et al., 2001a,b), providing supportive guidance around treatment selection, creating realistic expectations for treatment outcomes, and being available to address concerns and manage side effects (Brandes et al., 2009).

A Word about Those Diagnosed with Primary Progressive Multiple Sclerosis

As the number of treatment options for those with relapsing forms of MS continues to grow, so does the frustration of people diagnosed with primary progressive multiple sclerosis (PPMS), for whom no effective disease-modifying therapy is yet available. Referring to themselves as "orphans in the MS world" (Holland et al., 2010), they feel neglected and ignored by their doctors and forgotten by researchers. In order to set the stage for an effective, ongoing, and collaborative treatment relationship, it is essential for the diagnosing physician to explain what is known about PPMS and the ways it differs from relapsing forms of the disease; describe the challenges inherent in identifying and testing potential therapies in PPMS; emphasize the importance of effective symptom management; and state clearly that there is much that can be done on an ongoing basis to promote the person's health, wellness, and quality of life (Goodman, 2009). Fortunately, a number of excellent resources have recently become available for people diagnosed with this challenging form of MS (Coyle and Halper, 2008; National MS Society Web site, http://www.nationalMSsociety.org/PPMS).

Dealing with Invisible Symptoms

The invisible symptoms of MS—fatigue, visual impairment, dysesthesias, urinary urgency, and cognitive changes, to name just a few—create a disconnect between what the person with MS is feeling and what family members and colleagues can see and understand. The person may continue to look healthy and hearty in spite of significant discomfort. In the event that these symptoms significantly interfere with the person's ability to function optimally at home or at work, the changes in performance can easily be misinterpreted by family members and colleagues as laziness, disinterest, inattention, or lack of ability.

Deciding how best to respond to "But you look so good!" is a challenge shared by many recently diagnosed individuals—so much so that the National MS Society offers a publication on the subject (http://www.nationalmssociety.org/SpecialIssues). Although everyone likes to receive compliments on their appearance, the words may also convey a painful underlying message—"You look too good to have MS…you don't look sick… I don't understand why you're not doing the things I need you to do."

To address this disconnect between how he or she feels and what others perceive, the person needs to balance the need for privacy with the need for others to understand the variable, unpredictable, and often invisible nature of MS symptoms.

AS THE DISEASE PROGRESSES

Increasing disability brings several emotional and social challenges for people, beginning with the need to understand and acknowledge the progression of the disease. Adherence to treatment may falter as the disease continues to worsen in spite of immunomodulatory therapy, and people are attracted to alternative therapies and miracle "cures" that promise hope. This is also a time of significant role changes, at home and at work, as well as time when people need to come to terms with the use of adaptive equipment of various kinds.

Understanding Disease Progression

Prior to the clinical trials for the disease-modifying therapies, most patients were completely unaware of the four disease courses and spent little, if any, time worrying about them. Today, the transition from relapsing-remitting MS (RRMS) to secondary progressive MS (SPMS) has become a significant focus of attention and anxiety—in large part because most people are given little, if any, information about the natural history of the disease and what they might expect over time. In other words, clinicians are so intent on providing hope and reassurance for their newly diagnosed patients that they neglect to provide some critical information about MS progression.

Natural history data suggest that approximately one-half of the 80%–85% of people diagnosed with RRMS will transition to SPMS within about 10 years (Weinshenker, 1994). Although early treatment may delay this transition somewhat, the expectation is still that the disease will eventually become more steadily progressive for many people. When the transition occurs, however, many patients seem caught by surprise, wondering why it happened and whom to blame. Those for whom the adjustment is most challenging and painful tend to see the transition as a personal failure ("I didn't try hard enough…I wasn't strong enough…I didn't choose the right doctor or the right medicine…I didn't pray hard enough…I am being punished") (Kalb, 2007).

Clinicians can help ease this transition by taking the time to explain how and why it occurs, describing the treatments strategies that will be used to manage the disease course and symptoms, and directing their patients to information about the array of research studies (http://www.nationalMSsociety.org/Research_ProgressiveMS) and clinical trials (http://www.nationalmssociety.org/ClinicalTrials) currently underway to understand and address progressive MS.

Resisting Miracle "Cures"

Advertisements for complementary and alternative medicine (CAM) that offer quick cures, increased energy, improved health, and revitalization are very enticing—particularly for those whose MS is slowly but surely robbing them of their abilities. Even patients for whom the approved medications have helped to slow disease progression may be tempted by products or interventions that cost less, require no injections, and promise to work fast. As a person's disease becomes more progressive, he or she will benefit from an honest appraisal of treatment options. If the person is still a candidate for an immunomodulatory or immunosuppressive agent, adherence should be aided and encouraged by the health-care team and the pharmaceutical support program. If the person is no longer a suitable candidate for these medications, an open discussion of next steps is essential; in the absence of a proactive disease and symptom management plan, the promise of feeling better or being "cured"—even when it is false, expensive, or dangerous—becomes very alluring.

Although clinicians seldom have time during a busy office visit for prolonged conversations about CAM, some discussion is essential. Patients who perceive their doctors to be dismissive or critical of anything outside of mainstream medicine will simply stop talking about what they are doing or taking. Since studies indicate that more than 50% of people with MS are using some form of complementary or alternative medicine (Bowling, 2007), it is important to encourage the sharing of this information so that patients can be warned about potential side effects or harmful interactions, not to mention wasted money. The National MS Society can serve as a useful educational adjunct for the busy clinician; patients can be referred for information and educational materials designed to help them be cautious consumers.

Learning to Communicate One's Needs

An ongoing coping challenge for people disabled by MS involves finding a balance between the wish for autonomy and the need for assistance. A person who resents it when a family member or colleague seems to hover protectively or is too quick to provide assistance that *is not* needed may be equally resentful when those same individuals fail to recognize when assistance *is* needed. Ambivalence about the need for help often leads people to send mixed signals to family, friends, and colleagues, forgetting that even those closest to them cannot read their minds. Coming to terms with the need for occasional assistance—coupled with a comfortable strategy for requesting help when it is needed and politely refusing it when it is not—can help people negotiate this difficult hurdle.

Using Tools/Adaptations

As MS progresses, patients are challenged with the choice between giving up valued activities and roles and learning how to do them differently. Nowhere is the difference between the problem-focused and the emotion-focused coping strategy seen more clearly: The patients who are determined to stay active and involved will find an adaptive solution to every problem, embracing any and all forms of adaptive equipment as a welcome means to a variety of ends. Those who would rather retreat or retire than use any tool or strategy that would brand them as "disabled" or be perceived as "giving in to their MS," allow their world to grow smaller and smaller. The health-care team can encourage the problem-focused approach by helping patients reframe their thinking about assistive technology as a way to take charge of their MS rather than give in to it (Louise-Bender et al., 2002).

ADVANCED MULTIPLE SCLEROSIS

The advanced stages of MS pose some extraordinary psychosocial challenges (Kalb, 2008). Given the near-normal life expectancy for most people with MS, patients may live for many years with symptoms debilitating enough to threaten their sense of personal identity ("Who am I now that I can no longer live the way I used to live or do the things that helped to make me who I am?"); their ability to exert control over their environment ("I have lost my ability to manipulate my environment and do the things I need to do"); and their personal autonomy and independence ("All of my needs have to be met by someone else—I have lost the ability to function independently").

People with advanced disease often come to feel as though as every aspect of their life has been irrevocably distorted and diminished by MS. In reviewing these challenges and the ways in which clinicians can help patients to meet them, it is important to keep in mind that any person with significant cognitive impairment will require more extensive assistance.

Redefining Oneself

The grieving process continues into these later stages of the disease, complicated by the fact that there are fewer and fewer pleasures or gains to counterbalance the losses. The losses can be so extensive that the person begins to feel like a stranger to him- or herself and invisible to others— even to health-care providers. The severely disabled patient may be seen less and less frequently by the doctors for several reasons: the doctor may feel that he or she has little, if anything, to offer or the patient may feel there is nothing to be gained; the physician's office may not be sufficiently accessible for a motorized wheelchair or stretcher; the patient cannot afford the office visit; accessible transportation is not available; or no family member is able to attend or assist. Both patients and clinicians need to be reminded of the importance of ongoing care to provide hope, enhance function, prevent complications, and promote quality of life.

Counseling can facilitate the grieving process while also giving people the opportunity to talk about their lives, identify new interests or goals, and remind themselves of the qualities that make them unique. Support groups—virtual or in-person— can help people stay connected and involved. Clinicians are encouraged to refer patients with advanced MS to the National MS Society; individual chapters can provide information about helpful programs and resources for those with advanced disease, including care management services.

Redefining Control

When people can no longer carry out daily activities, manage their bodily functions, or perform their chosen roles, their sense of personal control is shattered. Regaining a sense of control over one's body, environment, and daily life involves learning to think about control in new and different ways. In addition to active symptom management to enhance comfort, continence, and quality of life, referrals to occupational therapy are extremely important at this time. Assistive technology—from the simplest tool to the most comprehensive environmental control system—can make it possible for people to re-establish their sense of mastery. The speech/language pathologist can suggest alternative communication strategies for people with severe dysarthria so that they can remain connected with others and interact with the world. By making these referrals to other members of the health-care team, the physician is also conveying to the patient with advanced MS that there is always more that can be done to manage symptoms and make life better and more manageable.

Redefining Independence

Like a person's feeling of control over his or her body and environment, the feeling of independence may be equally threatened. Those who must gradually come to depend on others for even the most basic—and personal activities—feel robbed of their adulthood. Once again, those individuals who approach their disease as a series of problems in search of solutions fare better than those whose coping strategies are more emotion focused. They are always on the lookout for any forms of assistance that will enable them to feel more independent, and they come to define independence as the ability to manage this assistance effectively. The cognitively intact patient is able to make decisions about care, hire and manage aides, modify his or her environment to maximize independent functioning, and maintain relationships and connections in ways that promote the feeling of independence.

Identifying the Multiple Sclerosis–Free Zone

A person with advanced MS can come to feel as though every aspect of living is compromised by the disease—that life apart from MS no longer exists. The concept of an *MS-free zone* can be very reassuring to people because it conveys the hopeful message that they are more than their disease

(Kalb, 2008). In conversation with family, friends, or a mental health professional, people with advanced disease can be reminded of those parts of themselves that MS has not touched or changed—perhaps their sense of humor, strong opinions, love of music or movies or soap operas, or faith in God. While each person's *MS-free zone* will be different, its importance lies in the potential for it to provide a much-needed source of positive emotional energy to deal with all the challenges of daily life. Although clinicians would do well to help patients (and their caregivers) identify and nurture their respective *MS-free zones* ("MS is a new part of your life but no need for it to be the center of your life") from the beginning, its role is especially critical as the disease becomes more advanced.

FAMILIES

Like any other illness, MS affects not only the person with the diagnosis but members of the family as well. The *uninvited guest* (Kalb, 2006) is a helpful metaphor for families, because almost anyone can relate to the intrusion of an unexpected visitor who arrives at the door, disrupts the household, and does not leave. The image also serves to convey the importance for each family member of getting to know the MS visitor and developing some kind of workable relationship with it. Against the backdrop of the uninvited guest, certain emotional and social challenges for family members, and the family as a whole, become very clear. Over time, the individuals in the family must find a way to meld their coping styles and strategies, communicate their feelings and needs, engage in effective planning and problem solving, and ensure that the needs of everyone in the family are met—not an easy set of challenges for any family (McDaniel et al., 1992).

Coping Is a Family Affair

The first part of this chapter described the feelings of grief, anxiety, anger, and guilt that ebb and flow for MS patients over the course of the disease. Not surprisingly, each family member experiences these emotions as well (McDaniel et al., 1992; Kalb, 2006). Just as the patient needs to redefine him- or herself as a person with MS, the family needs to redefine itself as well. For example, the family that is very active or sports-oriented may need to begin identifying itself in a somewhat different way, depending on how willing and able they are to adapt their activities to the needs of the person with MS. As the disease impacts each of their lives in different ways, family members will need to grieve over the changes or losses and deal with feelings of anger and guilt. The challenge for the family system is that these varied emotions do not emerge in any well-orchestrated way; each person will feel and express them in his or her own way and in his or her own time. The opportunities for hurt feelings, tension, and emotional upheaval are numerous, particularly if family members begin to "compete" over who has it worst—the person with the disease or those whose lives are turned topsy-turvy by a disease they do not even have.

Complicating the family's coping efforts is the fact that loved ones do not always share the same coping styles or strategies (Kalb, 2006). For example, while the person with a problem-focused coping style sets out to learn about MS, identify resources, and engage in planning and problem solving, the person with a more emotion-focused style is likely to want to think about it all as little as possible. When coping styles collide, communication and mutual support can be threatened.

Maintaining a Healthy Relationship

Maintaining a healthy relationship over time is a challenge for any couple; a chronic, progressive disease like MS adds to the challenge in a variety of ways. Although people are quick to assume that the rate of divorce among couples living with MS is very high, the data suggest that it hovers around the rate for the general population (Minden et al., 2006). Whether this means that marriages involving people with MS are no more or less difficult than other marriages is not clear. Some otherwise happy couples divorce in order to access entitlement programs for the partner with MS, and some couples that might otherwise separate stay together for financial reasons or to maintain insurance coverage for the partner with MS. In general, however, clinical experience has highlighted several common issues.

Maintaining closeness and intimacy

Although the potential impact of MS on sexual intimacy is dealt with extensively in the literature (see Chapter 16), the threat to emotional intimacy is equally important. Emotional intimacy depends on effective communication, mutual respect, shared goals and expectations, and trust, among other things.

Couples living with MS may find their ability to communicate hampered by a variety of factors, including the MS partner's cognitive or mood changes ("This isn't the same person I married"), as well as depression and/or anger in the non-MS partner. In addition, both partners may find themselves holding back for fear of upsetting or angering one another—for example: the partner with MS worrying about alienating the person he or she counts on the most ("How can I talk about what I feel or need right now when he's already doing so much for me—it may just drive him away"); the non-MS partner worrying about hurting or burdening the MS partner ("How can I talk about our finances when I know how upset she is about having to leave her job?"). Once communication patterns are disrupted or altered, the foundation of emotional intimacy is threatened.

Sustaining balance in the partnership

Likewise, when MS alters one partner's ability to carry out his or her identified roles or responsibilities, the partnership undergoes a shift. To the extent that roles can be successfully realigned to maintain balance in the relationship—with each person able to contribute in some way to the well-being of the other and of the household—the intimacy can be maintained. However, intimacy begins to suffer when one partner perceives him- or herself to be taking on more and more (and getting less and less), while the other no longer feels able to contribute in a meaningful way.

The intimate partnership also suffers when the unpredictable progression of MS forces a couple to alter its shared goals and dreams. To sustain the intimacy, they need to be able to grieve together over their losses and work toward building a different future—efforts made more challenging by

cognitive or emotional problems and communication difficulties.

Mental health professionals can facilitate a couple's efforts to maintain or enhance their intimacy by teaching effective communication strategies; encouraging them to identify and address any shifts in the balance of their relationship to ensure that each partner feels like a valued contributor; and helping them to share the grieving experience so that they can begin to revise their shared plans and goals. Physicians and nurses can support couples by asking routinely about changes in sexual function (see Chapter 16) that the person with MS may be hesitant to mention, and by referring couples to the National MS Society's education program entitled Relationship Matters (http://www.nationalMSsociety.org/RelationshipMatters), and for counseling, as needed, for help with their relationship issues. When initiating these conversations, clinicians need to keep in mind that all patients, regardless of their sexual orientation, whether they are in committed relationships or not, may have questions or concerns about intimacy and sexuality.

Managing resources

Multiple sclerosis is expensive not only in terms of health-care dollars but also in terms of other important resources, including time and physical and emotional energy. With everyone's attention focused on the needs of the person with MS, the needs of the other partner—and of their children—may be neglected, resulting in a disabled family rather than a family with one disabled member. Clinicians can help couples recognize and address this kind of imbalance in a variety of ways: Every couple should be encouraged by their health-care provider(s) to consult with a financial advisor about how best to manage their health-care and other expenses; rehabilitation specialists can recommend strategies to manage MS-related fatigue and enhance function in ways that benefit the whole family (equitable distribution of chores and responsibilities and enjoyable family recreation being prime examples); doctors and nurses can emphasize the importance of health and wellness for every family member; and mental health professionals can facilitate conversations about ways to meet each person's social and emotional needs. The goal of balancing family resources, as described by Gonzalez and colleagues (Gonzalez et al., 1989), is to "make a place for the illness while keeping the illness in its place."

Engaging in joint planning and problem solving

One of the most important messages to people living with MS—and one of the hardest for them to hear—is the importance of planning for the worst while hoping for the best. No one newly diagnosed with MS wants to think about the unthinkable, and no spouse or partner wants to be a doom forecaster; yet each of them is anxious about possible outcomes ("What if I can't walk? What if he has to leave his job? What if she can't drive anymore? What if my vision gets even worse?").

The health-care team can facilitate effective planning and problem solving by encouraging couples to learn about the disease and its potential impact; talk openly with one another about their concerns for the future; and work together with financial and vocational specialists to identify strategies they can implement today to protect themselves against future eventualities. For the majority who do not become severely disabled, nothing has been lost by going through this planning exercise, and much has been gained—the comfort of having taken some steps to mitigate the impact of future disability. Those who do become more disabled feel more prepared and more in control of their lives than if they had faced the future with no preparation or thought. The National MS Society offers financial planning resources (http://www.nationalmssociety.org/FinancialPlanning) as well as referrals to financial and employment specialists.

Managing risk tolerance levels

Risk tolerance has become an increasingly important issue as MS treatment options have expanded to include therapies that offer greater benefit with higher associated risks. It is not at all unusual for two members of a couple to have very different levels of tolerance for the associated risks; the MS partner may jump at the chance to take a medication that the other partner thinks should be avoided at all costs, or the non-MS partner may be less risk averse than the person with MS.

It is recommended that clinicians take the time to discuss the risks and benefits of a potential treatment with both members of the couple in order to make sure that they fully understand what is involved. Although the risk of serious problems may be small, patients and partners need to be encouraged to think carefully through the range of possible outcomes before coming to an informed decision. While the treatment decision is ultimately up to the patient, the partner's buy-in is critical to this process in order to avoid guilt and recrimination down the road.

Raising a Family

Raising a family is not easy for any parent in today's world. For couples in which one of the partners has MS, the usual challenges are further complicated by the progressive and unpredictable nature of the disease.

Making family planning decisions

Prior to 1950, women and men with MS were discouraged from having children. The research since that time—which has focused almost exclusively on women with MS—has determined that the disease has no significant impact on conception, pregnancy, delivery, or nursing and, conversely, that pregnancy, delivery, and nursing, have no long-term impact on a woman's MS (see Chapter 17). Armed with this important information, however, men and women still need to make informed family-planning decisions, taking into account a variety of factors: their relationship and feelings about having children; the progressive, unpredictable nature of MS; the genetic risk—albeit relatively small—for their children of developing MS; their financial resources; and the available support system (Birk and Giesser, 2006).

Clinicians can facilitate these important decisions by doing the following:

- Providing information about the disease and possible prognosis given the person's history and symptoms
- Explaining what is currently known about the genetic risk for children of a parent with MS

- Discussing the relative risks associated with interrupting immunomodulatory therapy for conception, pregnancy, and breastfeeding, given the woman's disease course
- Encouraging partners to share their feelings and concerns about parenting openly with one another, to think beyond the initial days or months of parenthood, and to talk with other parents with MS about their experiences
- Helping couples assess their ability to adapt, cope, and problem solve in the face of an unpredictable illness

The goal is to help couples reach the decisions that are right for them while taking into account the unpredictability of MS and the potential for disease worsening.

Parenting with multiple sclerosis

Children who have a parent with a chronic illness are considered to be at risk both emotionally and socially (Rutter, 1989). Although the impact of parental MS has been the focus of investigators in several countries (Australia, Canada, Israel, the United States, and Greece, among others), the variability in the samples and diversity of the cultures make it difficult to draw clear conclusions. Some investigators have looked primarily at behavioral issues and psychopathology in these children (Arnaud, 1959; De Judicibus and McCabe, 2004; Yahav et al., 2005; Diareme et al., 2006; Yahav et al., 2007), while others have focused more on delineating the factors that seem to promote adjustment (Pakenham and Bursnall, 2006) and identifying strategies to support these children's coping efforts (Cross and Rintell, 1999).

One study (Pakenham and Bursnall, 2006) found that compared to children of "healthy" parents, children of an MS parent reported greater family responsibilities, less reliance on problem solving and seeking social support as ways of coping, a greater tendency to somatization, and lower life satisfaction and positive affect. Among the children who had a parent with MS, better adjustment was associated with higher levels of social support, lower perceived stress, greater reliance on a more proactive coping style, and less reliance on avoidant coping strategies. They recommend that clinicians provide interventions for these children that target increased education about MS, social support, and adaptive, problem-solving coping strategies.

Cross and Rintell (1999) also emphasized the need for age-appropriate information about the disease, highlighting the importance of reassuring children that their behavior did not cause— and cannot worsen—a parent's MS, and that the likelihood of developing MS themselves is very small.

Several studies (Deatrick et al., 1998; Diareme et al., 2006) have reported the impact of parental depression on children's behavior and affect— which confirms the importance of diagnosing and treating depression and other affective disorders in people with MS (see Chapter 19). However, Steck and colleagues (2007) found that children's coping behavior was more closely related to the coping style of the parent without MS than the parent with MS—which highlights the importance for clinicians of providing support for the care partner as well as the patient.

Parents with MS routinely ask when they should begin talking to their children about it. Although many parents often postpone these discussions until they have obvious, visible symptoms or require a mobility aid, research (Cross and Rintell, 1999; Mutch, 2005) and clinical experience suggest that children are aware that something is wrong long before the physical symptoms become visible. They pick up on their parent's mood and worry, as well as any tension in the household. In the absence of clear information about what is happening, they will tend to fill in the blanks with whatever their active imaginations conjure up. For that reason, clinicians should encourage their patients to provide accurate, age-appropriate information about the disease (available from the National MS Society Web site at http://www.nationalmssociety.org/childrensinfo).

The benefits of talking to children about MS include the following: relieving them of the burden of having to imagine what is going on; ensuring that they hear the information from a parent rather than a well-meaning relative or neighbor; giving them tacit permission to voice their concerns and a vocabulary for doing so; and conveying the valuable message that family members share important information and help one another through difficult challenges. Clinicians can support this process by encouraging parents to bring their children to medical visits from time to time in order to meet the medical staff and ask their questions.

The Caregiving Role

Caregivers have long been known as the "invisible patients" (Andolsek et al., 1988). A caregiver is generally a family member who provides the majority of care for someone who needs assistance with activities of daily living and household management (Pandya, 2005). In this section, the primary focus will be on caregiving spouses, but the impact of caregiving on aging parents, adult children, and young children will also be addressed.

Caregiver burden, which has been defined as the strain or load borne by a person who cares for a chronically ill, disabled, or elderly family member (Stucki and Mulvey, 2000), is "…a multidimensional response to physical, psychological, emotional, social, and financial stressors associated with the caregiving experience" (Buhse, 2008). The burden can be objective (that which others can see and measure, such as hours spent, income lost, or number of tasks performed) or subjective (the individual's response to his or her caregiving role and activities), but it is the subjective experience that has been associated with higher risk of depression and reduced quality of life in caregivers of people with MS (Aronson, 1997).

Spouse caregivers

In their review of the literature on spousal caregivers of people with MS, McKeown et al. (2003) found reductions in quality of life, physical health, emotional well-being, financial security, and social activity—findings very similar to those for caregivers in the general population. However, the variability and unpredictability of MS, coupled with the fatigue, mood changes, and cognitive symptoms that are so common, create unique caregiving challenges for spouses of MS patients—often leading to a disruption of the partnership and an intense sense of loss (Aronson, 1997; Chipchase and Lincoln, 2001; Fivged et al., 20007; Buhse, 2008). And Pozzilli and colleagues (2004) found that depression in caregivers was associated with disease duration and severity in their partners.

In spite of these challenges, the research has shown that MS caregivers are often reluctant to engage community resources (Aronson et al., 1996). Just as MS patients differ in their readiness to initiate treatment (Holland et al., 2001a,b), MS caregivers differ in their readiness to acknowledge the need for support and assistance (McKeown et al., 2004). While their own denial about the diagnosis, and their wish to protect their loved one's privacy, may cause them initially to reject offers of support or assistance, the growing demands and stresses of caregiving eventually lead them to look for help from family, friends, and the community (O'Brien et al., 1995; McKeown et al., 2004). Similar to the MS patients themselves, caregivers who utilize problem-solving coping strategies may meet their challenges more adequately and comfortably than those who utilize more emotion-focused strategies; unfortunately, however, even the most determined caregivers can experience great difficulty navigating the system to find the resources they need (Cheung and Hocking, 1994).

Buhse (2008) offers the following recommendations to help clinicians address the needs of caregivers: *(1)* Stay alert to changes in a caregiver's behavior and signs of depression. *(2)* With the patient's permission, see the caregiver alone on occasion to talk about concerns. *(3)* Make sure that the caregiver has the necessary knowledge and skills to deal with the required caregiver tasks. *(4)* Emphasize to caregivers the importance of taking care of themselves (the flight attendant's message to passengers—to put on one's own oxygen mask before assisting another person with his or hers—is a very helpful metaphor for caregivers). *(5)* Teach caregivers the warning signs of caregiver burden, including depression, changes in appetite or sleep habits, increased alcohol or drug use, and anxiety.

Parent caregivers

In the event that young or middle-aged adults with MS become severely disabled, they may—by choice or not—need to rely on their parents for care and support. In a reversal of the expected pattern, the adult child returns to the parental home and the child role, while the older adults once again assume the parenting role. Along with all of the usual stresses and strains associated with caring for a person with a chronic, disabling illness is the added challenge of renegotiating a new, and very different, parent–child relationship (Kalb and Seidman, 2006).

The adult child who has lived independently for a number of years is likely to experience a deep sense of loss, even while being relieved and grateful for the loving care; the parents, who have been looking forward to retirement after successfully launching their children into the world, are likely to feel overwhelmed by fears for their child's future as well as their own. Clinicians may be called upon to help families problem solve around their new living arrangements in ways that respect the feelings and needs of all concerned.

Young child caregivers

Children growing up with a parent with MS report having more responsibilities than other children (Lackey and Gates, 2001; Yahav et al., 2005; Pakenham and Bursnall, 2006). Household chores and caregiving responsibilities that interfere with a child's age-appropriate activities or make demands on the child that are beyond his or her abilities or emotional resources can result in significant stress and distress. On the other hand, children report significant benefit and satisfaction from the experience of helping or caring for a parent (Lackey and Gates, 2001), particularly if they feel that they have had some choice in the type and amount of help they provide (Pakenham and Bursnall, 2006). Clinicians can help to ensure that children are not put in the position of having to take on responsibilities that are "bigger" than they are (e.g., hands-on physical assistance with feeding, bathing, dressing, toileting) by making every effort to connect their patients with community services and resources, including the National MS Society and other voluntary health agencies.

CONCLUSIONS

The psychosocial aspects of MS are no less complex or less important than the medical ones. Any reader of this book will appreciate the challenges facing individuals and families living with MS, as well as the clinicians providing their care. Healthcare professionals who are fortunate enough to work in a comprehensive care setting can work in a cohesive and collaborative way to address the myriad medical, social, and psychological needs of those affected by MS; others will need to reach into their communities to partner with colleagues to provide this multidisciplinary care. No clinician working in isolation has the time or ability to address all the issues. And without careful attention to the psychosocial needs of patients and the family members who help with their care, even the most powerful medications will not be enough to ensure a positive quality of life for all concerned.

REFERENCES

Ahlström G. Experiences of loss and chronic sorrow in persons with severe chronic illness. *J Clin Nurs.* 2007;16(3A):76–83.

Andolsek K, Clapp-Channing N, Gehlbach S, et al. Caregiving in elderly relatives: the prevalence of caregiving in a family practice. *Arch Neurol.* 1988;148:2177–2180.

Arnaud SH. Some psychological characteristics of children of multiple sclerotics. *Psychosom Med.* 1959;21(1):8–22.

Aronson KJ. Quality of life among persons with multiple sclerosis and their caregivers. *Neurology.* 1997;48(1):74–80.

Aronson KJ, Cleghorn G, Goldenberg E. Assistance arrangements and use of services among persons with multiple sclerosis and their caregivers. *Disabil Rehabil.* 1996;18:354–361.

Birk K, Giesser B. Fertility, pregnancy, and childbirth. In: Kalb R, ed. *Multiple Sclerosis: A Guide for Families.* 3rd ed. New York: Demos Medical Publishing; 2006:81–92.

Bowling A. *Complementary and Alternative Medicine and Multiple Sclerosis.* 2nd ed. New York: Demos Medical Publishing; 2007.

Brandes DW, Callender T, Lathi E, O'Leary S. A review of disease-modifying therapies for MS: Maximizing adherence and minimizing adverse events. *Curr Med Res Opin.* 2009;25(1):77–92.

Buhse M. Assessment of caregiver burden in families of persons with multiple sclerosis. *J Neurosci Nurs.* 2008;40(1):25–31.

Cheung J, Hocking P. The experience of spousal carers of people with multiple sclerosis. *Qual Health Res.* 2004;14:153–166.

Chipchase SY, Lincoln NB. Factors associated with carer strain in carers of people with multiple sclerosis. *Disabil Rehabil.* 2001;23:768–776.

Coyle P, Halper J. *Living with Progressive MS: Overcoming the Challenges.* 2nd ed. New York: Demos Medical Publishing; 2008.

Crawford P, Miller D. Parenting issues. In: Kalb R, ed. *Multiple Sclerosis: A Guide for Families.* 3rd ed. New York: Demos Medical Publishing; 2006: 93–110.

Cross T, Rintell D. Children's perceptions of parental multiple sclerosis. *Psychol Health Med.* 1999;4(4): 355–360.

Deatrick JA, Brennan D, Cameron ME. Mothers with multiple sclerosis and their children: effects of fatigue and exacerbations on maternal support. *Nurs Res.* 1998; 47(4):205–210.

De Judicibus MA, McCabe MP. The impact of parental multiple sclerosis on the adjustment of children and adolescents. *Adolescence.* 2004;39(155):551–569.

Dennison L, Moss-Morris R, Chalder T. A review of psychological correlates of adjustment in patients with multiple sclerosis. *Clin Psychol Rev.* 2009;9(2):141–153.

Diareme S, Tsiantis J, Kolaitis G, et al. Emotional and behavioural difficulties in children of parents with multiple sclerosis: a controlled study in Greece. *Euro Child Adolesc Psychiatry.* 2006;15(6):309–318.

Feinstein A, O'Connor P, Gray T, Feinstein K. The effects of anxiety of psychiatric morbidity in patients with multiple sclerosis. *Mult Scler.* 1999;5(5):323–326.

Fivged N, Myhr KM, Larsen JP, Aarsland D. Caregiver burden in multiple sclerosis: the impact of neuropsychiatric symptoms. *J Neurol Neurosurg Psychiatry.* 2007; 78(10):1097–1102.

Frohman EM, Havrdova E, Lublin F, et al. Most patients with multiple sclerosis or a clinically isolated demyelinating syndrome should be treated at the time of diagnosis. *Arch Neurol.* 2006;63(4):614–619.

Gonzalez S, Steinglass P, Reiss D. Putting the illness in its place: discussion groups for families with chronic medical illnesses. *Fam Process.* 1989;28(1):69–87.

Goodman A. Talking about primary progressive MS. National Multiple Sclerosis Society. 2009. Available at: http://www.nationalMSsociety.org/PRCPublications. Accessed on March 2, 2010.

Goretti B, Portaccio E, Zipoli V, et al. Coping strategies, psychological variables, and their relationship with quality of life in multiple sclerosis. *Neurol Sci.* 2009; 30(1):15–20.

Holland NJ, Burks, JS, Schneider DM. Primary Progressive Multiple Sclerosis: What You Need to Know. DiaMedica, New York, 2010.

Holland N, Wiesel P, Cavallo P, et al. Adherence to disease-modifying therapy in multiple sclerosis: part I. *Rehabil Nurs.* 2001a;26(5):172–176.

Holland N, Wiesel P, Cavallo P, et al. Adherence to disease-modifying therapy in multiple sclerosis: part II. *Rehabil Nurs.* 2001b;26(6):221–226.

Janssens AC, Buljevac D, van Doorn PA, et al. Prediction of anxiety and distress following diagnosis of multiple sclerosis: a two-year longitudinal study. *Mult Scler.* 2006;12(6):794–801.

Kalb R. When MS joins the family. In: Kalb R, ed. *Multiple Sclerosis: A Guide for Families.* 3rd ed. New York: Demos Medical Publishing; 2006: 1–10.

Kalb R. The emotional and psychological impact of multiple sclerosis relapses. *J Neurol Sci.* 2007;256(suppl 1): S29–S33.

Kalb R. Coping and adaptation: making a place for MS in your life. In: Kalb R, ed. *Multiple Sclerosis: The Questions You Have; The Answers You Need.* 4th ed. New York: Demos Medical Publishing; 2008: 255–269.

Kalb R, Holland N, Giesser B. *Multiple Sclerosis for Dummies.* Hoboken, NJ: Wiley; 2007.

Kalb R, Seidman F. Adults with MS and their parents. In: Kalb R, ed. *Multiple Sclerosis: A Guide for Families.* 3rd ed. New York: Demos Medical Publishing; 2006: 137–148.

Karussis D, Biermann LD, Bohlega S, et al. A recommended treatment algorithm in relapsing multiple sclerosis: report of an international consensus meeting. *Eur J Neurol.* 2006;13(1):61–71.

Korostil M, Feinstein A. Anxiety disorders and their clinical correlates in multiple sclerosis patients. *Mult Scler.* 2007;13(1):67–72.

Louise-Bender PT, Kim J, Weiner B. The shaping of individual meanings assigned to assistive technology: A review of personal factors. *Disabil Rehabil.* 2002; 24(1-3):5–20.

McCabe MP, McKern S, McDonald E. Coping and psychological adjustment among people with multiple sclerosis. *J Psychosom Res.* 2004;56(3):355–361.

McDaniel SH, Hepworth J, Doherty W. *Medical Family Therapy.* New York: Basic Books; 1992.

McKeown L, Porter-Armstrong A, Baxter D. The needs and experiences of caregivers of individuals with multiple sclerosis: a systematic review. *Clin Rehabil.* 2003; 17:234–258.

McKeown LP, Porter-Armstrong AP, Baxter GD. Caregivers of people with multiple sclerosis: experiences of support. *Mult Scler.* 2004;10(2):219–230.

Minden SL, Frankel D, Hadden L, et al. The Sonya Slifka longitudinal multiple sclerosis study: methods and sample characteristics. *Mult Scler.* 2006;12(1):24–38.

Minden SL, Orav J, Reich P. Depression in multiple sclerosis. *Gen Hosp Psychiatry.* 1987;9(6):426–434.

Mutch K. Information for young people when multiple sclerosis enters the family. *Br J Nurs.* 2005;14(14): 758–760.

National Multiple Sclerosis Society. Disease management consensus statement. 2007. Available at: http://www.nationalmssociety.org/ExpertOpinionPapers. Accessed on March 2, 2010.

O'Brien R, Wineman N, Nealon N. Correlates of the caregiving process in multiple sclerosis. *Sch Inq Nurs Pract.* 1995;9:323–338.

Pakenham KI. Adjustment to multiple sclerosis: application of a stress and coping model. *Health Psychol.* 1999; 18(4):383–392.

Pakenham KI, Bursnall S. Relations between social support, appraisal and coping and both positive and negative outcomes for children of a parent with multiple sclerosis and comparisons with children of healthy parents. *Clin Rehabil.* 2006;20(8):709–723.

Pandya S. Caregiving in the United States. 2005. Available at: http://www.directcareclearinghouse.org/download/AARP%20Family%20caregivers%20fact%20sheet.pdf. Accessed on March 31, 2010.

Pozzilli C, Palmisano L, Mainero C, et al. Relationship between emotional distress in caregivers and health status in persons with multiple sclerosis. *Mult Scler.* 2004;10:442–446.

Quesnel S, Feinstein A. Multiple sclerosis and alcohol: a study of problem drinking. *Mult Scler.* 2004; 10(2):197–201.

Rutter M. Pathways from childhood to adult life. *J Child Psychol Psychiatry.* 1989;30:23–51.

Steck B, Grether A, Amsler F, et al. Disease variables and depression affecting the process of coping in families with a somatically ill parent. *Psychopathology.* 2007; 40(6):394–404.

Stucki BR, Mulvey J. *Can Aging Baby Boomers Avoid the Nursing Home? Long-Term Care Insurance for Age in Place.* Washington, DC: American Council of Life Insurers; 2000.

Thrower BW. Clinically isolated syndromes: Predicting and delaying multiple sclerosis. *Neurology.* 2007;68(24 suppl 4):S12–S15.

Weinshenker BG. Natural history of multiple sclerosis. *Ann Neurol.* 1994;36(suppl):S6–S11.

Wingerchuk DM. Current evidence and therapeutic strategies for multiple sclerosis. *Sem Neurol.* 2008;28(1): 56–68.

Yahav R, Vosburgh J, Miller A. Emotional responses of children and adolescents to parents with multiple sclerosis. *Mult Scler.* 2005;11(4):464–468.

Yahav R, Vosburgh J, Miller A. Separation-individuation processes of adolescent children of parents with multiple sclerosis. *Mult Scler.* 2007;13(1):87–94.

Zorzon M, de Masi R, Nasuelli D, et al. Depression and anxiety in multiple sclerosis: a clinical and MRI study in 95 subjects. *J Neurol.* 2001;248(5):416–421.

RECOMMENDED RESOURCES

Professional Resource Center, National Multiple Sclerosis Society (healthprof_info@nmss.org; http://www.nationalMSsociety.org/PRC).

Talking with Your MS Patients about Difficult Topics—a National MS Society booklet series available at http://www.nationalMSsociety.org/PRCPublications.

Topics include the following:

- Communicating the diagnosis
- Initiating and adhering to treatment with an injectable disease-modifying agent
- Stress
- Family issues
- Sexual dysfunction
- Reproductive issues
- Role of rehabilitation
- Life planning
- Cognitive dysfunction
- Elimination problems
- Depression and other mood changes
- Progressive disease
- Primary progressive MS

27 Employment and Career Development Considerations

Phillip D. Rumrill, Jr. and Steven W. Nissen

Considering the wide-ranging medical and psychological symptoms of multiple sclerosis (MS), the unpredictable disease course and related adjustment issues, and the intrusion that the illness can cause in virtually every aspect of life—as described in other chapters of this book—it is not surprising that employment and career development are prominent concerns for people with MS. In this chapter, we describe the most prominent challenges facing people with MS as they attempt to maintain or resume their careers following diagnosis. We begin with a description of the contemporary employment scene for people with MS; then we discuss known determinants of employment status in an effort to explain the high jobless rate that has plagued the MS community for many years. We will also highlight two Federal laws, namely, the Americans with Disabilities Act and the Family and Medical Leave Act, that provide employment-related protections for Americans with MS, followed by a description of selected employment interventions and resources that can aid readers in addressing the needs of MS patients.

MULTIPLE SCLEROSIS AND THE WORLD OF WORK

In most societies of the world, who we are is determined in large measure by what we do for a living (Zunker, 1994; Rumrill, 2006; Wehman, 2006). When we are introduced to strangers at social functions, one of the first points of information we share is our occupation. Psychologically speaking, people often describe their jobs, their employers, and/or their career fields as defining attributes of their identities: "I'm a plumber," "I work at Sears," or "I'm in the restaurant business." Work

consumes a considerable portion of a person's sense of self, which stands to reason because experts estimate that American adults spend as much as 70% of their waking hours performing tasks related to their jobs (Wehman, 2006). This time commitment renders work the single most time-consuming social role for most people between the ages of 16 and 65—more time-consuming than the roles of parent, spouse or significant other, citizen, friend, and leisurite.

Not only does work occupy our time, it is the primary vehicle through which we earn money, procure goods and services, purchase homes, and save for retirement. Work also provides other, nonmonetary benefits, such as identity formation as previously mentioned, socialization, a sense of purpose and accomplishment, group membership (e.g., "I'm in the Teamsters Union"), and access to health care via employer-sponsored insurance (Dawis and Lofquist, 1984; Wehman, 2006). Sumner (1997) connected employment status to life satisfaction and general health, suggesting that people who work are healthier, happier, and more satisfied with their social lives in comparison to people who do not perform paid employment. In a study of Americans with MS, Roessler et al. (2004) reported that employed participants had lower levels of perceived stress and higher levels of overall quality of life than did unemployed participants.

From a developmental lens, the link between work and identity formation begins early in childhood and continues throughout the life cycle (Super, 1980; Hennessey, 2004). The onset of MS typically occurs between the ages of 20 and 50—a time that many people regard as the "prime of life." From a career development standpoint, those years are the most active decades of most people's lives. According to Super (1980), the period between ages 20 and 40 is marked by *(a)* exploration (gathering and processing occupational information to formulate career goals), *(b)* establishment (forging a plan for attainment of those goals and beginning a career), and *(c)* maintenance (advancing in one's career and attaining his or her goals) activities. For many people with MS, however, the career development process slows and, in many cases, stops after the illness begins to manifest itself.

More than 90% of Americans with MS have employment histories; that is, they have worked at some time in the past (LaRocca, 1995; Roessler et al., 2002). Some 60% of people with MS were still working at the time of diagnosis, even given the lengthy time period that often intervenes between the onset of initial symptoms and confirmed diagnosis (LaRocca, 1995; Rumrill, 1996). As the illness progresses, however, people with MS experience a sharp decline in employment; Fraser et al. (2002) estimated that only 20%–30% of Americans with MS are employed 15 years after diagnosis, and only 35%–45% of people with MS in the United States are currently employed (Roessler et al., 2002).

Not surprisingly, Americans with MS are concerned about the bleak employment prospects that await them following diagnosis. In a 2003 survey of 1310 adults with MS from 10 American states and Washington, DC, Roessler et al. (2003) found the majority of respondents dissatisfied with 29 out of 32 high-priority employment concerns. Majorities of people with MS were satisfied with only three items: their access to service providers (51%), the treatment they received from service providers (61%), and the encouragement they received from others to take control of their lives (56%). The employment concerns items with the highest dissatisfaction ratings clustered into three thematic categories: implementation and enforcement of the Americans with Disabilities Act, health care and health insurance coverage, and Social Security disability programs. Table 27-1 presents the 29 employment concerns items that were identified as problematic by the majority of respondents, in descending order of dissatisfaction ratings.

FACTORS ASSOCIATED WITH LABOR FORCE PARTICIPATION

For many years, medical, psychological, allied health, and rehabilitation researchers have sought to understand why people with MS make a wholesale departure from the labor force, usually of their own choosing and often before the disease has rendered them incapable of working. Among people with MS who are unemployed, 75% left their jobs voluntarily (Roessler et al., 2002), 80% believe that they retain the ability to work (Sumner, 1997), and 75% say that they would like to re-enter the work force (Rumrill, 2006). In the effort to explain the premature disengagement from work that often accompanies MS, the factors that predict employment and unemployment have been a primary focus. The medical and psychosocial accompaniments of MS, which, at first glance, might seem to be the most obvious culprits in the choice to stop working, fail to adequately explain the high rate of unemployment. The symptoms and course of MS have been linked to employment status, but so have a myriad of demographic and environmental variables such as gender, age, socioeconomic status, job type and working conditions, reactions of co-workers and employers, workplace discrimination, and disability benefits.

Gender

Although the unemployment rate among Americans with MS is disappointingly low for both sexes, women are significantly less likely to be employed than are men (LaRocca, 1995; Roessler et al., 2001). LaRocca et al. (1985) reported that 80% of women with MS were unemployed, as compared to 66% of men with the illness. Roessler et al. (2003) reported similar findings nearly two decades later, revealing jobless rates of 67% for women with MS and 51% for men with MS in their national survey. Roessler et al. (2004) found American women with MS nearly twice as likely to be unemployed as their male counterparts. Canadian citizens with MS appear to experience similar gender disparities when it comes to labor force participation; Edgley et al. (1991) reported unemployment rates of 58% and 70% for men and women, respectively.

TABLE 27-1 Priority Employment Concerns among People with Multiple Sclerosis, Ranked By Dissatisfaction Ratings

Item	Percent Dissatisfied
People with multiple sclerosis…	
have adequate financial help to stay on the job.	81
have access to reasonably priced prescription medications.	78
know their rights regarding job-related physical examinations.	77
have assistance in coping with stress on the job.	76
know about available employment and social services.	75
have their needs considered in the development of of Social Security programs.	74
have adequate health insurance so that they can recover and return to work.	73
are treated fairly by employers in the hiring process.	73
receive up-to-date, easily understood information about benefits and work incentives from the Social Security Administration.	72
have opportunities for home-based employment.	72
can work with employers and supervisors who understand the effects of multiple sclerosis.	71
have adequate help in comparing fringe benefits, particularly health insurance coverage, among different job options.	71
have adequate knowledge of the employment protections of Title 1 of the Americans with Disabilities Act.	70
have adequate information about short-and long-term disability.	70
have adequate information on provisions of the Family and Medical Leave Act.	69
can get retraining if it is required to return to work.	68
are considered for other jobs in the same company if their disabilities prevent them from going back to their own jobs	66
are prepared for real jobs in real work sites.	65
are helped to find employment for which they are prepared.	65
are treated fairly when they apply to work.	64
have transportation needed to travel to and from work.	64
are given support from employers and supervisors after returning to work.	63
can get help with the cost of assistive devices.	63
are encouraged to work part time, if full time is too difficult.	59
receive reasonable accommodations in the workplace.	58
have confidence in their potential to work.	58
can get help in identifying and designing workplace accommodations.	58
receive the same pay as would a nondisabled person.	53
have access to adequate information about Social Security programs.	52

Source: from Roessler et al., 2003, pp. 12–13.

Socioeconomic Status

Both men and women with MS are more likely to leave the work force if they have a spouse who is working (Genevie et al., 1987). People with MS who have higher levels of education and/or more money in savings and investments are more likely to be employed than are those in lower socioeconomic strata (Genevie et al., 1987; Edgley et al., 1991; Roessler et al., 2004). This finding may not be surprising given that people with higher levels of education tend to occupy positions that require less physical exertion, and that the physiological effects of MS therefore do not impose work impediments to the same extent as they do for those whose jobs require more physical exertion (Rumrill et al., 1998). Rumrill (2006) noted that higher level employees have more flexibility and autonomy in modifying their jobs to meet their MS-related needs. Indeed, employers are generally more likely to accommodate workers who are viewed as talented and essential to the operation of business than they are to meet the needs of less valued workers (Rumrill, 1993; Sumner, 1997).

Age

In a survey of 1180 Canadians with MS, Edgley et al. (1991) found unemployment to increase as a linear function of age. Respondents between the ages of 20 and 29 reported a 38% jobless rate, significantly lower than those rates indicated by their counterparts at ages 30–39 (57%), 40–49 (70%), 50–59 (84%), 60–69 (87%), and 70 and over (93%). The relationship between age and unemployment in people with MS has been upheld in several studies in the United States (Kornblith et al., 1986; Genevie et al., 1987). LaRocca et al. (1985) presented findings indicating a curvilinear direction of that relationship; they found middle-aged people with MS more likely to be employed than either younger or older ones. Rumrill (1999) reported similar findings in his survey of people with MS in Ohio.

Two factors related to MS and unemployment might help to explain why seasoned, older workers tend to leave the workforce before reaching retirement age. First, there is a significant relationship between age and MS-related functional disability (Wineman, 1990); as the years pass and

the illness progresses, the person becomes less able to meet the physical demands of employment. Second, age is positively associated with socioeconomic status; many older people with MS have the financial means to stop working and do so voluntarily to focus on other pursuits (Rumrill, 2006).

Physiological Symptoms

A number of studies have revealed the exacerbation and progression of physical symptoms to be strong predictors of job loss for people with MS. In denoting the most frequently cited reasons that people with MS leave the workforce, Rumrill (2006) and Fraser et al. (2002) noted that as many as 30% of unemployed people with MS attribute their jobless status to the physiological effects of the illness, especially fatigue. LaRocca et al. (1985) found scores on the Kurtzke Disability Status Scale (a measure for determining the severity of physical disability based on neurologic examination and functional assessment) to be significant predictors of employment status—the more severe the physical disability, the more likely people with MS were to be unemployed. Gulick, Yam, and Touw (1989) found mobility problems to be associated with unemployment in people with MS, as did Kornblith et al. (1986). Nearly half of unemployed respondents in the survey of people with MS conducted by Edgley et al. (2001) cited ambulation difficulties as the primary reason for leaving the workforce. Thirty-nine percent described fatigue as the most important contributing factor.

Course and Disease Progression

In their article on career development and MS, Gordon et al. (1994) noted that the most prominent impediment to vocational planning lies in the unpredictable, sometimes progressive course of the disease. Indeed, numerous characteristics of the disease process have been linked to employment status. Rumrill (1999) found people with chronic and progressive MS least likely to be employed. Roessler et al. (2004) found that people who experience MS symptoms most or all of the time, especially if the persistent symptoms are greater in number and more severe, are more likely to be unemployed than people with other symptom patterns. More symptoms, more persistent symptoms, and more severe symptoms are generally associated with primary or secondary progressive MS (once known as chronic-progressive MS; Schapiro, 2003), so it follows that people with progressive forms of the disease are at greater risk for job loss than people whose MS experience is more episodic and/or less intrusive.

Cognitive Dysfunction

Cognitive deficits associated with MS are, arguably, the most frustrating aspect of the illness (McReynolds and Koch, 2001; Fraser et al., 2002; Kalb, 2007). The rate at which one learns new information, skills, and procedures is often diminished (Franklin et al., 1989), as are short-term memory (Grant et al., 1984), long-term memory (Rao et al., 1989), and abstract reasoning abilities (Halligan et al., 1988). By their own reports, employees with MS identified significant career maintenance barriers resulting from thought-processing and memory deficits in Roessler and Rumrill's (1995) needs assessment study. Rao et al. (1991) reported that "cognitively impaired" people with MS were more likely to be unemployed than were "cognitively intact" MS patients. Roessler et al. (2004) found people with MS who reported cognitive impairments four times more likely to be unemployed than people with MS who did not report cognitive impairments. Edgley et al. (2001) indicated that the frequency of perceived cognitive problems was directly related to the rate of unemployment among people with MS in Canada. Respondents who indicated that they rarely experienced cognitive problems reported an unemployment rate of 53%, whereas the unemployment rates for people with MS who described the regularity of cognitive problems as sometimes (67%), often (73%), and almost always (86%) were significantly higher (Edgley et al., 2001).

Psychological and Emotional Factors

Although MS is often accompanied by emotional and/or psychological problems (e.g., depression, anxiety, bipolar disorder), people with MS do not generally equate them with job loss (Rumrill, 1996). LaRocca et al. (1985) found that only 2.8% of unemployed people with MS considered

emotional difficulties to be the primary reason for their job loss. Edgley et al. (2001) also noted that self-reported emotional problems had a much smaller impact on employment status than did such factors as gender, age, and physiological symptoms. On the other hand, Genevie et al. (1987) found that people with MS who identified problems with emotional lability were significantly less likely to be employed than were those who indicated stable emotional patterns.

Variability of Symptoms and Invisible Disability

Given the variability and unpredictability of symptoms, people with MS may wonder how they can ever be a reliable and consistent employee. Many symptoms of MS, such as fatigue, cognitive dysfunction, heat sensitivity, tingling, and numbness, are invisible in nature. This may lead the employee with MS to be very concerned about disclosure in the workplace. The employee may choose not to disclose in an attempt to protect his or her privacy. Or disclosing may cause that employee significant stress and anxiety. The decision to disclose is a very complicated one with both legal and practical ramifications. It is ultimately a personal decision to make and every effort should be made to connect that individual to resources and agencies available to provide guidance in the disclosure dilemma.

Workplace Discrimination

Technically, the choice to leave the workforce is most often made by the person with MS himself or herself. That said, it is often not clear to what extent the phenomenon of discrimination in the workplace "helps" people with MS to make that choice. Certainly, perceived discrimination is a major obstacle to continued employment following diagnosis with MS, and people with MS often believe that their employers treat them unfairly in comparison to nondisabled workers. Rumrill and Hennessey (2001) described workplace discrimination as the unifying feature of the employment experience for Americans with MS, suggesting that it is the number one underlying explanation for the high rate of workforce attrition that follows the onset of the illness.

In the national survey conducted by Roessler et al. (2002), no fewer than six items related to implementation of the Americans with Disabilities Act (ADA) and the Family and Medical Leave Act (FMLA) were reported among the 12 most prominent employment-related problems identified by people with MS. Specifically, the majority of respondents reported having been treated unfairly in the hiring process by employers (73%), having been denied reasonable accommodations (58%), having received lower pay than their nondisabled peers (53%), being refused schedule modifications that would have enabled them to continue working (59%), having received inadequate health insurance coverage (73%), and having received little or no information about their legal rights from employers (69%).

Between 1992 and 2003, the United States Equal Employment Opportunity Commission (EEOC) received and resolved 3669 allegations of employment discrimination from people with MS under Title I of the ADA. Allegations of unlawful termination constituted the most commonly cited form of workplace discrimination (29.9%), followed in descending order by complaints related to reasonable accommodations (21.9%), terms and conditions of employment (9.8%), harassment (6.7%), hiring (3.8%), discipline (3.4%), constructive discharge (i.e., creating a work environment that makes it impossible for the person to continue working; 3.0%), layoff (2.8%), and promotion (2.5%). People with MS filing ADA Title I allegations were mostly female (66.5%), predominantly Caucasian (76.1%), and of mid-career age on average (M = 42.47 years, SD = 8.54). Allegations were most often filed against employers in the South United States Census tracking region (35.7%), and employers in the service, financial, insurance, and real estate industries were most often the subjects of ADA Title I complaints.

In comparison to ADA Title I complainants with other disabilities, people with MS were more likely than people with other disabilities to allege discrimination in the areas of reasonable accommodations, terms and conditions of employment, constructive discharge, and demotion; less likely to allege discrimination in the area of hiring; and more likely to have their allegations of discrimination resolved in their favor by the United States EEOC (Unger et al., 2004; Rumrill et al., 2004, 2005). Even though people with MS do prevail in ADA Title I complaints to the EEOC at a higher rate than people with other disabilities, the troubling fact remains that 75% of all ADA Title I allegations filed by people with MS since 1992 have been found to have insufficient merit as to warrant a claim of discrimination.

Disability Benefits

It is well documented that people with MS who receive disability benefits from private insurers or from government agencies face extreme difficulties in restarting their careers. The benefits paid by most American long-term disability insurance carriers and the Social Security Administration's two disability programs (i.e., Social Security Disability Insurance [SSDI] and Supplemental Security Income [SSI]) are predicated on the beneficiary being too disabled to work (Marini, 2003). This requirement provides a powerful systemic disincentive that keeps thousands of Americans with MS from participating in the labor force. Once they have been adjudicated as too severely disabled to work by either long-term disability insurers or Social Security (or sometimes both), they integrate the external confirmation of their disabled status into their own self-concepts— self-concepts that do no include the role of worker (Roessler and Rumrill, 2003). From that point on in the vast majority of cases, unemployment and receipt of disability benefits conjoin in a self-fulfilling prophecy for people with MS (Rumrill and Hennessey, 2001). According to Fraser et al. (2004), people with MS progress from active employment to short-term disability insurance, long-term disability insurance, and, finally, SSDI at higher and faster rates than people with most other disabilities. Once on SSDI, the "too disabled to work" message has already registered loud and clear, and over time it would seem to become impervious to alternative messages of employability. According to Fraser et al. (2002), less than 1% of Americans with MS who receive SSDI benefits will ever resume gainful employment.

Lest readers conclude that archival data from insurance carriers and the Social Security Administration are the only bases for our assertion that disability benefits negatively impact employment, focus groups of people with MS identified work disincentives in SSDI, SSI, and long-term disability insurance among their three most important reasons for the low employment rate among adults with MS. Also in the voices of people with MS, no fewer than 52% of the 2411 people with MS who participated in Kent State University's nationwide MS Employment Assistance Service between 2001 and 2006 had concerns related to long-term disability insurance or Social Security programs (Rumrill, 2006).

FEDERAL LAWS THAT PROVIDE EMPLOYMENT-RELATED PROTECTIONS FOR AMERICANS WITH MULTIPLE SCLEROSIS

The prospect of obtaining or maintaining employment as a person with MS can be an exceedingly difficult one, but help is available in American federal law. Described in this section are the employment provisions of the ADA and the FMLA, both of which offer procedures to aid people with MS and other disabling conditions in balancing the effects of disability with the rigors of work.

The Americans with Disabilities Act

The ADA of 1990 and the ADA Amendments Act of 2008 were designed to eliminate discrimination on the basis of disability in the areas of employment, government services, public accommodations, and telecommunications. In fact, the ADA is the most comprehensive civil rights legislation passed since the Civil Rights Act of 1964. Title I of the ADA requires most employers to take proactive steps to ensure that people with disabilities are treated fairly in the workplace. Presented below are key Title l definitions and procedures drawn from ADA regulations (Rumrill et al., 2008).

Covered employers

All public and private employers with 15 or more employees must comply with the provisions set forth in Title I. The federal government, Native American tribes, and tax-exempt private membership clubs are not covered.

Reasonable accommodations

Reasonable accommodations are modifications to the job or to the work environment that enable qualified people with disabilities to perform the essential functions of their positions. Types of reasonable accommodations include the following: *(1)* restructuring of existing facilities, *(2)* restructuring of the job, *(3)* modification of work schedules, *(4)* reassignment to a vacant position, *(5)* modification of equipment, *(6)* installation of new equipment, *(7)* provision of qualified readers and interpreters, *(8)* modification of application and examination procedures or training materials, *(9)* flexible personal leave policies, and *(10)* use of supported employment programs. Reasonable accommodations do *not* include the following: *(1)* eliminating an essential job function; *(2)* lowering production standards that are applied to all employees (although an employer may have to provide reasonable accommodations to enable an employee with a disability to meet production standards); *(3)* providing personal use items such as prosthetic limbs, wheelchairs, eyeglasses, hearing aids, or similar devices; and *(4)* excusing a violation of uniformly applied conduct rules that are job-related and consistent with business necessity (e.g., violence, threats of violence, stealing, destruction of property).

For applicants or employees wishing to request a reasonable accommodation in the workplace, Title I regulations prescribe a collaborative, non-adversarial process involving the applicant or employee and the employer. The steps of this process are as follows (Rumrill et al., 2008):

1. The applicant/employee initiates a request for accommodation (preferably but not necessarily in written form).
2. The applicant/employee and employer collaborate to identify factors that limit the person's ability to perform the job's essential functions.
3. Using the applicant/employee as a resource, the employer identifies a variety of accommodations that would reduce or remove disability-related barriers to job performance.
4. The employer assesses the cost-effectiveness of each accommodation strategy to determine which one(s) could be implemented with the least economic hardship.

5. The employer implements an appropriate accommodation, considering the applicant/employee's preferences when two equivalent accommodations have been identified.

Given that the employee plays an active role in providing suggestions for accommodations, ideas may come from a variety of sources, including health professionals as well as the Job Accommodation Network (JAN), which will be discussed later in this chapter. Table 27–2 lists some common symptoms that individuals with MS may experience and some practical accommodations that might be helpful in the workplace. An individual might not experience all of the symptoms listed. These accommodations are not the only ones available but are provided as general suggestions to consider.

Disability

The ADA defines an individual with a disability as a person who *(1)* has a physical or mental impairment which substantially limits functioning in one or more *major life activities, (2)* has a record of such an impairment, or *(3)* is regarded as having such an impairment. Major life activities include, but are not limited to, walking, seeing, hearing, speaking, learning, working, and self-care. Individuals who are *not* protected by Title l of the ADA include *(1)* people with disabilities who pose a direct threat to the health or safety of themselves or others in the workplace; *(2)* active abusers of illegal substances; *(3)* employees who use alcohol during work; *(4)* people who are homosexual, transvestites, bisexual, or transsexual (sexual orientation is not considered a disabling condition); *(5)* voyeurs or people who have other sexual disorders; *(6)* people who have the disorders of kleptomania, compulsive gambling, or pyromania; and *(7)* people whose medical conditions can be mitigated by assistive technology, medication, or surgery. Under the ADA Amendments Act of 2008, it clarified that a condition that is in remission or episodic, which is how MS oftentimes presents itself, is considered a disability if it would substantially limit a major life activity when it is active. This offers individuals with MS significantly more protection given the variability and unpredictable nature of MS.

Qualified

Under Title I of the ADA, a qualified person with a disability is one who satisfies the primary requirements of the position and who can perform the fundamental duties (i.e., essential functions) of the job, with or without reasonable accommodations. The employer is not required to give preference to applicants with disabilities or to hire or retain an employee with a disability who does not have the required training, skills, and/or experience. The ADA offers no protection for employees whose disabilities have progressed to the point where they are unable to perform the essential functions of their jobs.

Essential functions

Essential job functions are those primary duties which the worker must be capable of performing, with reasonable accommodations if required. A function is considered essential when *(1)* the position exists to perform the function; *(2)* there are a limited number of other employees available to perform the function, or among whom the function can be distributed; and/or *(3)* the function is highly specialized, and the person in the position is hired for his or her special expertise and ability to perform the function. Essential functions do not include tasks that are marginal or unnecessary to performing the primary duties of the job (e.g., requiring a driver's license when driving is not required to carry out work-related tasks (Rumrill et al., 2008). Essential functions can be identified in a job analysis conducted by a trained rehabilitation professional, and they should be delineated on the written job description, which is given to all applicants.

Undue hardship

An employer is not required to make an accommodation if it would impose an undue hardship on the operation of the business or agency. Undue hardship refers to any accommodation that exceeds the bounds of practicality (e.g., it costs more than alternatives that are equally effective, requires extensive or disruptive renovations, or negatively affects other employees and/or customers). Undue hardships are determined on a case-by-case basis

TABLE 27-2 Accommodations Chart

Multiple Sclerosis Symptom/Limitation	Accommodation Strategies
New diagnosis	• Flexible medical leave/sick time policies that allow time off for diagnostic tests or treatment • Flexible or reduced work hours • Re-assignment of nonessential tasks to another employee
Medical treatment/ exacerbation	• Flexible medical leave policies that allow time off for medical treatments • Pooled sick leave or sick leave hours donated by other employees • Flexible or reduced work hours • Job sharing with another employee • Part-time options • Home-based work • Re-assignment of nonessential tasks to another employee
Fatigue	• Flexible work hours, especially to avoid rush-hour commuting • Use of the health office cot or a couch in a quiet and private location for a rest period • Combining of morning and afternoon breaks in order to take one longer rest break • Situating desk and workspace near supplies, equipment, and restroom • Ergonomic workstation design • Accessible space for using and/or storing a scooter or other mobility aid if walking is required • Home-based work • Telecommuting opportunities
Visual symptoms	• Readers: computerized or human • Temporary re-assignment of tasks • Halogen lights rather than fluorescent • Job modifications such as tape recorders, readers, large-print materials, and adaptive computer equipment or software (enlarged fonts/icons, scanners, antiglare screen, voice recognition software, talking computers)
Mobility and dexterity	• Wheelchair-level access to all workstations and/or adjustable workstations that allows for physical changes • Carts with wheels for transporting equipment and supplies • Assigning some or all walking, lifting, and carrying duties to others • Adaptive telephone equipment, including telephone headsets, speakerphone, and automatic dial • "Fat" pens and adapted computer keyboards • Flexible schedules that allow for open start and quit times to adjust to hazardous travel/weather times • Proper ergonomic furniture and workstation design

TABLE 27-2 (continued)

Multiple Sclerosis Symptom/Limitation	Accommodation Strategies
	• Parking spaces close to the worksite entrance
	• Automatic door openers
	• Accessible toilet facilities
	• Adjustable desk heights to accommodate a scooter or wheelchair
	• Note takers or tape recorder
	• Alternate phone access (e.g., headphone, etc.).
	• Enlarged or levered door knobs
Bladder/bowel	• Flexible work schedules.
	• Workspaces close to the restroom.
	• Accessible bathrooms
	• Frequent breaks
Cognitive (difficulty concentrating, remembering, learning new tasks)	• Assistance to simplify and organize workstation and tasks
	• Written job instructions
	• Self-paced workload
	• Assistance to divide work into specific sequential tasks
	• Telephone logs, notes/minutes from meetings with recorded directions and supervision instructions
	• Calendar diaries or day planners
	• Electronic diaries and planners that provide auditory and visual
	• reminders of meetings and appointments
	• Elimination of distractions such as background music
	• Allowing more time to learn new information
	• Providing new information through a variety of senses; vision, speech, hearing
	• Hand-held personal assistant devices
Slurred speech	• Speech amplification devices
	• Speech enhancement or simulation software
	• Written communication as much as possible, e.g., e-mail, fax
	• Reassignment of tasks that require significant verbal communication
Heat sensitivity	• Air conditioning or a fan to lower the ambient air temperature
	• Home-based work during very hot or humid spells or if the office air conditioning goes out
	• Indirect lighting
	• Refrigerators for storing a cooling vest or gel pack neck scarves

Source: From *Providing Information about MS to Employers.* National Multiple Sclerosis Society, 2005. Reproduced with permission.

using criteria such as the cost and nature of the requested accommodation, the overall financial resources of the facility, and the type of operation of the employer (Rumrill et al., 2008).

Other employment protections in Title I of the Americans with Disabilities Act

Although reasonable accommodations are an important part of the ADA, the employment protections available to people with disabilities go far beyond on-the-job accommodations. Under Title I, people with disabilities have the civil right to enjoy the same benefits and privileges of employment as their nondisabled co-workers. This means that personnel decisions (e.g., hiring, promotion, layoff, termination) must be made without regard to the person's disability status. Workers may not be harassed or intimidated on the basis of their disabilities, and the compensation they receive must be commensurate with their qualifications and productivity irrespective of disability. It should also be noted that many American states' fair labor and human rights statutes provide employment protections that are more comprehensive than those set forth in Title I of the ADA.

Enforcement of the Americans with Disabilities Act

Title I of the ADA is enforced by the U.S. Equal Employment Opportunity Commission (EEOC). Job applicants and employees (i.e., plaintiffs) are required to file claims with the EEOC within 300 days of the alleged violation. If it is determined by the EEOC that discrimination has likely occurred, one of two courses of action is taken: the EEOC may either prosecute or issue the plaintiff a "right to sue" letter. The right to sue letter allows the plaintiff to retain an attorney and proceed in federal civil court with a jury trial. If the employer is found to have discriminated against the applicant or employee, remedies available to the plaintiff include hiring, reinstatement, court orders to stop discriminatory practices, and punitive and compensatory damages.

The Family and Medical Leave Act

Another law with important implications to the employment of people with MS is the Family and Medical Leave Act (FMLA) of 1993. The FMLA has enabled thousands of American employees to retain their jobs while taking unpaid leaves of absence to attend to important family health concerns. The law requires employers in the public and private sectors to hold workers' jobs open and continue paying health insurance premiums while employees take time off to treat and/or recover from illnesses or injuries. It also provides leave for employees who must attend to the healthcare needs of their family members.

A covered employer under the FMLA is one who has 50 or more employees residing within a 75-mile radius of the work location. Employees are eligible for protection if they have at least 1 year of seniority on the job (i.e., at least 1250 hours worked within the 12 months preceding the requested leave date) *and* have a serious health condition.

The FMLA defines a serious health condition as any illness, injury, impairment, or regimen of treatment that renders one unable to perform any essential function of his or her job. The term *serious health condition* is broader and more inclusive than the ADA's definition of disability. This means that a worker with MS could be a person with a serious health condition as per the FMLA but not meet the ADA's standard as a person with a disability. Unlike the ADA's term *disability*, which includes only those impairments that are not alleviated by time or medical intervention, serious health conditions pertain to both temporary and permanent impairments. Examples of commonly invoked serious health conditions under the FMLA include pregnancy, birth or adoption of a child, surgery, chemotherapy, and chronic illnesses.

The FMLA requires covered employers to provide up to 12 weeks of unpaid leave per calendar year for an eligible employee. The employee may take all accrued, paid sick leave before requesting unpaid time off. The 12 weeks of unpaid leave need not be taken consecutively, and the employer must allow the worker to return to the same or a similar, equivalent position. Return to work following FMLA-covered leave may be denied only to "key" employees—those earning the highest 10% of salaries. This exception applies only when holding open those employees' jobs would create substantial and grievous long-term economic harm to the employer's operations. The employer's burden of proof for this exception is more stringent than for the ADA's defense of undue hardship.

Eligible employees may take time off to attend to their own serious health conditions or to assist in the care and treatment of family members who have serious health conditions. Family members are defined as spouses, children, and parents. For example, a person whose wife has MS and needs transportation to weekly appointments with her neurologist could request unpaid time off to accompany her to doctor's visits.

In the event that the need for leave is foreseeable (e.g., pregnancy, elective surgery), the employee must give the employer 30 days advance notice. If the need for leave is unforeseeable (e.g., an exacerbation of MS, accident), employees are required to give reasonable notice (undefined in FMLA regulations). Once the employee has filed a request for leave, the employer has 2 business days to determine the employee's eligibility for the requested time off. Failure on the employer's part to respond within 2 business days automatically renders the employee eligible for the leave that he or she has requested. Of course, an employer may request that the employee document his or her serious health condition or the condition of a family member. If requested, the employee must provide verification from a health-care provider, with the following conditions:

1. The provider should verify only the need for a medical leave and not disclose the underlying medical condition.
2. The information reported should be job related (e.g., need for, length of, and timing of the medical leave).
3. Inquiry into the possible future effects of the serious health condition should be avoided.
4. On the employer's part, leave requests should be processed by a designated, knowledgeable person so that discussion with the employee's supervisors and co-workers is kept to a minimum.
5. Supervisors should be notified only of facts related to the circumstances of the requested leave, not about specific aspects of the employee's (or a family member's) serious health condition.

6. Records related to medical leave must be maintained in a separate file from the employee's personnel records.

Vocational Interventions And Employment-Related Resources For People With Multiple Sclerosis

Over the past 30 years, there has emerged a wealth of resources, demonstration projects, research, direct services, and advocacy efforts to promote the employment and career advancement of people with MS and other disabling conditions. Some of these interventions and resources are designed specifically for people with MS, whereas others target people with all types of disabilities. Some of these interventions are delivered by rehabilitation professionals, and others are of the "self-help" variety. Some of these interventions are delivered in-person, and others can be accessed via telephone or the Internet. Some of these interventions focus on job acquisition (i.e., getting a job), and others focus on job retention (i.e., keeping and advancing in the job one has).

As different as these programs and projects are in design and implementation, together they form a powerful set of tools and strategies for combating the deleterious impact that MS too often exacts on a person's employment status. In this section, we describe the essential elements and outcomes of employment interventions and resources that have proven efficacious or could be helpful to people with MS in their career-related pursuits. We begin by highlighting MS-specific interventions, then we follow with descriptions of several national-scale programs that address the employment needs and concerns of Americans with various disabilities. Health-care providers should be confident and comfortable referring patients to these resources.

Multiple Sclerosis–Specific Interventions

Multiple Sclerosis Employment Assistance Service: Kent State University

Since 1999, the Center for Disability Studies at Kent State University in Ohio has offered employment assistance and career counseling services to adults with MS (Rumrill et al., 2008). The MS

Employment Assistance Service is staffed by nationally certified rehabilitation counselors who provide a wide range of vocational services, including the following:

- Career counseling
- Assessments of vocational interests and aptitudes
- Transferable skills analysis
- Resume preparation
- Interview skills training
- Targeted job placement assistance
- Social Security advocacy
- Self-advocacy training
- Benefits planning
- Referrals to legal resources
- On-the-job accommodation planning
- Consultation in employment litigation

All services are provided via telephone or e-mail, and each participant develops a customized plan of services and assistance from the "menu" just described. Some participants use the MS Employment Assistance Service over an extended time period, whereas others call or e-mail for specific, point-in-time answers to employment-related questions and concerns. The service is supported by subscriptions from individual chapters of the National Multiple Sclerosis Society, and 2411 people with MS representing 16 chapters of the Society have taken part in the project as of this writing (Rumrill et al., 2008). The most common employment-related issues raised by people with MS inquiring to the service include job search (46% of participants), workplace discrimination and employer relations (42%), short- and long-term disability (40%), Social Security (38%), on-the-job accommodations (37%), disclosure of disability (34%), the Family and Medical Leave Act (27%), and home-based employment (19%). The percentages in the preceding list total more than 100% because most participants inquire to the MS Employment Assistance Service with more than one issue or concern.

Operation Job Match

Founded in 1980 as a job-readiness training program, Operation Job Match (OJM) is the employment assistance and support program of the National Capital Chapter of the National Multiple

Sclerosis Society in Washington, DC. The program addresses a variety of employment- and disability-related issues, including job-seeking skills components and a selective job development component. Topics include disability management, stress management, assertiveness training, disclosure issues, accommodation strategies, interview skills, resume and cover letters, and networking. Operation Job Match maintains a job bank of positions available in the metropolitan Washington, DC area, and the staff match program participants to available positions. Job bank participants are private-sector employers, federal government agencies, colleges and universities, and nonprofit organizations. Though originally designed for individuals with MS, the program was expanded to include participants with other adult-onset physical disabilities such as lupus, arthritis, diabetes, and spinal cord injury. Originally offered as a multiweek group, program components are now offered individually, specifically tailoring services and supports to the individual's needs.

Operation Job Match increases the job-seeking proficiency of participants by enlisting assistance from the employer community to generate a wide range of career options. The initial program proved to be so successful that it has been replicated at National Multiple Sclerosis Society chapters throughout the United States.

Career Crossroads: Employment and Multiple Sclerosis

In 2004, the National Multiple Sclerosis Society produced a comprehensive employment program, Career Crossroads: Employment and MS, geared primarily toward individuals who are currently working and seeking to retain employment. This program consists of a video/DVD, an accompanying participant manual, and a leader manual. The program is designed to be implemented in a small-group setting over several weeks. It can also be offered as a self-paced program, with the individual being paired with an employment advisor from their local National MS Society chapter. In the video, a fictional character, Claire, is struggling with challenging MS symptoms that are beginning to affect her job performance as a graphic designer. She has been recently diagnosed but has not disclosed her MS at work or requested any accommodations from her employer. Her friend, fictional character Vanessa, who is a librarian, assists Claire with researching the appropriate steps to request accommodations and access available resources to maintain her employment. In doing so, actual clients, rehabilitation professionals, attorneys, employers, and medical professionals are interviewed. Topics covered in Career Crossroads include the following:

- The importance of work
- The impact work has on MS and the impact MS has on work
- Legal protections: Americans with Disabilities Act (ADA), Family and Medical Leave Act (FMLA), Health Insurance Portability and Accountability Act (HIPAA), and Consolidated Omnibus Budget Reconciliation Act (COBRA)
- Disclosure: including a disclosure script "formula" and a description of the advantages and disadvantages of disclosing
- Accommodations: practical strategies for managing symptoms in the workplace and the relationship to disclosure
- Resources: including the National Multiple Sclerosis Society, Job Accommodation Network (JAN), United States Equal Employment Opportunity Commission (EEOC), and Disability and Business Technical Assistance Centers (DBTAC)
- Information on tax incentives for hiring people with disabilities
- Work–life balance and planning ahead

Local chapters of the National MS Society can be reached at 1-800-344-4867 or online at http://www.NationalMSSociety.org. In addition to Career Crossroads, the National MS Society offers a variety of employment publications, resources, and personnel to offer employment assistance, guidance, and to make referrals to community-based employment assistance programs. Information geared toward employers is also available.

Programs Available to People with All Types of Disabilities

The State-Federal Vocational Rehabilitation program

Within each U.S. state, there is an agency that provides comprehensive vocational rehabilitation (VR) services to individuals with disabilities. These agencies may have slightly different names in different states and may offer slightly different services, but each one is part of a nationwide program to promote employment opportunities for people with disabilities. The VR program combines federal and state funds and, though federally mandated, is carried out by individual state agencies. Vocational rehabilitation services are an eligibility program rather than entitlement program (Rumrill et al., 2008). This means that one must demonstrate eligibility for VR services by having a physical or mental impairment that results in a substantial impediment to employment. There must be a reasonable expectation that vocational rehabilitation services can help the individual to gain or maintain employment. Many state VR agencies work under an "Order of Selection" mandate, which means that services are prioritized for individuals with the most significant disabilities.

Services may vary from state to state. Some of the services that may be available include the following:

- Vocational evaluation and assessment to determine skills, abilities, interests, and the impact of disability on employment
- Specialized assessments addressing computer/assistive technology needs
- Vocational guidance and counseling
- Medical appliances and prosthetic devices, to increase the individual's ability to work
- Vocational training and education
- Occupational tools and equipment
- Job development and placement services
- Follow-along services
- Postemployment services

Vocational rehabilitation services are available for people who are looking to gain or maintain employment. A person does not have to be unemployed to apply for services. For the individual with MS, one of the challenges may be demonstrating significant enough symptoms under the Order of Selection mandate given invisible symptoms or symptoms that come and go. It is important to discuss all of the symptoms that a person presently experiences, the symptoms experienced in the past, how the course of the disease may change over time, and the impact symptoms may have in the workplace. In addition, most states take financial criteria into account when funding services. Many of the specialized assessments and vocational guidance and counseling services, however, can be performed regardless of an individual's financial situation. In some situations, the individual may be expected to contribute financially toward the cost of his or her program, with the state VR agency contributing a portion as well. A listing of state VR agencies can be found at http://askjan.org/cgi-win/TypeQuery.exe?902.

Disability and Business Technical Assistance Centers

The Disability and Business Technical Assistance Centers (DBTACs), also known as the ADA and IT Technical Assistance Centers, were established by the U.S. Department of Education, National Institute on Disability and Rehabilitation Research (NIDRR) to provide information, training, and technical assistance to employers, people with disabilities, and other entities with responsibilities under the ADA. There are 10 regional centers throughout the United States. Though the regional centers may vary somewhat in their provisions, all centers provide the following:

- Technical assistance
- Education and training
- Materials dissemination
- Information and referral
- Public awareness
- Local capacity building

Information and assistance are available on issues regarding the various titles or sections of the ADA, including employment, public accommodations, public services, and communications. Centers may also be able to address other key legislation, including the Family and Medical Leave Act and the Rehabilitation Act of 1973. Local DBTACs can be contacted by calling 1-800-949-4232 (voice/TTY) or online at http://www.adata.org.

The Job Accommodation Network

The Job Accommodation Network (JAN) is a free service of the United States Department of Labor, Office of Disability Employment Policy (ODEP). Its mission is to facilitate the employment and retention of workers with disabilities by providing employers, employment service providers, people with disabilities, their family members, and other interested parties with information on job accommodations, self-employment, and small business opportunities. Consultants of JAN can assist employers to determine appropriate accommodations for employees, gain a better understanding of their responsibilities under the ADA and the Rehabilitation Act, and obtain answers to accessibility questions. For people with disabilities, JAN consultants can help identify accommodation strategies given particular symptoms and job duties, educate individuals about their rights and responsibilities under the ADA and other disability-related legislation, address the connection between disclosure and effective ways of requesting accommodations, and provide contact information for state VR and community agencies. JAN also makes its services available to rehabilitation and health-care professionals. JAN can be contacted online at http://askjan.org/ or by telephone at 1-800-526-7234 (voice) or 1-877-781-9403 (TTY). This free service provides excellent resources and technical assistance in implementing reasonable accommodations in the workplace. Research has demonstrated that the majority of accommodations used by people with MS in the workplace cost little or nothing to implement (Rumrill et al., 2008).

SUMMARY

Extant research, clinical observations, and reports from people with MS bear witness to the differences that people with MS encounter as they attempt to seek, secure, and maintain employment. Certainly, the fact that more than half of these qualified, seasoned, and productive workers disengage from the workforce before reaching retirement age indicates significant gaps in research, program development, and service delivery—gaps that, left unfilled, will continue to deprive society of the vast labor resource that exists within the MS community.

The disappointing employment prospects that currently await people with MS as the disease progresses continue to be problematic, but solutions lie in the numerous laws, programs, services, and interventions that have been implemented over the past three decades to promote employment opportunities for people with MS. Some of these initiatives are specific to the needs of people with MS, others include people with various types of adult-onset chronic illnesses, and still others are available to people with disabilities in general. Taken in aggregate these initiatives provide a formidable array of legal protections, information, technical assistance, advocacy, and direct services that can greatly aid people with MS in continuing their careers after this highly intrusive disease begins to manifest itself.

REFERENCES

Dawis R, Lofquist L. *A Psychological Theory of Work Adjustment.* Minneapolis: University of Minnesota Press; 1984.

Edgley K, Sullivan M, Dehoux E. A survey of multiple sclerosis, part 2: determinants of employment status. *Can J Rehabil.* 1991;4(3):127–132.

Franklin G, Nelson L, Filley C, Heaton R. Cognitive loss in multiple sclerosis: case reports and review of the literature. *Arch Neurol.* 1989;46(2):162–167.

Fraser, R, Clemmons, D, Bennett, F. *Multiple Sclerosis: Psychosocial and Vocational Interventions.* New York: Demos; 2002.

Fraser R, McMahon B, Dancyzk-Hawley C. Progression of disability benefits: a perspective on multiple sclerosis. *J Vocational Rehabil.* 2004;19(3):173–179.

Genevie L, Kallos J, Struenig E. Job retention among people with multiple sclerosis. *J Neurol Rehabil.* 1987; 1:131–135.

Gordon PA, Lewis MD, Wong D. Multiple sclerosis: strategies for rehabilitation counselors. *J Rehabil.* 1994;60(3):34–38.

Grant I, McDonald WI, Trimble M, Smith E, Reed R. Deficient learning and memory in early and middle phases of multiple sclerosis. *J Neurol Neurosur Psychiatry.* 1984;47:250–255.

Gulick EE, Yam M, Touw MM. Work performance by persons with multiple sclerosis: conditions that impede or enable the performance of work. *Int J Nurs Stud.* 1989;26(4):301–311.

Halligan FR, Reznikoff M, Friedman H, LaRocca NG. Cognitive dysfunction and change in multiple sclerosis. *J Clin Psychol.* 1988;44(4):540–548.

Hennessey M. *An Examination of the Employment and Career Development Concerns of Postsecondary Students with Disabilities: Results of a Tri-Regional Survey* [dissertation]. Kent, OH: Kent State University; 2004.

Kalb R. *Multiple Sclerosis: The Questions You Have, the Answers You Need.* New York: Demos Medical Publishing; 2007.

Kornblith AB, LaRocca NG, Baum HM. Employment in individuals with multiple sclerosis. *Int J Rehabil Res.* 1986;9:155–165.

LaRocca NG. *Employment and Multiple Sclerosis.* New York: National Multiple Sclerosis Society; 1995.

LaRocca NG, Kalb R, Scheinberg LC, Kendall P. Factors associated with unemployment of patients with multiple sclerosis. *J Chron Dis.* 1985;38:203–210.

Marini I. What rehabilitation counselors should know to assist Social Security beneficiaries in becoming employed. *Work.* 2003;21(1):37–44.

McReynolds C, Koch L. Psychological issues. In: Rumrill R, Hennessey M, eds. *Multiple Sclerosis: A guide for Rehabilitation and Health Care Professionals.* Springfield, IL: Charles C. Thomas; 2001: 44–78.

National Multiple Sclerosis Society. *Providing Information about MS to Employers.* Denver, CO: National Multiple Sclerosis Society Programs and Services Department; 2005.

Rao S, Leo G, Ellington L, Nauertz T, Bernardin L, Unverzagt F. Cognitive dysfunction in multiple sclerosis: impact on employment and social functioning. *Neurology.* 1991;41(5):692–696.

Rao S, Leo G, St. Aubin-Faubert P. A critical review of the Luria-Nebraska neuropsychological literature. *Int J Clin Neuropsychol.* 1989;11(3):137–142.

Roessler R, Fitzgerald S, Rumrill P, Koch L. Determinants of employment status among people with multiple sclerosis. *Rehabil Counsel Bull.* 2001;45(1):31–39.

Roessler R, Rumrill P. The relationship of perceived work-site barriers to job mastery and job satisfaction for employed people with multiple sclerosis. *Rehabil Counsel Bull.* 1995;39(1):2–14.

Roessler R, Rumrill P. Multiple sclerosis and employment barriers: a systemic approach. *Work.* 2003;21(1):17–23.

Roessler R, Rumrill P, Fitzgerald S. Predictors of employment status for people with multiple sclerosis. *Rehabil Counsel Bull.* 2004;47(2):97–103.

Roessler R, Rumrill P, Hennessey M. *Employment Concerns of People with Multiple Sclerosis: Building a National Employment Agenda. Report Submitted to the National Multiple Sclerosis Society.* Kent, OH: Kent State University Center for Disability Studies; 2002.

Roessler R, Rumrill P, Hennessey M, Vierstra C, Pugsley E, Pittman A. Perceived strengths and weaknesses in employment policies and practices among people with multiple sclerosis: results of a national survey. *Work.* 2003;21(1):25–36.

Rumrill P. *Increasing the Frequency of Accommodation Requests Among Employed People with Multiple Sclerosis* [dissertation]. Fayetteville, AR: University of Arkansas; 1993.

Rumrill P. *Employment Issues and Multiple Sclerosis.* New York: Demos; 1996.

Rumrill P. Effects of a social competence training program on accommodation request activity, situational self-efficacy, and Americans with Disabilities Act knowledge among employed people with visual impairments and blindness. *J Voc Rehabil.* 1999;12(1):25–31.

Rumrill P. Help to stay at work: vocational rehabilitation strategies for people with multiple sclerosis. *Mult Scler Foc.* 2006;7:14–18.

Rumrill P, Hennessey M. eds. *Multiple Sclerosis: A Guide for Rehabilitation and Health Care Professionals.* Springfield, IL: Charles C. Thomas; 2001.

Rumrill P, Hennessey M, Nissen S. *Employment Issues and Multiple Sclerosis.* 2nd ed. New York: Demos; 2008.

Rumrill P, Koch L, Reed C. Career maintenance and multiple sclerosis. *J Job Placement Dev.* 1998;14(1):11–17.

Rumrill P, Roessler R, McMahon B, Fitzgerald S. Multiple sclerosis and workplace discrimination: the National Equal Employment Opportunity Commission, Americans with Disabilities Act research project. *J Voc Rehabil.* 2005;23(3):179–188.

Rumrill P, Roessler R, Unger D, Vierstra C. Title I of the Americans with Disabilities Act and Equal Employment Opportunity Commission case resolution patterns involving people with multiple sclerosis. *J Voc Rehabil.* 2004;20(3):171–176.

Schapiro R. *Managing the Symptoms of Multiple Sclerosis.* New York: Demos Medical Publishing; 2003.

Sumner G. *Project Alliance: A Job Retention Program for Employees with Chronic Illnesses and Their Employers.* New York: National Multiple Sclerosis Society; 1997.

Super D. A life-span, life-space approach to career development. *J Voc Behav.* 1980;16:282–298.

Unger D, Rumrill P, Roessler R, Stacklin R. A comparative analysis of employment discrimination complaints filed by people with multiple sclerosis and individuals with other disabilities. *J Voc Rehabil.* 2004;20(3):165–170.

Wehman P. *Life beyond the Classroom: Transition Strategies for Young People with Disabilities.* Baltimore: Paul H. Brookes; 2006.

Wineman NM. Adaptation to multiple sclerosis: the role of social support, functional disability, and perceived uncertainty. *Nurs Res.* 1990;39:294–299.

Zunker VG. *Foundations of Career Counseling: Applied Concepts of Life Planning.* Pacific Grove, CA: Brooks/Cole; 1994.

28 Legal Planning Issues*

Laura D. Cooper

The physician's view of his or her professional role in the lives of patients often will not correspond to the view held by the patients of the physician's role. The disparity arises from the natural tendency of patients to view the physician's office as "ground zero" for all of the problems attendant to their disease. Thus, it is not unusual for frustrated and desperate patients who have a whole range of problems to "spill" those issues over into the conversations during their medical appointments. However, by doing so, such patients implicitly yield authority to their physicians over the entire range of discussed problems despite the fact that the role of the physician does not necessarily include expertise to address those "spillover" problems. Physicians must be *strictly* on guard for that tendency, and they should graciously but gently refuse to undertake inappropriate social roles; furthermore, when such opportunities arise, the physician should also iterate the importance of the relative contributions in the patient's life of other appropriate professionals, *including nonmedical professionals.*

However, it is precisely because of that natural tendency of patients that a physician is also in a

unique position to encourage those patients to obtain professional help for those "spillover" issues especially when the patient does not realize that such help may even exist. It is important for referring physicians to understand that legal advocacy and planning are inextricably related in the sense that issues that trigger the need for legal planning include all issues which, if left unaddressed, would likely require the services of a lawyer to resolve. In that respect, legal planning simply requires an individual to take immediate steps to ameliorate issues that might otherwise arise in the absence of that planning, and it involves *changing outcomes.* In essence, therefore, any good legal advisor is essentially an expert *planner* on the theory that it is better to get "ahead" of the issue through legal advice than to chase after the limited solutions that may be available once the legal problem has thoroughly erupted. In fact, the optimal strategy is usually the one that obviates the need for further lawyering on the issue at all.

Therefore, as a general rule, a physician should seriously consider making a legal *planning* referral for any patient at the earliest possible moment on *any* issue that—if left unaddressed—could eventually require the assistance of a lawyer. Such issues do not necessarily appear at first blush to constitute strictly legal issues and may merely present as "social" conflicts. For example, a patient who is experiencing disease-related employment concerns may not seem to have an immediate need for a lawyer; however, that situation presents an entire matrix of potential disease-related legal concerns, ranging from discrimination or job action claims to filing disability claims.

As an example, it is not uncommon for a patient to seek from his or her physician vocational

---

* This Chapter was written before the introduction and passage of the 2010 federal health insurance bill. As of the time of this writing, the legal status of that legislation is too tenuous to make any reasonable predictions about how the subject of health insurance and health security planning in the United States will change in its wake. For that reason, the reader is cautioned that any planning endeavors based on the materials herein should take into account the fluid nature of current federal health insurance law, and understand that this Chapter was written for planning to be undertaken in the absence of such federal provisions.

counseling or direction about insurance or disability benefits, including seeking advice on whether it is appropriate to apply for Social Security Disability. Despite the tendency of many physicians to view that question as inherently medical, *it is not*. Medical information is merely *evidence* from which a primarily *vocational functional* assessment is made by the federal agency. Similarly, private disability insurance claims also rely on a matrix of vocational/functional assessments with an overlay of medical *evidence*. Thus, an enlightened physician would refer such a patient for an expert professional vocational assessment *along with relevant supporting medical evidence* in order to give the patient all the relevant data from which an informed *vocational* decision could be made.

In addition to professionals, another valuable resource that should be included in the physician's referral rolodex are nonprofit or charitable organizations which offer resource and referral services. For example, a Center for Independent Living is an excellent resource for local information for individuals with various forms of disabilities. Some of the practical spillover issues that are likely to be brought to a physician's office by a patient with significant neurological illness are likely to include life circumstance issues—or practical issues arising out of the deteriorating physical functioning of the patient. Those issues are likely to be accentuated by diminishing mobility but ameliorated by the adoption of mobility aids. However, if the patient's own residence is inhospitable to the use of a mobility aid because of existing barriers, adoption of the mobility aid itself is likely to present a housing crisis, which will require the daunting challenge of locating accessible local housing on short notice. In those circumstances, understanding the prohibitions against discrimination based on disability contained in federal Fair Housing requirements can make that task considerably easier because that law also specifies design and construction accessibility provisions for certain residential structures. Thus, a local organization armed with basic scoping information about federal fair housing laws as well as knowledge of the local real estate market should be able to readily identify residential options that are likely to accommodate even the most significant mobility impairment.

In summary, two key scoping provisions exist within that federal law: *(1)* accessibility requirements pertain only to residential structures that contain four or more dwelling units (other than townhouses); and *(2)* accessibility requirements only apply to units that were developed for first occupancy on or after March 1991. Thus, in short, all apartment or condominium complexes (excluding townhomes) with four or more dwelling units that were built in the United States after 1991 should incorporate sufficient accessible features by design so as to accommodate the mobility needs of most individuals, including those who necessarily rely on wheelchairs or other mobility aids. A local Center for Independent Living (organized through the National Council on Independent Living, available online at http://www.ncil.org/) should be able to identify specific accessible housing options within the local community.

Other nonprofit organizations may also serve a critical link for a physician to meet his or her own obligations under federal law. For example, a physician's office is considered a "public accommodation" under Title III of the Americans with Disabilities Act ["ADA"], and as such it is prohibited from discriminating based on disability in the provision of services to the public. The ADA does not prohibit a physician from terminating an individual with a disability from a practice as long as that termination is for appropriate, non-disability-related reasons (such as failure to pay the bill or disruptive behavior unrelated to the disability). However, as proprietors or operators of places of public accommodation, physicians are also required to make "reasonable accommodation" for people with disabilities, which includes accommodating auxiliary aids such as service animals or wheelchairs, as well as creating effective communication for deaf or hard-of-hearing patients. The affirmative accommodation obligations of a "public accommodation" are based on relative resources; a solo practitioner is not expected to provide the same level of accommodations as a large, multispecialty group. For example, although a deaf patient is usually allowed to select the method of communication that serves his or her needs, an interpreter is more likely to be considered an "undue burden" (imposing a significant difficulty or expense) to the solo physician. In any event, the physician cannot charge the patient for any extra expenses related to such accommodation. Nonprofit organizations may provide local resources for sign interpreters, including a national society, the National Registry of Interpreters for the Deaf at (703) 838-0030, or the local center for the deaf.

More generally, the ADA protects an "individual with a disability" against discrimination. An "individual with a disability" is defined in the law as a person with *(1)* a physical or mental impairment that substantially limits one or more of the major life activities, *(2)* a record of such impairment, or *(3)* being regarded as having such impairment. A "major life activity" can include self-care activities or other things such as breathing, learning, or working. However, not everything that restricts a person's major life activities is considered an "impairment" under the ADA. Exclusions include such things as obesity (unless there is an underlying physiological disorder), hepatitis A, and side effects from certain drugs.

The best source for information about obligations under the ADA, or for further assistance in solving problems that may arise under that Act, are attorneys who specialize in civil rights cases. However, a person who believes that he or she may have a claim under the ADA needs to be aware of specific legal constraints presented under the law. For example, a discrimination claim based on employment must be presented to the federal Equal Employment Opportunity Commission or its state agency equivalent within 180 days of the date the discriminatory act occurred or the claim will be waived. Even if the agency agrees with the complainant, the most likely action they will take is to simply issue a "right to sue" letter, which still requires the individual to file a private lawsuit. A "right to sue" letter is a prerequisite for suit in federal court on the employment claim; however, the time limit for filing after the letter is issued is 90 days. These ADA time limits are strict and compliance is crucial to enforcing rights. Thus, it is critical to consult a lawyer as quickly as possible once the situation arises.

In addition to complying with nondiscrimination requirements, most physicians are also required to have a plan for obtaining English language interpretive services under federal law if they are recipients of federal HHS payments (Medicaid or Medicare other than Part B). A sole practitioner should investigate technological services or resource sharing with other providers to meet these requirements. Family member interpreters are recommended only as a last resort. Local hospitals should maintain a list of qualified interpreters. Additionally, physicians should have consent forms, especially those for invasive procedures, translated into the applicable non-English languages by a certified translator.

Additionally, physicians with 15 or more employees may be covered under Title I of the ADA, which prohibits discrimination by an employer against a qualified applicant or employee with a disability. (Note: some state laws cover employers with fewer employees under state nondiscrimination provisions.)

It is important to iterate that it is *not* appropriate for a physician to make a universal referral to a "social worker" to resolve all nonmedical referral issues. Social workers fulfill a specific professional function, which is to resolve conflicts between the patient and the social systems to which he or she belongs. Like all professionals, social workers will naturally undertake tasks that are assigned to them through the prism of their own training. However, the "toolbox" of social workers is composed entirely of *social* resources, notably those available through government or charitable entities. Unfortunately, when social workers are utilized as a catchall referral, that professional bias necessarily limits the universe of "solutions" a patient will likely be offered such that the solutions will inevitably be composed primarily or strictly based upon nonprivate, social resources. As a consequence, those solutions primarily rely on government entitlements. While some planning situations are better served with entitlements, that is a decision that should not be made at the outset by the physician's selection of a referral source. Even when entitlements are available, their rules almost invariably require stifling economic constraints such that once the quest to qualify for a government entitlement program becomes a paramount impetus, a once productive citizen may find the entitlement rules horse often driving the life choices cart.

For example, to ameliorate noncontinuous group employer-sponsored health coverage, social workers will often counsel people with serious conditions to try to establish eligibility for Medicaid (which requires persistent poverty) or Medicare. However, for the latter, a nonelderly claimant must first qualify for Social Security Disability (which *seriously* limits productive work or income) and maintain that eligibility for at least *29 months* before Medicare kicks in. While COBRA health insurance extensions my be available from an employer to provide "gap" health benefits coverage until Medicare eligibility occurs, a rational financial "plan" for a family, which is constructed around Medicare eligibility, must nevertheless presume that the insured will refrain from producing gainful *income* for almost *3 years*. A rational plan for a middle class family based on Medicare coverage as the primary source of health coverage must therefore either presume net savings sufficient for the qualification period or income replacements of some kind for that entire period. If neither is available, and the insured is eligible for neither Veterans assistance nor workers compensation, the quest for Medicare can easily become a social road to poverty.

A far better approach would be to refer the patient to a planner who will take a more global view of financial planning and resources. Such planners will take explicit account of government entitlements, but only rely on them when the planner cannot otherwise develop an adequate plan without them. In the circumstance described earlier, for example, a better strategy would be to locate and lock in continuous health coverage that is not connected to employment status, such as through a non-employer group high-deductible catastrophic excess major medical plan (discussed later), which does not force the choice between income or health coverage that government entitlements require. Such group insurance policies can still be obtained through some large associations on a guaranteed issue basis for preexisting conditions, and they are quite affordable.

Therefore, if a patient expresses to his or her physician some concerns about present or future finances or insurance coverage or similar *resource* issues (including concerns regarding continuing employment), it would be more advisable to refer the patient to a professional with suitable overall life planning expertise (such as a life planner or elder law attorney) rather than resorting to a reflexive social worker referral.

If that patient is also a primary breadwinner, the referral becomes even more urgent. That planning process also takes on greater significance as the severity of the neurological disease increases because the social and financial future for persons with severe illnesses or disabilities are so tenuous—meaning that they have greater *known* risks. In the face of such potential risk, the fewer resources an individual has, the *more important* it is that they plan wisely.

If the primary breadwinner in a family becomes disabled, he may jeopardize the continuation of the *family's* entire health insurance package. And, while he is laid up, he somehow has to provide income replacement for the time he is not working, including finding income supplements for additional expenses attributable to any disability he may incur. He may find it difficult or impossible after a significant diagnosis to increase his life insurance to provide ample financial security for his loved ones. And, even upon returning to work (assuming that he is able, and that he is able to obtain adequate health insurance coverage from his employer), he may find that he is not as productive as he was before his disability occurred, and therefore he will not be able to produce the same income he was previously able to garner. All of these possibilities are daunting, to say the least. If the patient had planned for all of them, he might be able to salvage whatever lifestyle his family had before his disability occurred. If he had adequately planned for none or only part of them, and was forced to endure a significant disability for a substantial period of time, his family's quality of life would probably forever be diminished as a result.

Understandably, the subject of planning for serious illness or disability is one that most people find distressing; however, it has been my professional experience that the distress caused by the planning exercise pales in comparison to the everyday problems faced by individuals who failed to engage in that process at all. Moreover, by constructing a long-range plan that incorporates preselected solutions for otherwise unforeseen but potentially catastrophic problems, the client can feel secure about his or her family's well-being regardless of what the disease might ultimately bring.

Given the wide range of potential legal problems involved in these circumstances, lawyers are among the professionals who can either assist individuals in accomplishing planning goals or refer them for other specialized assistance as appropriate.

In fact, certain legal specialists have practices that are mostly composed of planning (notably tax lawyers, elder lawyers, estate lawyers, and some specialized family lawyers). While this chapter highlights some of the principal components in a legal planning process, because each family's situation is unique and the complex laws pertaining to these issues vary considerably from state to state, the information provided here should in no way be considered comprehensive. Instead, individuals must be encouraged to seek out and consult with qualified professionals to construct their own plan based on specific individual needs.

Regardless of who is called upon to accomplish it, the "nub" of the planning issue with serious neurological diseases is that the medical future is typically both *unknown* and simultaneously potentially *devastating*. Although disease-modifying drugs have completely changed the overall risk profile for people with many formerly untreatable diseases such as multiple sclerosis, there is nevertheless no way to predict with any certainty what an individual's *particular* future will bring with respect to specific symptoms or potential disability or incapacity. From that standpoint, neurological illness still presents a patient with the same "great unknown" that it has always provided—nobody knows who will become severely disabled and who will not.

From a professional planner's standpoint, however, that lack of knowledge is not an insoluble problem. The point of planning is to take steps now so that even a catastrophic outcome need not prevent the individual or her family from achieving important life goals. In other words, without engaging in planning both the individual and her family effectively subject their own most important life goals to the dictates of *chance*. Unfortunately, the intrusion of a serious diagnosis increases the prospect that *chance* will not be very kind.

INTRODUCTION TO PLANNING

The driving concerns for any legal planning process should be *fundamental life goals*—those things that provide "meaning" to an individual's life. In its most basic form, the overall planning process required after serious diagnosis is a process that encourages a person to set life goals and to formulate a workable plan for ensuring that those goals remain achievable no matter what life may bring. Such a plan simply represents a concerted effort to coordinate life goals with current and future choices as well as available resources.

In reality, the life planning task is not to *construct* a plan (which already exists even if not recognizable), but to *improve on the one that already exists*. The particular existing "plan" may simply be to take things as they come, to live from paycheck to paycheck, and to presume, therefore, that the planner will not become old, sick, or disabled. That is a poor plan, but it is a plan nonetheless. As another example, if the planner has health coverage based strictly on a spouse's employment, then the inferred "plan" *presumes* both the spouse's eligibility for continuous health coverage as well as the existence of that marital relationship into perpetuity.

Thus, the planning process described here is simply a concerted effort to recognize the plan that is actually in place and either make it "workable" or replace parts of it altogether with a more reasoned approach. Some form of planning, whenever it occurs, is almost always more likely to produce better outcomes than pure chance. It goes without saying that serious illness or disability is a circumstance that no one would opt for; however, when it does occur, the key to a rich and fulfilling life lies in knowing that no matter what may happen, the most important aspects of life—the *fundamental life goals*—will still be preserved.

The success of the plan in preserving such goals will depend upon how the plan addresses "risk." In that sense, "risk" is the possibility—any possibility—that things will not go exactly as the planner had planned or hoped. Other than bad outcomes from bad financial market performance (which a good financial planner can ameliorate or buffer against through structuring a financial portfolio), most "risk" falls into one of two categories. First, risk may consist of things that occur by virtue of individual conduct or choices; a second form of risk includes things that happen that are in no way related to anything the individual has done (and which could not have been prevented in any event). To the extent that risk is due to an individual's choices, it is controllable and *avoidable*. Exposure to that form of risk can be heightened or lessened depending upon individual choices, and "planning" for this kind of risk simply requires consciousness of the choices the individual is making. However, when a risk occurs in spite of choices and cannot be avoided, it must either be assumed or protected against.

A well-developed plan must therefore be viewed as a scheme designed to address *unavoidable* contingencies so that the possibility of its not being implemented approaches zero. The more comprehensive the plan, the fewer items are left to chance and unavoidable risk. A good overall plan therefore includes many different aspects of formal individual legal and other planning, including financial, estate, and vocational plans. The planning process requires a consideration of everything that is important to the individual for whom the plan is being developed, and the specific components will depend on the individual's personal goals and situation.

Regardless of when planning begins, the fundamental approach required for good planning following significant neurological illness is the same and begins with analysis of a worst-case scenario in order to assess what options would exist should that occur. When an overall risk plan provides acceptable options even in the face of a worst-case scenario, then that plan may be deemed "bullet-proof"—that is, achievable despite the potential occurrence of the worst contingencies.

LIFE PLANNING

The necessity to consider the worst-case scenario casts a shadow of potential severe or lifelong disability for the person diagnosed with a serious condition. In that respect, the planning process required of a family with a member who has such a condition is not unlike the planning required of a family with a member with a developmental disability. The "life planning" process developed and extensively used within the developmental disability community can be of significant assistance to people with serious illnesses or disabilities in evaluating their own long-term issues.

The developmental disability life planning process includes four major types of planning:

1. Life circumstances planning, or planning for nonnegotiable personal needs

2. Planning and implementing an ample financial portfolio or set of financial strategies to fund the nonnegotiable personal needs attendant to the life goals that have been set

3. Planning for advocacy and directives by choosing professional and personal representatives or guardians in advance, as well as formulating advance directives

4. Preparing estate plans that include financial strategies to fund any obligations that may survive death

A fifth activity includes following through with the plan by organizing all critical records in order to permit continuity of administration of affairs throughout any period of disability, as well as after death. Regulations and penalties for medical providers who share medical information have become daunting and provide incentives for providers to dispose of older medical records. As a consequence, it may be more difficult for an individual to keep a complete, long-term medical record by relying on medical providers to do so. Given the complexities of the information age, it is now in *each individual's own interest* to keep a thorough record of his or her own health history, and the physician should encourage his or her patients to create and maintain a complete, private medical record, including copies of imaging reports, lab reports, and any other record critical to the individual's own long-term health care.

Life Circumstances Planning

The first step a planning attorney (or other professional) would take in developing a "bullet-proof" strategy is to know exactly what long-term options will exist to deal with the worst catastrophe; for example, what are the precise nature of any "holes" that actually exist in the current plan? Strategy recommendations will therefore be completely dependent upon the current resources and risks, and no easy "formula" or algorithm can be written to accomplish this task.

Despite the primacy of financial concerns, the nature and extent of risks and related financial needs will be largely determined by the circumstances in which an individual chooses to live. From that standpoint, the financial and life circumstances plan go hand in hand. Traditionally, life circumstances planning includes planning for housing, living arrangements, education, employment, transportation, long-term services, and other social objectives. Life circumstances planning is the most important early step because it will determine the overall setting in which the life plan will be implemented.

For example, a person who chooses to live in an isolated, rural area will certainly find efforts to obtain necessary personal services and transportation to present a substantial challenge. Similarly, that old Victorian or new townhome may seem "quaint" but their "vertical" architecture may impede independence, accentuate disability, and enforce social isolation from neighbors living in similarly inaccessible structures. On the other hand, accessible housing on reliable public transportation lines in a metropolitan area may be difficult to find as well as expensive to procure. However, despite the basic cost of living, a person who lives in an area where cooperative long-term care is available may require a fraction of the resources over the long haul that would be required by an individual who desires private long-term care in their home.

Despite social norms and customs to the contrary, it has been my experience that the wisest choices for people with serious illness are to adopt a "planning" mindset insisting on universal access from the very beginning of the disease—even before any mobility issues may exist. An able-bodied person can function quite well in an accessible dwelling, but a person with a mobility impairment may find her own home quite literally constitutes a form of "jail" if it is not accessible. By insisting on accessible housing options along transportation lines with accessible options from the beginning, neither housing nor mobility will ever become limiting social problems. Moreover, chances are that the family will not have to make a drastic—and expensive—decision to "solve" any such problem at the most inconvenient time (when a loved one is coping with serious illness). Practical home access is far less expensive than personal assistance, and an accessible transportation system is also far less expensive than one of those $50,000 lift-equipped vans. By taking *circumstances out of the equation at the beginning* most other practical problems can be addressed. Location and housing type will tend to dictate the price and availability of various forms

of long-term services, as well as educational and employment opportunities. Moreover, the cost of almost every element of the life plan will be strongly influenced by the location and type of residence you select. The ideal housing location will allow an individual to take advantage of educational, community, and employment opportunities that meet his or her personal goals and afford access to all the long-term services needed (and affordable) in case of severe illness or disability.

The most effective means of performing this life circumstances planning is to construct a "letter of intent." This informal document is a way for an individual to communicate important information about himself to individuals who might provide care or exercise judgment on their behalf in the future. A letter of intent encourages an individual to sit down and think about what factors are critical for life goals. Although it is not legally binding, a letter of intent is a useful document. It should include information about the author, the author's family members, other relationships, advocates, medical history and care, housing, religious values, other systems of values, final arrangements, education, daily living skills, work life, government or private benefits available, hobbies and interests, and anything else that comprises an important personal life factor.

The letter of intent also serves as the organizing core of the life circumstances planning process and provides important information regarding necessary or available types and amounts of financial resources for both the financial and estate planning processes. Before a person with a disability begins working up a financial or estate plan, he or she is well advised to complete a thorough life circumstances plan and make decisions about housing, transportation, education, and other social circumstances upon which all other elements of a well-constructed life circumstances plan will be based.

Financial Planning

Financial planning is the methodical process of evaluating an individual's total assets, liabilities, and future income potential, and then using that information to determine the individual's best options for meeting future needs and wants. Plans should be made as soon as possible for the family members or friends who provide support, as well as the person who has the serious diagnosis. The plans should then be revised periodically or as new circumstances dictate. The planning process may include the assessment of a myriad of financial options, including insurance, annuities, pensions, home equity, and availability of government benefits. Certified financial planners and lawyers may be valuable in sorting through the options and identifying the possible legal and tax consequences of various choices and choice combinations.

The normal process of financial planning requires a sequential series of steps, including the following:

1. Determining one's financial situation
2. Setting goals
3. Developing a plan
4. Keeping simple records
5. Making an informal budget
6. Dealing with shortfalls, credit, and debt
7. Reviewing your progress

However, financial planning for families with members who have a disability is fundamentally different. Families with a member who has a disability that could become severe enough to require long-term services cannot normally be expected to earn enough to meet their own financial needs. Therefore, these families may be required to develop alternative financial (and estate) plans that explicitly incorporate available government benefits. The resources required for long-term services are significantly lower if the person with a disability stays at home, has a disability that is less severe, or requires less assistance or supervision. Beyond this, the topic of financial planning is so situation specific that very few generalities can be stated in a presentation of this type beyond the preliminary insurance discussion already provided previously.

The traditional financial model in America assumes that an individual will begin working as a young adult and continue—essentially uninterrupted—until retirement age. Serious illness can dramatically alter that model in several fundamental ways: a disease could cause work life to be substantially shortened, thereby reducing the number of years in which an individual is able to accrue resources; the disease could also cause an individual to start drawing upon savings at a premature age, and also cause an individual to have to draw upon those savings for a longer time than

the typical retirement period; additionally, the disease could easily *increase overall expenses.*

Because it is unrealistic to think that a typical middle class person will be able to save sufficient resources to allow him or her to retire prematurely, stay retired longer, and have higher overall health-related expenses for any length of time in retirement, the *most* critical element of the plan for a middle class person will be construction of the risk or insurance plan. In fact, the insurance plan may drive all of the other components of an overall life plan; if there is a *shortage* of life, health, or disability coverage, the possible resulting limited financial resources if disability were to intrude could require a fundamental retooling of the entire life plan, including altering of life goals.

An insurance policy is simply a type of contract. Insurance is essentially a means of transferring financial risk to an outside party. Rather than risk all the consequences of a particular occurrence, the insured instead pays a premium and transfers that defined risk to an insurance company. For example, in such a contract the consumer agrees to pay an insurer a particular amount in exchange for which the insurer agrees to compensate the consumer for particular expenses the consumer incurs in connection with certain health problems. In that sense, health insurance can be thought of as a form of casualty insurance. Like other forms of casualty insurance, the contract will specify the types of problems that are covered, under what circumstances, and what exactly the insurer has agreed to pay when the casualty occurs. Of course, as the probability increases of that risk coming to fruition, the cost to the insurance company will increase correspondingly.

Health Insurance

The purpose of health insurance is to protect an insured against the potentially catastrophic costs of medical expenses that can accompany a serious illness. Thus, in the overall scheme of things, health insurance is simply a means of protecting an individual's *other assets* from the enormous expenses that can accompany a serious illness. Insurance companies are able to undertake the risk because they "spread" that risk over large groups of people.

Because the only reasonable way to finance the enormous costs of catastrophic health conditions is to do so in large insurance pools that include a large number of young and healthy people, Congress has encouraged the creation of large insurance groups through employer-sponsored insurance. However, the typical provider of employer-sponsored benefits is the *employer* and a break between the employee and the employer can eventually cause a break with the *coverage*.

However, in the Employment Retirement Security Act of 1974 ("ERISA") and subsequent amendments thereto, Congress imposed *legal limits* on the time period that equivalent group health insurance benefits must be made available for individuals who cease employment due to illness or disability. Instead of bringing more high-risk people into the pools of mostly healthy people, Congress has instead created specific rules designed to force some of the sickest people out of employer insurance groups.

If an employer is large enough (at least 20 employees), it will usually be covered by federal ERISA law and an insured will have to make a determination whether to accept "COBRA" continuation coverage when eligibility for the group ceases. Federal law sets the premium, which is the *entire* premium plus a 2% administrative charge. However, federal law limits "COBRA" health continuation coverage to a typical period of 18 months, and only under certain circumstances is that period longer.[1] Consequently, employer-based coverage can accurately be described as *noncontinuous as a matter of federal law and by specific Congressional design.*[2]

To create the perception of having addressed this glaring inequity, Congress passed the 1996 law entitled the "Health Insurance Portability and Accountability Act" (HIPAA), which requires insurers for a limited time to offer "guaranteed issue" conversion plans to individuals whose COBRA eligibility ends. However, that HIPAA "solution" is illusory: there is no requirement that a HIPAA conversion plan bear any reasonable resemblance to the former group plan because HIPAA contains neither coverage nor cost requirements. Since only people who have difficulty finding other coverage tend to accept HIPAA policies, the coverage tends to degrade quickly and premiums can rise dramatically in short order. Thus, there is no guarantee that any particular HIPAA plan will provide reasonable coverage at a reasonable cost unless

state law requires such provisions through its own regulation. While some individual HIPAA plans may be good as a consequence of an individual employer's decision or state law, as a matter of federal law the coverage offered by insurers under these plans need not provide any better risk coverage for the sick individual than the overall individual marketplace is likely to provide on its own. Consequently, a thorough insurance and financial plan must include specific strategies that can be implemented when or if employer-sponsored insurance becomes unavailable or insufficient.[3]

In evaluating employer-based options, an individual should check to make sure what premium would have to be paid for COBRA benefits. If COBRA is bypassed, then the individual should make sure that any coverage in lieu of COBRA would *itself* be continuous.[4] Additionally, it is essential to check renewability and cancellation provisions in individual policies; for group policies in order to confirm the basis for eligibility, and that it is something for which there is satisfactory assurance that is likely to continue *throughout life.*[5] Because COBRA is only for *limited duration*, an individual should *have a workable* plan for continuation coverage once the COBRA is over before the COBRA is undertaken. If the HIPAA plan is adopted, the insured should make sure of the exact terms of the plan, including any limitations in the benefits, and the extent to which the insurer can raise premiums over the long term.[6] Most states have taken steps to provide some mechanism for individuals who cannot obtain insurance in the individual marketplace to get coverage. However, in some states, eligibility for a HIPAA plan—no matter how inferior—will disqualify an individual for any state insurance risk pool. Thus, a critical set of steps in evaluating continuity is to determine—before making the COBRA decision—what other options for insurance exist. If the choice to select COBRA disqualifies the individual from state HIPAA options, COBRA may not be the best choice.

Another reality about insurance coverage that must inform the astute planner is that insurer recalcitrance is inversely proportional to the strength of legal remedies that may be used to enforce an insurance contract. The more likely an insurer will suffer deleterious consequences from failure to enforce policy provisions, the more likely the insurer will abide by contract terms. Conversely, if there are few penalties for questioning claims or reading the policy in extraordinarily narrow ways, the more likely an insurer will attempt to reduce claims losses through such behavior. Employer-sponsored coverage governed by federal ERISA law has the least effective set of legal remedies available, and is therefore the *most* likely to result in recalci-trant insurer behavior—and significantly more so than for any other type of private health insurance contracts available in the United States. On the other hand, coverage that is not employer spon-sored is governed by state law, which can include remedies for breach of contract or consumer protec-tion and in some cases bad faith tort remedies. For that reason, the likelihood of recalcitrant insurer behavior is *greatest* among employer-sponsored health insurance plans and relatively less under non-employer association–issued group plans. Yet few people are ever educated about this crucial dif-ference. In fact, a series of Supreme Court rulings has completely exempted "self-insured" employers from state insurance regulation altogether.

Unfortunately, most people only discover the lack of enforcement "teeth" in employer-sponsored health insurance only after they have sustained a serious illness or injury. To make matters worse, Congress has not mandated private or govern-ment solutions when discontinuity or coverage gaps occur: only the poorest of the poor qualify for Medicaid, and individuals who apply for Social Security Disability Insurance benefits, must wait 29 months from the date of application before Medicare coverage becomes available (assuming they eventually qualify for SSDI benefits). Even when Medicare does become available, in some states no federally regulated "Medigap" insurance plans are available to non-elderly Medicare benefi-ciaries with disabilities or chronic illnesses, so Medicare can become the *only* coverage available apart from the (temporary) COBRA and the (illu-sory) HIPAA employer-based options.

Thus, the options that will be available for most individuals who leave an employer group after a ratable diagnosis will largely be dependent *upon state law.*[7]

For information about specific state law, go to http://www.healthinsuranceinfo.net, a website maintained by Georgetown University's Health Policy Institute. States offer various approaches;

in some states, there is a designated "insurer of last resort" (such as Blue Cross) that offers specific plans at specific times of the year for open enroll-ment. The most common approach, taken by more than half of the states, is the offering of a "high-risk pool." States understandably discour-age reliance on high-risk pools; these pools are far from a panacea and their characteristics vary greatly from state to state. Some states cap enroll-ment, and most do not advertise their programs.[8] Over time, these pools are likely to become more financially squeezed and less reliable. All such pools of necessity operate at a loss. Only limited revenues are available to states to operate these pools because self-insured employers are exempt from paying into them. A good long-term strategy, therefore, should not rely exclusively upon a state high-risk pool as a source for health coverage, if at all possible.

Some state alternatives to a high-risk pool that have been developed have included small busi-ness guarantee issue requirements (i.e., to sell to all applicants of a certain minimum size, some-times as low as one employee) and to restrict the extent to which premium rates can vary based on health status or age. Thus, another strategy for obtaining insurance, depending upon your state guarantee issue law, would be to start your own small business.

Unfortunately, in the absence of strong state law, market-based options after a significant "rat-able" diagnosis typically leave only two alterna-tives: the individual must either plan to assume all eventual risks involving health issues with cash and no reliable risk-spreading insurance products; or qualify for a government-mandated program under state or federal law.

Despite this limitation, a number of general strat-egies can still be outlined. For persons who cannot obtain insurance through traditional employer or individual sources, if the "ratable" diagnosis can be considered "benign," then a local insurance agent may be able to find coverage by consulting the book annually published by National Underwriters entitled *Who Writes What.*

On the other hand, if the "ratable" condition is not benign, then the individual might have other options under state law. If coverage can become available by excluding one individual or condition, then one way to deal with other health needs is to take a "waiver" or exclusion for the ratable condition.[9] In that way, it may be possible to obtain good, thorough, long-term coverage for the person with the ratable condition (*without* that condition coverage) and other members of the family. This strategy requires payment for more than one health policy by the family, but the improvement in coverage should make the investment very worthwhile.

Yet another strategy is to find coverage on the groups market by locating a large association with a "guarantee issue" provision to obtain group coverage that is *not* based on employment. In other words, these are not policies available from an individual insurance agent. Instead, the potential insured should seek out an association of some kind that offers insurance benefits to its members (such as a fraternal, religious, or other large association; large college alumni associations are among the more common insured groups). The larger that association and its insured membership is, the more likely they will be able to offer underwriting for serious health issues; the largest associations may even offer "guaranteed issue" coverage for the preexisting ratable condition, or as an alternative to medical underwriting a large group may only impose a waiting period for preexisting conditions.

Congress prefers employer-sponsored insurance for one simple reason: employer sponsorship provides a legal mechanism for Congress to regulate the national health insurance market. However, as of this writing, individual citizens do *not* have to adopt the inequitable Congressional scheme, and perhaps the best way to ameliorate the effects of our national two-tiered system is to acquire catastrophic coverage that is not employer sponsored. These policies are known variously as a "catastrophic excess major medical" or sometimes just as "excess major medical." These products are *only* available in the group insurance market, and due to their enormous underwriting exposure are only sold to large groups. They are readily identifiable by the size of their deductibles, which begin at the low end with $25,000.[10] Fortunately, when the sponsoring group is large enough, the coverage may be available on either a guaranteed issue basis or simply subject to a waiting period as an alternative to medical underwriting for preexisting conditions. In that way, people with ratable conditions may still be able to obtain

coverage even *after* diagnosis. In fact, such plans might enable clients to avoid Medicare as the only long-term health insurance prospect, or even to re-enter the job market following a period of disability.

What is most astonishing about these policies, however, is their *affordability*: in fact, a *very good* catastrophic major medical policy can be obtained from non-employer groups for a person in their twenties or thirties for as little as $10/month with a catastrophic deductible of $25,000; as the deductible increases, the premiums are reduced even further. Even though such a policy would not pay first-dollar expenses of any kind aside from a serious health event, such a policy would nevertheless create a stop-loss that could prevent medical bankruptcy from *ever occurring* for mere pennies a day and also provide good, comprehensive coverage in the event a truly significant health event arises. (For example, many such policies explicitly cover transplants, as well as transplant *donor* expenses, as well as comprehensive forms of therapy and care options.) In fact, this is likely a wiser choice for a young and healthy person than *much* more expensive, first-dollar coverage in any event. If every uninsured person knew about these large-deductible catastrophic policies, we might be able to make dramatic inroads into the number of so-called uninsured Americans who believe that insurance is too expensive and reduce the attendant social problems that accompanies a significant uninsured illness.

Planning for Advocacy and Directives

This portion of the planning process requires consideration for the possibility of *legal incompetence*. Every *competent* adult has the legal right to make decisions about his or her own medical care, including the decision to accept or refuse that care. Sometimes illness interferes with a person's ability to exercise that legal right. This occurs, for example, when a person becomes too cognitively impaired to make competent decisions. As a result, the person who is judged legally incompetent can no longer carry out his or her personal wishes. Unfortunately, this may occur at precisely the moment when those wishes would need to be followed *because of the effects of illness*. Under these circumstances, the person does not actually lose the right to make a decision; rather, the *ability* to carry out those wishes is lost due to legal incapacity to make the relevant decisions. To make matters even more difficult, health-care providers need not abide by the decisions of an individual who has been judged legally incompetent if those decisions conflict with the health-care provider's own judgment.

The way to enforce an individual's wishes about medical care decisions, even in the event of legal incompetence, is to make those decisions *ahead of time* and place them in a set of legally enforceable "advance directives."[11] Doing so preserves an individual's legal ability to carry out his or her wishes as stated in the advance directive, even after the individual becomes incapacitated. If an individual has a legally enforceable advance directive, health-care providers must be directed by those wishes regardless of whether they agree with them.

Advance directives are the generic description for written documents in which competent persons state their anticipated medical decisions for the future. Directives can be communicated in one of two ways: *(1)* by making express written directives to health-care providers, as in a *living will*, or *(2)* by designating another person who knows and would be sympathetic to the desires of an individual when the time for decision making arrived, if that individual were too incapacitated to make his or her wishes known. This second form of advance directive is known as a *health-care proxy* or *power of attorney for health-care decision making*.

Although the living will and health-care proxy are both advance directives, many standardized forms for directives only incorporate one of these two types. No matter which standardized form may be offered, a complete set of advance directives should include both a living will *and* a health-care proxy. The basic distinction between a living will and a health-care proxy is the type of directive involved. A living will establishes certain treatment guidelines that are to be followed in the future. A health-care proxy does not establish treatment guidelines directly. Rather, it appoints a trusted person to act as the agent (proxy) in making health-care decisions if the appointer becomes too incapacitated to make them himself. A health-care proxy can incorporate provisions of a living will by requiring that the proxy follow any directives stated in a separate living will, or by incorporating the living will directly into the health-care proxy

(in which case, the authority of the chosen proxy would be limited by the living will conditions stated in the health-care proxy). Because it is almost impossible to predict all circumstances that might arise during any future illness, it would be difficult to place all advance directives in a living will. A health-care proxy in conjunction with a living will is necessary to safeguard an individual's complete right to self-determination. Consequently, a good set of advance directives will include both a living will and a health-care proxy.

If an individual becomes incapacitated without leaving any specific directives, the individual's family members will generally be considered suitable substitute decision makers. In theory, most courts agree that family members are the appropriate decision makers, even in the absence of a proxy. In practice, however, family member decisions that are made without an enforceable health-care proxy are not followed by health-care providers if the providers question the good faith of the family members or strongly disagree with the medical decision. On the other hand, if an enforceable health-care proxy specifically appoints the family member as proxy, health-care providers must treat the decisions made by the proxy as if the individual had made them himself, and providers would not be able to deviate from those decisions even if they happened to disagree with them. Advance directives that specifically appoint a proxy therefore provide protection against health-care providers who would be hesitant to follow an individual's personal values (as understood by the proxy). Thus, health-care proxies are critical devices for people who hold any values that differ substantially from those within the health-care community.

An important legal distinction should here be made between a *proxy* and a *surrogate*. A proxy implies that a person is designated in an advance directive and is therefore someone appointed directly by the incapacitated patient. A surrogate is someone who is legally appointed outside of an advance directive. For example, if no valid health-care proxy exists, a surrogate may be appointed to make decisions for the incapacitated patient. A family member appointed without an enforceable advance directive is a surrogate. This surrogate may become empowered either by a legal relationship that automatically gives rise to the right to make surrogate decisions (such as a family member) or by appointment as guardian by a court. Decisions by proxies are almost invariably followed with respect to quality-of-life decisions, in keeping with an individual's right of self-determination. However, decisions made by surrogates are examined with close scrutiny to make sure that they conform to the incapacitated individual's desires or best interests. Again, the best way to ensure that an individual's wishes are followed is for that person to execute a complete set of advance directives.

Estate Planning

A cohesive estate plan accomplishes the following things: *(1)* designates who will get estate property after death; *(2)* sets up procedures and devices to make estate property pass to others free from probate; *(3)* sets up ways to pass estate property to others while reducing or avoiding taxes; and *(4)* sets up trust management for estate property who might need outside help to manage that property.

Generally, the method an individual will choose to dispose of assets will involve a will, a trust, or both a will and a trust. In using estate planning tools to protect loved ones, it is advisable to consult an experienced attorney because the law is complex and a mistake might have irrevocable and unfortunate consequences for their future. For example, a common problem overlooked in estate plans is the effect inheritances or gifts can have on eligibility for public benefits. For that reason family members who are trying to provide for a loved one who may need long-term care or other long-term services may need to be careful not to jeopardize eligibility for public benefits by leaving assets directly in that person's name. In certain circumstances, it may be preferable to limit or eliminate the transfer of assets, so that the beloved beneficiary is not put in the position of missing out on valuable social services.

NOTES

1. The essential provisions of COBRA extending beyond 18 months are as follows:

    - If you die or divorce, your spouse can get 36 months of COBRA.
    - Dependent children who become too old to qualify under the parent's policy can get 36 months of COBRA.
    - If you apply for Social Security Disability, you can get 29 months of COBRA.

    - If you become eligible for Medicare, but your spouse is too young to do so, the spouse can get 36 months of COBRA.
    - You reduce your hours from full time to part time and the employer benefits would not otherwise be available in that status, you can get 18 months of COBRA.

2. A recent U.S. Supreme Court ruling also allows employers to change retiree health benefits, so there is no guarantee that those benefits will be available throughout retirement despite what an employer may promise.

3. When an employee moves between employer ERISA groups, a certificate of prior credible coverage prevents an insurer from imposing a preexisting condition. However, a continuity problem still arises when an individual is no longer qualified and must leave the employer group.

4. The older you get, the harder it will be to find alternative coverage until you are Medicare eligible. In some states, Medicare supplement insurance—or "Medigap"—is not available at all to individuals who are younger than retirement age. So if your plan is to get Medicare, make sure you understand whether—or what kind—of supplement would be available to you in your state. If no Medigap is available, then you need to have a plan to meet your expenses that are not covered by Medicare. Again, a catastrophic policy is a good idea.

5. Most master group insurance contracts have a provision called the "Class of Eligibles" that defines the exact characteristics of the group the insurer has agreed to underwrite. If you are unsure of the basis for your eligibility, you should consult the master contract and look at the language within this provision.

6. You may find that your choice to take the COBRA—and therefore be eligible for HIPAA—limits some of your other choices under state law. This is a serious issue for any person who, for any reason, loses his or her health coverage because of a medical condition.

7. If your employer is not large enough to be covered by ERISA, you may live in a state that provides similar rights for employees of smaller firms, through what is called a "mini-COBRA" law. Some states offer other approaches, and these are often termed "portability" rules.

8. State risk pools often charge premiums that are high relative to incomes, and they typically include sizeable deductibles and copayments and often restrict annual and lifetime benefits. Even though these pools are designed for people with serious or chronic illnesses, the pools still try to limit enrollment by imposing pre-existing condition exclusions; some are closed to new applicants (including Florida); and some impose long waiting times (including California and Illinois). While some states ban HIPAA-eligibles from participating in the pool, other states use the hig-risk pools to comply with the federal HIPAA, so that the pool becomes the "guaranteed issue" option when COBRA expires. Some states use their high-risk pools as a means of providing Medicare-eligible individuals with a

Medicare Supplement, while a few ban enrollment of Medicare eligibles. Because the rules and suitability of the state insurance pools vary tremendously, you should make sure you understand exactly how your own state's pool works.

9. Unfortunately, in an effort to "help" individuals with ratable health conditions, some states may not make this option available because of underwriting limitations imposed by law.

10. Many people are put off by the high deductible; but that is a mistake. Even though that amount may sound like a lot, it is important to keep in mind that "deductible" is a contract term defined within the contract itself. In most of these policies, the "deductible" is not renewable annually, nor is it typically limited to amounts spend "out of pocket." Instead, in most of these policies, there is a contractually specified revolving term—usually between 36 and 48 months—in which the deductible must be accrued. Additionally, these deductibles are not ordinarily measured by the amount that the beneficiary of the policy pays out of pocket; instead they often include amounts that any other insurer has paid toward a given condition (including, for example, Medicare, Veterans Administration, worker's compensation, or private insurance). For example, a $25,000 revolving 36-month deductible simply requires that $25,000 be paid toward a given health condition within a 36-month period by any accepted payor (including another insurance company). If your multiple sclerosis has cost an accumulation of the policy deductible in expenses to all of your payers, you might qualify under the catastrophic plan. In that case, your condition could be declared catastrophic and would be covered (usually at 100% coverage) by the catastrophic plan. The deductible under these policies are instituted to make sure that claims are only filed for truly catastrophic expenses and in so doing they exclude well care altogether but provide significant coverage for that truly catastrophic condition.

11. Advance directive requirements vary greatly from state to state. A lawyer should be consulted in your own state properly to execute these documents.

Part 7 **Research**

29 Issues in the Design and Interpretation of Multiple Sclerosis Clinical Trials

Stephen Krieger, Svenja Oynhausen, and Aaron Miller

Multiple sclerosis (MS) is a disease whose heterogeneity poses unique challenges in making the diagnosis, offering prognosis, and deciding about treatment. The heterogeneity may pose even greater challenges in the design of clinical trials because it leads to problems of operational definitions, ascertainment of clinical data, and selection of meaningful outcomes as they pertain to characterizing the disease course. Applying the results of clinical trials to individual patients adds an additional degree of difficulty.

The natural history of MS has been well characterized over the past several decades. Although there are numerous methodological problems with the direct use of natural history controls, the entire enterprise of designing clinical trials for MS begins with applied natural history. Assumptions about the expected behavior of the disease are implicated in trial design, outcome selection, entrance criteria, and power calculations. Clinical trials of MS treatments are typically short term, relapse, or magnetic resonance imaging (MRI)-based studies; long-term benefits assessed utilizing robust clinical measures remain to be definitively established. As the disease course typically spans several decades, it is particularly difficult to draw firm conclusions about the consequence of treatments that have been available for only a fraction of this duration. Indeed, it is not clear how best to determine whether, and to what degree, current medications are influencing the long-term course of the disease (Noseworthy, 2007).

A discussion of MS clinical trial design and interpretation must begin with a critical review of the operational definitions used to characterize the disease. The broad range of MS disease course has been delineated into four subtypes, relapsing-remitting MS (RRMS), secondary progressive MS (SPMS), primary progressive MS (PPMS), and progressive-relapsing MS (PRMS). It should be emphasized that the names for the clinical subtypes are of limited, mostly descriptive applicability. As they are based solely on the effects of the disease that cross the clinical threshold, the categories do not necessarily reflect the true underlying pathological heterogeneity. In RRMS, for instance, the formation of new T2 lesions is far more common than the occurrence of clinical attacks, indicating that even during periods of clinical quiescence, tissue damage continues to accumulate. The subtypes also vary in their definition as they apply to the temporal course of MS: PPMS is a discrete subtype, but RRMS and SPMS can both occur in the same individual at different points in his or her disease course. In addition, the transition from RRMS to SPMS is indistinct and can only be definitively identified in retrospect. One, therefore, cannot know whether a patient with RRMS has already begun to progress at the time of enrollment into an RRMS trial.

Nonetheless, these categories are most useful in the context of clinical trials, where homogenous populations are desirable to most clearly discern a therapeutic effect, and much of the successful work in the field, as well as the focus of this chapter, pertains to relapsing-remitting disease. Although necessary from a trial design perspective, the use of categories that are not biologically defined imposes several assumptions on the planning of a trial. As Randy Schapiro (personal communication) has noted, "There is no relapsing-remitting MS or secondary progressive MS—there is only MS."

While MS experts debate whether MS is one disease or many, confining clinical trials to a particular disease state not defined by distinct pathophysiologic mechanisms may increase both false-positive and false-negative results for clinical research. The reliance on these classifications for clinical trials limits the generalizability of the results across the entire MS spectrum, and it typically restricts approval and licensure of an agent to the subtype of MS in which it has been studied. An era in which the subtype-delineations are likely to be updated, as genetics and biomarkers become available to better elucidate the pathological substrates for clinical patterns, is likely beginning.

Clinical trials in MS have, since the early 1980s, followed a traditional "double-blind, placebo-controlled, randomized paradigm" (McFarland and Reingold, 2005) and have led to the approval of six agents for the treatment of MS. The widespread use of these treatments has transformed the management of MS and has significantly impacted the design of clinical trials that are needed to find safer and more effective therapies for relapsing MS and to test new therapies for other as yet untreatable forms of the disease (McFarland and Reingold, 2005). Despite the extraordinary advancements in neuroimmunology, rational drug development, and clinical trial design and analyses, clinical trials are hampered by an incomplete basic understanding of the MS disease process, the mechanism of action of the agents under investigation, and the ideal way to gauge their clinical effectiveness. The hope is that early treatment will impact long-term course and the subsequent development of disability, but there is, as yet, little convincing evidence that our current agents affect this outcome (Noseworthy, 2007). In addition, the currently available therapies are only partially effective, have side effects, are difficult to deliver, and are expensive. However, the widespread availability and clinical acceptance of these agents has led to a transformation in the design of modern MS clinical trials, one that is both ethically and practically based (McFarland and Reingold, 2005). Currently, more than ever, a dynamic pipeline of parenteral and oral agents is already in phase III testing so that several new agents may reach the market in the next few years. This new landscape of MS therapeutics presents novel challenges to future clinical trials, and this chapter will review the assumptions and design considerations of pivotal and recent MS trials to provide a historical perspective on how we have arrived at the present moment in considering the future of MS research. It will conclude with an evaluation of the current state of ethics of placebo-controlled trials, as well as an overview of new approaches to the study of MS that take a more holistic approach than that of the traditional clinical trial.

CLINICAL TRIAL OUTCOMES MEASUREMENT: AN OVERVIEW

Multiple sclerosis clinical trials must be designed to capture the broad array of potential disease manifestations across individuals, but they must do so in a way that is reproducible and standardized. Outcome measures must be multidimensional in order to adequately encompass the myriad ways MS effects patients both in the short and long term. To this end, clinical trials focus on the two hallmark characteristics of MS: the occurrence of relapses and the accrual of disability. Choice of the outcome measure depends on the presumed mechanism of action of the investigated treatment and its anticipated clinical effect. It is important to choose the most appropriate primary outcome measure for each individual trial (D'Souza et al., 2008). In addition, a study must be of sufficient duration to allow the benefit of the agent to become evident and have a subject population large enough to power the study adequately. As long-term disability cannot be adequately assessed directly in a short-term clinical trial, all of our clinical measures from relapse-based assessments to measures of sustained disability in the short term can be considered surrogate markers of our ultimate long-term therapeutic goals.

Short-Term, Relapse-Based Outcomes

Clinical trials of disease-modifying agents for MS typically utilize relapse-based endpoints to demonstrate therapeutic effect. As short-term trials (usually between 1 and 3 years in duration) are often underpowered to demonstrate effect on long-term disability, endpoints such as the annualized relapse rate, time to first relapse, and percent of patients relapse free serve as surrogate markers of disease suppression. These trials, and in particular their placebo arms, provide an instructive data source to characterize the short-term behavior of relapsing MS.

A relapse may be operationally defined as an objectively, clinically ascertainable, new or seriously worsening neurological deficit that persists for more than 24 hours, that develops at an interval of at least 30 days after a previous relapse, and is not related to infections. This 1-month window does not necessarily correspond with the actual biology of the disease, where often more than one area of active inflammation in the central nervous system (CNS) exists, each of which runs an independent time course (D'Souza et al., 2008). Short-lived aggravation of the symptoms related to elevations in body temperature (e.g., with fever, physical exercise, hot showers, warm weather) are referred to as Uthoff phenomena or "pseudoexacerbations." They result from an unmasking of subclinical lesions or worsening of chronic symptoms by transient elevations in temperature, and they do not constitute new inflammatory CNS activity. Patients cannot always distinguish a true exacerbation from a pseudoexacerbation, which is significant given that many trials rely on patients to report the occurrence of a relapse.

Problems comparing the efficacy of various treatments are amplified by trial-to-trial variation in relapse definition in terms of duration (24 or 48 hours) and whether a change on the neurological exam (as noted by a blinded evaluator) is present. Furthermore, trials are inconsistent about whether the objective change in the neurological examination must correspond with the clinical symptoms as described by the patient. The more narrow the definition, the lower the recorded relapse rate. Additionally, changes on the neurological examination (particularly changes in reflexes or subtle sensory changes) may be noted by the examiner in the absence of new symptoms to qualify as a relapse. Even with the most rigorous relapse criteria, borderline events will always be left to the investigators' judgment to interpret. If the expectations of the trial's sponsor are apparent to the investigators and their patients, the relapse rate in one group of patients might be underestimated in nonblinded studies (Sørensen, 2008).

Beyond the issues of ascertainment, relapse rate is a useful, but flawed, measure of MS disease activity.

Suppressing relapses benefits patients both immediately in terms of functional status, and potentially in the long term, as relapses are associated with significant residual deficits (Lublin et al., 2003). In addition, the relapse rate early in the disease is an important determinant of accumulation of disability later in the disease course. Although lower relapse rates in the early years of the disease may portend less eventual disability, whether a reduction in relapse rate imposed by treatment provides the same effect on long-term disability as would a relatively relapse-free experience as part of an individual's natural history remains unknown (Noseworthy et al., 2006).

Long-Term Observational Studies and Disability-Based Outcomes

The maximum clinical variability of MS is seen in the short term after disease onset; the illness becomes more predictable upon long-term observation. Much of the data on long-term outcomes in MS comes from several longitudinally followed cohorts and not from randomized clinical trials. As natural-history studies, these are largely comprised of patients who did not receive disease-modifying treatments; because of the availability of treatment, it is no longer feasible to follow such cohorts prospectively in the modern era. Three cohorts that provide large-scale, prospective analyses of untreated populations are those from Lyon, France (Confavreux et al., 2000), Sweden (Runmarker and Andersen, 1993), and London, Ontario (Weinshenker et al., 1991). Long-term prognosis is often described using time to development of disability landmarks in the Expanded Disability Status Score (EDSS). These include EDSS 4, the development of moderate disability with preserved gait; EDSS 6, the need for assistance with ambulation; and EDSS 7, the need for a wheelchair for mobility. While these classifications are limited by their focus on mobility, they provide a meaningful window into the time course of accrual of disability and reflect particular outcomes of great concern to patients diagnosed with MS.

The EDSS remains the criterion standard by which disability is measured in both the long and the short term. In short-term studies lasting from 1 to several years, "sustained disability" as an outcome variable requires a measured change on the EDSS being reproduced at two points separated in time, usually by 6 months. If a patient "changes by 1 point on the EDSS," however, this could mean a variety of things depending on where along the scale the patient is, and vary even further depending on what functional system brought about the change in EDSS step. In addition, persistent or sustained increases in physical impairment may occur because of a failure to completely recover from a relapse or from the slow accrual of disability that characterizes progressive MS. The use of "sustained disability" as a clinical endpoint fails to elucidate this distinction. As these processes are likely based on varying pathophysiology, lumping them together as a single clinical endpoint may not adequately capture the biologic response to a therapeutic agent.

The EDSS has a number of limitations that bear mention when considering its use in clinical trials. It is weighted toward ambulatory disability but is insensitive to other aspects of MS-related impairment, in particular cognitive dysfunction. Although a numerical scale, it is ordinal and categorical in nature and neither quantitative nor linear. The EDSS is thus not ideally suited to the deltas and changes in the "mean" that are frequently used as outcome variables. As an assessment tool, the EDSS has only moderate inter-relater reliability particularly at the lower range, is not entirely objective, and can have great fluctuation particularly at the lower levels. In its highest levels, the scale becomes a subjective description of a patient's home care needs, and thus patients in the upper strata of EDSS are rarely included in clinical trials.

ISSUES IN CLINICAL TRIAL DESIGN AND INTERPRETATION

Reconsidering the Evolution of Pivotal Trials

The 1990s saw the publication of large clinical trials evaluating the three brands of interferon beta and glatiramer acetate as disease-modifying drugs in MS, and their subsequent regulatory approval and evolution into standard of care. Although the individual disease-modifying agents are discussed in previous chapters, some of the implications of the pivotal trials on the design and interpretation of subsequent and recent studies will be reviewed here.

The randomized, placebo-controlled paradigm of the pivotal trials demonstrated not only efficacy of the agents studied but pronounced placebo effects on relapse rates when comparing prestudy with on-study exacerbation rates in the placebo group (D'Souza et al., 2008). The results of the interferon β-1b pivotal trial reported in 1993 (IFN β Multiple Sclerosis Study Group, 1993) are an archetype for this period in MS clinical research, and they demonstrated an annualized relapse rate of 0.78 in the interferon group versus 1.27 in the placebo group. The study was criticized for issues of relapse-ascertainment and confirmation, as relapses were self-reported and not universally confirmed by an examining neurologist. Three years later, in the weekly interferon β-1a study (Jacobs et al., 1996), the placebo group had an annualized relapse rate of 0.82, which was comparable to that of the rate of 0.84 in the placebo group of the pivotal trial of glatiramer acetate (Johnson et al., 1995). It was already clear that although there was a comparable degree of relative relapse rate reduction between the agents, the actual annualized relapse rates varied considerably between trials. All the values are likely to be skewed toward higher attack rates, as patients were selected for these studies on the basis of high prestudy clinical disease activity. The relapse rate may then "regress towards the mean" once these patients have been enrolled in the trial, in part explaining the extent of the apparent placebo effect. The efficacy of placebo may also reflect the impact of the comprehensive care provided to trial participants (D'Souza et al., 2008). The pivotal trials' placebo group results underscore the importance of randomized, placebo-controlled trials and why positive head-to-head equivalency studies alone cannot be used to prove an agent's efficacy, nor have they been considered sufficient evidence for regulatory approval.

The interferon β-1b pivotal trial did not demonstrate a statistically significant effect on disability, and as the trial enrolled ambulatory, relapsing-remitting patients it was likely underpowered to assess this outcome. In contrast, the pivotal trial of weekly intramuscular interferon β-1a (Jacobs et al., 1996) utilized disability as the primary outcome measure and demonstrated a slower rate of accumulation of disability for the treated group, which was defined in advance as deterioration by ≥ 1 point on the EDSS for ≥ 6 months. In the subsequent pivotal trials of natalizumab, AFFIRM (Polman et al., 2006) and SENTINEL (Rudick et al., 2006), disability endpoints were also met, with sustained disability defined as persisting for ≥ 3 months.

A significant issue in the pivotal trials was that of the success of the blinding. Type and degree of blinding play an important role in the adjudication of patient-reported symptoms and their ascertainment by an evaluator. As the majority of treatments tested including glatiramer acetate, interferons, and mitoxantrone have easily recognized side effects or hallmarks such as injection site reactions, it is likely that the patients were able to correctly guess whether they were receiving placebo or active drug, which can confound the results given the subjective nature of relapses as assessed in these trials. Unscheduled symptom-initiated study visits and the methods of ascertainment of relapses at these visits should be equal across treatment arms to ensure that relapse assessment is not affected by systematic ascertainment bias. Modern double-blind studies have employed both a treating-neurologist and blinded evaluating neurologist to conduct the trial assessments. However, as oral and parenteral agents now in development have distinct modes of administration from the self-injected therapies with which they are being compared, this has necessitated using single-blind designs where maintenance of evaluator blinding is of paramount importance. Nonetheless, the lack of a double-blind design must be considered when interpreting these trials, which include the phase II and III trials of alemtuzumab (Coles et al., 2008).

Extension Trials and Long-Term Observational Studies

Given that clinical trials must establish efficacy in a short time frame, extension trials and open-label follow-up can provide a greater window into the benefit and safety profile of a therapeutic agent in the long term. In addition, there are ethical reasons to design an extension study, as it ensures continued access of an agent to the study population.

Typically, at the conclusion of a randomized controlled study, patients in the treatment group continue on the study drug, and patients initially randomized to the control group are offered the active drug and continue to be followed, albeit usually with a reduced frequency of assessments than during the randomized phase of the trial.

Although extension trials are frequently cited as evidence of the long-term efficacy of an agent, the quality of the data obtained in such an investigation is clearly inferior to that of the randomized phase, as the extension is open-label, uncontrolled, and the study population may exhibit self-selection by the patients who responded to the drug in the initial trial. Thus, extension trials may exhibit a significant selection bias toward "responders" and are of limited value in obtaining data that can be generalized overall regarding drug efficacy. In addition, extension trials are of limited impact with regard to outcome measures as they are generally no longer blinded, although to address this concern more recent trials have re-randomized the placebo group into a dose-blinded extension.

To provide even longer term assessments of the impact of a therapeutic agent, nonrandomized long-term observational studies have been undertaken lasting over a decade. These are in essence interminable extension trials, and their data suffer, at best, from similar methodological limitations. Large, long-term observational data sets for both the interferons and glatiramer have been analyzed (Ebers and Traboulsee, 2009; Rovaris et al., 2007) and are of greatest value in providing information about safety and long-term survival, while the "sustained efficacy" described in these data sets is confounded by enormous dropout rates, the unavoidable bias favoring responders, and the lack of an effective intention-to-treat analysis. These observational studies blur the distinction between research and clinical practice, and while they may attempt to quantify outcomes seen in "real world" standard of care, they lack the rigor and generalizability of well-performed clinical trials. That said, carefully designed long-term observational studies with specific hypotheses and preplanned analyses have the potential to provide valuable information that cannot be captured during the short-term randomized clinical trials of agents currently in testing.

The Problem of Cross-Trial Comparison

The reduction in relapse rate in the pivotal trial of weekly interferon β-1a (Jacobs et al., 1996) at 18% was more modest than that seen in the interferon β-1b pivotal trial. In the weekly interferon β-1a trial, the relapse rate declined from 1.2 to 0.61 in the treatment group versus 1.2 to 0.82 in the placebo group. These two trials underscore the problems of cross-trial comparison even for studies done in the same era, as the raw annualized relapse rate outcome would appear to favor weekly interferon β-1a as opposed to the 0.78 seen with interferon β-1b, while the relative reduction versus placebo favors the latter. Which drug is "better?" As discussed later in this chapter, this issue becomes all the more pronounced when one compares the results of the pivotal trials to those done in the "postmillennial" or "McDonald era" where an on-drug relapse rate of 0.78 or 0.61 would be considered an utter failure in the context of the current standard of efficacy.

Another example of the difficulties in comparing between two trials comes from the studies of the effect of subcutaneous interferon β–1b on disease progression in SPMS. The initial European study demonstrated that treatment with interferon β–1b was associated with a higher probability of stabilization of progression of disability compared to placebo. The therapeutic effect on this outcome measure, however, was not replicated in a North American study using a comparable but not identical study design (Panitch et al., 2004). Given the heterogeneity of MS in terms of clinical course and variable outcome, subtle variations in such factors as inclusion criteria, matching of study cohorts, selection of outcome variables, and statistical analyses are sufficient to render study results incomparable.

In the pivotal trial era, however, head-to-head studies were not performed. The Food and Drug Administration (FDA) does not accept "equivalency trials" as sufficient evidence for licensing approval, particularly as one could reasonably conclude from equivalence in a head-to-head study either that an agent is equally as effective or equally as ineffective as its comparator. This position favored the use of placebo-controlled trials, particularly as it statistically easier to demonstrate superiority of an investigational drug, with a smaller sample size, when compared with an ineffective placebo than versus a partially-effective comparator.

The head-to-head trial era in MS began with the development of subcutaneous interferon β–1a given three times a week. As it is the same molecule as once-weekly interferon β-1ba, in order to expedite regulatory approval as Rebif, the FDA required positive head-to-head superiority studies before it could enter the market in the United States. Head-to-head comparisons of the relative efficacy of high- and low-dose interferon β–1a used as their relapse-based outcome the proportion of relapse-free and MRI activity–free patients. While both the INCOMIN (Durelli et al., 2002) and EVIDENCE studies (Panitch et al., 2002) demonstrated an advantage of high-dose interferon, by choosing as the primary outcome measure the "proportion of relapse-free patients" rather than the overall relapse rate, these trials evaluate the number of optimal responders and may not reflect a differential of general effectiveness across the population. They nonetheless were sufficient to justify the licensure of subcutaneous interferon β-1a in the United States, and they established a head-to-head trial paradigm that not all subsequent such studies were able to replicate.

The McDonald-Era Clinical Trials: Head-to-Head and Clinically Isolated Syndrome Trial Designs

Head-to-head studies

The successful implementation of active-comparator trials, including the head-to-head studies of high- versus low-dose interferon in the EVIDENCE and INCOMIN trials, led to the design and recruitment of several head-to-head trials of high-dose interferon β versus glatiramer acetate (Copaxone). Recruiting during the McDonald era, the BEYOND and REGARD trials (Mikol et al., 2008; see also Achiron and Fredrikson, 2009) failed to show a difference on relapse-based outcomes between either of the interferon β products and glatiramer acetate. These trials differ considerably in design, but the common factor involved in both trials' failure to reach their relapse-based primary endpoints was the low event rate observed in all groups. The REGARD study was a 2-year, randomized, open-label, head-to-head comparative study of subcutaneous interferon β-1a 44 μg three times a week and glatiramer acetate, which showed no difference in the primary outcome measure, time to first relapse, or the proportion of patients who were relapse free. The sample size and power calculations, as previously described in the example above, are predicated on assumptions of an expected event rate. Although the annualized relapse rates in the REGARD study were almost identical (0.30 for interferon β-1a and 0.29 for glatiramer acetate), they were much lower than those reported in landmark trials (0.87 for interferon β-1a and 0.59 for glatiramer acetate) (Sørensen, 2008). The revised McDonald criteria allowed for the use of MRI to establish the diagnosis of MS; since many lesions detectable on MRI are clinically silent, these revised criteria allow a diagnosis of confirmed MS to be made earlier than would have been possible using clinical manifestations of relapses alone (Lublin, 2005). The inclusion of this new population in the postmillennial trials shifted the curve toward patients less likely to experience relapses in the short term.

A second consideration in the REGARD trial was the selection of time to first relapse as the primary outcome variable. Time to first relapse on treatment is a robust parameter, even in trials with high dropout rates. However, it does not make use of the second and subsequent relapses in the course of a trial, and thus it is particularly sensitive to differences in time course of therapeutic onset. It favors drugs with rapid onset, as compared to those with a more delayed but perhaps in the long run an equivalent or better-sustained effect (D'Souza et al., 2008). There are competing influences on trial design, where the goal is to assess a meaningful benefit in as little time as possible, but to be done in such a way as to demonstrate efficacy for a product intended for long-term use in a lifelong disease. It is of particular note that REGARD failed to demonstrate the purported more rapid time of onset of interferon β over glatiramer acetate.

Clearly the use of historical controls, particularly in the modern era of across-the-board decrease in observed relapse rates, imparts an unacceptably high degree of false-positive error. But what are the other implications of the relapse rates of the McDonald era on clinical trial design and interpretation? One consideration is how to interpret the results of the AFFIRM trial (Polman et al., 2006) conducted at the outset of the McDonald era, which demonstrated the 68% reduction in relapse rate that natalizumab (Tysabri) established, approximately twice as great a reduction as the existing injectable therapies achieved in their pivotal trials. These same injectable agents, however, demonstrated approximately an 80% reduction in relapse rate in the BEYOND and REGARD trials of the past few years. Is AFFIRM the last trial of the pivotal era or the first of the McDonald era? There have been no head-to-head studies to elucidate this.

Either way, for most patients with MS, relapses are a relatively infrequent event. In studies planned for short duration, only a small percentage of patients will experience a relapse. It may be difficult to ascertain which of these patients respond optimally and which experienced either a more mild form of the disease, or just a period of disease quiescence unrelated to the therapeutic intervention (Walton, 2007). If most patients with RRMS experience either one or no relapses during a 2-year trial, the trial may be underpowered because of the low event rate, and it further calls into question the utility of the relapse outcome measure in trials of this duration. To maximize the expected event rate, some trials have employed clinical or radiographic entrance criteria (i.e., recent pre-enrollment relapses or enhancing lesions, respectively) during a specified time period. While this technique may increase the chances that an investigational drug will demonstrate a significant impact on a primary outcome variable, it further constrains the trial participants in a manner that further reduces the broad application of trial outcomes across the MS population and, of course, makes the trial more difficult to enroll.

In the pivotal trials of the 1990s, MRI outcomes were utilized to supplement the clinical data and provide further evidence supporting the drug's effectiveness. This was done to alleviate concerns about subjectively influenced efficacy findings such as effect on the relapse rate (Walton, 2007). Agents being tested in the treatment era have a higher standard of clinical efficacy to achieve and, to make matters more difficult, lower observed relapse rates on which to demonstrate their benefit.

Thus, surrogate markers like MRI are now utilized not to prove overall efficacy, which must be demonstrated clinically and convincingly, but rather to suggest a study subpopulation that may have a greater response. Magnetic resonance imaging and other surrogate markers can be used either as selection criteria or as a planned subgroup analysis to improve the risk–benefit ratio of an agent by identifying the population with the maximal response. The results of BEYOND and REGARD may have established clinical equipoise between interferon β and glatiramer acetate; however, these were both open-label, single-blind trials. We will have to wait for CombiRx, a large, ongoing, randomized, double-blind, double-dummy study that compares intramuscular interferon β-1a given weekly, glatiramer acetate given daily, and the combination of the two drugs given together to provide the highest-possible quality head-to-head evaluation of these agents (Sørensen, 2008). The CombiRx trial will also provide biomarker data to better identify patient characteristics that predict response to one of the therapeutic two modalities.

Clinically isolated syndrome trials

From a design perspective, clinically isolated syndrome (CIS) trials can be considered as RRMS trials recruiting after the first episode, where the outcome measures based on relapse occurrence are recast as time to "conversion to MS." These trials have been implemented largely to satisfy regulatory requirements for an approved indication in CIS. Just as use of MRI in the McDonald criteria (McDonald et al., 2001; Polman et al., 2005) has allowed for the determination of dissemination in time sooner than would be found with clinical episodes alone, so, too, has the use of MRI in CIS trials provided radiographic outcome measures that dramatically raise the event rate of "conversion to MS."

Building on the knowledge that MRI lesions at the time of a first demyelinating event are predictive of recurrence, large clinical trials of CIS patients have required clinically silent lesions as entrance criteria. Examining the data from the placebo arms of these trials lends support to the capacity of MRI lesions to predict conversion to MS. These trials include the Optic Neuritis Treatment Trial (ONTT), Controlled High Risk Subjects Avonex

Multiple Sclerosis Prevention Study (CHAMPS), the Early Treatment of Multiple Sclerosis Study (ETOMS), and more recently, the study of interferon β-1b in CIS, known as BENEFIT. The cumulative probability of developing a second attack in 2 years was 18% in the ONTT (Beck et al., 1995), 38% in CHAMPS (Jacobs et al., 2000), and 45% in ETOMS (Comi et al., 2001). The increased rates of conversion to MS in CHAMPS and ETOMS are attributable to the presence of clinically silent lesions on MRI as an enrollment criterion, underscoring the utility of initial MRI appearance to predict short-term outcomes. In BENEFIT (Kappos et al., 2006), after 2 years, 45% of placebo patients had experienced a second attack, but 85% fulfilled the McDonald criteria, demonstrating the increased sensitivity conferred by the radiographic diagnostic criteria and underscoring the hazards of evolving diagnostic criteria for cross-trial comparisons. Glatiramer acetate and intramuscular weekly interferon β-1a and interferon β-1b have demonstrated efficacy and garnered FDA approval for use at CIS, as would be anticipated from their established effect in relapsing remitting disease. A very low weekly dose of subcutaneous interferon β-1a also resulted in a statistically significant reduction in relapse rate, but this preparation is not currently approved by the FDA for the treatment of CIS.

Progressive Multiple Sclerosis and the Emerging Focus on Neuroprotection

In SPMS greater uncertainty exists regarding the short-term benefits of treatment; and the different results between the European and North American IFN trials in SPMS (Panitch et al., 2004) highlight the role that continued relapses and inflammatory activity play in the extent to which treatments have a "disease-modifying" effect on this form of the disease. This also highlights the continuum that exists between RRMS and SPMS, and how, even with restrictive inclusion criteria, trial populations differ in their range of pathophysiology such that one may reach its endpoint while the other fails to do so.

In addition, even those SPMS trials that do reach disability endpoints may not reflect the true risk–benefit profile of the agent. For example, the European trial of mitoxantrone in SPMS (see Martinelli et al., 2005) demonstrated a decreased number of patients with EDSS progression, but at 188 patients it was too small to adequately predict the rare but serious potential consequences that have come to limit its use, including secondary leukemias. The issue of estimating such rare but potentially lethal side effects of the disease-modifying therapies was highlighted by the emergence of PML with natalizumab after the SENTINEL trial was completed. While this was initially estimated to be a "one in a thousand" risk potentially confined to its use in combination with interferon, the occurrence of PML in natalizumab monotherapy in post-marketing is a salient example of the difficulty of basing these estimates on the comparatively small population of a clinical trial.

Negative trials also provide valuable information for our understanding of the protean manifestations of the disease. The PROMiSe study, evaluating the effect of glatiramer acetate on accumulation of disability in PPMS, failed to reach its endpoint despite a sample size of over 900 patients and was halted after planned interim analysis. Akin to the methodological problem that caused REGARD and BEYOND to fail to reach their endpoints, the observed annual progression rate on the Expanded Disability Status Scale was only 36%, which was markedly lower than the 50% annual progression rate estimate used in the power calculations for sample size (Kieseier et al., 2007). Future clinical trial methodologies in progressive forms of MS are likely to focus on neuroprotection, which refers to targeting mechanisms of neuronal injury to prevent destruction, rather than the upstream efforts at immunomodulation that have shown minimal effect in progressive disease (Kapoor, 2006).

IMPLICATIONS FOR CURRENT AND FUTURE STUDY DESIGNS

Oral and Parenteral Agents

The goals of current MS clinical trials have evolved based on the successes that have preceded them. The pivotal trials established efficacy of the existing agents and assured their regulatory approval. These were followed by trial designs that confirmed the utility of treatment at first event and subsequently by direct head-to-head and trials of comparative dosing strategies. Agents currently in clinical trials will be judged not only on the basis of reaching their study endpoints but also on what they add to the current armamentarium. To this end, there are several oral and parenteral drugs that are in phase III testing, and while it is as-yet unknown which will come to fruition, there are several paradigm changes in the current research era that bear mention.

Alemtuzumab is a monoclonal antibody given by annual cycles of IV infusion for which the results of a successful phase II trial were published in October 2008 (Coles et al., 2008). The alemtuzumab study was a bold design in two ways: instead of a placebo-control, the investigators used an active-comparator design, comparing two doses of alemtuzumab against subcutaneous interferon β-1a; and they chose sustained accumulation of disability as the primary endpoint. As discussed earlier, both of these design decisions decrease the likelihood of a positive trial, particularly when studied in a typical phase II sample size of 334 patients. Nonetheless, compared to interferon β-1a, relapses were reduced by 75% and sustained disability by 60% in patients receiving alemtuzumab. Importantly, the positive effects persisted at comparable magnitudes after 3 years (Kleinschnitz et al., 2008). These results have provided a considerably better understanding of how the novel treatment compares to current standard of care. While placebo-controlled trials have historically been the criterion standard, in the modern era comparator trials will be essential for clinicians and patients to make informed choices with regard to therapy (McFarland, 2009).

The encouraging results of the alemtuzumab trial were, however, tempered by six cases of idiopathic thrombocytopenic purpura (ITP), one with a fatal outcome leading to interruption of administration of study drug during the trial (Kleinschnitz et al., 2008). There were significant risks of autoimmune thyroid and renal diseases associated with this agent as well. Alemtuzumab can be viewed as a long-lasting form of selective immune ablation (Kleinschnitz et al., 2008), but the emergence of secondary autoimmune conditions may indicate that more powerful immunomodulatory agents aimed at acting more incisively on MS may entail unwanted life-threatening perturbations of the immune system elsewhere, as was previously seen with the occurrence of PML with natalizumab (Lublin, 2005). The phase III alemtuzumab trials known as CARE-MS are currently ongoing, and they are slated to enroll approximately 2000 patients. They follow the same general paradigm as in phase II, comparing alemtuzumab against subcutaneous interferon β-1a; however, superior efficacy is all but a foregone conclusion on the basis of the phase II results. The phase III trials will thus largely serve to evaluate the incidence of adverse events such as ITP and autoimmune thyroid disease in a much larger study population. Unlike the pivotal phase III trials of the 1990s that were intended to establish an agent's clinical benefit, these phase III trials will enhance our ability to estimate the amount of risk in alemtuzumab's risk–benefit profile.

Rare but potentially lethal opportunistic infections have also been reported in the ongoing phase III studies of FTY720, or fingolimod, one of the promising oral agents in development. As new agents emerge that address the limited modes of administration and effectiveness of the current generation of therapeutics, this new potential for serious adverse effects mandates very close monitoring. With 15 years of experience with the current FDA-approved medications, physicians will face difficult decisions about whether and how to use new drugs that may be more efficacious but may also carry greater risks. New drugs in development must be designed with the understanding of the relatively modest benefit, but very substantial safety profile of the current era in MS therapeutics in mind.

Ethical and Practical Challenges to Placebo-Controlled Clinical Trials

While randomized, placebo-controlled clinical trials have been the mainstay and criterion standard for testing new drugs in MS, there are several challenges facing this design paradigm in the current era (McFarland, 2009). Because of the recent successes in developing new therapies for MS, placebo-controlled trials face three important hurdles: decreasing number of patients who qualify for studies; ethical concerns regarding the use of placebo when approved therapies are available;

and limited applicability of placebo-controlled results given the availability of several effective agents.

The ethics and future of placebo-controlled trials in MS have received considerable attention and have been the subject of a consensus opinion most recently revised in 2008. This resulted from a meeting of an international group of clinicians, ethicists, statisticians, regulators, and representatives from the pharmaceutical industry that convened under the auspices of the National MS Society's International Advisory Committee on Clinical Trials of New Agents in MS to reexamine the ethics of placebo-controlled clinical trials (Polman et al., 2008). The ethical conduct of placebo-controlled trials in MS rests upon the concept of clinical equipoise, which states that the lack of consensus among experts regarding preferred treatment justifies the need for clinical trials to further knowledge in the area. Even in the age of multiple approved drugs for MS, the condition still fits this definition, insofar as the medications are all incompletely effective, none halts relapses or progression, and all have problematic side effect profiles that affect tolerability and adherence (Polman et al., 2008). The number needed to treat (NNT) measure derived from published trials provides insight into the limitations of the current therapies: in patients with CIS, seven must be treated to prevent one patient from developing CDMS at 3 years. In RRMS, nine have to receive interferon to prevent a single relapse at 1 year, and eight must be treated for 2 years to prevent one patient from worsening by a single EDSS point during this interval (Noseworthy et al., 2006). Clearly much work remains to be done to discover and evaluate potentially better therapies. Despite these limitations, however, the use of placebo controls in clinical trials cannot be justified for those patients willing to initiate treatment with one of the approved medications (Miller, 2007).

The National MS Society Task Force (Polman et al., 2008) maintains that for patients with relapsing MS for which established effective therapies exist, placebo-controlled trials should only be offered with rigorous informed consent if the subjects refuse to use these treatments, have not responded to them, or if these treatments are not available to them for other reasons (e.g., economics) (Polman et al., 2008). Use of placebo-controlled trials is ethical for patients whose disease falls outside the regulatory or regionally accepted criteria for treatment with available agents. This category has been taken to include PPMS, for which no treatment has been shown to be effective, and to some degree SPMS, for which there is limited consensus on the true risk–benefit ratio of the approved disease-modifying therapies (Miller, 2007).

Despite the requirements for "rigorous informed consent," obtaining consent from a potential study subject may not be sufficient to ensure truly informed decision making. Contemporary informed consent documents are complex and voluminous. As an example, at the time of this writing the informed consent form for the current phase III trial of alemtuzumab is 13,000 words, or roughly the length of this chapter. Furthermore, these documents are often presented to patients with worsening disease, whose condition sometimes makes them feel greater pressure for potential trial participation (Polman et al., 2008).

Independent of the ethical issues, it is increasingly difficult to recruit and retain patients for placebo-controlled trials. Many recent trials have recruited subjects from Eastern European and Asian countries where treatment availability is variable; this raises further concerns regarding the provision of therapy to the participants at the conclusion of a trial. In addition, as discussed earlier with regard to the alemtuzumab trials, in this competitive treatment era, placebo-controlled trials fail to provide increasingly important information about comparative efficacy among available agents (McFarland and Reingold, 2005). Is it meaningful to know simply that a new agent is more effective than placebo when there are six agents already approved for the treatment of MS?

Alternatives to placebo-controlled designs

Particular focus has been placed on trials that either avoid the use of a placebo because of the ethical considerations or on designs that allow new therapies to be studied more rapidly or with fewer patients than would be needed in a conventional placebo-controlled trial (McFarland and Reingold, 2005). Such alternative trial designs include dose-finding strategies, where a placebo arm may be replaced by a lowest-dose arm not expected to confer maximal benefit but still conceptually an improvement over placebo. Some have argued that it may be possible to conduct shorter, and therefore perhaps ethically and practically more acceptable trials. But the concept of a short-term study of an agent intended for a lifelong disease is controversial and even trials of 2 or 3 years' duration may be insufficient (McFarland and Reingold, 2005). Indeed, the major critique of the currently approved disease-modifying agents is that their long-term efficacy remains unproven.

Another alternative to monotherapy placebo-controlled trials are add-on trials, in which the investigational agent or placebo is added on to an existing therapy to evaluate whether the investigational drug will confer increased efficacy. This is best suited for use when the two agents have different and potentially synergistic mechanisms of action. Methodological issues arise owing to our often incomplete understanding of the drugs' molecular mechanisms of action, and consequent difficulty in predicting how the combination of agents will behave clinically. There is a potential for unexpected antagonism, as was recently seen in a small trial evaluating statins added on to interferon (Birnbaum et al., 2008), as well as unexpected synergistic consequences, as with the incidence of PML when natalizumab was added on to interferon in the SENTINEL trial (Rudick et al., 2006). In addition, success of an agent in an add-on trial yields subsequent ethical and practical challenges when considering whether the new agent should be approved and prescribed as monotherapy if it was never tested in such a manner.

A further strategy is a deferred treatment/crossover design, where after an initial randomization to placebo or active drug, the placebo patients are switched to active treatment either at a prespecified interval or after they reach a clinical endpoint. This was the premise of the BENEFIT trial of interferon β-1b in CIS, whereby at conversion to CDMS the CIS patients on placebo were switched to interferon. This design addressed the ethical concerns inherent in keeping patients who now met McDonald criteria off of an approved therapy, and allowed for a comparison between early- and delayed-treatment in the CIS population. This trial was able to demonstrate both a significant risk reduction by interferon β on conversion from CIS to MS (Kappos et al., 2006), as well as a modest but significant decrease in risk of sustained disability at 3 years (Kappos et al., 2007). If, however, one takes this study as incontrovertible evidence of the need for early treatment, it ethically precludes the further use of this placebo-controlled CIS design. This presents a paradigmatic example of the changing landscape of MS research: as existing treatments are shown to be superior to placebo in more numerous contexts, the study of new agents in the same manner is no longer ethically permissible.

As placebo-controlled trials can be performed with smaller populations than active-comparator or add-on trials, they potentially could expose fewer patients to a novel agent of unknown risk and unclear benefit than the larger trials required to test an investigational drug against an existing treatment. The deaths of patients in recent MS clinical trials of such agents as natalizumab (Goodin et al., 2008), alemtuzumab (Coles et al., 2008), and fingolimod (Leypoldt et al., 2009) are humbling reminders that every patient who agrees to participate in a trial of an experimental medication assumes not just foreseeable risks and those risks associated with placebo, but unforeseeable risks associated with novel therapeutics as well.

The conundrum in which the field of MS finds itself is that while randomized, controlled clinical trials are necessary to demonstrate efficacy on short-term, relapse-based outcomes, and are designed to conform to the standards of proof required by regulatory agencies for licensure, these 2–3 year trials are unlikely to ever answer the question as to whether long-term use of these agents dramatically alters the ultimate natural history of the disease. There are thus ethical and practical reasons to shorten the standard 2-year clinical trial paradigm while conceptual and theoretical reasons argue to study these agents long term.

Alternative outcomes for MS trials include composite outcome measures to reduce sample size and potentially shorten the duration of these studies. Composite outcomes comprise measures of multiple clinical domains and can thus increase the "event rate" as recorded in a trial. The EDSS and MSFC are themselves composite measures; however, by generating more comprehensive composite outcomes rather than a single primary outcome measure, the overall sensitivity of clinical measures can be increased. In addition, results derived from composite outcomes could potentially be more clinically meaningful than such single outcome measures as "proportion of patients relapse free." An example of an interesting possible future alternative to grading disability and mobility according to the artificial confines of the EDSS could be the use of a mobile device for long-term continuous measurement of physical activity. One such device, the ACTIBELT system, is currently being evaluated at the Sylvia Lawry Centre for Multiple Sclerosis Research. This wearable electronic device is integrated into the buckle of a clothing belt and provides quantitative information about patients' physical activity under real-life conditions (D'Souza et al., 2008).

BEYOND THE CLINICAL TRIAL: CONSIDERATIONS FOR MULTIPLE SCLEROSIS HEALTH CARE AND ALTERNATIVE OUTCOMES

In addition to individual heterogeneity of symptoms, their severity, and their timing, the consequence of neurological impairment on a patient's degree of functional disability varies considerably. A patient could be significantly neurologically impaired but not functionally disabled (e.g., a computer programmer who is wheelchair confined), while another can be vocationally disabled with minimal findings on neurological examination (e.g., a concert pianist with impaired right-hand proprioception). The former patient has an EDSS of 8, and the latter an EDSS of 2. Evaluating disability from a patient-centric perspective must take into account both objective impairment and its meaningful impact on the patient, including his or her coping strategies and quality of life. The focus in the field of MS has been for many years on the impact that investigational agents have on the commonly used rating scales; there has recently been a renewed emphasis on finding validated measures and performing well designed-studies on our ability to improve patients' lives.

Psychosocial, Quality of Life, and Vocational Impact Studies

Measuring the clinical impact of MS is a critical issue for judging experimental therapies in clinical trials. To this end, outcomes are being developed that take a more holistic view of patient well-being and response to a variety of modalities of care beyond just those agents aimed at "modifying the disease." A formal investigative approach to the psychosocial consequences and emotional aspects of MS has become a major focus of research in recent years. The field of MS research has moved beyond the rating scales that are solely based on the neurological examination such as the EDSS, which are associated with weak psychometric properties. More patient-oriented measures like the Guy's Neurological Disability Scale (GNDS) and a wide range of disease-specific quality-of-life (QOL) instruments are character-ized by high clinical relevance as they reflect the patient's perspective on the overall impact of medi-cal intervention. Some of the examples of these metrics include the 36 Item Short Form Health Survey (SF 36), the Self-Rated Abilities for Health Practices Scale (SRAHP), the Health Promoting Lifestyle Profile II, and the MS Impact Scale (MSIS-29) (Amato and Portaccio, 2007).

The problems of access to care and services have also been increasingly addressed. Several studies provide evidence that MS patients benefit from rehabilitation and health promotion inter-ventions. Exercise programs have been shown to improve strength, endurance, fatigue and func-tional abilities, mental and physical health, and health-related QOL. Access to these interventions is, however, oftentimes difficult for the physically disabled MS patients who need them the most. To overcome logistic barriers, a study by Bombardier and colleagues (2008) evaluated telephone coun-seling for Health Promotion in MS patients by using the HPLP II as a primary outcome measure and the SF 36 as a secondary outcome measure. The trial supports that telephone-based motiva-tional interviewing is an effective method of health promotion in people with MS. Ennis and colleagues (2006) also found similar effective-ness of a health-promotion education program (the OPTIMISE program) among MS patients.

Evaluating the efficacy of rehabilitation interven-tions, however, is a challenging issue as patients in trials are not easily blinded and control groups are not readily established. Defining an outcome measure is of particular difficulty because of the individual variation of functional deficits and rehabilitation needs. As an example of the diffi-culty in proving the efficacy of rehabilitation, Storr and colleagues developed a trial methodology with a double-blinded design for evaluating the short-term efficacy of multidisciplinary, inpatient rehabilitation among MS patients. Impairment was evaluated by the MSIS 29, and activity was assessed by the GNDS (Storr et al., 2006). Despite the use of the modern methodology, the study was unable to prove a significant advantage of rehabili-tation for stable MS patients (Storr et al., 2006).

Vocational impact studies focus on the conse-quences of MS on patients during their employ-ment years. Employment is not only an important factor in QOL of MS patients, but, by influencing aspects such as insurance status and means of access to health care, it can also be an important factor in their overall health (Wilson and Walker, 1993; Aronson, 1997). Early in the disease, patients with MS may be impaired in finding and main-taining a workplace not only due to obvious physical handicaps but also because of "hidden disabilities" such as subtle cognitive impairments, fatigue, coping problems, and even workplace discrimina-tion (Johnson et al., 2004). Up to 50% of patients with MS lose their job, retire early, reduce their work hours, or change workplaces for less demand-ing but often also less-well-paid jobs (Kornblith et al., 1986; Jackson et al., 1991). This is especially a problem in persons suffering from a disease that in itself causes a major financial burden. A substantial part of the cost of MS relates to losses in earnings due to vocational problems (Whetten-Goldstein et al., 1998).

In a recent systematic review, Khan and col-leagues (2009) reported that they found only two interventional studies focused on vocational reha-bilitation for MS patients with enough internal validity to be regarded as meaningful enough to be included in their review. LaRocca and colleagues (1996) investigated job retention in employed MS patients, and Rumrill et al. (1998) focused on career entry in unemployed patients. Both of these studies still had major limitations such as small sample sizes, no blinding of participants, care providers, or assessors, and unclear intention to treat analyses. Nevertheless, they showed that vocational rehabilitation in MS was feasible and revealed that many patients tended to ignore or neglect possible future problems in finding and main-taining employment until they reached a crisis. Enabling persons with MS to achieve, maintain, or return to a status of employment and economic self-sufficiency is therefore one of the main aspects of rehabilitation, whether it is provided by general

MS rehabilitation or specialized MS vocational rehabilitation.

Multiple Sclerosis Databases and Resource Utilization Studies

The MS International Federation (MSIF) was established in 1967 as an international network targeted on a global linking of the activity of the national MS Society around the world. The Atlas of MS database by the MSIF provides a variety of data on the epidemiology of MS and the availability and accessibility of resources for the diagnosis, treatment, rehabilitation, and support for MS patients; it is aimed at improving life quality of people affected by MS. Another example of a useful database for MS is the New York State MS Consortium (NYSMSC), a regional alliance consisting of 15 MS centers throughout New York State. The NYSMSC developed a clinical long-term follow-up centralized MS patient registry, to offer a potential tool for interdisciplinary research. Similar to the MSIF Atlas, the NYSMSC database collection system is based on registry questionnaires and follow-up forms acquired at participating MS centers. In 1996, the North-American Consortium of MS Centers initiated the NARCOMS (North American Research Committee on Multiple Sclerosis) MS Patient Registry as a long-term project to promote and facilitate clinical and epidemiological research in MS. NARCOMS is a patient-driven, self-reported database with information collected semi-annually. Between 1996 and 2004, more than 28,000 participants were registered (Flachenecker and Stuke, 2008).

Resource utilization studies have examined the costs incurred by a diagnosis of MS, which is a topic of considerable importance to individual patients as well as the health-care delivery system in light of the annual expense of the disease-modifying agents. Kobelt and colleagues estimated the average total cost per American MS patient at $47,000 per year in 2006, an increase of $12,000 since 1995 (Kobelt et al., 2006). These numbers include direct costs such as medication and hospitalization, as well as indirect costs such as reduced working time and income or early retirement. Notably, the costs per person correlate very significantly with the number of relapses and stage of disability. Another study (O´Brien et al., 2003) determined the direct medical cost of managing MS relapses in the United States, including the costs of hospitalization, ER, and physician office visits. The authors found that the majority of costs were attributable to hospital stays and concluded that the care of relapsing MS patients should be provided in the patients' homes as much as possible, while at the same time treatments that reduce the relapse frequency and thus the rate of hospital admissions may decrease patients' total financial burden.

Conclusions

The philosophy of early therapeutic intervention has begun to alter the natural course of MS, allowing patients to remain optimistic and play an active part in their disease management. Clinical trials for MS have been forever changed by the rapid development of disease-modifying agents, which raises both practical and ethical issues for the study of future agents targeted at the same outcomes. Clinical research has thus evolved to include both new agents and new outcome measures, including those that capture the impact of the disease in a patient-specific way not encapsulated by the standard neurologic exam–based metrics and arbitrary relapse definitions. As our current therapies do not result in an elimination of relapses or halt the accrual of disability, it is essential for a clinician to be aware of the widespread psychosocial impact of MS in terms of their patients' social involvement, partnership, family roles, and employment. The development of new effective agents for MS will require both a better biologic understanding of the disease's pathophysiology, likely with a focus on biomarkers, and the study of neuroprotection, as well as close attention to the risk/benefit profile of new agents based on an increasingly patient-centric approach. In the treatment era, there is an ongoing need for this work to broaden the perspective of neurologists and MS specialists on improving the care for patients with MS.

REFERENCES

Achiron A, Fredrikson S. Lessons from randomised direct comparative trials. *J Neurol Sci*. 2009;277(suppl 1): S19–S24.

Amato MP, Portaccio E. Clinical outcome measures in multiple sclerosis. *J Neurol Sci*. 2007;259(1-2):118–122.

Aronson KJ. Quality of life among persons with multiple sclerosis and their caregivers. *Neurology.* 1997;48: 74–80.

Beck RW, Trobe JD. The Optic Neuritis Treatment Trial. Putting the results in perspective. The Optic Neuritis Study Group. *J Neuroophthalmol.* 1995;15(3):131–135.

Birnbaum G, Cree B, Altafullah I, Zinser M, Reder AT. Combining beta interferon and atorvastatin may increase disease activity in multiple sclerosis. *Neurology.* 2008;71(18):1390–1395.

Bombardier CH, Cunniffe M, Wadhwani R, et al. Counseling for Health Promotion in People With Multiple Sclerosis: A Randomized Controlled Trial. *Arch Phys Med Rehabil.* 2008; 89 (10):1849–1856.

Coles AJ, Compston DA, Selmaj KW, et al. for the CAMMS223 Trial Investigators. Alemtuzumab vs. interferon beta-1a in early multiple sclerosis. *N Engl J Med.* 2008;359(17):1786–1801.

Comi G, Filippi M, Barkhof F, et al. Early treatment of Multiple Sclerosis Study Group. Effect of early interferon treatment on conversion to definite multiple sclerosis: a randomised study. *Lancet.* 2001;357(9268): 1576–1582.

Confavreux C, Vukusic S, Moreau T, Adeleine P. Relapses and progression of disability in multiple sclerosis. *N Engl J Med.* 2000;343(20):1430–1438.

D'Souza M, Kappos L, Czaplinski A. Reconsidering clinical outcomes in Multiple Sclerosis: relapses, impairment, disability and beyond. *J Neurol Sci.* 2008; 274(1-2):76–79.

Durelli L, Verdun E, Barbero P, et al. Independent comparison of Interferon (INCOMIN) Trial Study Group. Every-other-day interferon beta-1b versus once-weekly interferon beta- 1a for multiple sclerosis: results of a 2-year prospective randomised multicentre study (INCOMIN). *Lancet.* 2002;359.9316:1453–1460.

Ebers GC, Reder AT, Traboulsee A, et al., Investigators of the 16-Year Long-Term Follow-Up Study. Long-term follow-up of the original interferon-beta1b trial in multiple sclerosis: design and lessons from a 16-year observational study. *Clin Ther.* 2009 Aug;31(8):1724–1736.

Ennis M, Thain J, Boggild M, Baker GA, Young CA. A randomized controlled trial of a health promotion education programme for people with multiple sclerosis. *Clin Rehabil.* 2006;20(9):783–792.

Flachenecker P, Stuke K. National MS registries. *J Neurol.* 2008;255(suppl 6):102–108.

Goodin DS, Cohen BA, O'Connor P, Kappos L, Stevens JC, Therapeutics and Technology Assessment Subcommittee of the American Academy of Neurology. Assessment: the use of natalizumab (Tysabri) for the treatment of multiple sclerosis (an evidence-based review): report of the Therapeutics and Technology Assessment Subcommittee of the American Academy of Neurology. *Neurology.* 2008;71(10):766–773.

IFNB Multiple Sclerosis Study Group. Interferon beta-1b is effective in relapsing-remitting multiple sclerosis. Clinical results of a multicenter, randomized, double-blind, placebo-controlled trial. *Neurology.* 1993;43(4): 655–661.

Jackson MF, Quaal C, Reeves MA. Effects of multiple sclerosis on occupational and career patterns. *Axone.* 1991;13:16–17, 20–22.

Jacobs LD, Beck RW, Simon JH, et al. Intramuscular interferon beta-1a therapy initiated during a first demyelinating event in multiple sclerosis. CHAMPS Study Group. *N Engl J Med.* 2000;343(13):898–904.

Jacobs LD, Cookfair DL, Rudick RA, et al. Intramuscular interferon beta-1a for disease progression in relapsing multiple sclerosis. The Multiple Sclerosis Collaborative Research Group (MSCRG). *Ann Neurol.* 1996;39(3): 285–294.

Johnson K, Amtmann D, Yorkston K, Klasner ER, Kuehn CM. Medical, psychological, social and programmatic barriers to employment for people with multiple sclerosis. *J Rehabil.* 2004;70:38–50.

Johnson KP, Brooks BR, Cohen JA, et al. Copolymer 1 reduces relapse rate and improves disability in relapsing-remitting multiple sclerosis: results of a phase III multicenter, double-blind placebo-controlled trial. The Copolymer 1 Multiple Sclerosis Study Group. *Neurology.* 1995;45(7):1268–1276.

Kapoor R. Neuroprotection in multiple sclerosis: therapeutic strategies and clinical trial design. *Curr Opin Neurol.* 2006;19(3):255–259.

Kappos L, Freedman MS, Polman CH, et al. Effect of early versus delayed interferon beta-1b treatment on disability after a first clinical event suggestive of multiple sclerosis: a 3-year follow-up analysis of the BENEFIT study. *Lancet.* 2007;370(9585):389–397.

Kappos L, Polman CH, Freedman MS, et al. Treatment with interferon beta-1b delays conversion to clinically definite and McDonald MS in patients with clinically isolated syndromes. *Neurology.* 2006;67(7):1242–1249.

Khan F, Ng L, Turner-Stokes L. Effectiveness of vocational rehabilitation intervention on the return to work and employment of persons with multiple sclerosis. *Cochrane DB Sys Rev.* 2009;1:CD007256.

Kieseier BC, Wiendl H, Hemmer B, Hartung HP. Treatment and treatment trials in multiple sclerosis. *Curr Opin Neurol.* 2007;20(3):286–293.

Kleinschnitz C, Meuth SG, Wiendl H. The trials and errors in MS therapy. *Int MS J.* 2008;15(3):79–90.

Kobelt G, Berg J, Lindgren P, Jönsson B. Costs and quality of life in multiple sclerosis in Europe: method of assessment and analysis. *Eur J Health Econ.* 2006; 7(suppl 2):S5–S13.

Kornblith AB, LaRocca NG, Baum HM. Employment in individuals with multiple sclerosis. *Int J Rehabil Res.* 1986;9:155–165.

LaRocca NG, Kalb RC, Gregg K. A program to facilitate retention of employment among persons with multiple sclerosis. *Work.* 1996;7:37–46.

Leypoldt F, Münchau A, Moeller F, Bester M, Gerloff C, Heesen C. Hemorrhaging focal encephalitis under fingolimod (FTY720) treatment: a case report. *Neurology.* 2009;72(11):1022–1024.

Lublin F. Multiple sclerosis trial designs for the 21st century: building on recent lessons. *J Neurol.* 2005;252: V46–V53.

Lublin FD, Baier M, Cutter G. Effect of relapses on development of residual deficit in multiple sclerosis. *Neurology*. 2003;61(11):1528–1532.

Martinelli Boneschi F, Rovaris M, Capra R, Comi G. Mitoxantrone for multiple sclerosis. *Cochrane DB Sys Rev*. 2005;4:CD002127.

McDonald WI, Compston A, Edan G, et al. Recommended diagnostic criteria for multiple sclerosis: guidelines from the International Panel on the diagnosis of multiple sclerosis. *Ann Neurol*. 2001;50(1):121–127.

McFarland HF. Alemtuzumab versus interferon beta-1a: implications for pathology and trial design. *Lancet Neurol*. 2009;8(1):26–28.

McFarland HF, Reingold SC. The future of multiple sclerosis therapies: redesigning multiple sclerosis clinical trials in a new therapeutic era. *Mult Scler*. 2005; 11(6):669–676.

Mikol DD, Barkhof F, Chang P, et al. Comparison of subcutaneous interferon beta-1a with glatiramer acetate in patients with relapsing multiple sclerosis (the REbif vs Glatiramer Acetate in Relapsing MS Disease [REGARD] study): a multicentre, randomised, parallel, open-label trial. *Lancet Neurol*. 2008;7(10):903–914.

Miller AE. Ethical considerations in multiple sclerosis clinical trials. In: Cohen JA, Rudick RA, eds. *Multiple Sclerosis Therapeutics*. 3rd ed. Boca Raton, FL: CRC Press; 2007: 343–356.

Noseworthy JH. The challenge of long-term studies in multiple sclerosis: use of pooled data, historical controls, and observational studies to determine efficacy. In: Cohen JA, Rudick RA, eds. *Multiple Sclerosis Therapeutics*. 3rd ed. Boca Raton, FL: CRC Press; 2007: 319–330.

Noseworthy JH, Miller D, Compston A. Disease modifying treatments in multiple sclerosis. In: Compston A, McDonald IR, Noseworthy J, Lassmann H, eds. *McAlpine's Multiple Sclerosis*. London: Churchill Livingstone Elsevier; 2006: 729–802.

O'Brien JA, Ward AJ, Patrick AR, Caro J. Cost of managing an episode of relapse in multiple sclerosis in the United States. *BMC Health Serv Res*. 2003;3(1):17.

Panitch H, Goodin DS, Francis G, et al. Evidence of interferon dose-response: European North American Comparative Efficacy; University of British Columbia MS/MRI Research Group. Randomized, comparative study of interferon beta-1a treatment regimens in MS - The EVIDENCE trial. *Neurology*. 2002;59(10):1496–1506.

Panitch H, Miller A, Paty D, Weinshenker B, North American Study Group on Interferon beta-1b in Secondary Progressive MS. Interferon beta-1b in secondary progressive MS: results from a 3-year controlled study. *Neurology*. 2004;63(10):1788–1795.

Polman CH, O'Connor PW, Havrdova E, et al. A randomized, placebo-controlled trial of natalizumab for relapsing multiple sclerosis. *N Engl J Med*. 2006;354(9): 899–910.

Polman CH, Reingold SC, Barkhof F, et al. Ethics of placebo-controlled clinical trials in multiple sclerosis: a reassessment. *Neurology*. 2008;70(13 pt 2):1134–1140.

Polman CH, Reingold SC, Edan G, et al. Diagnostic criteria for multiple sclerosis: 2005 revisions to the "McDonald Criteria". *Ann Neurol*. 2005;58(6):840–846.

Rovaris M, Comi G, Rocca MA, et al. Long-term follow-up of patients treated with glatiramer acetate: a multicentre, multinational extension of the European/Canadian double-blind, placebo-controlled, MRI-monitored trial. *Mult Scler*. 2007;13(4):502–508.

Rudick RA, Stuart WH, Calabresi PA, et al. Natalizumab plus interferon beta-1a for relapsing multiple sclerosis. *N Engl J Med*. 2006;354(9):911–923.

Rumrill PD, Roessler RT, Cook BG. Improving career re-entry outcomes for people with multiple sclerosis: a comparison of two approaches. *J Voc Rehabil*. 1998; 10(3):241–252.

Runmarker B, Andersen O. Prognostic factors in a multiple sclerosis incidence cohort with twenty-five years of follow-up. *Brain*. 1993;116(pt 1):117–134.

Sørensen PS. REGARD: what can we learn from randomised, open-label, head-to-head studies? *Lancet Neurol*. 2008; 7(10):864–866.

Storr LK, Sørensen PS, Ravnborg M. The efficacy of multidisciplinary rehabilitation in stable multiple sclerosis patients. *Mult Scler*. 2006;12(2):235–242.

Walton MK. Selection and interpretation of end-points in multiple sclerosis clinical trials. In: Cohen JA, Rudick RA, eds. *Multiple Sclerosis Therapeutics*. 3rd ed. Boca Raton, FL: CRC Press; 2007: 295–308.

Weinshenker BG, Rice GP, Noseworthy JH, Carriere W, Baskerville J, Ebers GC. The natural history of multiple sclerosis: a geographically based study. 3. Multivariate analysis of predictive factors and models of outcome. *Brain*. 1991;114(pt 2):1045–1056.

Whetten-Goldstein K, Sloan FA, Goldstein LB, Kulas ED. A comprehensive assessment of the cost of multiple sclerosis in the United States. *Mult Scler*. 1998; 4(5):419–425.

Wilson SH, Walker GM. Unemployment and health: a review. *Pub Health*. 1993;107(3):153–162.

Basic Science in Multiple Sclerosis Research: Progress and Promise

Wendy Gilmore and Leslie P. Weiner

This chapter provides an overview of basic science research in multiple sclerosis (MS), with a focus on features of neurobiology, immunology, genetics, environmental factors, and gender associated with this highly complex neurological disease. To set the stage, we will first highlight characteristics of disease that inform and challenge our understanding of MS pathogenesis and our ability to achieve the overall goals of basic research, which are to develop new insights into the causes, triggers, and mechanisms of disease activity in MS and to translate them into strategies to prevent, treat, and ultimately cure this enigmatic disease. A condensed perspective of MS pathogenesis will then be offered, accompanied by a discussion of several directions in ongoing research.

There have been many excellent review articles that provide thorough descriptions of MS pathogenesis and insightful discussions of key questions in MS research, especially in recent years. A partial list is included in the reference section (Trapp, 2004; Hafler et al., 2005; Dhib-Jalbut et al., 2006; Frohman et al., 2006; Gold et al., 2006; Hauser and Oksenberg, 2006; Hemmer et al., 2006; Dutta and Trapp, 2007; Lassmann et al., 2007; Hauser, 2008; Trapp and Nave, 2008; Bennett and Stuve, 2009; Weiner, 2009), as well as throughout the text as appropriate to specific subjects. In addition, many of the chapters in this book provide an important source of more detailed information concerning specific basic and clinical research topics in MS, such as neuropathology, immunology, genetics, epidemiology, and the influences of gender. However, the reader is encouraged to conduct searches on his or her own and to read original source publications for additional information.

PROGRESS AND CHALLENGES INHERENT IN MULTIPLE SCLEROSIS RESEARCH

Multiple sclerosis is generally described as an autoimmune demyelinating disease of the central nervous system (CNS) in which an abnormal immune response against central myelin is triggered by an environmental factor, perhaps an infectious agent, in genetically susceptible individuals. More recently, strong evidence has emerged to indicate that tissue damage is not restricted to inflammation and demyelination but also involves axonal damage, axonal loss, neuron loss, and CNS atrophy (Trapp et al., 1998; Bjartmar et al., 2003; Trapp, 2004; Hauser and Oksenberg, 2006; Pirko et al., 2007; Bennett and Stuve, 2009; Wegner and Stadelmann, 2009). This has prompted re-evaluation of MS as a neurodegenerative disease, informed in part by insights gained from the study of classical neurodegenerative diseases, such as Alzheimer disease and Parkinson disease. Such descriptions speak to the complex nature of MS and justify the fact that basic science in MS research involves investigations in fields as broad as neurobiology, immunology, autoimmunity, genetics, epigenetics and molecular biology, developmental biology, microbiology, virology, environmental biology and epidemiology, and numerous subspecialties within them.

The complexity in MS is especially evident in the heterogeneity and variability inherent in clinical and pathological characteristics of disease (Lucchinetti et al., 2000; Confavreux et al., 2003; Hauser and Oksenberg, 2006; Confavreux and Vukusic, 2006, 2008; Weiner, 2009). Several distinct, but overlapping clinical subtypes are recognized, including relapsing-remitting MS (RRMS), secondary progressive MS (SPMS), and primary progressive MS (PPMS), but an early stage of disease, referred to as clinically isolated syndrome (CIS), and benign or fulminant forms of MS also occur. Approximately 85% of MS patients present with RRMS, characterized by attacks of neurological dysfunction (relapses) followed by periods of remission. Relapsing-remitting MS (RRMS) is more common in women, with at least a 2:1 female to male ratio, and is generally diagnosed in young adulthood. Relapses represent development of new inflammatory lesions dominated by a variable mixture of T cells, B cells, macrophages, and their pro-inflammatory products, though inflammatory lesions can also occur in the absence of obvious clinical signs or disability. A large percentage of patients with RRMS will develop SPMS, though the time to "conversion" to this clinical subtype is variable and difficult to predict. Fifteen percent of MS patients present with PPMS, in which disability accumulates rapidly from onset. Primary progressive MS (PPMS) tends to occur in older individuals, without a female prevalence. However, most patients with active MS of any form will show some degree of clinical progression over time, confirming the presence of a persistent, insidious disease process. In addition, although inflammation is a consistent finding in all forms of MS, it is not clearly linked to neurological deficits and disability observed in PPMS and SPMS. Instead, cumulative neurological disability in progressive MS, including cognitive deficits, correlate with axonal dysfunction and loss, neuron loss, and atrophy. In addition, perivascular lesions in late stages of MS lack a dominant lymphocyte infiltrate, but they retain activated microglia, macrophages, and astrocytes, suggesting a different role for inflammation in disease progression. Moreover, findings in the last decade, primarily from imaging and neuropathology, indicate that neurodegenerative changes are not limited to progressive forms of MS but also occur early in the disease course, even in RRMS. The picture is further complicated by evidence from longitudinal magnetic resonance imaging (MRI) studies that inflammatory lesions in normal-appearing white matter appear and regress throughout the course of RRMS disease, and that most lesions, referred to as "pre-active" lesions, do not develop into classical, clinically significant demyelinating lesions

(van der Valk and Amor, 2009). These findings indicate that some form of intrinsic mechanism exists to "select" lesions for further development or to regulate their progression into more advanced pathological stages. Intrinsic regulation may reflect a genetically determined, endogenous capacity to repair or remyelinate early lesions or to control various features of autoimmunity or inflammation. Indeed, remyelination is observed at all stages of MS, and it may be extensive in subsets of MS patients, occurring side by side with demyelination (Prineas and Connell, 1979; Raine and Wu, 1993; Bruck et al., 2003; Patrikios et al., 2006; Albert et al., 2007; Patani et al., 2007). Ultimately, however, it is destined to fail in the majority of patients (Franklin, 2002; Bruck et al., 2003; Piaton et al., 2009), and progression ensues.

Research efforts are also challenged by limited access to CNS tissue for the study of pathological features of MS, and by the fact that histopathological studies represent a snapshot of disease at a single point in time, rather than the dynamic changes that occur in disease pathogenesis over time. Thus, it has been difficult to establish a clear understanding of the relative contribution of white or gray matter demyelination and atrophy, axonal damage, axonal loss, and specific types of inflammation to clinical disease subtypes or activity over time.

Adding to the complexity, MS exhibits many features of autoimmune diseases (Whitaker and Snyder, 1984; De Keyser, 1988; Hohlfeld et al., 1995; Hafler et al., 2005; Hemmer et al., 2006; Lassmann, 2006; Lassmann et al., 2007; McFarland and Martin, 2007), including an overall female prevalence, presence of persistent inflammation in the target tissue (i.e., the CNS), evidence of clonal expansion of myelin-specific pro-inflammatory T and B cells in the CNS, cerebrospinal fluid (CSF) or peripheral blood, and association with human leukocyte antigen (HLA) and other immune response genes. As is the case for autoimmune diseases in general, immune regulatory mechanisms are impaired in MS (Antel and Owens, 2004; Viglietta et al., 2004; Haas et al., 2005; Astier et al., 2006; Venken et al., 2008; Fletcher et al., 2009), resulting in lack of tolerance for self-antigens including myelin proteins or peptides, and perhaps other CNS antigens. This shifts the balance in the peripheral immune system toward myelin-specific pro-inflammatory immune cells capable of gaining entry to the CNS and initiating or promoting a cascade of deleterious inflammatory processes. However, the precise nature of the dysfunction in immune regulation is not clear, and to date, no single myelin protein or peptide has been convincingly identified as the quintessential target antigen of autoreactivity in MS. Moreover, the relative contribution of pathogenic effector T cell subsets, B cells, plasma cells, natural killer cells and other leukocyte populations to clinical subtypes and pathological features of MS is not understood.

The complexity inherent in MS is also reflected in studies of genetic factors (Oksenberg and Hauser, 2005; Hauser and Oksenberg, 2006; Sadovnick, 2006; Ramagopalan et al., 2007; Oksenberg et al., 2008). Although it has been well documented that MS aggregates in families and varies with ethnicity, there is no clear pattern of inheritance, and the "MS-prone genotype" most likely consists of modest contributions, by multiple polymorphic genes, to the risk of developing MS. Genes associated with MS susceptibility appear to interact with environmental factors, such as infectious pathogens (primarily viruses), sunlight, vitamin D, toxins and others (Kalman et al., 2002; Ebers et al., 2004; Herrera et al., 2007; Lincoln and Cook, 2009; Ramagopalan et al., 2009b), and gender (Ramagopalan et al., 2009a; Sadovnick, 2009) to trigger or modify clinical and pathological disease activity.

Environmental influences on MS have been long recognized in the form of distinct clusters, or outbreaks of disease, in migration studies that support the concept of critical periods for exposure to environmental factors, and in the influence of latitude on MS susceptibility (Hauser and Oksenberg, 2006; Ascherio and Munger, 2007a, 2007b, 2008; Kampman and Brustad, 2008; Dickinson et al., 2009; Lincoln and Cook, 2009). A large number of environmental factors have been implicated, including infectious pathogens (viruses and bacteria), exposure to sunlight, dietary factors, toxins, and more. The strongest evidence supports a role for Epstein-Barr virus (EBV) (Ohga et al., 2002; Ascherio, 2008; Bagert, 2009; Lunemann and Munz, 2009), which causes infectious mononucleosis and a variety of other disease entities. Individuals who develop infectious mononucleosis

in childhood are significantly more likely to develop MS than individuals exposed to EBV but who have not developed infectious mononucleosis. The underlying mechanisms of EBV-associated risk for developing MS have yet to be identified. Exposure to sunlight may contribute to MS susceptibility (Islam et al., 2007; Hayes et al., 2008) via its ability to stimulate synthesis of vitamin D following activation of the vitamin D receptor, a member of the nuclear receptor superfamily that includes peroxisome proliferator-activated receptors and corticosteroid, sex steroid, and thyroid hormone receptors. All act as anti-inflammatory transcription factors and may function in synergy to influence MS risk or disease activities. Circulating vitamin D levels have been reported to be reduced in patients with MS (Munger et al., 2006), but it is not clear what constitutes concentrations sufficient to provide some measure of protection against disease activity.

Sex differences in MS provide an additional layer of complexity to disease pathogenesis in MS and may interact with both genes and environmental factors to modify the risk for developing MS (Eikelenboom et al., 2009; Sadovnick, 2009). New evidence indicates that the increase in MS incidence that has occurred over the last half-century in Canada is primarily due to an increase in women, and it implicates an association with environmental factors (Orton et al., 2006; Ramagopalan et al., 2009a). Similar findings have been published for other regions of the world (Pugliatti et al., 2009). However, the influence of sex differences is not limited to modification of risk for developing MS but also involves poorly understood effects on disease phenotypes and activities. For example, there is evidence that men with MS progress more rapidly than women, and that disease activity and underlying pathological processes are affected by hormones and reproductive states, such as puberty (Ramagopalan et al., 2009b) and pregnancy (Damek and Shuster, 1997; Confavreux et al., 1998).

Currently approved disease-modifying treatments, such as the beta-interferons (Avonex, Betaseron, and Rebif) and glatiramer acetate (Copaxone) have significantly improved management of RRMS, acting to suppress general inflammatory mechanisms, reduce overall relapse rates, and inhibit new inflammatory lesions detected by MRI

(Martin et al., 2001; Goodin, 2005, 2008; Kieseier et al., 2009). Unfortunately, clinical efficacy has stalled at approximately 35%–40%, and many patients are treatment nonresponders for reasons that are unclear. In addition, progressive MS is notoriously resistant to immunosuppressive treatment strategies. Although disease-modifying drugs may act indirectly as neuroprotective agents via anti-inflammatory properties, none appear to be capable of promoting remyelination and repair. There is a great need for new insights into disease mechanisms that will lend themselves to the development of new and more effective strategies to promote a healthy balance between autoreactive and regulatory immune mechanisms; limit inflammation; prevent axonal damage, neuron loss, and disease progression; and promote remyelination and repair.

It is important to note that the cause of MS is unknown, and it is not clear when the disease process starts. It only becomes apparent when it generates symptoms that prompt an individual to seek medical attention. Since MS is increasingly recognized to occur in children (Yeh et al., 2009), it is possible that the disease process is triggered earlier than the average age of diagnosis in young adulthood.

In summary, MS presents many challenges to basic research, including a high degree of complexity, heterogeneity, and variability in multiple features of the disease, from the influence of genes, environment, and gender to clinical and pathological disease activities and endogenous repair capacity. Despite these challenges, the progress that has been made in our understanding of MS, especially in the last 15–20 years, serves as an excellent platform for posing specific research questions and designing experiments to answer them.

TOOLS FOR BASIC RESEARCH

A discussion of basic research in MS would not be complete without mention of the tools available for use. Briefly, they include advanced neuroimaging techniques; high-resolution histopathological and microscopic methods; conventional and high-throughput genetic screening and molecular techniques; sophisticated flow cytometry techniques to evaluate cell surface and functional phenotypes

of immune and neural cell types; in vitro cell culture techniques to model functional interactions among and between immune and neural cells, including stem cells; sensitive assays for soluble factors such as cytokines, chemokines, growth factors, neurotranmsitters, and hormones; and animal models.

Innovations in the development of research tools are critical to meet the challenges inherent in MS research. For example, advances in MRI techniques and their use in longitudinal studies have contributed to the understanding that axonal and neuronal damage and loss correlate with irreversible neurological disability in MS (Fisher et al., 2007; Tomassini and Palace, 2009). Optical coherence tomography (OCT), a noninvasive rapid imaging technique, is currently under intense investigation as a tool to assess retinal nerve fiber layer thickness as a measure of neurodegeneration over time (Kallenbach and Frederiksen, 2007; Frohman et al., 2008). It is also possible to image inflammation in real time on a cellular level in MS patients with the use of radiolabeled positron emission tomography (PET) ligands specific for the peripheral benzodiazepine receptor, which is expressed on activated microglia, macrophages, and astrocytes (Banati et al., 2000; Raivich and Banati, 2004). As experience with neuroimaging techniques and protocols expands, there is promise that they will yield more specific information about the nature of CNS injury and a more precise understanding of the sequence of inflammatory and neurodegenerative events in MS pathogenesis, especially in combination with sophisticated histopathological approaches.

High-throughput experimental techniques, such as genomics and genetic screening, gene and protein expression arrays, pharmacogenomics, and flow cytometry facilitate comprehensive approaches to the study of MS in human subjects, as well as in relevant animal models. In addition, sophisticated data analysis tools, such as bioinformatics, statistics, data mining, and network analysis methods make it possible to combine multiple approaches to identify molecular signatures of disease activity, especially in combination with CNS imaging techniques and assays to assess changes in immune cell types and functions over time. These comprehensive approaches show promise for the development of biomarkers to track disease activity and response to treatment, as well as for the identification of new targets for future treatment strategies (Bielekova and Martin, 2004; O'Connor et al., 2006; Fossey et al., 2007; Harris and Sadiq, 2009; Sellebjerg et al., 2009).

Although no single animal model of MS faithfully reproduces pathological and clinical MS, most are useful for the study of specific features of MS (Fleming, 1985; Friese et al., 2006; Mix et al., 2008; Furlan et al., 2009; Lassmann, 2009). For example, the most commonly used animal model, collectively referred to as experimental autoimmune encephalomyelitis (EAE), is especially useful for studies of the autoimmune components of MS but also exhibits several features of demyelination and neurodegeneration that can be mined for pathogenic insights and testing of new treatment strategies (Steinman and Zamvil, 2006; Furlan et al., 2009). Experimental autoimmune encephalomyelitis (EAE) can be induced by immunization against myelin proteins such as myelin basic protein (MBP), proteolipid protein (PLP) or myelin oligodendrocyte glycoprotein (MOG), or by adoptive transfer of myelin-specific T cells to cause acute or chronic relapsing-remitting and progressive forms of inflammatory demyelinating disease. It is also useful for the study of mechanisms involved in inflammation of the CNS by immune cells from the periphery, that is, extrinsic inflammation. The cuprizone model of myelin injury is particularly useful for the study of the sequence of cellular and molecular interactions involved in demyelination and remyelination (Matsushima and Morell, 2001; Torkildsen et al., 2008). This information is essential to future studies designed to reveal mechanisms underlying demyelination and remyelination in MS. When added to the diet, cuprizone, a copper chelating agent, selectively kills myelin-producing oligodendrocytes, followed by a robust remyelination phase upon withdrawal from the diet. Since demyelination and remyelination occur in the relative absence of inflammation by T cells and B cells, this model facilitates a focus on intrinsic infiltration of demyelinating lesions by microglia and astrocytes, and extrinsic infiltration by peripheral macrophages. Additional animal models include virus-induced demyelinating diseases (e.g., Theiler murine encephalomyelitis virus and murine coronaviruses such as JHMV) (Drescher and Sosnowska,

2008; Hosking and Lane, 2009), myelin-deficient, dysmyelinating myelin mutant or transgenic mice (Lunn et al., 1995; Campagnoni and Skoff, 2001), and "humanized" mice, in which the mouse immune system is replaced with various cellular or molecular components of the human immune system to model specific features of CNS inflammation, immune regulation, demyelination, remyelination, and neurodegeneration in MS (Taneja and David, 1998; Kaushansky et al., 2009).

All of these research tools have strengths and limitations that should be carefully considered when applying them to MS as a disease entity, especially when evaluating new strategies for treatment.

MULTIPLE SCLEROSIS PATHOGENESIS: PERSPECTIVES, KEY QUESTIONS, AND PROMISE IN BASIC RESEARCH

Numerous models of MS pathogenesis have been offered over the years to illustrate what is known about MS and to frame questions for ongoing and future research efforts. It is useful to think of pathology and dysfunction in MS as occurring in two primary systems, the central nervous system, and the immune system, each subject to modifying influences of genetic factors, environmental factors, and factors associated with gender. Essential goals in basic MS research are to identify the sequence of events that leads to the formation of CNS lesions and onset of clinical disease, and to determine the relative contribution of immune and CNS dysfunction, genetic and environmental factors, and gender to disease susceptibility, expression of clinical disease subtypes, and disease outcomes. To accomplish these goals, currently active research efforts address a large variety of questions relevant to each topic. The following section will focus primarily on questions concerning CNS and immune dysfunction in MS.

Perhaps one of the most important questions in MS research is whether the primary injury arises in the CNS itself (i.e., an intrinsic defect in oligodendrocytes or structural or functional characteristics of myelin, resulting in myelin instability), followed by secondary damage induced by a misguided and poorly controlled immune response to CNS antigens in individuals who have inherited a genetic background of autoimmune susceptibility.

Since MS is most likely diagnosed long after the initial CNS injury, a definitive answer to this question may be difficult to achieve, especially with limited access to tissue at the early stages of disease.

Is there evidence of a structural or functional defect in myelin, oligodendrocytes, or oligodendrocyte precursor cells in MS? In general, the answer is "yes." Studies by Moscarello et al. suggest that the myelin obtained from MS patients may be less developmentally mature and more susceptible to degradation (Moscarello et al., 1994), primarily due to an increase in citrullinated myelin basic protein (MBP)(Moscarello et al., 1986), and perhaps other modifications of myelin proteins. The possibility that this could have consequences for a secondary immune response is indicated by the detection of enhanced T cell responses to citrulline-containing MPB in MS patients (Tranquill et al., 2000). In addition, Lund et al. (2006) have reported that MPB peptides isolated from normal-appearing white matter in MS brains associate with heat shock protein 70 (Hsp70) and significantly enhance in vitro proliferation in MBP-specific T cell lines. Although changes in myelin lipid composition and metabolism in normal-appearing white matter have also been observed (Wheeler et al., 2008; Podbielska and Hogan, 2009), it is not clear if they occur in the absence of active inflammation. Oligodendrocyte death may occur in early MS in the absence of inflammation (Barnett and Prineas, 2004), suggesting a primary insult to or intrinsic defect in oligodendrocytes, but the consistency of this finding has not yet been established. Longitudinal studies of individuals at risk for developing MS or with CIS, in combination with sensitive neuroimaging protocols, high-throughput molecular screening, and assessment of immune responses to lipid or altered protein components of myelin may provide some clues to the putative existence of intrinsic myelin/oligodendrocyte defects, capable of inducing secondary pathogenic immune responses in MS.

If intrinsic defects in myelin structure, stability, or function were to be identified, one can then ask whether they only become apparent upon exposure to one or more extrinsic challenges, imposed either by a direct insult to the CNS, such as by a neurotropic virus, or indirectly, by a misguided immune response to that insult. An affirmative answer to this question may explain findings that multiple environmental factors contribute to MS susceptibility, but none have emerged as a single determinant of disease susceptibility or as a cause of MS. It is also consistent with variability in the ability to mount healthy, adaptive responses to limit and repair CNS damage and regulate the misguided immune response. Finally, it may also explain observations that robust, myelin-specific, pro-inflammatory T cell responses exist in healthy individuals or individuals with other autoimmune diseases who show no evidence of MS or susceptibility to MS (Pelfrey et al., 2000; Sospedra and Martin, 2005).

In this scenario, the MS-susceptible CNS might be compared with a poorly built wood frame house that is susceptible to damage induced by multiple threats, such as termites, bad weather, daily wear and tear, and a myriad of other factors. In addition, if the homeowners cause damage themselves, or fail to maintain or repair the home due to lack of appropriate expertise or access to resources, damage accumulates over time until repair is no longer possible.

Intrinsic instability in myelin structure and function may also be evident in the cellular and molecular processes involved in myelin formation during critical postnatal developmental periods, and in myelin maintenance throughout life. Although very little is understood about these processes, there is interest in using new neuroimaging strategies (Miller et al., 2003; Hesseltine et al., 2006; Terajima et al., 2007; Fox, 2008), especially diffusion tensor imaging (DTI) protocols, to characterize normal and abnormal myelination patterns in white matter tracts in MS patients, healthy control subjects, and animal models (Budde et al., 2008; Baloch et al., 2009).

What is responsible for axonal damage and neuron death in MS? This is an area of intense investigation by multiple laboratories. Several possibilities exist, including myelin dysfunction prior to demyelination, exposure of axons to inflammatory damage following demyelination, glutamate excitotoxicity, and mitochondrial damage (Smith and Lassmann, 2002; Pitt et al., 2003; Hauser and Oksenberg, 2006; Mahad et al., 2008). A better understanding of the molecular mechanisms responsible for axonal dysfunction, axonal transection, and neuron death may lead to identification of new targets for neuro-protective treatment strategies.

What limits myelin repair in MS? As previously indicated, remyelination is a common occurrence in MS, but it eventually fails to keep up with cumulative damage. Damaged axons may not be able to provide appropriate signals to oligodendrocytes to stimulate myelin formation. Oligodendrocyte precursor cells may also be resistant to differentiation as a consequence of abnormal activation, or timing of activation, of key signaling or regulatory molecules, such as LINGO-1 and Notch1 (Miller and Mi, 2007; Zhang et al., 2009). More recently, data have been published to indicate abnormal activation of a developmental pathway, known as the "wnt" signaling pathway, in CNS tissue from MS patients (Fancy et al., 2009). Wnt signaling is an essential regulator of cell decisions to either maintain proliferative capacity, which is necessary to support a pool of pluripotent stem cells, or to differentiate, which is required for specialized cell functions, such as myelin formation by mature oligodendrocytes (McMillan and Kahn, 2005; Marson et al., 2008). Both are essential for normal repair processes. Strategies to correct abnormal wnt signaling, as well as additional signaling pathways, may lead to stimulation of endogenous myelin repair. In addition, oligodendrocytes or oligodendrocyte precursor cells may not be able to effect myelin repair in the pro-inflammatory environment in the CNS of MS patients. For this reason, stem cell transplantation and other strategies to induce endogenous repair may need to include treatment with anti-inflammatory agents.

What is the nature of immune dysfunction in MS? Information is emerging to implicate at least three "new" types of pro-inflammatory effector cell types in MS, including interleukin-17-producing CD4+ T cells Th17 cells (Hedegaard et al., 2008; Montes et al., 2009), myelin-specific CD8+ T cells (Jacobsen et al., 2002; Crawford et al., 2004; Friese and Fugger, 2005) and myelin glycolipid-specific NK T cells (Blewett, 2008). Th17 cells have been demonstrated to be primary effectors of autoimmunity in EAE (Aranami and Yamamura, 2008), but have only recently been isolated from MS patients. Moreover, oligoclonal Th17 cells were isolated from normal-appearing white matter from the brain of one MS patient, providing proof of concept that Th17 cells infiltrate the CNS

in MS (Montes et al., 2009). Of interest is that myelin-specific CD8+ T cells, which have been somewhat neglected in favor of CD4+ T cells in MS, show clear associations with axonal dysfunction (Skulina et al., 2004; McDole et al., 2006; Haegele et al., 2007; Friese and Fugger, 2009).

As previously indicated, immune regulatory mechanisms are defective in MS, contributing to the lack of a healthy balance between effector and regulatory lymphocytes in MS. At least three types of regulatory T cells (Tregs) have been examined: classical CD4+CD25^{hi}, foxP3+ Tregs (Viglietta et al., 2004; Haas et al., 2005), IL-10-producing CD46+ T cells (Astier et al., 2006), and CD39+ foxP3+ CD4+ Tregs (Fletcher et al., 2009). Our understanding of the cellular and molecular basis of regulatory dysfunction in MS depends upon further analysis of these, and additional regulatory cell subsets.

The effects of genes, environmental factors, and gender on CNS and immune dysfunction in MS are intense areas of ongoing investigation in patients and animal models. Data emerging from these efforts should help to define whether specific types of CNS damage and dysfunction, or key indicators of immune imbalance and autoimmunity segregate with ethnicity and/or gender, whether some environmental factors exert weak or strong influences on CNS and immune damage based on specific genotypes, and finally, whether specific hormones play protective or deleterious roles in MS susceptibility, disease activity, or clinical disease outcome.

CONCLUDING REMARKS

Basic science is generally defined as the study of a subject simply to yield knowledge and understanding, regardless of immediate practical application (Stevens, 2002). In this context, the quest for basic knowledge is generally motivated by curiosity, rather than the search for solutions to specific problems. However, in medicine, basic research is more like applied science; that is, it is conducted specifically to build the foundation of knowledge and understanding required for development of new conceptual and technical tools to diagnose, treat, prevent, and ultimately cure diseases. It is highly dependent upon a strong partnership between basic and physician scientists.

The effort to translate scientific discoveries into clinical applications, known as the bench-to-bedside approach, is a two-way street; it involves an exchange of tools and knowledge between basic and clinical scientists. Clinicians provide critical observations about disease activities to drive experimental approaches and discovery in the laboratory, while basic scientists provide insights into normal and pathological processes that can then be applied to disease management and treatment strategies. The importance of this partnership has been recognized in the form of funding opportunities for translational and interdisciplinary research, initiated by the National Institutes of Health (NIH), the Department of Defense (DOD), the National Multiple Sclerosis Society (NMSS), and many academic institutions. For example, the NIH Roadmap for Medical Research was launched in 2004 to establish a common fund to support innovative and interdisciplinary research programs to foster high-risk/high-reward research, to develop tools and methodologies to transform the way biomedical research is conducted, to fill fundamental gaps in our knowledge, and to encourage collaboration in academia (McLellan, 2003; NIH releases roadmap for medical research, 2004). Similarly, the NMSS has established flexible funding resources for collaborative research centers to combine laboratory and clinical studies between MS investigators and those from other fields and diseases.

This is an exciting time for research in MS, full of promise for significant advances in the understanding of MS pathogenesis and potential for treatment as interdisciplinary, collaborative partnerships mature and new data emerge.

ACKNOWLEDGMENTS

We wish to thank Drs. Luisa Raijman and Brett Lund for helpful discussions in the preparation of this chapter.

REFERENCES

Albert M, Antel J, Bruck W, Stadelmann C. Extensive cortical remyelination in patients with chronic multiple sclerosis. *Brain Pathol.* 2007;17(2):129–138.

Antel J, Owens T. Multiple sclerosis and immune regulatory cells. *Brain.* 2004;127(pt 9):1915–1916.

Aranami T, Yamamura T. Th17 cells and autoimmune encephalomyelitis (EAE/MS). *Allergol Int.* 2008;57(2): 115–120.

Ascherio A. Epstein-Barr virus in the development of multiple sclerosis. *Expert Rev Neurother.* 2008;8(3): 331–333.

Ascherio A, Munger K. Epidemiology of multiple sclerosis: from risk factors to prevention. *Semin Neurol.* 2008; 28(1):17–28.

Ascherio A, Munger KL. Environmental risk factors for multiple sclerosis. Part I: the role of infection. *Ann Neurol.* 2007a;61(4):288–299.

Ascherio A, Munger KL. Environmental risk factors for multiple sclerosis. Part II: noninfectious factors. *Ann Neurol.* 2007b;61(6):504–513.

Astier AL, Meiffren G, Freeman S, Hafler DA. Alterations in CD46-mediated Tr1 regulatory T cells in patients with multiple sclerosis. *J Clin Invest.* 2006;116(12):3252–3257.

Bagert BA. Epstein-Barr virus in multiple sclerosis. *Curr Neurol Neurosci Rep.* 2009;9(5):405–410.

Baloch S, Verma R, Huang H, et al. Quantification of brain maturation and growth patterns in C57BL/6J mice via computational neuroanatomy of diffusion tensor images. *Cereb Cortex.* 2009;19(3):675–687.

Banati RB, Newcombe J, Gunn RN, et al. The peripheral benzodiazepine binding site in the brain in multiple sclerosis: quantitative in vivo imaging of microglia as a measure of disease activity. *Brain.* 2000;123(pt 11):2321–2337.

Barnett MH, Prineas JW. Relapsing and remitting multiple sclerosis: pathology of the newly forming lesion. *Ann Neurol.* 2004;55(4):458–468.

Bennett JL, Stuve O. Update on inflammation, neurodegeneration, and immunoregulation in multiple sclerosis: therapeutic implications. *Clin Neuropharmacol.* 2009; 32(3):121–132.

Bielekova B, Martin R. Development of biomarkers in multiple sclerosis. *Brain.* 2004;127(pt 7):1463–1478.

Bjartmar C, Wujek JR, Trapp BD. Axonal loss in the pathology of MS: consequences for understanding the progressive phase of the disease. *J Neurol Sci.* 2003; 206(2):165–171.

Blewett MM. Hypothesized role of galactocerebroside and NKT cells in the etiology of multiple sclerosis. *Med Hypotheses.* 2008;70(4):826–830.

Bruck W, Kuhlmann T, Stadelmann C. Remyelination in multiple sclerosis. *J Neurol Sci.* 2003;206(2):181–185.

Budde MD, Kim JH, Liang HF, Russell JH, Cross AH, Song SK. Axonal injury detected by in vivo diffusion tensor imaging correlates with neurological disability in a mouse model of multiple sclerosis. *NMR Biomed.* 2008;21(6):589–597.

Campagnoni AT, Skoff RP. The pathobiology of myelin mutants reveal novel biological functions of the MBP and PLP genes. *Brain Pathol.* 2001;11(1):74–91.

Confavreux C, Hutchinson M, Hours MM, Cortinovis-Tourniaire P, Moreau T. Rate of pregnancy-related relapse in multiple sclerosis. Pregnancy in Multiple Sclerosis Group. *N Engl J Med.* 1998;339(5):285–291.

Confavreux C, Vukusic S. Accumulation of irreversible disability in multiple sclerosis: from epidemiology to treatment. *Clin Neurol Neurosurg.* 2006;108(3):327–332.

Confavreux C, Vukusic S. The clinical epidemiology of multiple sclerosis. *Neuroimaging Clin N Am.* 2008; 18(4):589–622, ix–x.

Confavreux C, Vukusic S, Adeleine P. Early clinical pre-
    dictors and progression of irreversible disability in
    multiple sclerosis: an amnesic process. *Brain*. 2003;
    126(pt 4):770–782.

Crawford MP, Yan SX, Ortega SB, et al. High prevalence
    of autoreactive, neuroantigen-specific CD8+ T cells in
    multiple sclerosis revealed by novel flow cytometric
    assay. *Blood*. 2004;103(11):4222–4231.

Damek DM, Shuster EA. Pregnancy and multiple sclerosis.
    Mayo Clin Proc. 1997;72(10):977–989.

De Keyser J. Autoimmunity in multiple sclerosis.
    Neurology. 1988;38(3):371–374.

Dhib-Jalbut S, Arnold DL, Cleveland DW, et al.
    Neurodegeneration and neuroprotection in multiple
    sclerosis and other neurodegenerative diseases. *J Neuro-
    immunol*. 2006;176(1–2):198–215.

Dickinson JL, Perera DI, van der Mei AF, et al. Past envi-
    ronmental sun exposure and risk of multiple sclerosis:
    a role for the Cdx-2 Vitamin D receptor variant in this
    interaction. *Mult Scler*. 2009;15(5):563–570.

Drescher KM, Sosnowska D. Being a mouse in a man's
    world: what TMEV has taught us about human disease.
    Front Biosci. 2008;13:3775–3785.

Dutta R, Trapp BD. Pathogenesis of axonal and neuronal
    damage in multiple sclerosis. *Neurology*. 2007;68
    (22 suppl 3):S22–S31, S43–S54.

Ebers GC, Sadovnick AD, Veith R. Vitamin D intake and
    incidence of multiple sclerosis. *Neurology*. 2004;
    63(5):939.

Eikelenboom MJ, Killestein J, Kragt JJ, Uitdehaag BM,
    Polman CH. Gender differences in multiple sclerosis:
    cytokines and vitamin D. *J Neurol Sci*. 2009;286(1–2):
    40–42.

Fancy SP, Baranzini SE, Zhao C, et al. Dysregulation
    of the Wnt pathway inhibits timely myelination and
    remyelination in the mammalian CNS. *Genes Dev*.
    2009;23(13):1571–1585.

Fisher E, Chang A, Fox RJ, et al. Imaging correlates of
    axonal swelling in chronic multiple sclerosis brains.
    Ann Neurol. 2007;62(3):219–228.

Fleming JO. Animal models of multiple sclerosis. *Mayo
    Clin Proc*. 1985;60(7):490–492.

Fletcher JM, Lonergan R, Costelloe L, et al. CD39+Foxp3+
    regulatory T Cells suppress pathogenic Th17 cells and
    are impaired in multiple sclerosis. *J Immunol*. 2009;
    183(11):7602–7610.

Fossey SC, Vnencak-Jones CL, Olsen NJ, et al.
    Identification of molecular biomarkers for multiple
    sclerosis. *J Mol Diagn*. 2007;9(2):197–204.

Fox RJ. Picturing multiple sclerosis: conventional and
    diffusion tensor imaging. *Semin Neurol*. 2008;28(4):
    453–466.

Franklin RJ. Why does remyelination fail in multiple scle-
    rosis? *Nat Rev Neurosci*. 2002;3(9):705–714.

Friese MA, Fugger L. Autoreactive CD8+ T cells in multi-
    ple sclerosis: a new target for therapy? *Brain*.
    2005;128(pt 8):1747–1763.

Friese MA, Fugger L. Pathogenic CD8(+) T cells in multi-
    ple sclerosis. *Ann Neurol*. 2009;66(2):132–141.

Friese MA, Montalban X, Willcox N, Bell JI, Martin R,
    Fugger L. The value of animal models for drug

development in multiple sclerosis. *Brain*. 2006;129
    (pt 8):1940–1952.

Frohman EM, Fujimoto JG, Frohman TC, Calabresi PA,
    Cutter G, Balcer LJ. Optical coherence tomography: a
    window into the mechanisms of multiple sclerosis.
    Nat Clin Pract Neurol. 2008;4(12):664–675.

Frohman EM, Racke MK, Raine CS. Multiple sclerosis:
    the plaque and its pathogenesis. *N Engl J Med*. 2006;
    354(9):942–955.

Furlan R, Cuomo C, Martino G. Animal models of multi-
    ple sclerosis. *Methods Mol Biol*. 2009;549:157–173.

Gold R, Linington C, Lassmann H. Understanding patho-
    genesis and therapy of multiple sclerosis via animal
    models: 70 years of merits and culprits in experimental
    autoimmune encephalomyelitis research. *Brain*. 2006;
    129(pt 8):1953–1971.

Goodin DS. Treatment of multiple sclerosis with human
    beta interferon. *Int MS J*. 2005;12(3):96–108.

Goodin DS. Disease-modifying therapy in multiple scle-
    rosis: update and clinical implications. *Neurology*.
    2008;71(24 suppl 3):S8–S13.

Haas J, Hug A, Viehover A, et al. Reduced suppressive
    effect of CD4+CD25high regulatory T cells on the
    T cell immune response against myelin oligodendro-
    cyte glycoprotein in patients with multiple sclerosis.
    Eur J Immunol. 2005;35(11):3343–3352.

Haegele KF, Stueckle CA, Malin JP, Sindern E. Increase
    of CD8+ T-effector memory cells in peripheral blood
    of patients with relapsing-remitting multiple sclerosis
    compared to healthy controls. *J Neuroimmunol*. 2007;
    183(1–2):168–174.

Hafler DA, Slavik JM, Anderson DE, O'Connor KC, De
    Jager P, Baecher-Allan C. Multiple sclerosis. *Immunol
    Rev*. 2005;204:208–231.

Harris VK, Sadiq SA. Disease biomarkers in multiple
    sclerosis: potential for use in therapeutic decision
    making. *Mol Diagn Ther*. 2009;13(4):225–244.

Hauser SL. Multiple lessons for multiple sclerosis. *N Engl
    J Med*. 2008;359(17):1838–1841.

Hauser SL, Oksenberg JR. The neurobiology of multiple
    sclerosis: genes, inflammation, and neurodegeneration.
    Neuron. 2006;52(1):61–76.

Hayes CE, Donald Acheson E. A unifying multiple sclerosis
    etiology linking virus infection, sunlight, and vitamin D,
    through viral interleukin-10. *Med Hypotheses*. 2008;
    71(1):85–90.

Hedegaard CJ, Krakauer M, Bendtzen K, Lund H,
    Sellebjerg F, Nielsen CH. T helper cell type 1 (Th1):
    Th2 and Th17 responses to myelin basic protein and
    disease activity in multiple sclerosis. *Immunology*.
    2008;125(2):161–169.

Hemmer B, Nessler S, Zhou D, Kieseier B, Hartung HP.
    Immunopathogenesis and immunotherapy of multi-
    ple sclerosis. *Nat Clin Pract Neurol*. 2006;2(4):
    201–211.

Herrera BM, Cader MZ, Dyment DA, et al. Multiple scle-
    rosis susceptibility and the X chromosome. *Mult Scler*.
    2007;13(7):856–864.

Hesseltine SM, Law M, Babb J, et al. Diffusion tensor
    imaging in multiple sclerosis: assessment of regional
    differences in the axial plane within normal-appearing

cervical spinal cord. *AJNR Am J Neuroradiol.* 2006; 27(6):1189–1193.

Hohlfeld R, Londei M, Massacesi L, Salvetti M. T-cell autoimmunity in multiple sclerosis. *Immunol Today.* 1995;16(6):259–261.

Hosking MP, Lane TE. The biology of persistent infection: inflammation and demyelination following murine coronavirus infection of the central nervous system. *Curr Immunol Rev.* 2009;5(4):267–276.

Islam T, Gauderman WJ, Cozen W, Mack TM. Childhood sun exposure influences risk of multiple sclerosis in monozygotic twins. *Neurology.* 2007;69(4): 381–388.

Jacobsen M, Cepok S, Quak E, et al. Oligoclonal expansion of memory CD8+ T cells in cerebrospinal fluid from multiple sclerosis patients. *Brain.* 2002;125(pt 3): 538–550.

Kallenbach K, Frederiksen J. Optical coherence tomography in optic neuritis and multiple sclerosis: a review. *Eur J Neurol.* 2007;14(8):841–849.

Kalman B, Albert RH, Leist TP. Genetics of multiple sclerosis: determinants of autoimmunity and neurodegeneration. *Autoimmunity.* 2002;35(4):225–234.

Kampman MT, Brustad M. Vitamin D: a candidate for the environmental effect in multiple sclerosis - observations from Norway. *Neuroepidemiology.* 2008; 30(3):140–146.

Kaushansky N, Altmann DM, Ascough S, David CS, Lassmann H, Ben-Nun A. HLA-DQB1*0602 determines disease susceptibility in a new "humanized" multiple sclerosis model in HLA-DR15 (DRB1*1501; DQB1*0602) transgenic mice. *J Immunol.* 2009; 183(5):3531–3541.

Kieseier BC, Wiendl H, Hartung HP, Stuve O. The future of multiple sclerosis therapy. *Pharmacol Res.* 2009; 60(4):207–211.

Lassmann H. Genetic predisposition for autoimmunity in multiple sclerosis? *Lancet Neurol.* 2006;5(11): 897–898.

Lassmann H. Axonal and neuronal pathology in multiple sclerosis: what have we learnt from animal models. *Exp Neurol.* 2009 October 17; Epub ahead of print.

Lassmann H, Bruck W, Lucchinetti CF. The immunopathology of multiple sclerosis: an overview. *Brain Pathol.* 2007;17(2):210–218.

Lincoln JA, Cook SD. An overview of gene-epigenetic-environmental contributions to MS causation. *J Neurol Sci.* 2009;286(1–2):54–57.

Lucchinetti C, Bruck W, Parisi J, Scheithauer B, Rodriguez M, Lassmann H. Heterogeneity of multiple sclerosis lesions: implications for the pathogenesis of demyelination. *Ann Neurol.* 2000;47(6):707–717.

Lund BT, Chakryan Y, Ashikian N, et al. Association of MBP peptides with Hsp70 in normal appearing human white matter. *J Neurol Sci.* 2006;249(2):122–134.

Lunemann JD, Munz C. EBV in MS: guilty by association? *Trends Immunol.* 2009;30(6):243–248.

Lunn KF, Fanarraga ML, Duncan ID. Myelin mutants: new models and new observations. *Microsc Res Tech.* 1995;32(3):183–203.

Mahad D, Lassmann H, Turnbull D. Review: mitochondria and disease progression in multiple sclerosis. *Neuropathol Appl Neurobiol.* 2008;34(6):577–589.

Marson A, Foreman R, Chevalier B, et al. Wnt signaling promotes reprogramming of somatic cells to pluripotency. *Cell Stem Cell.* 2008;3(2):132–135.

Martin R, Sturzebecher CS, McFarland HF. Immunotherapy of multiple sclerosis: where are we? Where should we go? *Nat Immunol.* 2001;2(9):785–788.

Matsushima GK, Morell P. The neurotoxicant, cuprizone, as a model to study demyelination and remyelination in the central nervous system. *Brain Pathol.* 2001; 11(1):107–116.

McDole J, Johnson AJ, Pirko I. The role of CD8+ T-cells in lesion formation and axonal dysfunction in multiple sclerosis. *Neurol Res.* 2006;28(3):256–261.

McFarland HF, Martin R. Multiple sclerosis: a complicated picture of autoimmunity. *Nat Immunol.* 2007; 8(9):913–919.

McLellan F. NIH director reviews first year on the job. "Roadmap" calls for reorganisation of basic and clinical research. *Lancet.* 2003;362(9381):381–382.

McMillan M, Kahn M. Investigating Wnt signaling: a chemogenomic safari. *Drug Discov Today.* 2005;10(21): 1467–1474.

Miller JH, McKinstry RC, Philip JV, Mukherjee P, Neil JJ. Diffusion-tensor MR imaging of normal brain maturation: a guide to structural development and myelination. *AJR Am J Roentgenol.* 2003;180(3):851–859.

Miller RH, Mi S. Dissecting demyelination. *Nat Neurosci.* 2007;10(11):1351–1354.

Mix E, Meyer-Rienecker H, Zettl UK. Animal models of multiple sclerosis for the development and validation of novel therapies - potential and limitations. *J Neurol.* 2008;255(suppl 6):7–14.

Montes M, Zhang X, Berthelot L, et al. Oligoclonal myelin-reactive T-cell infiltrates derived from multiple sclerosis lesions are enriched in Th17 cells. *Clin Immunol.* 2009;130(2):133–144.

Moscarello MA, Brady GW, Fein DB, Wood DD, Cruz TF. The role of charge microheterogeneity of basic protein in the formation and maintenance of the multilayered structure of myelin: a possible role in multiple sclerosis. *J Neurosci Res.* 1986;15(1):87–99.

Moscarello MA, Wood DD, Ackerley C, Boulias C. Myelin in multiple sclerosis is developmentally immature. *J Clin Invest.* 1994;94(1):146–154.

Munger KL, Levin LI, Hollis BW, Howard NS, Ascherio A. Serum 25-hydroxyvitamin D levels and risk of multiple sclerosis. *JAMA.* 2006;296(23):2832–2838.

NIH releases "roadmap for medical research". *J Investig Med.* 2004;52(2):86–87.

O'Connor KC, Roy SM, Becker CH, Hafler DA, Kantor AB. Comprehensive phenotyping in multiple sclerosis: discovery based proteomics and the current understanding of putative biomarkers. *Dis Markers.* 2006;22(4):213–225.

Ohga S, Nomura A, Takada H, Hara T. Immunological aspects of Epstein-Barr virus infection. *Crit Rev Oncol Hematol.* 2002;44(3):203–215.

Oksenberg JR, Baranzini SE, Sawcer S, Hauser SL. The genetics of multiple sclerosis: SNPs to pathways to pathogenesis. *Nat Rev Genet.* 2008;9(7):516–526.

Oksenberg JR, Hauser SL. Genetics of multiple sclerosis. *Neurol Clin.* 2005;23(1):61–75, vi.

Orton SM, Herrera BM, Yee IM, et al. Sex ratio of multiple sclerosis in Canada: a longitudinal study. *Lancet Neurol.* 2006;5(11):932–936.

Patani R, Balaratnam M, Vora A, Reynolds R. Remyelination can be extensive in multiple sclerosis despite a long disease course. *Neuropathol Appl Neurobiol.* 2007;33(3):277–287.

Patrikios P, Stadelmann C, Kutzelnigg A, et al. Remyelination is extensive in a subset of multiple sclerosis patients. *Brain.* 2006;129(pt 12):3165–3172.

Pelfrey CM, Rudick RA, Cotleur AC, Lee JC, Tary-Lehmann M, Lehmann PV. Quantification of self-recognition in multiple sclerosis by single-cell analysis of cytokine production. *J Immunol.* 2000;165(3):1641–1651.

Piaton G, Williams A, Seilhean D, Lubetzki C. Remyelination in multiple sclerosis. *Prog Brain Res.* 2009;175:453–464.

Pirko I, Lucchinetti CF, Sriram S, Bakshi R. Gray matter involvement in multiple sclerosis. *Neurology.* 2007; 68(9):634–642.

Pitt D, Nagelmeier IE, Wilson HC, Raine CS. Glutamate uptake by oligodendrocytes: Implications for excitotoxicity in multiple sclerosis. *Neurology.* 2003;61(8): 1113–1120.

Podbielska M, Hogan EL. Molecular and immunogenic features of myelin lipids: incitants or modulators of multiple sclerosis? *Mult Scler.* 2009;15(9):1011–1029.

Prineas JW, Connell F. Remyelination in multiple sclerosis. *Ann Neurol.* 1979;5(1):22–31.

Pugliatti M, Cossu P, Sotgiu S, Rosati G, Riise T. Clustering of multiple sclerosis, age of onset and gender in Sardinia. *J Neurol Sci.* 2009;286(1–2):6–13.

Raine CS, Wu E. Multiple sclerosis: remyelination in acute lesions. *J Neuropathol Exp Neurol.* 1993;52(3): 199–204.

Raivich, G, Banati R. Brain microglia and blood-derived macrophages: molecular profiles and functional roles in multiple sclerosis and animal models of autoimmune demyelinating disease. *Brain Res Brain Res Rev.* 2004;46(3):261–281.

Ramagopalan SV, Byrnes JK, Orton SM, et al. Sex ratio of multiple sclerosis and clinical phenotype. *Eur J Neurol.* 2009a November 24; Epub ahead of print.

Ramagopalan SV, Dyment DA, Herrera BM, et al. Clustering of autoimmune disease in families at high risk for multiple sclerosis? *Lancet Neurol.* 2007;6(3): 206–207.

Ramagopalan SV, Valdar W, Criscuoli M, et al. Age of puberty and the risk of multiple sclerosis: a population based study. *Eur J Neurol.* 2009b;16(3): 342–347.

Sadovnick AD. The genetics and genetic epidemiology of multiple sclerosis: the "hard facts". *Adv Neurol.* 2006;98:17–25.

Sadovnick AD. European Charcot Foundation Lecture: the natural history of multiple sclerosis and gender. *J Neurol Sci.* 2009;286(1–2):1–5.

Sellebjerg F, Krakauer M, Hesse D, et al. Identification of new sensitive biomarkers for the in vivo response to interferon-beta treatment in multiple sclerosis using DNA-array evaluation. *Eur J Neurol.* 2009;16(12): 1291–1298.

Skulina C, Schmidt S, Dornmair K, et al. Multiple sclerosis: brain-infiltrating CD8+ T cells persist as clonal expansions in the cerebrospinal fluid and blood. *Proc Natl Acad Sci USA.* 2004;101(8):2428–2433.

Smith KJ, Lassmann H. The role of nitric oxide in multiple sclerosis. *Lancet Neurol.* 2002;1(4):232–241.

Sospedra M, Martin R. Immunology of multiple sclerosis. *Annu Rev Immunol.* 2005;23:683–747.

Steinman L, Zamvil SS. How to successfully apply animal studies in experimental allergic encephalomyelitis to research on multiple sclerosis. *Ann Neurol.* 2006; 60(1):12–21.

Stevens LM. JAMA patient page. Basic science research. *JAMA.* 2002;287(13):1754.

Taneja V, David CS. HLA transgenic mice as humanized mouse models of disease and immunity. *J Clin Invest.* 1998;101(5):921–926.

Terajima K, Matsuzawa H, Tanaka K, Nishizawa M, Nakada T. Cell-oriented analysis in vivo using diffusion tensor imaging for normal-appearing brain tissue in multiple sclerosis. *Neuroimage.* 2007;37(4):1278–1285.

Tomassini V, Palace J. Multiple sclerosis lesions: insights from imaging techniques. *Expert Rev Neurother.* 2009; 9(9):1341–1359.

Torkildsen O, Brunborg LA, Myhr KM, Bo L. The cuprizone model for demyelination. *Acta Neurol Scand Suppl.* 2008;188:72–76.

Tranquill LR, Cao L, Ling NC, Kalbacher H, Martin RM, Whitaker JN. Enhanced T cell responsiveness to citrulline-containing myelin basic protein in multiple sclerosis patients. *Mult Scler.* 2000;6(4):220–225.

Trapp BD. Pathogenesis of multiple sclerosis: the eyes only see what the mind is prepared to comprehend. *Ann Neurol.* 2004;55(4):455–457.

Trapp BD, Nave KA. Multiple sclerosis: an immune or neurodegenerative disorder? *Annu Rev Neurosci.* 2008; 31:247–269.

Trapp BD, Peterson J, Ransohoff RM, Rudick R, Mork S, Bo L. Axonal transection in the lesions of multiple sclerosis. *N Engl J Med.* 1998;338(5):278–285.

van der Valk P, Amor S. Preactive lesions in multiple sclerosis. *Curr Opin Neurol.* 2009;22(3):207–213.

Venken K, Hellings N, Thewissen M, et al. Compromised CD4+ CD25(high) regulatory T-cell function in patients with relapsing-remitting multiple sclerosis is correlated with a reduced frequency of FOXP3-positive cells and reduced FOXP3 expression at the single-cell level. *Immunology.* 2008;123(1):79–89.

Viglietta V, Baecher-Allan C, Weiner H. L, Hafler DA. Loss of functional suppression by CD4+CD25+ regulatory T cells in patients with multiple sclerosis. *J Exp Med.* 2004;199(7):971–979.

Wegner C, Stadelmann C. Gray matter pathology and multiple sclerosis. *Curr Neurol Neurosci Rep.* 2009;9(5):399–404.

Weiner HL. The challenge of multiple sclerosis: how do we cure a chronic heterogeneous disease? *Ann Neurol.* 2009;65(3):239–248.

Wheeler D, Bandaru VV, Calabresi PA, Nath A, Haughey NJ. A defect of sphingolipid metabolism modifies the properties of normal appearing white matter in multiple sclerosis. *Brain.* 2008;131(pt 11):3092–3102.

Whitaker JN, Snyder DS. Studies of autoimmunity in multiple sclerosis. *CRC Crit Rev Clin Neurobiol.* 1984; 1(1):45–82.

Yeh EA, Chitnis T, Krupp L, et al. Pediatric multiple sclerosis. *Nat Rev Neurol.* 2009;5(11):621–631.

Zhang Y, Argaw AT, Gurfein BT, et al. Notch1 signaling plays a role in regulating precursor differentiation during CNS remyelination. *Proc Natl Acad Sci USA.* 2009;106(45):19162–19167.

Index

Note: Page references followed by *"f"* and *"t"* denote figures and tables, respectively.